CAROTENOID CHEMISTRY AND BIOCHEMISTRY

Some Other IUPAC Titles of Interest from Pergamon Press

Books

BENOIT & REMPP: Macromolecules

BROWN & DAVIES: Organ-Directed Toxicity—Chemical Indices and Mechanisms

CIARDELLI & GIUSTI: Structural Order in Polymers

FRANZOSINI & SANESI: Thermodynamic and Transport Properties of Organic Salts

FREIDLINA & SKOROVA: Organic Sulfur Chemistry

FUWA: Recent Advances in Analytical Spectroscopy

GEISSBÜHLER: Advances in Pesticide Science, 3 volume set

GOETHALS: Polymeric Amines and Ammonium Salts

HÖGFELDT: Stability Constants of Metal-Ion Complexes
Part A: Inorganic Ligands

IRVING, FREISER & WEST: Compendium of Analytical Nomenclature

IUPAC: Nomenclature of Inorganic Chemistry, 2 volume set

JEMMALI: Mycotoxins in Foodstuffs—3

KORNHAUSER, RAO & WADDINGTON: Chemical Education in the Seventies

MIYAMOTO: 5th International Congress of Pesticide Chemistry

LAIDLER: Frontiers of Chemistry

PERRIN: Stability Constants of Metal Ion-Complexes
Part B: Organic Ligands

RIGAUDY & KLESNEY: Nomenclature of Organic Chemistry

TROST & HUTCHINSON: Organic Synthesis—Today and Tomorrow

WHIFFEN: Manual of Symbols and Terminology for Physicochemical Quantities and Units

Journals (a free specimen copy gladly sent on request)

CHEMISTRY INTERNATIONAL, the news magazine for chemists in all fields of specialization in all countries of the world.

PURE AND APPLIED CHEMISTRY, the international research journal publishing proceedings of IUPAC conferences, nomenclature rules and technical reports.

INTERNATIONAL UNION OF PURE AND APPLIED CHEMISTRY
(Organic Chemistry Division)

CAROTENOID CHEMISTRY AND BIOCHEMISTRY

Proceedings of the 6th International Symposium on Carotenoids
Liverpool, UK, 26-31 July 1981

Edited by

GEORGE BRITTON and TREVOR W. GOODWIN

University of Liverpool, UK

PERGAMON PRESS

OXFORD · NEW YORK · TORONTO · SYDNEY · PARIS · FRANKFURT

U.K.	Pergamon Press Ltd., Headington Hill Hall, Oxford OX3 0BW, England
U.S.A.	Pergamon Press Inc., Maxwell House, Fairview Park, Elmsford, New York 10523, U.S.A.
CANADA	Pergamon Press Canada Ltd., Suite 104, 150 Consumers Rd., Willowdale, Ontario M2J 1P9, Canada
AUSTRALIA	Pergamon Press (Aust.) Pty. Ltd., P.O. Box 544, Potts Point, N.S.W. 2011, Australia
FRANCE	Pergamon Press SARL, 24 rue des Ecoles, 75240 Paris, Cedex 05, France
FEDERAL REPUBLIC OF GERMANY	Pergamon Press GmbH, 6242 Kronberg-Taunus, Hammerweg 6, Federal Republic of Germany

First edition 1982

Library of Congress Cataloging in Publication Data

International Symposium on Carotenoids (6th :
1981 : Liverpool, Merseyside)
Carotenoid chemistry and biochemistry.
At head of title: International Union of
Pure and Applied Chemistry (Organic Chemistry
Division).
Includes index.
1. Carotinoids—Congresses. I. Britton,
George. II. Goodwin, T.W. (Trevor Walworth)
III. International Union of Pure and Applied
Chemistry. Organic Chemistry Division.
IV. Title.
QD441.I57 1981 574.19'218 82-3875

British Library Cataloguing in Publication Data

International Symposium on Carotenoids *(6th : 1981 : Liverpool)*
Carotenoid chemistry and biochemistry.
1. Carotenoids—Congresses
I. Title II. Britton, George III. Goodwin,
T.W. IV. International Union of Pure and
Applied Chemistry. *Organic Chemistry Division*
547.8'69 QP671.C35
ISBN 0-08-026224-4

In order to make this volume available as economically and as rapidly as possible the authors' typescripts have been reproduced in their original forms. This method unfortunately has its typographical limitations but it is hoped that they in no way distract the reader.

Printed in Great Britain by A. Wheaton & Co. Ltd., Exeter

CONTENTS

Organizing Committee

Chairman

T. W. Goodwin

Secretary

G. Britton

Assistant Secretary

S. Pollard

Members

B. H. Davies
F. J. Leuenberger
G. P. Moss
B. C. L. Weedon

Sponsors & Contributors

International Union of Pure and Applied Chemistry
F. Hoffmann-La Roche & Co Ltd, Roche Products Ltd
The University of Liverpool
The Royal Society
BASF (UK) Ltd
The University College of Wales, Aberystwyth

INTERNATIONAL UNION OF PURE AND APPLIED CHEMISTRY

**IUPAC Secretariat: Bank Court Chambers, 2-3 Pound Way,
Cowley Centre, Oxford OX4 3YF, UK**

PREFACE

The International Symposium on Carotenoids other than Vitamin A, held at Trondheim, Norway, in 1966 became the first of a triennial series which visited Las Cruces (New Mexico, U.S.A.), Cluj (Romania), Bern (Switzerland) and Madison (Wisconsin, U.S.A.) before reaching the United Kingdom in 1981. The 6th International Symposium on Carotenoids took place at Liverpool, 26th-31st July, 1981, and was attended by two hundred scientists from 25 countries. Whereas the first Symposium was devoted largely to carotenoid chemistry, the Liverpool programme reflected the increasing interest in biochemical and biological topics. This book contains the texts of the main lectures presented at the Symposium. In addition, around one hundred original papers and posters were presented, an indication of the healthy state of the carotenoid field.

In this book we have maintained tradition by including sections on carotenoid chemistry - new structures, synthesis and physical methods - all of which place much emphasis on stereochemistry. The chemistry of complexes between carotenoids or retinoids and protein - the novel blue carotenoproteins, the visual pigments and the nutritionally important retinol-binding proteins - is also included. Animal carotenoids are well covered; animals have provided many new carotenoid structures, and there is much new information about carotenoid metabolism and transformations, including interesting stereochemical findings. Biosynthesis has always been covered in these meetings, but we have introduced a substantial section on carotenoids in photosynthesis, reflecting current interest in this area. More applied aspects are not neglected. The industrial importance of carotenoids is discussed, and medical aspects now include not only nutrition but also the use of carotenoids in treatment against skin photosensitivity and their possible role in protection against cancer. The effects of chemicals on carotenoid biosynthesis is also reviewed as an area relevant to herbicide design. The twentyfive chapters of this book thus present a wide and up to date picture of the expanding carotenoid field.
We are most grateful to Dr. Susan Pollard for painstaking work in the preparation of the comprehensive Index.

If the Symposium has been considered a success, this is due in no small part to the tremendous efforts of our local secretariat, to whom we and the Organizing Committee are deeply indebted.

We are also most grateful to F. Hoffmann-La Roche and Co. Ltd., and Roche Products Ltd. for their continued interest in and support for the carotenoid field and the Symposium, to all other sources, notably BASF (U.K.) Ltd., The Royal Society and The University of Liverpool, whose contributions helped to make the Symposium possible, and for the support of IUPAC.

We now look forward to Munich 1984 and wish Professor Rau and his colleagues every success, and as much enjoyment and pleasure as we derived from Liverpool, 1981.

G. Britton

T. W. Goodwin

Liverpool, 1981.

NEW CAROTENOID STRUCTURES AND STEREOCHEMISTRY

Conrad Hans Eugster

Institute of Organic Chemistry, University of Zurich, Winterthurerstrasse 190, CH-8057 Zurich, Switzerland

Abstract - A review is presented on progress made since the 5th International Symposium on Carotenoids, Madison, USA, 1978, in the following areas:

- diastereo- and enantio-selectively deuterated carotenes and conformation of substituted ε-endgroups,
- new carotenoids having ε-endgroups,
- carotenes with vic. diolgroups,
- carotene-5,6- and 5,8-epoxides,
- structure of Z/E-isomeric carotenes and carotenoids,
- chirality of selected carotenoids,
- new findings on carotenoids from rose flowers.

INTRODUCTION

The organizers of this symposium have delegated me with the task of informing you about new carotenoid structures which have been published since my summary in Madison (Ref. 1). The term "structure" always includes information about the spacial arrangement of a molecule, and hence with chiral molecules also about their absolute configuration.

On briefly characterising the period of my report, I can observe the following:

- many absolute configurations have been published, but few really new structures have been discovered,
- the problem of Z/E isomerism in carotenoids has been the subject of particularly extensive research,
- great activity was prevalent on the synthesis of optically active carotenoids,
- analytical methods such as HPLC and spectroscopy have been refined.

I will take the liberty of not only referring to published works, but of also presenting unpublished results from my own group.

Let me begin with the problem of the stereochemistry of the ring closure in the carotene series.

1. DIASTEREO- AND ENANTIO-SELECTIVELY DEUTERATED CAROTENES

Analysis of the absolute configurations has revealed, as all of you know, that, in nature, different kinds of foldings are employed (Refs. 1 & 2), so that we find diverse absolute configurations at C(2) and C(6) (see Scheme 1). This has certain analogies in other classes of terpenes e.g. diterpenoids, where the cyclisation is similarly triggered off by protons (see Note a).

Note a. The striking uniformity in the squalene cyclisations, at least in the case of triterpenes from eukaryotes, is attributable to the enantioselective epoxidation which determines the folding.

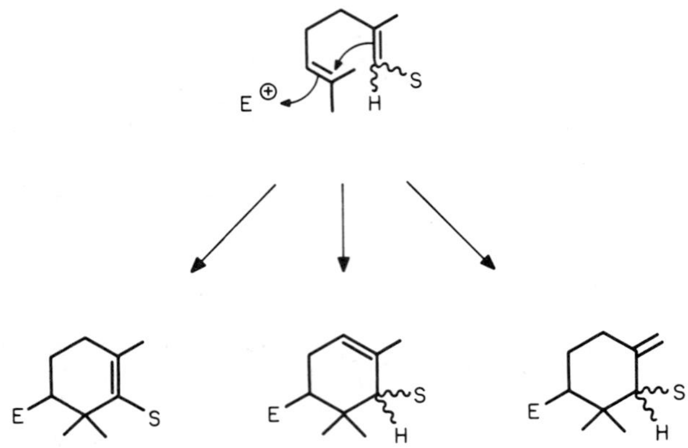

β ε γ

Scheme 1

Scheme 2 takes into consideration the different chair- and boat-foldings and the configuration of the C(5)- C(6)-double bond (Ref. 1). The ten different

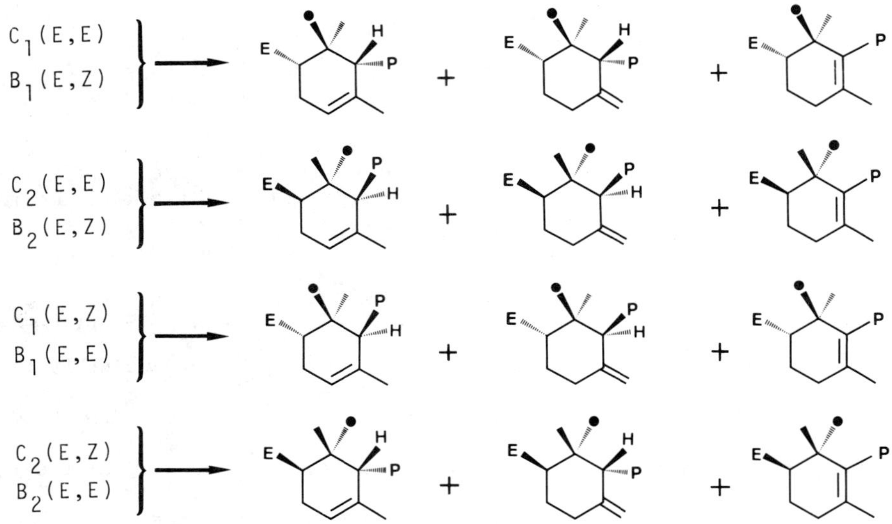

Scheme 2

stereoisomers drawn here result from four conformations of the E/Z-isomeric alicyclic precursors, assuming an overall trans-addition of electrophile and 5,6-double bond.

Thus, one can draw conclusions about the folding of the acyclic precursor if the absolute configuration at C(1), C(2) and C(6) of the cyclisation product is known. This assumes, of course, that no subsequent inversions have occurred in the organism.

As chemists we have selected a method for the unequivocal characterisation of the products of a cyclisation, such that few NMR- and CD-measurements suffice. The work mentioned in Madison has now been fully concluded (Refs. 3 & 4)(see Scheme 3).

It deals with the degradation of abietic acid to the deuterated homocyclogeranic acids (C_{11}) and the building up of the carotenes according to the scheme

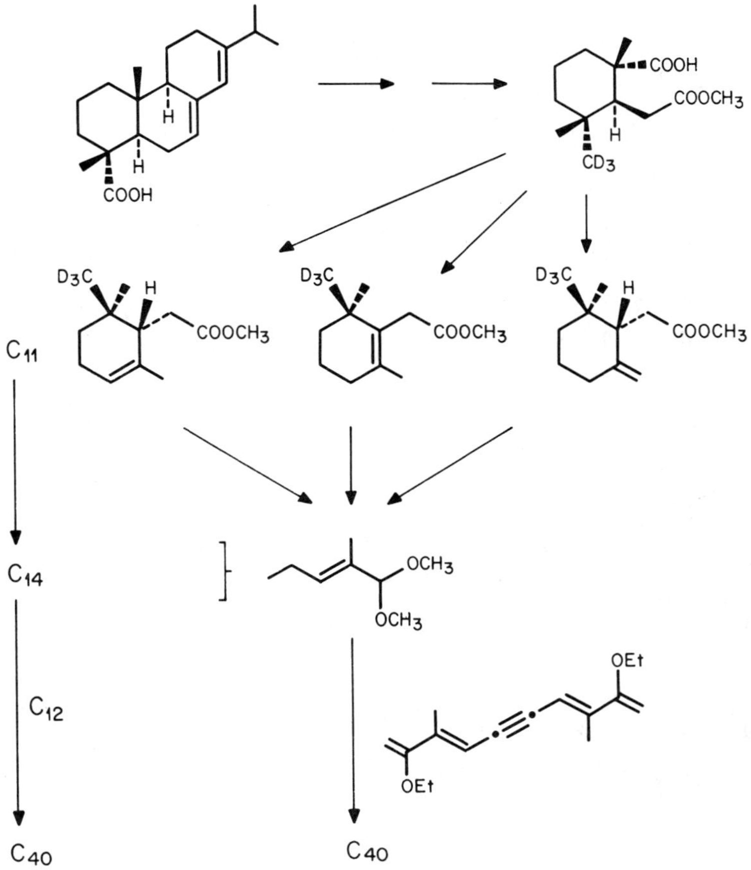

Scheme 3

$C_{11} \longrightarrow C_{14} \xrightarrow{C_{12}} C_{40}$ in accordance with the little used procedure of Isler et al. (Ref. 5). It presented considerable difficulties, by the way, on changing to the milligram scale.

The following carotenes were synthesised:

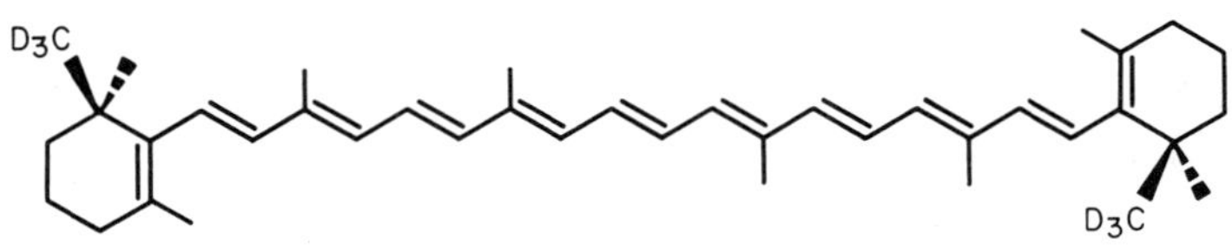

1 (1R,1'R)-d_6-β,β m.p. 176-177^0

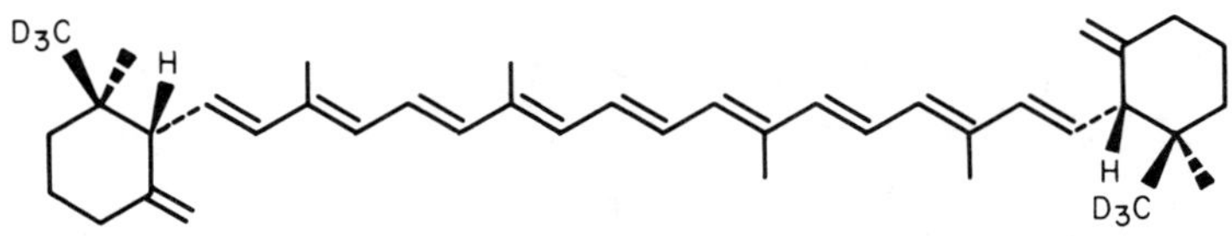

2 (1R,1'R,6S,6'S)-d_6-γ,γ m.p. 203-203,5^0

($\pm$) m.p. 183^0 (Ref. 6)

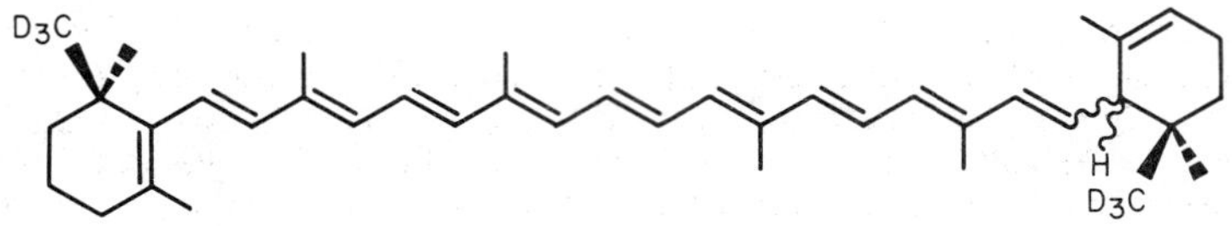

3 (1R,1'R,6'R,S)-d_6-β,ε m.p. 152,5-153°

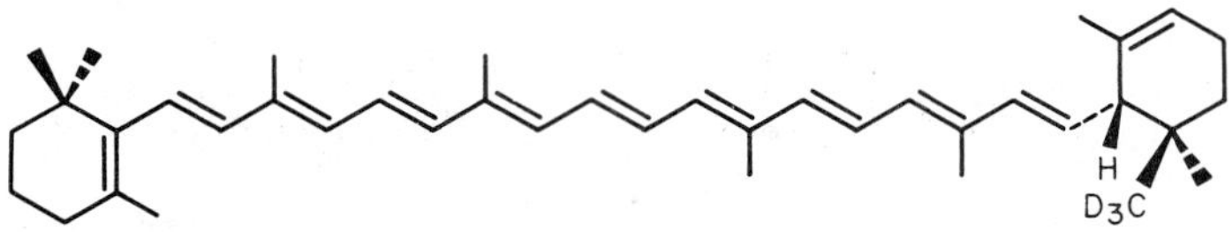

4 (1'R,6'S)-d_3-β,ε m.p. 181-182°

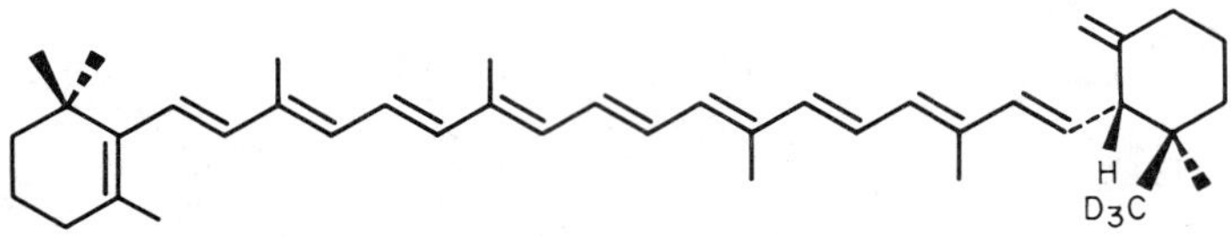

5 (1'R,6'S)-d_3-β,γ m.p. 174,5-175,5°

Scheme 4

γ,γ-carotene (<u>2</u>) has thus, to my knowledge, been synthesised for the first time in an enantiomerically pure form.

I will now mention a few properties of the deuterated carotenes which are of general importance for the carotene chemistry; firstly the NMR-data:

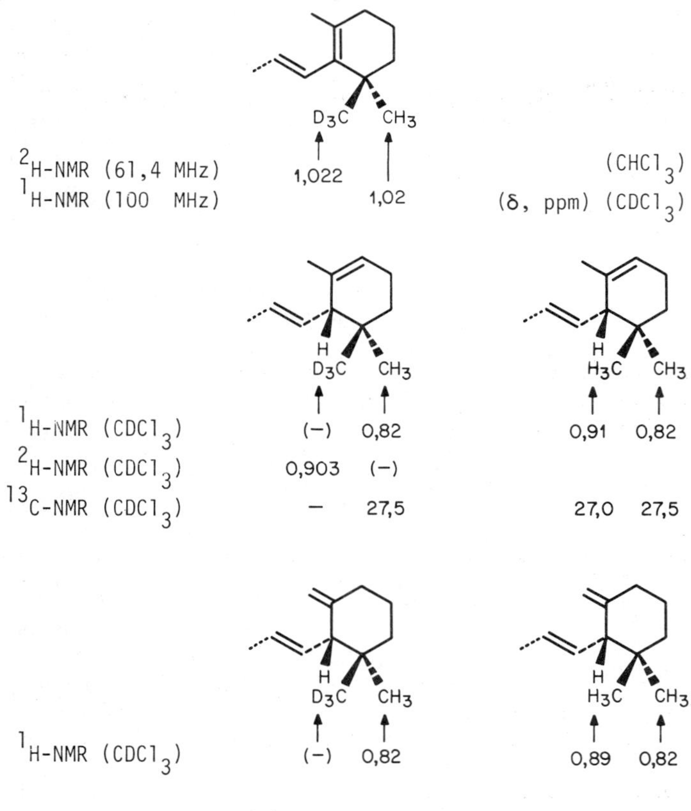

Scheme 5

This is an extension of the NMR-signal assignments, previously made in Madison, of diastereotopic methyl groups at C(1) of ε- and γ-endgroups by ^{1}H- and ^{13}C-NMR-measurements. The rule states: the methyl groups at C(1) <u>cis</u> to the polyene chain absorb in the ^{1}H-NMR at higher field, in the ^{13}C-NMR at lower field (see Note a). There are, however, exceptions in compounds with polar side chains and with substituted ε-rings.

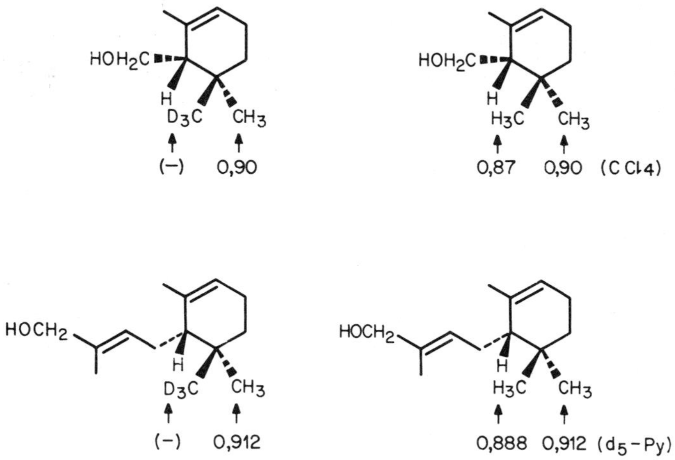

Scheme 6

I think that one can draw conclusions on the conformational equilibrium from these data.

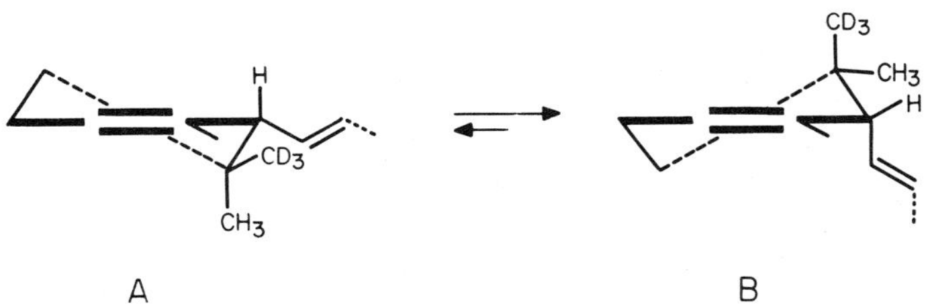

Scheme 7

The conformation with pseudo-axial polyene side chain and axial CD_3-group is more strongly populated (B); the CH_3-group is preferentially equatorial and absorbs in the ^{13}C-NMR at lower field (see Note b). When the corresponding ^{13}C-NMR-data for the γ-endgroup have been analysed, conclusions regarding the preferred conformation should likewise result.

Now to the CD-data of <u>1</u> to <u>5</u>. Those with the ε-endgroup are in agreement with the non-deuterated compounds. For the β,γ-compound <u>5</u>, a good agreement with data from Prof. Jensen (Ref. 11) has been found. The Δε-values for the γ,γ-carotene

Note a. Is valid for the unsubstituted ε-endgroup. As yet, we have no ^{13}C-data available for the γ-endgroup. The assignment of the ^{1}H-NMR-signals made by Bingham et al. (Ref. 7) with no citation of arguments is wrong.

Note b. Compare analogous shift arguments for isophorol (3,5,5-trimethyl-2-cyclohexen-1-ol) (Ref. 8), lutein (Ref. 9) and zeaxanthin (Ref. 10).

lie almost twice as high. Thus, the chirality of the γ,γ-carotene (Ref. 12), hitherto found only in traces in nature, can also be determined. The d_6-β,β-carotene 1 is chiral because of the isotope substitution next to the chirality centre. The effect of this chirality only came to light at the end of this ca. three year work.

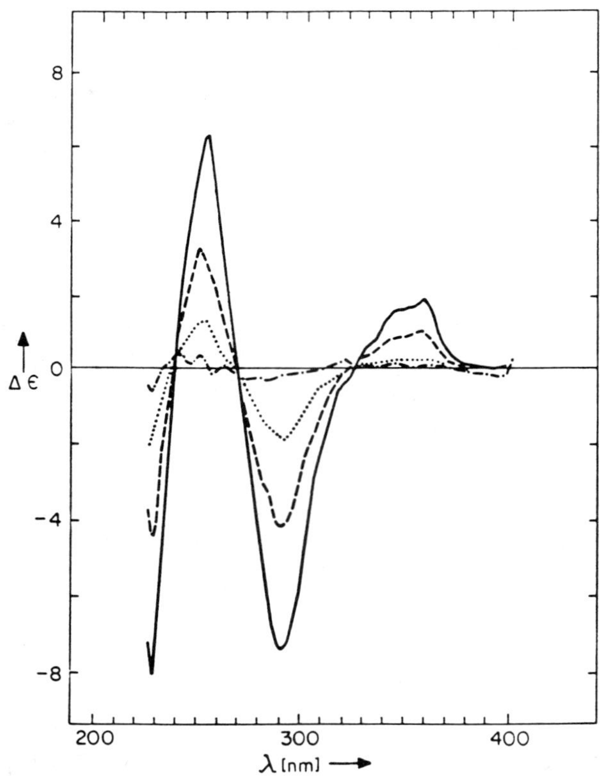

CD-spectra of all-(E)-(1R,1'R)-[16,16,16,16',16',16'-d_6]-β,β-carotene (1) in ether-isopentane-ethanol (5:5:2); –·–·– +25°, ········ -100°, ---- -150°, —— -180°C.

Fig. 1

Exact analysis shows that a zeaxanthin conformation with pseudo-equatorial CD_3-group is present.

With the syntheses of the deuterated carotenes 1 to 5 it would seem that all chemical-spectroscopic requirements have been met for in vivo cyclisation experiments on suitable deuterated precursors. The chirality of the products expected can be determined on milligram fractions of isolated carotene by ^{1}H-NMR- and CD-measurements. Should the deuterated carotene content fall below 10-20% because of dilution effects, ^{2}H-NMR-spectroscopy can be applied with a good chance of success.

2. NEW FINDINGS ON CAROTENOIDS WITH ε-ENDGROUPS

In the literature numerous statements about the occurrence of "lutein" in animal organs can be found (Ref. 13). When we investigated the so-called lutein from goldfish (Ref. 14), we established that it was in fact 3'-epilutein (3'R,6'S-lutein) (Ref. 15).

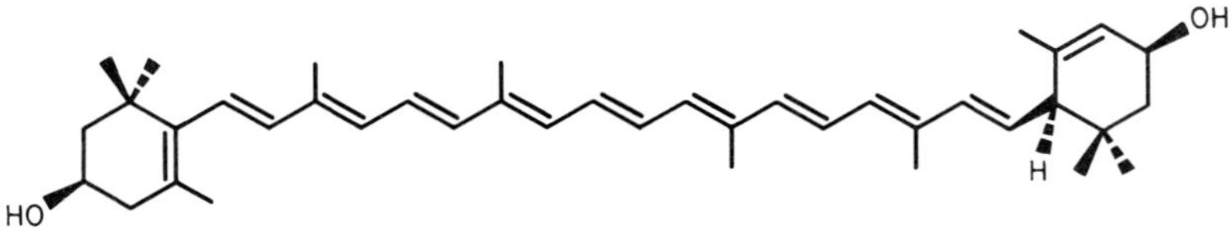

6 Goldfish (Ref. 15); Caltha palustris (Refs. 16 & 17)

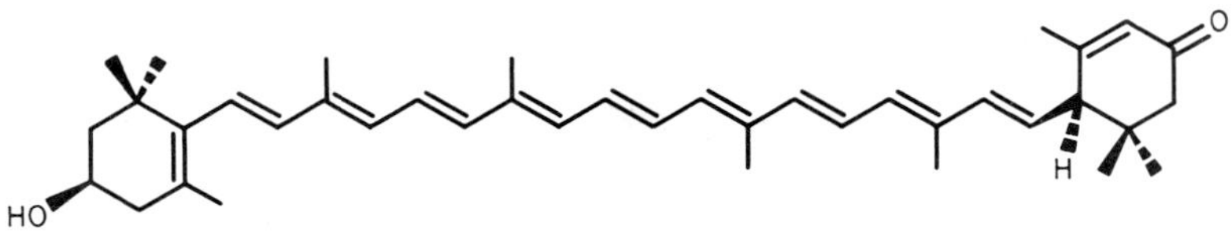

7 Egg yolk (Ref. 16); Caltha palustris (Ref. 16)

Scheme 8

We postulated that this 3'-epilutein arises by dehydrogenation of lutein to 3'-O-didehydrolutein (7) followed by diastereoselective reduction to 6.

In this connection, both carotenoids were synthesised with very high purity (see Note a) and exhaustively characterised. This enabled us to discover them at a later date in egg yolk and in blossoms from Caltha palustris (Ref. 16), which substantiated the earlier assumption that "calthaxanthin" (Ref. 17) is an epimer of lutein.

Oxolutein (7) is very labile to alkali and can therefore not be traced after standard isolation procedures which include an alkaline hydrolysis. One will have to take this fact into account in future if one wishes to isolate such oxocarotenes from natural products.

In our view, oxolutein (7) is a key product for the understanding of carotenoid metabolism in animals. I will dispense with a discussion and simply refer to the lecture by Dr. Buchecker.

Now to the assignment of the geminal methyl groups in lutein, 3'-epilutein (6) and oxolutein (7) (see Scheme 9). ASIS experiments on lutein (Refs. 9, 19 & 20) have shown that the hydroxyl group at C(3') exerts hardly any influence on the chemical shift of the CH_3-group at C(1'). However, it determines the conformational equilibrium in favour of a half-chair with pseudo-equatorial 3'-OH and 6'-polyene side chain (see Note b) (conformation C). This is not the case with epilutein: the preferred conformation D has a pseudo-equatorial hydroxyl group, but now a pseudo-axial side chain. In oxolutein it may be again the side chain which determines the preferred conformation (E) if a half-chair conformation is assumed. The assignments of the ^{1}H- and ^{13}C-NMR-signals for the

---

Note a. First synthesis of oxolutein (7), see Ref. 18.

Note b. Compare the detailed analysis of the epimeric 3-methoxy-α-ionones (Ref. 21).

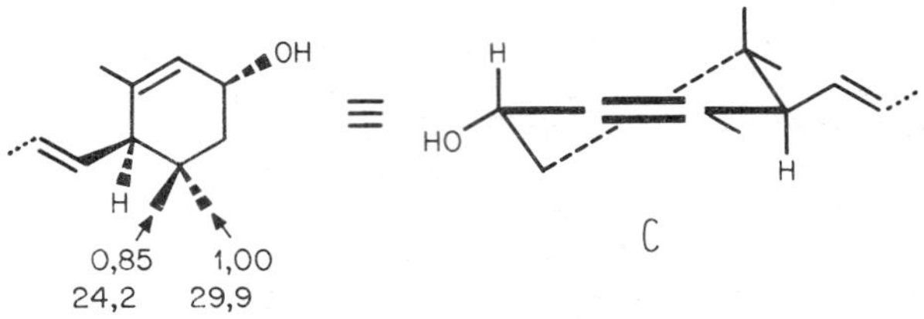

(3'R,6'R)-Lutein

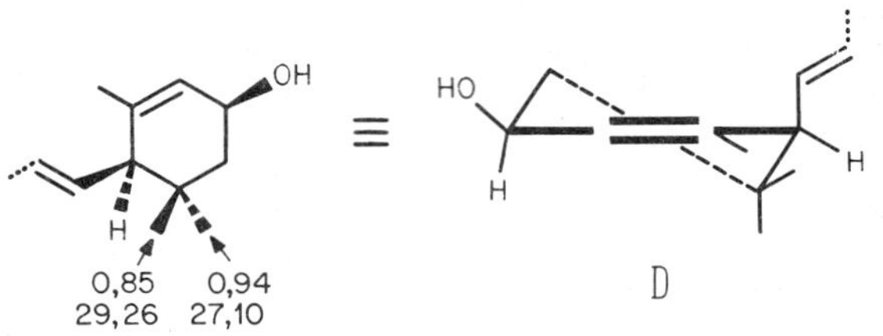

(3'S,6'R)-Lutein (3'-Epilutein)

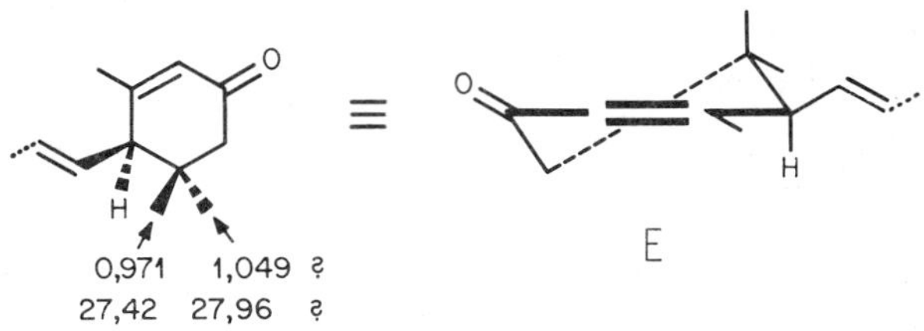

(6'R)-3'O-Didehydrolutein (Oxolutein)

Scheme 9

geminal methyl groups (see Note a) follow on the basis of these arguments. Now to the ε,ε-carotene-3,3'-diols.

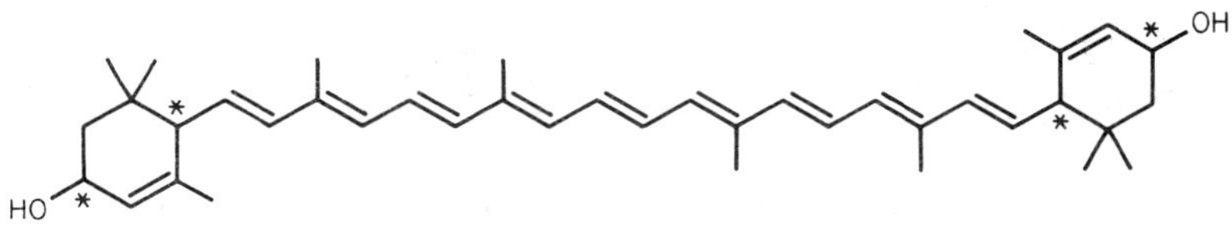

(3R,6S,3'R,6'S)	cis-cis	dissymm.	Tunaxanthin (=Oxyxanthin-58)	(**8**)
(3S,6R,3'S,6'R)	cis-cis	dissymm.	Chiriquixanthin B	(**9**)
(3R,6S,3'S,6'R)	cis-cis	meso	unknown	
(3R,6R,3'R,6'R)	trans-trans	dissymm.	Lactucaxanthin	(**10**)
(3S,6S,3'S,6'S)	trans-trans	dissymm.	Tunaxanthin (=Oxyxanthin-45)	(**11**)
(3R,6R,3'S,6'S)	trans-trans	meso	unknown	
(3R,6S,3'S,6'S)	cis-trans	asymm.	Tunaxanthin (=Oxyxanthin-51)	(**12**)
(3S,6R,3'S,6'S)	cis-trans	asymm.	unknown	
(3R,6S,3'R,6'R)	cis-trans	asymm.	unknown	
(3R,6R,3'S,6'R)	trans-cis	asymm.	Chiriquixanthin A (=Flavidxanthin-55)	(**13**)

Scheme 10

Note a. For earlier ^{13}C-NMR-data on lutein see Refs. 22 and 23.

Of the ten possible stereoisomers (four centres of chirality, each pair showing the same constitution) a total of six have so far been isolated from natural sources. I have already reported on the chiriquixanthins in Madison (Ref. 1). Since then the research groups of Prof. Jensen and Prof. Mosher have isolated and clarified four new stereoisomers, namely the tunaxanthins 8, 11 and 12 (Refs. 7 & 24) and the lactucaxanthin (10) (Ref. 25). The tunaxanthins are the main carotenoids in marine fish, but are rarely found in freshwater fish. Earlier "taraxanthin"-like carotenoids are doubtless tunaxanthins. *Sebastes flavidus* contains 13; *Oxyjulis californica* contains 8, 11 and 12. 12 was found in *Thunnus thynnus*, *Amanses modestus*, *Seriola quinqueradiata* etc. 10, on the other hand, originates from Compositae (*Lactuca sativa*, *Prenanthes*, *Cicerbita*, *Mycelis*; Ref. 25). Isolated compounds such as 13 are strongly racemised (or contain unseparated meso-compounds).

The structural assignments are based on known arguments: aliphatic nonaene chromophore, MS, ^{1}H-NMR-data (symmetry, *cis*- or *trans*-substituted ε-endgroups) and CD-comparison with the enantiomeric ε,ε-carotenes (Refs. 26 & 27). However, I would like to sound out a warning here on the extensive use of shift differences of the C(1')-methyl groups in *cis*- and *trans*-3'-hydroxy-ε- endgroups (see Note a).

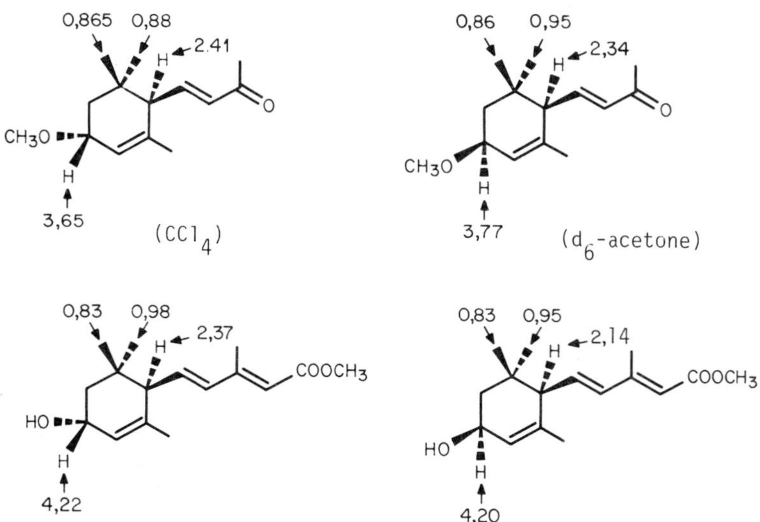

14 **15**

Scheme 11

In both these optically active diastereoisomers 14 and 15, about which Dr. Eschenmoser will further comment, the shift argument for the geminal methyl groups failed. Of more general usefulness is the interpretation of the signal for H-C(6'): in the *trans* isomer it lies at lower field than in the *cis* isomer; the coupling constants are also clearly different due to the differing ring conformations. These observations can also be applied to the carotenoids. I would therefore recommend that, in order to avoid potential mistakes in future structural elucidations, one should not only observe the shift differences of the geminal methyl groups but also the shift of H-C(6), which is especially dependent on the conformation of the ε-ring!

Note a. These shift differences were first determined on the isomeric 3-methoxy-α-ionones (Ref. 21), but were not employed for the structural assignment. In this case, the sign and size of long-range couplings of the ring protons served. Shift differences in the ^{13}C-NMR - spectra are also of use (Refs. 22 & 28) but, as yet, find no general application.

3. CAROTENE GLYCOLS

Professor Jensen's research group has published new investigations on the distribution and chirality of oscillaxanthin (16) (Refs. 29 & 30).

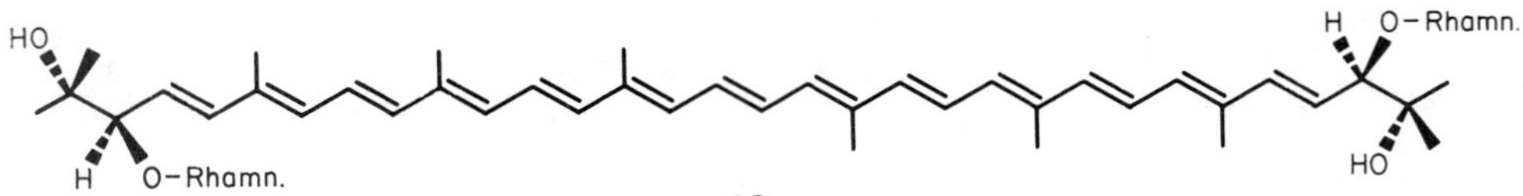

16

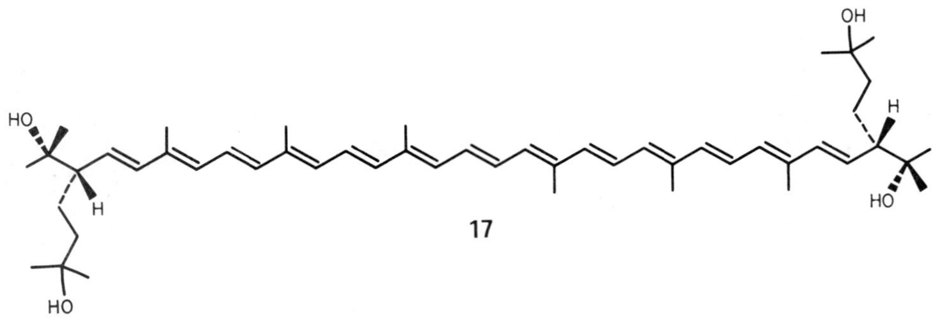

17

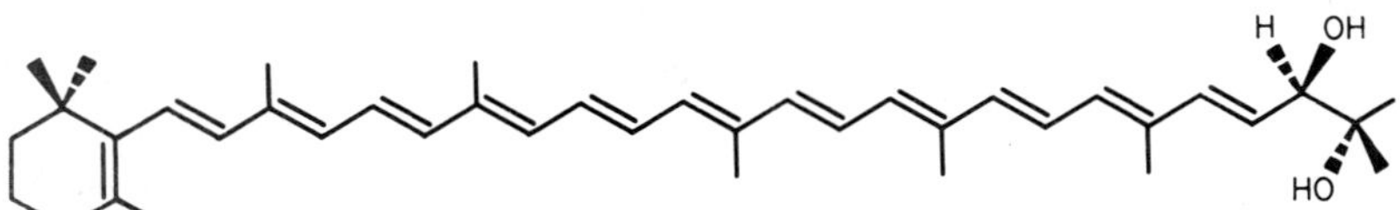

18

Scheme 12

The hexa-O-acetate of 16 was chiroptically compared with (2S,2'S)-bacterioruberin (17) and plectaniaxanthin (18) as its β-D-glucoside, respectively. From the fact that 16 and 17 show similar but opposite Cotton effects whilst 18 similar Cotton effects with the same sign, the absolute configuration given in 16 was deduced (see Note a).

The aglycone of 16, i.e. ent-16, oscillol is unstable (Refs. 29 & 30, and earlier works) and presents a particularly tough problem for its synthesis.

Since, to my knowledge, optically active glycols of acyclic carotenes have not been prepared, we began to synthesise and characterise such compounds (Ref. 32) (see Scheme 13 and 14).

Starting from the inexpensive L-tyrosine we synthesised the diol 20. After protection of the glycol function the ring was degraded to the compound 21 already been described by Terashima et al. (Ref. 76). From 22 the C_{10}-ester 23 was built up via the addition of the cuprate-derivative to tetrolic ester. Using conventional steps the carotenoid glycol 25 was obtained as the 2,2'-di-O-acetyl compound; m.p. $143-145^{o}$, λ_{max} (ether) 446 (111300), 468 (150300), 499 (124600). As expected, at roomtemperature, compound 25 shows only a weak CD-effect which increases after cooling and is very similar to that of oscillaxanthin hexaacetate despite the fact that 25 does not have an allylic oxygen function.

Note a. In the dissertation by H. Rønneberg (Ref. 30), however, new arguments were compiled which assign to oscillaxanthin the enantiomeric configuration (ent-16). For the absolute configuration of bacterioruberin see Refs. 1 & 31 and earlier communications.

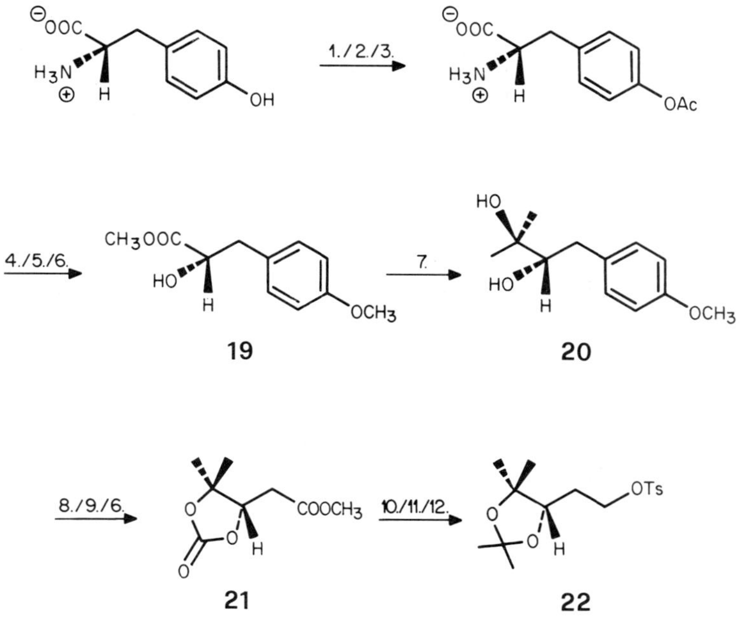

19 20 21 22

1. $HClO_4$/HOAc; 2. Ac_2O; 3. $C_8H_{17}NH_2$; 4. $C_5H_{11}NO$/HOAc; 5. 2% $HCl/H_2O/\Delta$; 6. CH_2N_2; 7. 2 CH_3MgBr; 8. $(EtO)_2CO/NaOCH_3$; 9. O_3(HOAc); 10. $LiAlH_4$; 11. TosOH/acetone; 12. TosCl/py.

Scheme 13

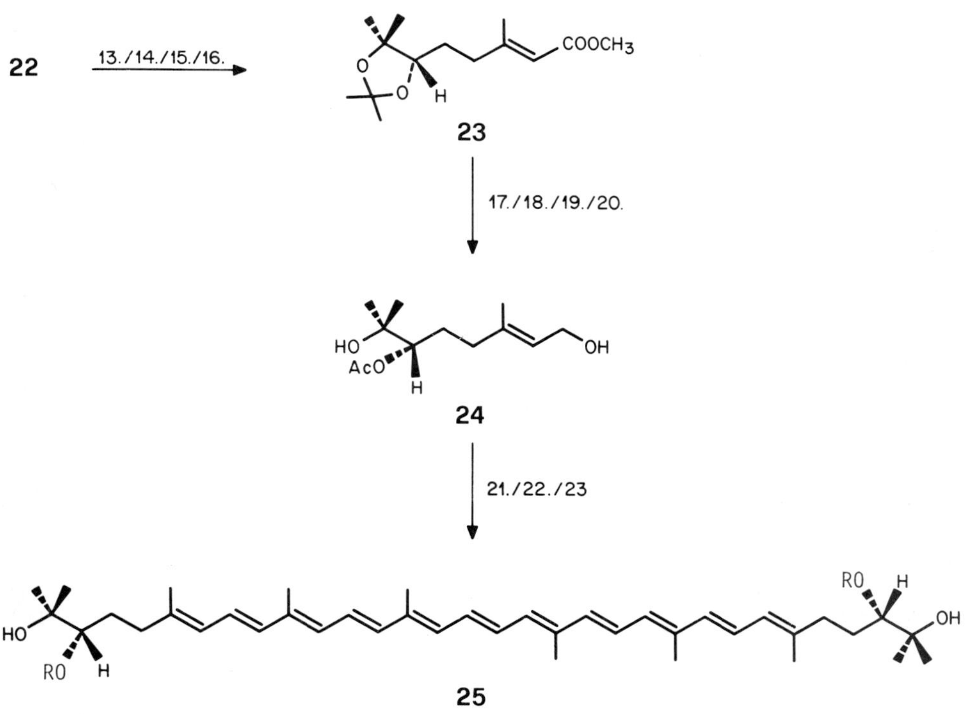

23 24 25

13. LiBr/dimethoxyethane; 14. Mg/ether; 15. CuCl/pyrrolidine; 16. CH_3-C≡C-$COOCH_3$; 17. Dibah; 18. 90% HOAc; 19. Ac_2O/pyridine; 20. $KHCO_3/H_2O/CH_3OH$; 21. N-bromo-succinimide/CH_3SCH_3; 22. $(C_6H_5)_3P$; 23. 50% KOH/CH_2Cl_2/crocetin-dial/Δ.

Scheme 14

The optically active cyclic endgroups with glycol structure, on which Dr. Eschenmoser lectured, have now also been used as building blocks to various apocarotenoids with glycol endgroups (Ref. 33):

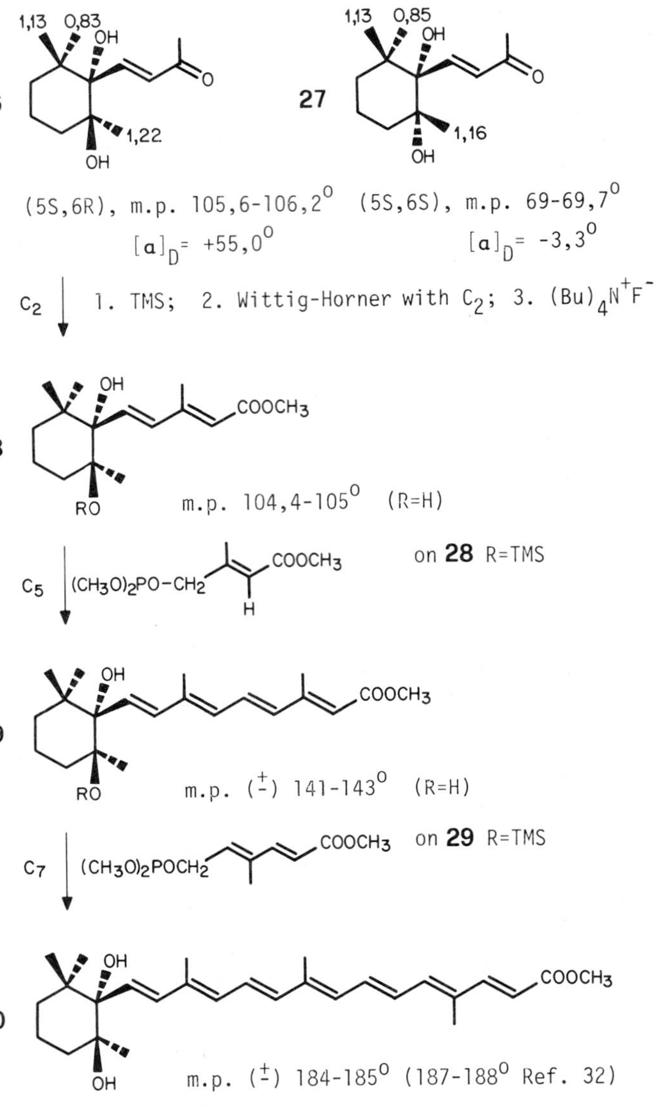

Scheme 15

The syntheses employ the two optically active ionone glycols 26 and 27. They have to be protected as the monosilyl ethers, in order to avoid side reactions. In three conventional olefinations with C_2, C_5 and C_7, we obtained the C_{15}-, C_{20}- and C_{27}-compounds of interest to us. The reaction steps involve in each case reduction of the esters and oxidation to the aldehyde, and with 28 separation into the (9Z/9E)-isomers. The deprotected C_{15}-, C_{20}- and C_{27}-esters 28, 29 and 30 are given.

An initial synthesis of rac. azafrin ester (30) using another building-up sequence was first published by Prof. Weedon et al. (Ref. 34). Here, the synthesis of (±)-azafrin methyl ester was realised by a different route.

Of importance is the determination of the absolute configuration of a series of apocarotene glycols, which have been isolated by Kulkarni (Ref. 35) and Endo (Ref. 36) from *Aeginetia* and *Rehmannia*, respectively (see Scheme 16).

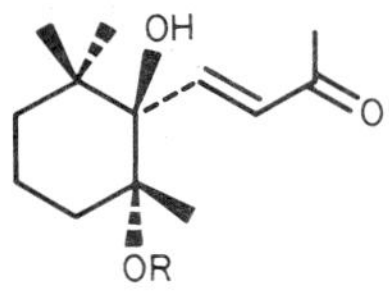

31 R=H
R=β-D-glucose
(Rehmannia-glucoside)

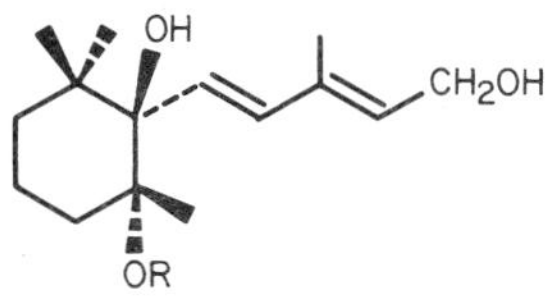

32 R=H
R=β-D-glucose
(Aeginetoside)

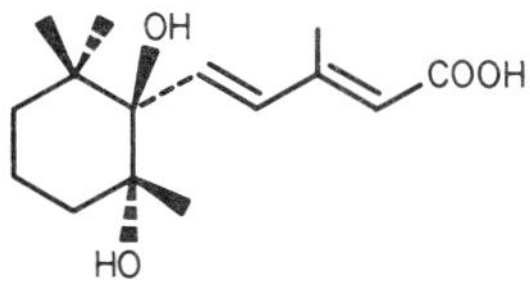

33 Aeginetic acid

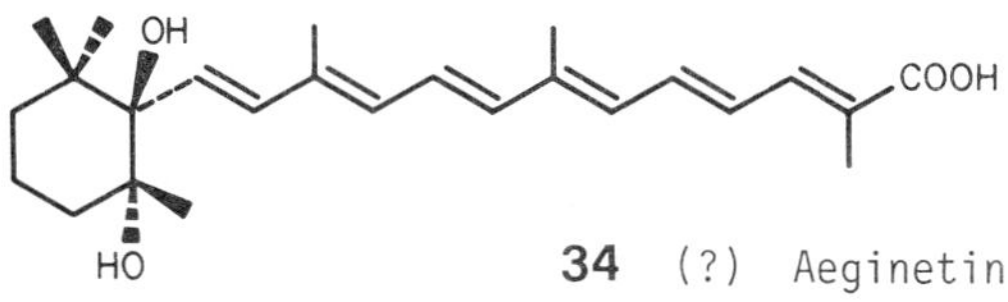

34 (?) Aeginetin

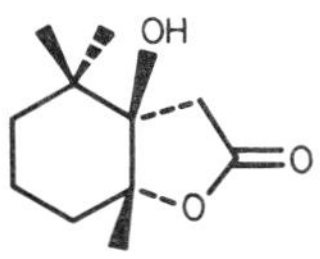

35 (?) Aeginetolide

Scheme 16

The absolute configurations of 31, 32 and 33 (see Note a) result from comparison of their spectroscopic and chiroptical data with published values (and partly by comparison with authentic reference substances), whilst those for 34 and 35 have not yet been rigorously proved. The splendid uniformity with regard to the stereochemistry at the glycol group should not obscure the fact that there also exist carotene glycols with different stereochemistry (Ref. 1). If the starting materials are 5,6-epoxides, the outcome of the acid-catalysed epoxide hydrolysis can be influenced by the neighbouring group effect of hydroxyl groups, e.g. at C(3). Up till now too few investigations have been made in this context.

I would, however, like to point out the interesting work of Behr et al. (Ref. 38) in which such a neighbouring group participation has been found (see Scheme 17).

Note a. 31 R=H: isolated from rhizomes of Rehmannia glutinosa var. purpurea (Ref. 36) as well as from tea oil (Ref. 37); R=β-D-glu from Aeginetia indica var. gracilis (Ref. 36). 32 R=β-D-glu: from Ae. indica (Ref. 36). 33, 34 and 35 from Ae. indica (Ref. 35).

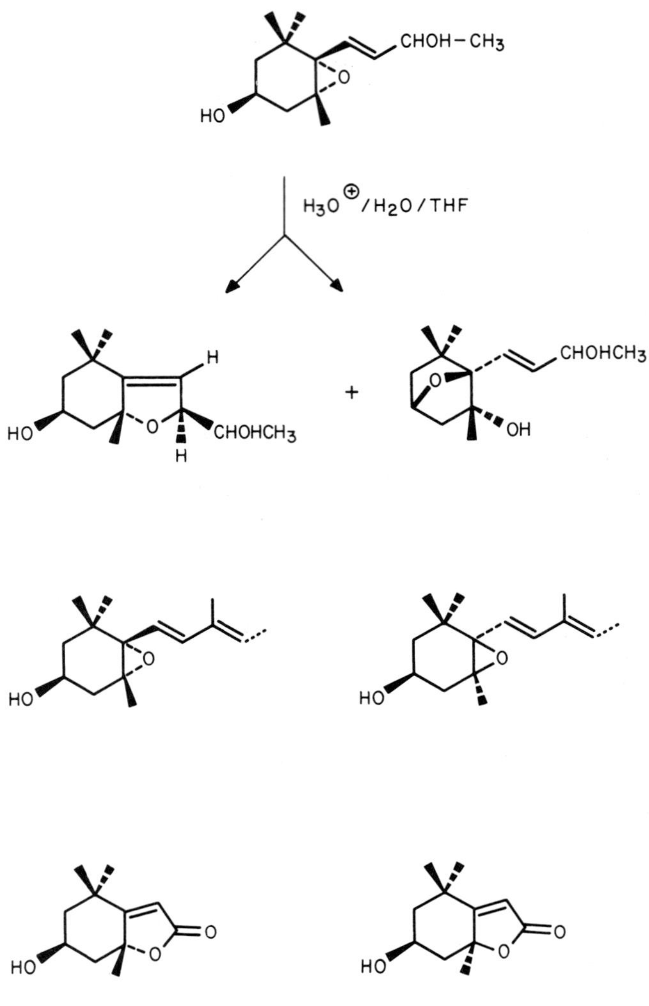

(-)-loliolide (+)-isololiolide

Scheme 17

4. 5,6- AND 5,8-EPOXYCAROTENOIDS

All xanthophyll epoxides hitherto elucidated exhibit a trans-relationship between OH(3) and the epoxide group. This is preserved as was shown by Prof. Weedon on acid-catalysed rearrangement to 5,8-epoxides. The (-)-loliolide discovered in many plants may have arisen by degradation reactions from furanoid carotenoids. Recently, now also (+)-isololiolide has been isolated from tobacco (Ref. 38) and from the marine sponge *Tedania ignis* (Ref. 39). Perhaps this is a pointer to the rearrangement of a 5,6-epoxide to a 5,8-epoxide with inversion of configuration at C(5) or, yet again, to the occurrence of still unknown isomeric xanthophyll epoxides (also compare Ref. 40) (see Scheme 17).

During the structural elucidation of mimulaxanthin (36) (see Note a) and de-epoxyneoxanthin (37) (see Note b) we came up against the old problem of a clean de-epo-

---

Note a. From *Lamium montanum* (Ref. 41).

Note b. From *Mimulus guttatus* and *M. tigrinus* (Ref. 41).

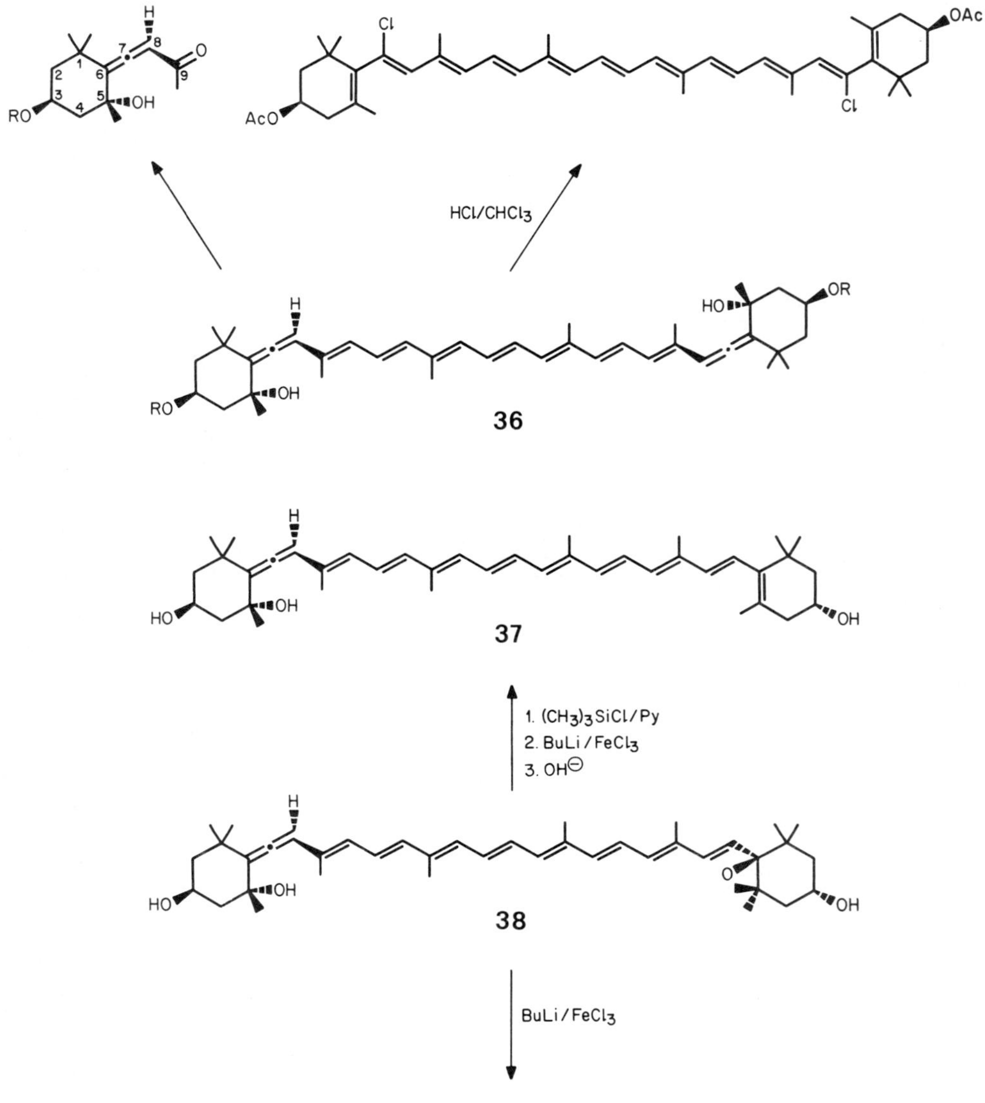

(3R,3'R)-Zeaxanthin (**39**)

Scheme 18

xidation reaction in order to prove the chirality of the basic carotenoid. Since previously used methods (see Note a) could not be considered for allenic carotenoids, e.g. 36, 37 and 38, we worked with the BuLi/$FeCl_3$ system (Ref. 45) and obtained good results by suitable modification: with no silylation of the hydroxyl groups of neoxanthin (38), reduction of the epoxide function is also accompanied by a reduction and elimination at the allene group to give zeaxanthin (39); on silylation only the epoxide group is removed and de-epoxyneoxanthin (37) is formed in good yield; thus its absolute configuration is established.

Note a. Propyl-MgBr/$FeCl_3$ (Ref. 42); $LiAlH_4$/ether/infrared (Refs. 43 & 44).

(3R,3'R)-Zeaxanthin (**39**)

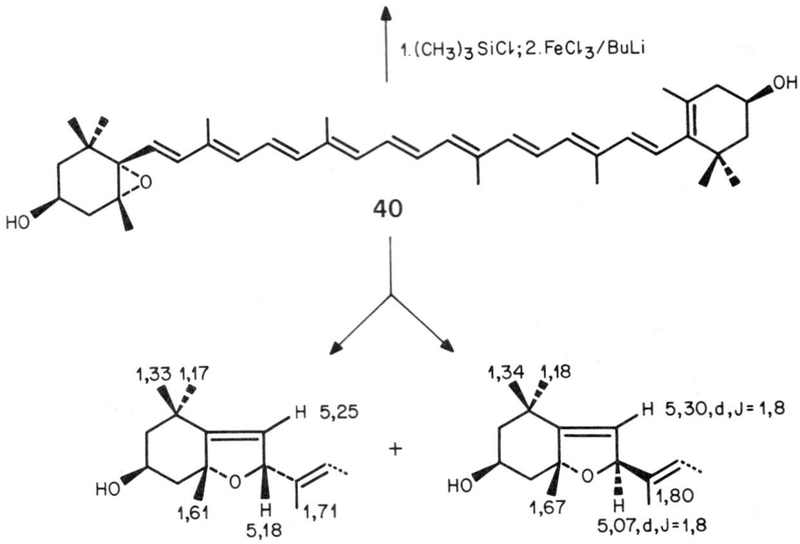

41 Mutatoxanthin a
m.p. 203^0

42 Mutatoxanthin b
m.p. 159^0

δH(7) > δH(8)

trans: H(7) & H(8) s br.

cis: H(7) & H(8) d, J=∿2Hz

Scheme 19

Structure 40 for antheraxanthin (see Note a) is based on known firm argumentation so that the de-epoxidation to (3R,3'R)-zeaxanthin (see Note b) was predictable.

We have also separated the stereoisomeric mutatoxanthins, which arise by acid catalysed rearrangement of *cis*- and *trans*-antheraxanthin, and structurally traced back to flavoxanthin and chrysanthemaxanthin (Refs. 9 & 19), respectively. The crucial points in our assignment concern: the chemical shifts of H-C(7) and H-C(8) and the coupling constants. Our conclusions were later independently confirmed by Jeger et al. (Ref. 47). They allow further assignments to be made than so far recorded in the literature (see Scheme 20): Prof. Jensen's team has now published the complete arguments for the absolute configuration of peridinin and dinoxanthin (43) (Ref. 48; see also Ref. 1). "Sulcatoxanthin" isolated from *Anemonia sulcata* and *Phycobrachia douglasii* is identical with peridinin (Ref. 49).

Comparison of the data published for both dinochromes (44 & 45) with our own data, enables us to draw conclusions as to the structure of these dinochrome,

---

Note a. ORD and partial synthesis from zeaxanthin (antheraxanthin A with OH(3) and epoxide *trans*; antheraxanthin B with OH(3) and epoxide *cis*) (Ref. 46); de-epoxidation with $LiAlH_4$ giving zeaxanthin (Ref. 43).

Note b. The reaction was performed on the (9Z)-stereoisomer ("*cis*-antheraxanthin").

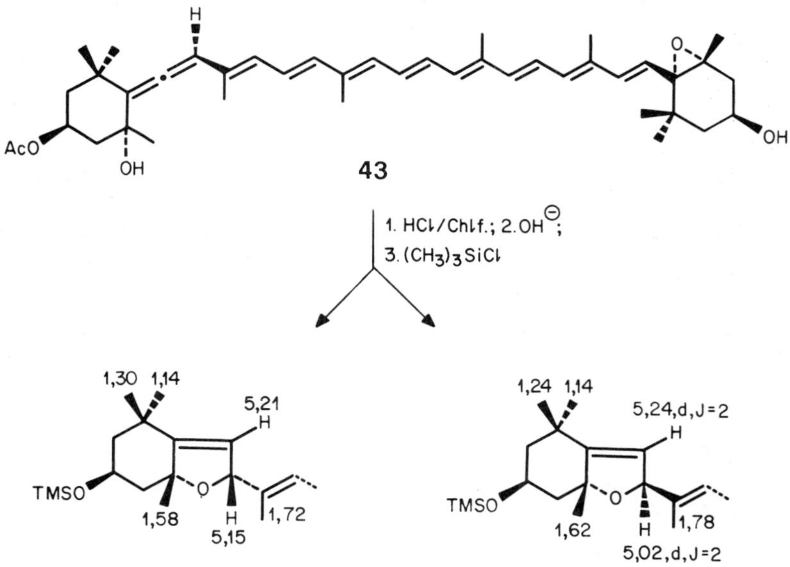

44 Epimer 1 (Note a)
(Dinochrome b, Neochrome b)

45 Epimer 2 (Note a)
(Dinochrome a, Neochrome a)

Scheme 20

(=3-O-acetyl-neochrome) epimers, respectively (see Note b).

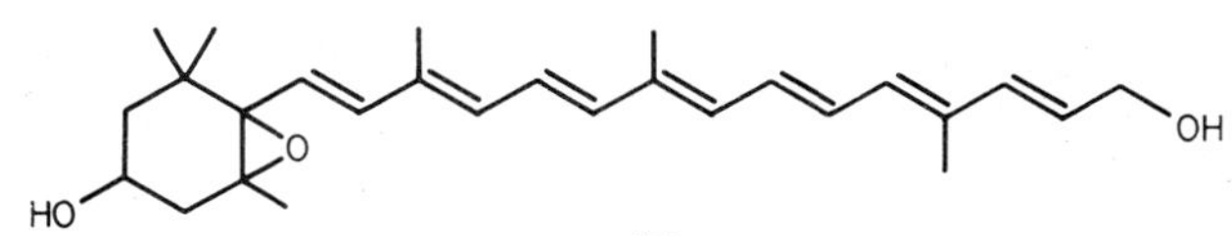

46

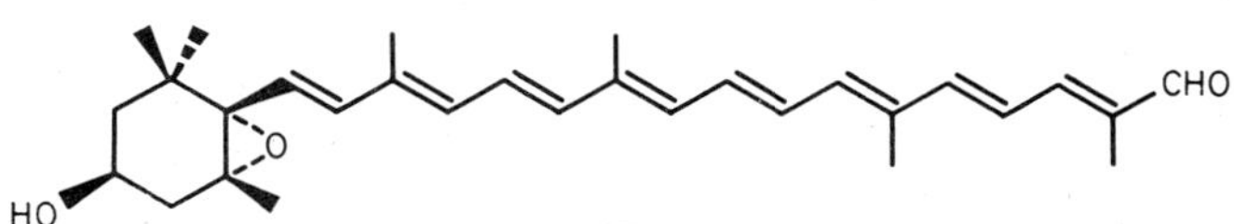

47

Scheme 21

In the more recent literature various apocarotenoids with 5,6- and 5,8-epoxide functions have been described, e.g. 46 from "Golden Delicious" apples (Ref. 51). Unfortunately, lack of data prevents conclusions on the stereochemistry. A great number of apocarotenals were synthesised by Molnar and Szabolcs by controlled $KMnO_4$ oxidation of 5,6- and 5,8-epoxycarotenoids (Ref. 52). Apo-8'-violaxanthal (47) (5,6-epoxy-citraurin) has been newly discovered in Valencia oranges (Ref. 53).

Note a. Assignment changed with respect to Ref. 48 (Scheme 20).

Note b. Similar assignments can now be made for fucochrome a and fucochrome b on the basis of the published ^{1}H-NMR-data (Ref. 50).

5. Z/E-ISOMERIC CAROTENES AND CAROTENOIDS

The facile (Z/E)-isomerism, the separation of the isomers and the localisation of the (Z)-bond is a fundamental problem in carotene chemistry. As Dr. Moss in Bern (Ref. 22) illustrated, ^{13}C-NMR-spectroscopy supplies us with very distinct information. Using this method, the configurations of four stereoisomeric luteins and four capsanthins have been clarified (Ref. 23): neo-A'-lutein has the (13'Z)-, neo-A" (13Z)-, neo-B'(9'Z)- and neo-B" (9Z)-configuration. Similar results were obtained for the capsanthin series.

The following new natural products were isolated and structurally elucidated: (15,15'Z)-violaxanthin (m.p. 107°) from Viola tricolor (Ref. 54), (9Z,9'Z)-antheraxanthin from Valencia oranges (Ref. 53), (13Z)- and (15,15'Z)-zeaxanthin as well as several (Z)-rubixanthins from hips of Rosa pomifera (Ref. 55).

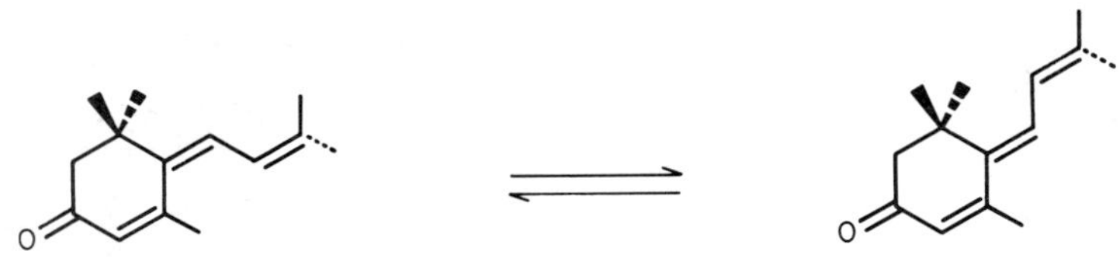

(6Z)- (6E)-

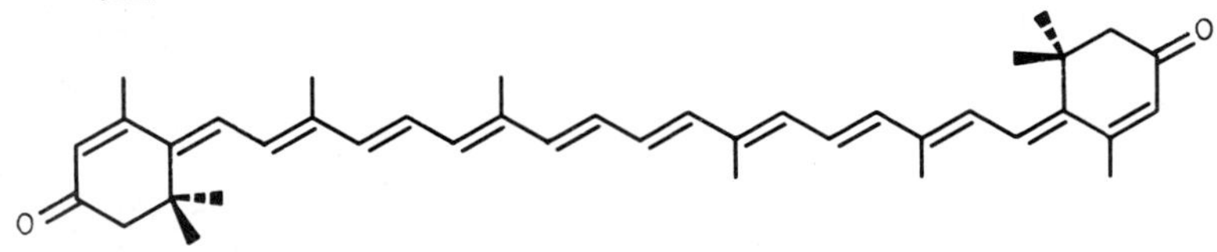

48

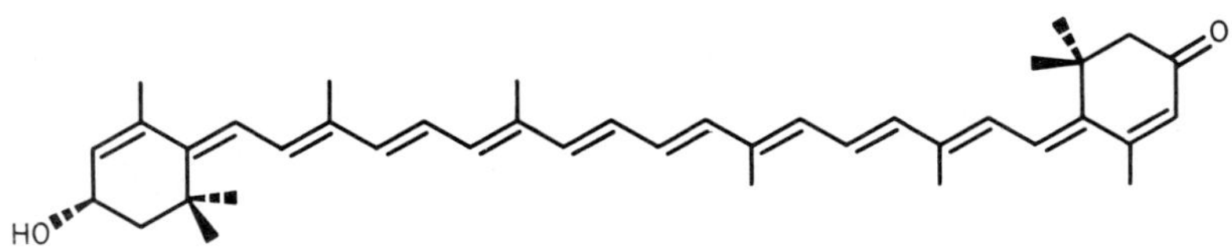

49

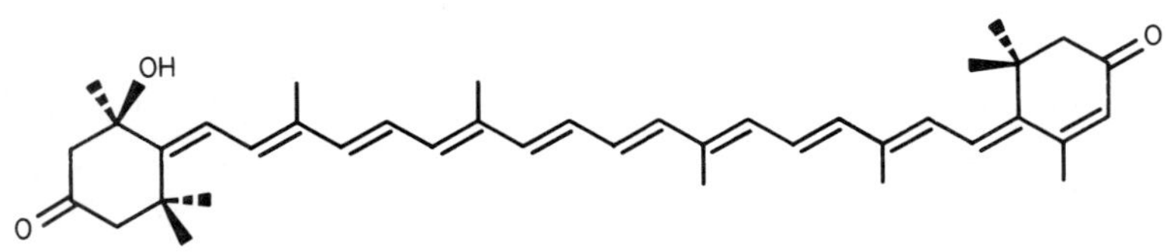

50

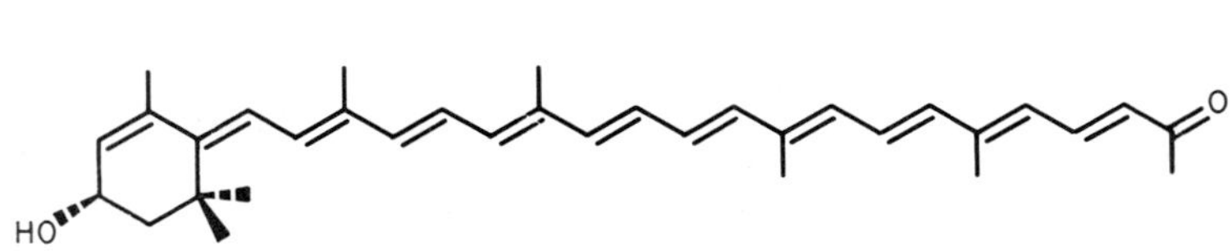

51

Scheme 22

The extensive spectroscopical investigations by Andrewes et al. (Ref. 56) provided an important clarification of the stereochemical characteristics of retro carotenoids. NOE-experiments show that rhodoxanthin exists in solution to 90% in the (6E)-configuration. Model compounds with retro structure show about 70% of the (6E)- and 30% of the (6Z)-form. Similarly, eschscholtzxanthin (48) prefers the (6E)-configuration. The mechanism of the E/Z-isomerisation in retro compounds is not known. It is assumed that eschscholtzxanthone has structure 49, loniceraxanthin structure 50 and tangeraxanthin structure 51 (Ref. 56).

Acetylenic carotenoids isomerise particularly easily. Fiksdahl et al. (Ref. 57) have carried out new extensive investigations using HPLC separation techniques. It seems that not only sterical but also electronic effects exert an influence on the position of the (Z/E)-isomer equilibria.

The most important advancement in the localisation of (Z)-double bonds has been provided by high-field ^{1}H-NMR-spectroscopy, since much smaller amounts of substance are required than for ^{13}C-NMR-spectra. As Dr. Englert will be lecturing himself and he is one of the pioneers of this method, I can limit myself to a few comments.

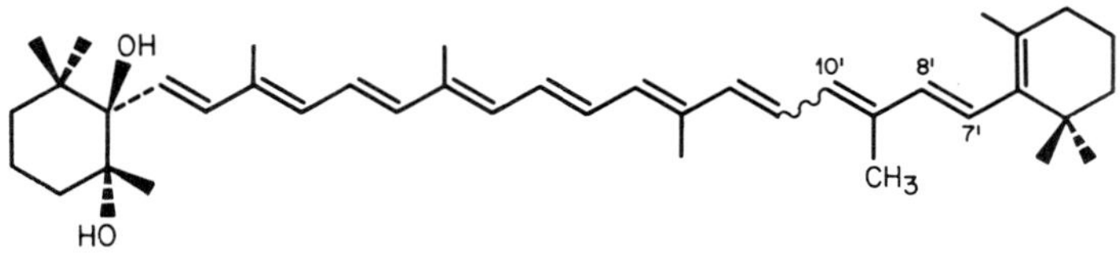

52

	CH_3(5')	H(7')	H(8')	CH_3(9')	H(10')	H(11')
Δδ(10Z-10E)	+0,03	0	+0,55	0	-0,08	+0,16

(360 MHz; Ref. 58)

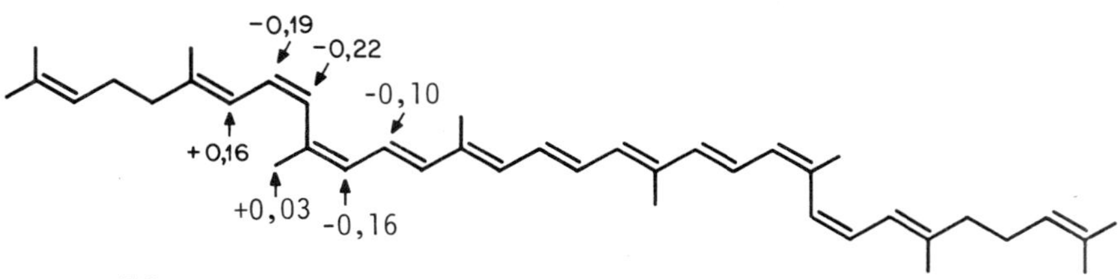

53 Prolycopene (Ref. 59) (Δδ Z-E)

Scheme 23

360 MHz-spectra led Dr. Eschenmoser to clarify the (Z/E)-isomerism in the carotene glycol 52 (Ref. 58). The shift differences found show that H(8') and H(11') in the (9'Z)-isomer undergo strong shifts to lower field.

The structure of the so-called prolycopene, isolated from tomatoes by Zech--meister (1941), was deduced simultaneously by two research groups to be 53 (Refs. 59 & 60). Furthermore, Clough & Pattenden (Ref. 60) have elucidated the structures of (15,15'Z)-, (9'Z)-phytofluene, (9Z,9'Z)-ζ-carotene and (9Z,9'Z,7'Z)-neurosporene from tangerine tomatoes.

On the basis of careful isomerisation experiments, Szabolcs and co-workers have postulated the (9Z)-configuration as being very probable in the so-called cis-antheraxanthin from species of *Lilium* (Ref. 61). Dr. Englert very kindly measured the ^{1}H-NMR-spectra (400 MHz) of the three antheraxanthin isomers 54 (9Z), 55 and 56 and confirmed the structures given (see Scheme 24). The (9Z)-configuration is easy to recognize by the strong shift to low field of H(8) (see Note a). The all-E-antheraxanthins 55 and 56 show unexpectedly small differences in their ^{1}H-NMR-spectra, chiroptical and chromatographical variations being more characteristic.

Note a. Compare Ref. 62 and tables 6, 7 & 8 in this Ref.

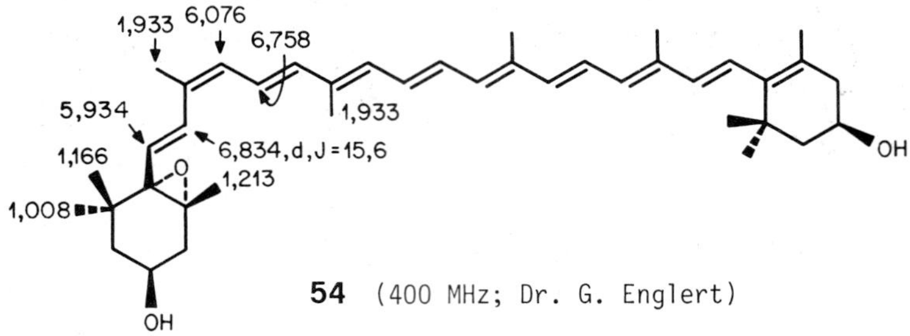

54 (400 MHz; Dr. G. Englert)

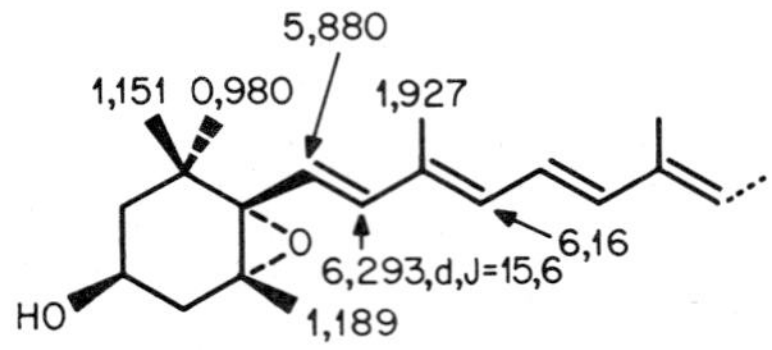

55 (400 MHz; Dr. G. Englert)

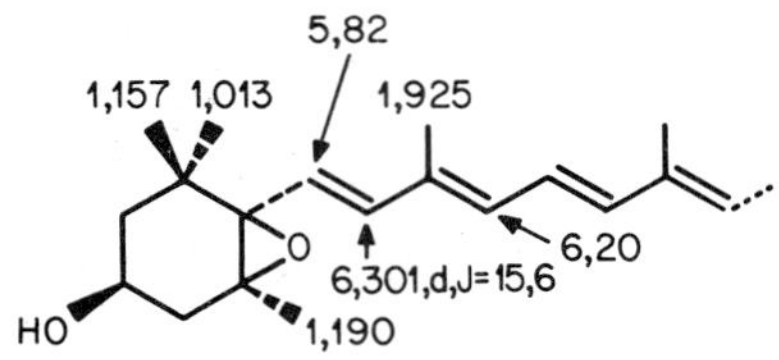

56 (400 MHz; Dr. G. Englert)

Scheme 24

6. A FEW FURTHER CAROTENOIDS WHOSE CHIRALITY HAS BEEN DETERMINED

Since most of the carotenoids to be discussed here have been isolated from marine organisms and will be dealt with in other lectures, I will limit myself to a short enumeration.

(R)-β-Citraurin, (R)-β-citraurol and (R)-β-citraurinene have been synthesised (Ref. 63). Physoxanthin from Physalis alkekengi is identical with α-cryptoxanthin (Ref. 64). It also occurs in blossoms of Caltha palustris (Ref. 41). CD-comparisons have confirmed the structure as being (3R,6'R)-β,ε-caroten-3-ol (Refs. 41 & 64).

Tedanin (57), agelaxanthin A (58) and tethyatene (59) have been synthesised (Refs. 65 & 66) (see Scheme 25). The critically commented structure of "tedaniaxanthin" (Ref. 1) has now been changed to the more plausible 3-hydroxy-7,8-didehydro-β,χ-carotene (Ref. 67). Its absolute configuration 60 was derived by Litchfield & Jensen (Ref. 68). These authors suggest the more logical name of allopurpurin for 60. Further new carotenoids isolated from Micronia prolifera are (Ref. 68): 3,4- or 2,3-didehydro-γ,χ-carotene (61), trikentriophidin (3-hydroxy-κ,φ-carotene-6,8-dione; 62), and allobetaxanthin (7,8-didehydro-β,β-caroten-3-ol; 63). The isomer of 60 with a φ-endgroup (=isotedaniaxanthin; 3-hydroxy-7,8-didehydro-β,φ-carotene) has now also been discovered in Tedania digitata (Ref. 69).

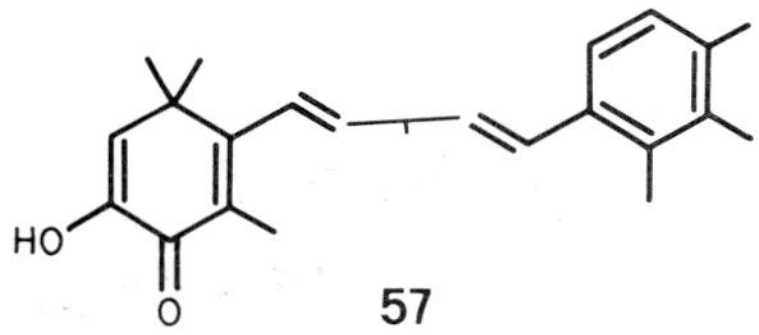

57

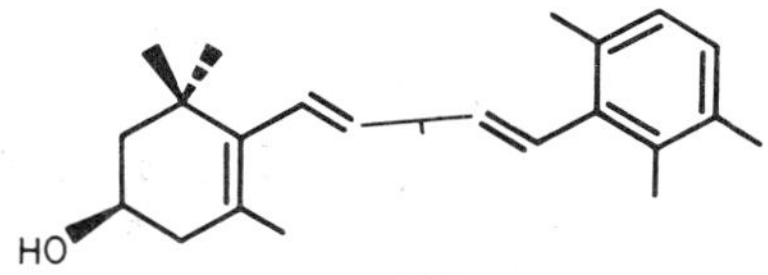

58

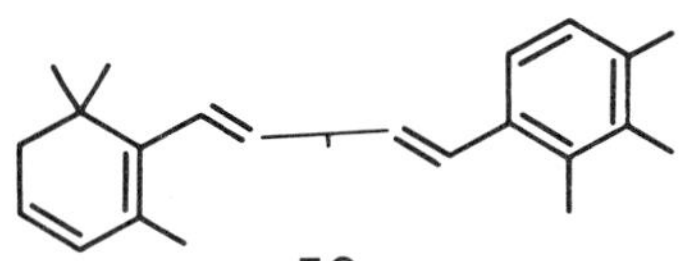

59

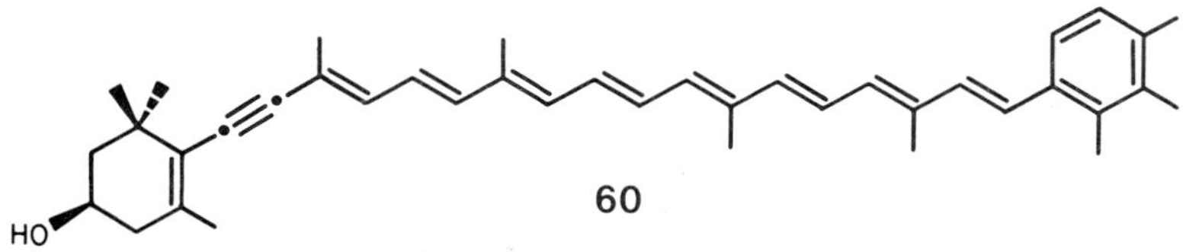

60

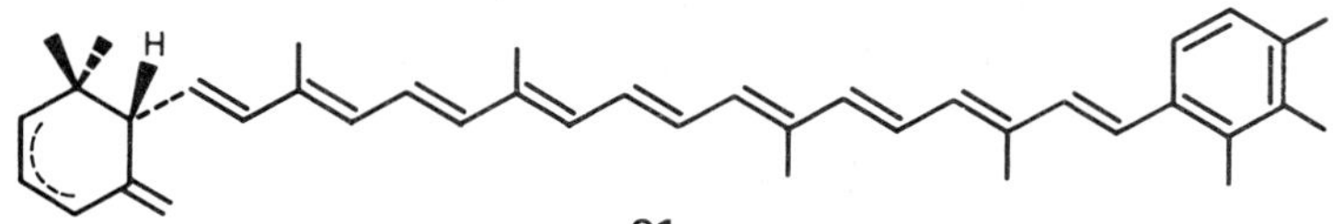

61

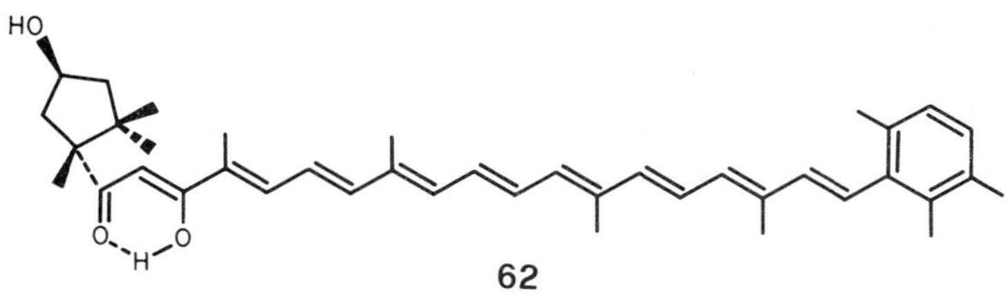

62

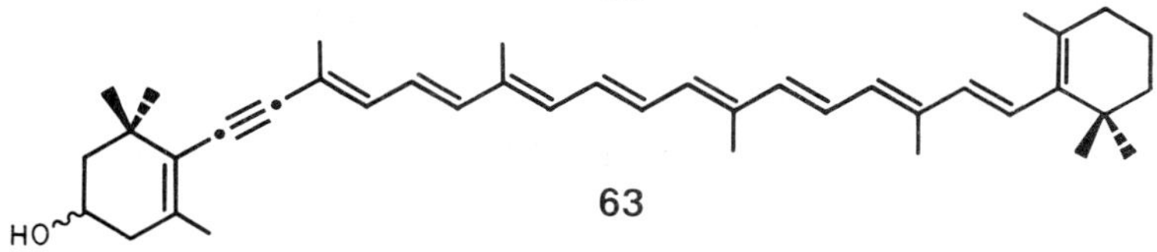

63

Scheme 25

The absolute configuration of actinioerythrin (64) (a mixture of fatty acid esters of the di-nor-carotenoid actinioerythrol), isolated from the red variation of the sea anemones *Actinia equina* and *A. tenebrosa*, has been independently determined by two research teams to be (3S,3'S) (Refs. 70 & 71) (see Scheme 26). Foss et al. degraded it to (+)-(S)-dimethyl-2-hydroxy-3,3-dimethylsuccinate (65) and obtained the absolute configuration by comparison with the enantiomers which they prepared from (-)-(R)- and (+)-(S)-pantolactone (Ref. 70).

Müller et al. (Ref. 71) synthesised the diastereomeric camphanic acid esters 66, separated them by crystallisation and chromatography and determined their absolute configuration by X-ray analysis on the (2S)-isomer of 66. The syntheses of 64 and ent-64 were accomplished via the enantiomeric phosphonium salts 67 and 68. It is important to note that both research groups came to the same result regarding the chirality of natural actinioerythrin (64) by completely different routes.

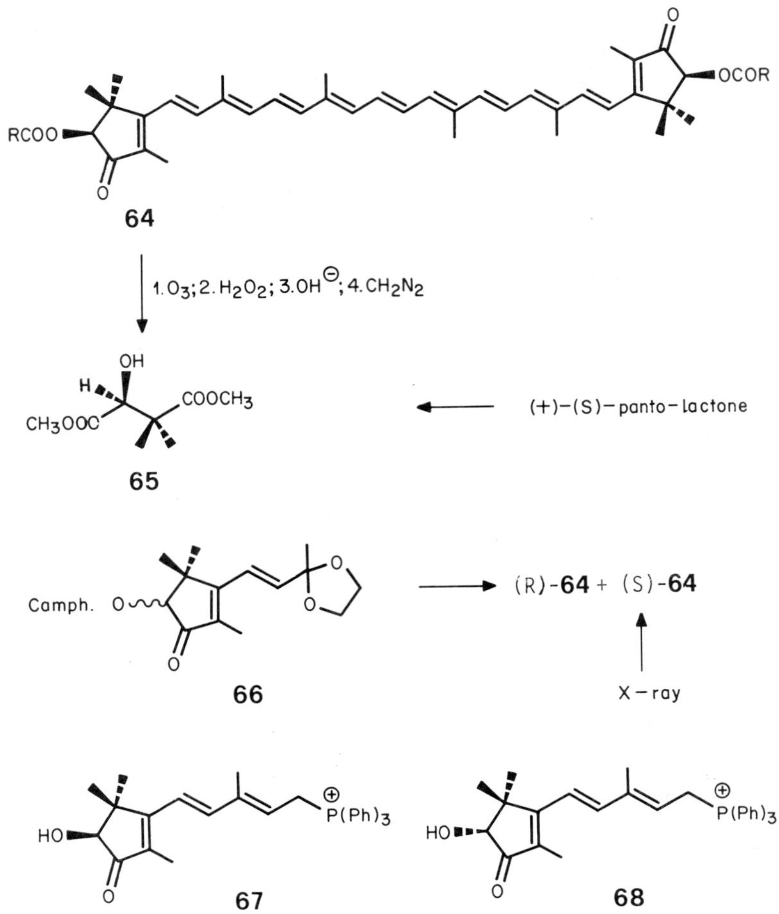

Scheme 26

7. A FEW NEW OBSERVATIONS ON CAROTENOIDS FROM ROSES

In my report in Madison in 1978 (Ref. 1), I presented an analysis of the carotenoids from Rosa foetida. This is the species whose intercrossing around 1900 has led to our modern garden roses with countless colour shades of yellow, salmon, apricot and copper.

Of course there were also yellow garden roses before 1900. They can be traced back to the intercrossing of "Parks Yellow-Tea-scented China" (Rosa X odorata ochroleuca) from about 1830. The colour "yellow", however, only really came into existence in Tea- and Noisette-roses from about 1840 ("Safrano" 1839, "Chromatella" 1843, "Gloire de Dijon" 1853, "Maréchal Niel" 1864 etc.) (see Note a).

The flowers are endowed with a characteristic soft butter-yellow colour which strongly fades outdoors. This instability of the yellow shades is typical for most of the yellow roses before 1900. A preliminary analysis of the carotenoids in "Maréchal Niel" gave the following results (Ref. 55): (15Z)-phytoene (64%), (15Z)- and all-E-phytofluene (7%), ζ-carotene (3%), neurosporene (2%), a (Z)-lycopene (trace), lycopene (0,4%), polar, aliphatic epoxides with λ_{max}

Note a. For history on the origination of the classical roses (i.e. the hybrids before 1900) compare Refs. 72, 73, 74 & 75.

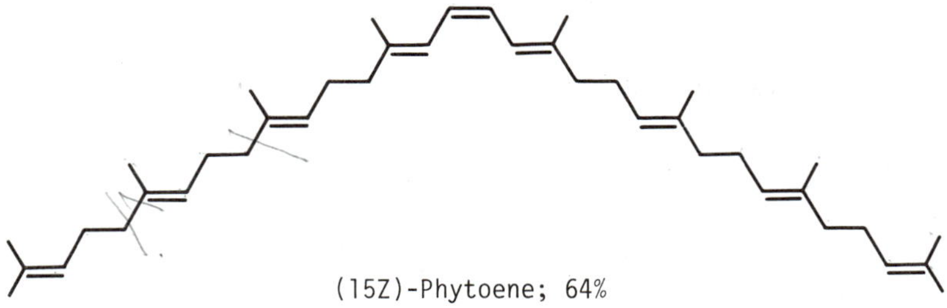

(15Z)-Phytoene; 64%

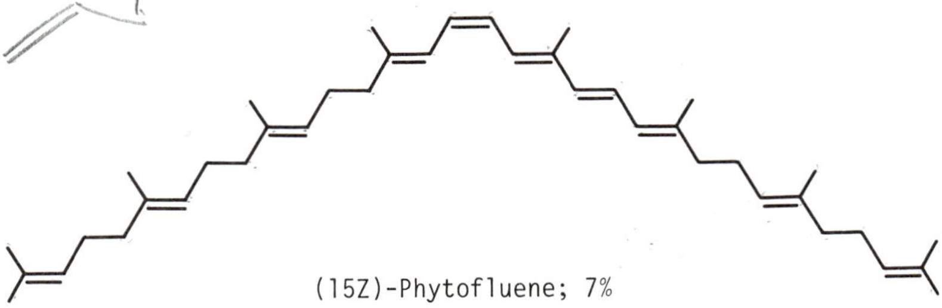

(15Z)-Phytofluene; 7%

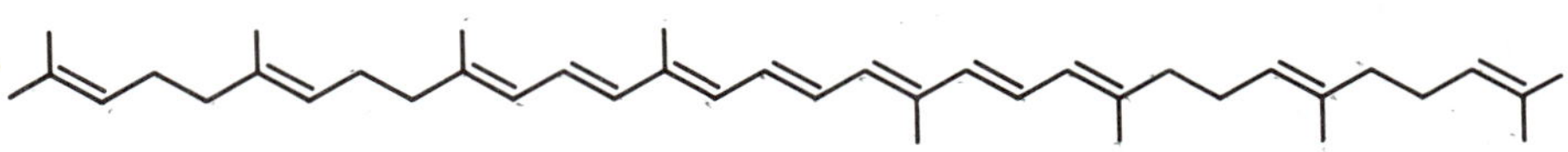

ζ-Carotene; 3%

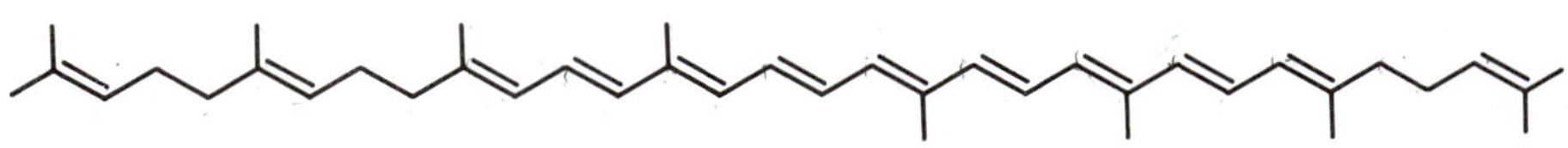

Neurosporene; 2%

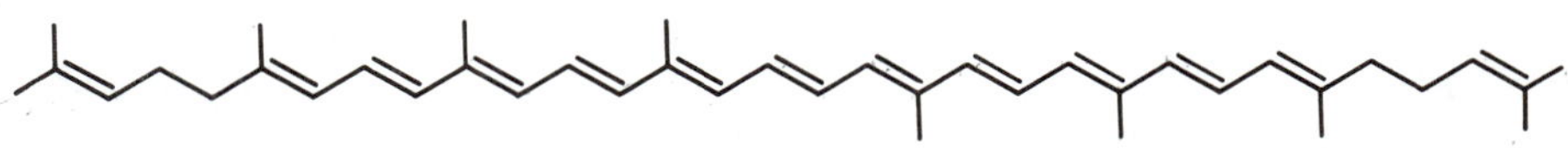

Lycopene; 0,4%

Scheme 27

< 430 nm (23%).

"Maréchal Niel" is rich in carotenes. All those identified so far are acyclic and to a small degree dehydrogenated. It seems that only ζ-carotene, neurosporene and perhaps also traces of lycopene contribute to the colour.

If one compares these results with analyses on modern roses, differences are immediately noticeable in the degree of unsaturation and the content of cyclic carotenes and epoxides thereof.

We suspect that the yellows of the classical yellow Tea roses and Noisettes were unstable because those carotenes responsible for the colour remained at early stages in the Porter-Lincoln pathway, were not cyclised and hardly epoxidised. They were, therefore, essentially lacking active carotene cyclases!

If this supposition is correct, then only a small step is required to comprehend the white roses. Analysis of one of the most famous white tea hybrids Virgo (Mallerin 1947) showed the following: (15Z,15'Z)-phytoene (83%), (15Z)- + all-E-phytofluene (9%), ζ-carotene (1%), β,β-carotene (0,5%), others (zeaxanthin, lutein, neochrome etc. (6%)).

The more strongly coloured carotenes presumably originate from the weakly yellow base of the petals or were extracted from carried over anthers.

We have obtained similar results from several classical and modern white roses (Ref. 55). This leads to the surprising fact that white roses are characterised not only by the absence of anthocyanins but also by the presence of relatively large amounts of carotenes which have remained at a very early stage in the Porter-Lincoln pathway.

I am convinced that a deeper analysis of the carotenes in roses will contribute a great deal to the understanding of their pigment formation as well as their geneological connections.

Acknowledgement - For their own contributions to this review I would like to thank the following coworkers: Dr. Hans Peter Märki, Dr. Walter Eschenmoser, Peter Uebelhart, Dr. Arnold Hofer, Miss Heidi Meier, Dr. Richard Buchecker and Mrs. Edith Märki-Fischer. For financial support I would like to thank the Swiss National Foundation for scientific research and the Ministry of Education in canton Zurich.

REFERENCES

1. C.H. Eugster, Pure Appl. Chem. 51, 463 (1979).
2. S. Liaaen-Jensen, "Stereochemistry of Naturally Occurring Carotenoids", Progress Chem. Org. Nat. Prod. 39, 123 (1980).
3. H.P. Märki and C.H. Eugster, Helv. Chim. Acta 64 (1981), in press.
4. H.P. Märki, "Synthesen von stereoselektiv deuterierten Carotinen", Ph. D. Thesis, University of Zurich (1980).
5. O. Isler, M. Montavon, R. Rüegg and P. Zeller, Liebigs Ann. Chem. 603, 129 (1957).
6. A.G. Andrewes and S. Liaaen-Jensen, Acta Chem. Scand. 27, 1401 (1973).
7. A. Bingham, D.W. Wilkie and H.S. Mosher, Compar. Biochem. Physiol. B 62, 489 (1979).
8. J. Lessard, Phan Viet Minh Tan, R. Martino and J.K. Saunders, Canad J. Chem. 55, 1015 (1977).
9. H. Cadosch, U. Vögeli, P. Rüedi and C.H. Eugster, Helv. Chim. Acta 61, 783 (1978).
10. G. Britton, T.W. Goodwin, W.J.S. Lockley, A.P. Mundy, N.J. Patel and G. Englert, Chem. Commun. 1979, 27.
11. M. Hallenstvet, R. Buchecker, G. Borch and S. Liaaen-Jensen, Phytochem. 16, 583 (1977); N. Arpin, J.-L. Fiasson, M.P. Bouchez-Dangye-Caye, G.W. Francis and S. Liaaen-Jensen, ibid. 10, 1595 (1971).
12. A.G. Andrewes, H. Kjøsen, S. Liaaen-Jensen, K.H. Weisgraber, R.J.J.C. Lousberg and U. Weiss, Acta Chem. Scand. 25, 3878 (1971).
13. D.L. Fox, "Animal Biochromes and Structural Colours", Univ. California Press, Berkeley (1976).
14. T. Katayama, H. Yokoyama and C.O. Chichester, Int. J. Biochem. 1, 438 (1970); M. Hata and M. Hata, ibid. 2, 11 (1971); T. Katayama, K. Shintani and C.O. Chichester, Compar. Biochem. Physiol. B 44, 253 (1973).
15. R. Buchecker, C.H. Eugster and A. Weber, Helv. Chim. Acta 61, 1962 (1978).
16. R. Buchecker and C.H. Eugster, Helv. Chim. Acta 62, 2817 (1979).
17. A.G. Dabbagh and K. Egger, Z. Pflanzenphysiol. 72, 177 (1974).
18. S. Liaaen-Jensen and S. Hertzberg, Acta Chem. Scand. 20, 1703 (1966).
19. H. Cadosch, U. Vögeli, P. Rüedi and C.H. Eugster, Helv. Chim. Acta 61, 1511 (1978).

20. H. Cadosch, "Struktur und Eigenschaften von Carotinoid-5,8-epoxiden (Flavoxanthin und Chrysanthemaxanthin)", Ph. D. Thesis, University of Zurich (1979).
21. R. Buchecker, P. Hamm and C.H. Eugster, Helv. Chim. Acta 57, 631 (1974).
22. G.P. Moss, Pure Appl. Chem. 47, 97 (1976).
23. M. Baranyai, P. Molnár, J. Szabolcs, L. Radics and M. Kajtár-Peredy, Tetrahedron 37, 203 (1981).
24. H. Rønneberg, G. Borch, S. Liaaen-Jensen, H. Matsutaka and T. Matsuno, Acta Chem. Scand. B 32, 621 (1978).
25. D. Siefermann-Harms, S. Hertzberg, G. Borch and S. Liaaen-Jensen, Phytochem. 20, 85 (1981).
26. C.H. Eugster, R. Buchecker, Chr. Tscharner, G. Uhde and G. Ohloff, Helv. Chim. Acta 52, 1729 (1969); R. Buchecker, R. Egli, H. Regel-Wild, Chr. Tscharner, C.H. Eugster, G. Uhde and G. Ohloff, ibid. 56, 2548 (1973).
27. R. Buchecker and C.H. Eugster, Helv. Chim. Acta 56, 1124 (1973).
28. D. Behr, I. Wahlberg, T. Nishida and C.R. Enzell, Acta Chem. Scand. B 32, 391 (1978).
29. H. Rønneberg, P. Foss, Th. Ramdahl, G. Borch, O.M. Skulberg and S. Liaaen-Jensen, Phytochem. 19, 2167 (1980).
30. H. Rønneberg, "Syntese og Stereokjemi for utvalgte Carotenoider, og Karakterisering av nye Carotenoproteiner", Ph. D. Thesis, University of Trondheim (1980).
31. J.E. Johansen and S. Liaaen-Jensen, Acta Chem. Scand. B 33, 551 (1979).
32. A. Hofer, Heidi Meier and C.H. Eugster, unpublished (1980/1981).
33. W. Eschenmoser, P. Uebelhart, A.B. Kulkarni and C.H. Eugster, unpublished (1981).
34. M. Akhtar, A.E. Faruk, C.J. Harris, G.P. Moss, S.W. Russell and B.C.L. Weedon, J. Chem. Soc. Perkin I 1978, 1511.
35. S.S. Dighe and A.B. Kulkarni, Indian J. Chem. 11, 404 (1973), 12, 413, 414 (1974), B 15, 546, 550 (1977).
36. T. Endo, H. Taguchi, H. Sasaki and I. Yosioka, Chem. Pharm. Bull. Japan 27, 2807 (1979).
37. H. Etoh, K. Ina and M. Iguchi, Agr. Biol. Chem. 44, 2999 (1980).
38. D. Behr, I. Wahlberg, T. Nishida and C.R. Enzell, Acta Chem. Scand. B 33, 701 (1979).
39. F.J. Schmitz, Y. Gopichand, D.P. Michaud, R.S. Prasad, S. Remaley, M.B. Hossain, A. Rahman, P.K. Sengupta and D. van der Helm, Pure Appl. Chem. 53, 853 (1981).
40. A.J. Aasen, S.-O. Almquist and C.R. Enzell, Beiträge Tabakforsch. 8, 366 (1966).
41. R. Buchecker and C.H. Eugster, Helv. Chim. Acta 63, 2531 (1980).
42. L. Jaeger and P. Karrer, Helv. Chim. Acta 46, 683 (1963).
43. L. Cholnoky, J. Szabolcs and G. Tóth, Liebigs Ann. Chem. 708, 218 (1967).
44. B.P. Schimmer and N.I. Krinsky, Biochem. 5, 3649 (1966).
45. T. Fujisawa, K. Sugimoto and H. Ohta, Chem. Letters 1974, 883.
46. L. Bartlett, W. Klyne, W.P. Mose, P.M. Scopes, G. Galasko, A.K. Mallams, B.C.L. Weedon, J. Szabolcs and G. Tóth, J. Chem. Soc. C 1969, 2527.
47. A.P. Alder, H.R. Wolf and O. Jeger, Helv. Chim. Acta 61, 2681 (1978), 63 1833 (1980).
48. J.E. Johansen, G. Borch and S. Liaaen-Jensen, Phytochem. 19, 441 (1980).
49. A. Fiksdahl, M. Hallenstvet, L. Béress and S. Liaaen-Jensen, Biochem. System. Ecol. 7, 173 (1979).
50. K. Bernhard, G.P. Moss, G. Tóth and B.C.L. Weedon, Tetrahedron Letters 1976, 115.
51. J. Gross and G. Eckhardt, Phytochem. 17, 1803 (1978).
52. P. Molnár and J. Szabolcs, Acta Chim. Acad. Sci. Hung. 99, 155 (1979).
53. P. Molnár and J. Szabolcs, Phytochem. 19, 633 (1980).
54. P. Molnár and J. Szabolcs, Phytochem. 19, 623 (1980).
55. E. Märki-Fischer, R. Buchecker and C.H. Eugster, unpublished (1981).
56. A.G. Andrewes, G. Englert, G. Borch, H.H. Strain and S. Liaaen-Jensen, Phytochem. 18, 303 (1979).
57. A. Fiksdahl, J.D. Tauber, S. Liaaen-Jensen, G. Saucy and G.F. Weber, Acta Chem. Scand. B 33, 192 (1979).
58. W. Eschenmoser, "Synthese und absolute Konfiguration von optisch aktiven 5,6-Epoxy- und 5,6-Dihydroxy-carotinoiden", Ph. D. Thesis, University of Zurich (1979).
59. G. Englert, B.O. Brown, G.P. Moss, B.C.L. Weedon G. Britton, T.W. Goodwin, K.L. Simpson and R.J.H. Williams, Chem. Commun. 1979, 545.

60. J.M. Clough and G. Pattenden, Chem. Commun. 1979, 616.
61. G. Tóth, J. Kajtár, P. Molnár and J. Szabolcs, Acta Chim. Acad. Sci. Hung. 97, 359 (1978).
62. W. Vetter, G. Englert, N. Rigassi and U. Schwieter, "Carotenoids" (ed. by O. Isler, H. Gutmann and U. Solms), Birkhäuser, Basel (1971).
63. H. Pfander, A. Lachenmeier and M. Hadorn, Helv. Chim. Acta 63, 1377 (1980).
64. C. Bodea, A.G. Andrewes, G. Borch and S. Liaaen-Jensen, Phytochem. 17, 2037 (1978).
65. A. Shimada, Y. Ezaki, J. Inanaga, T. Katsuki and M. Yamaguchi, Tetrahedron Letters 22, 773 (1981).
66. M. Yasuhara, K. Inanaga, T. Kumae, H.R. Brahmana, N. Okukado and M. Yamaguchi, Bull. Chem. Soc. Japan 53, 1629 (1980).
67. Y. Tanaka and T. Katayama, Bull. Jap. Soc. Sci. Fisheries 45, 633 (1979).
68. C. Litchfield and S. Liaaen-Jensen, Compar. Biochem. Physiol. B 66, 359 (1980).
69. Y. Tanaka and T. Katayama, Bull. Jap. Soc. Sci. Fisheries 46, 381 (1980).
70. P.S. Foss, P.J. Green and R.W. Rickards, Austr. J. Chem. 31, 1981 (1978).
71. R.K. Müller, H. Mayer, K. Noack, J.J. Daly, J.D. Tauber and S. Liaaen-Jensen, Helv. Chim. Acta 61, 2881 (1978).
72. R.E. Shepherd, "History of the Rose", Macmillan, New York (1954).
73. A.P. Wylie, Endeavour 14, 181 (1956) (German Edition).
74. G.S. Thomas, "The old Shrub roses", J.M. Dent, London (1971).
75. L.A. Wyatt, The Rose Annual 1975, 38.
76. S. Terashima, M. Hayashi, C.C. Tseng and K. Koga, Tetrahedron Letters 1978, 1763.

RECENT ADVANCES IN THE SYNTHESIS AND ANALYSIS OF 3,4-OXYGENATED XANTHOPHYLLS

Robert K. Müller, Kurt Bernhard and Max Vecchi*

Department of Vitamin and Nutritional Research and Central Research Units*, F. Hoffmann-La Roche & Co., Ltd., CH-4002 Basle, Switzerland

Abstract - The progress made within the last three years in the synthesis and analysis of astaxanthin and of other related 3,4-oxygenated xanthophylls is reviewed. This includes preparatively attractive routes to all optical isomers of adonirubin, 3-hydroxy echinenone, and of adonixanthin.

(3R,3'R)-, (3S,3'S)-, as well as meso-(3R,3'S)-astaxanthin could be separated by HPLC when (3RS,3'RS)-astaxanthin (a 1:1 mixture of racemate and meso-form) was first converted into the corresponding diastereomeric di-(-)-camphanates. The usefulness of this accurate analytical method for the separation of optical isomers of astaxanthin was demonstrated by the analysis of various astaxanthin samples from different natural sources. Surprisingly, some of these were found to be mixtures of the three optical isomers. The extension of this separation technique to other 3-hydroxy-4-oxo carotenoids provided, in combination with spectroscopic data, an excellent analytical method for the determination of the constitution, chirality and purity of these carotenoids.

INTRODUCTION

In his "Key to Carotenoids", Straub (Ref. 1) mentions 33 3,4-oxygenated xanthophylls possessing at least one of the end groups shown in Fig. 1. Some well known carotenoids of this class are adonirubin, astacene, adonixanthin, 3-hydroxyechinenone, crustaxanthin, actinioerythrin and violerythrin. The best known and most important of all 3,4-oxygenated xanthophylls is undoubtedly the symmetrically functionalized astaxanthin which is found in many crustaceans, such as the common lobster (Hommarus gammarus), in salmon, in the plumage of birds and in numerous other organisms. It is also the pros-

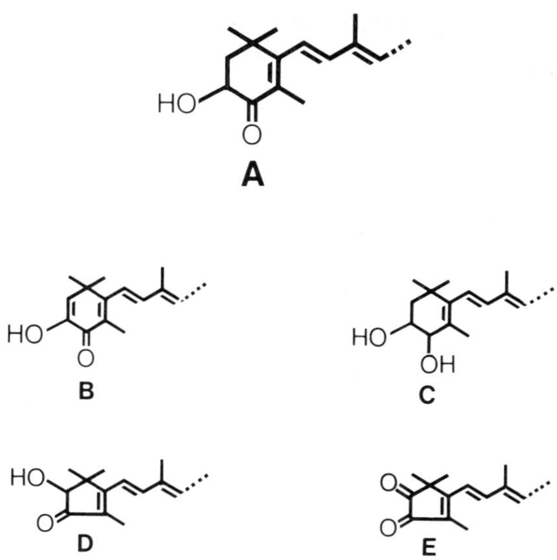

Fig. 1 End groups of 3,4-oxygenated xanthophylls.

thetic group in many carotenoproteins. Diesters with fatty acids are also common, e.g. in the skin of goldfish (Carassius auratus) and trout (Salmo trutta).

The whole field of the natural occurrence of 3,4-oxygenated xanthophylls has been reviewed by Weedon (Ref. 2); stereochemical aspects have recently been discussed by Liaaen-Jensen (Ref. 3).

The structure of astaxanthin was elucidated by Kuhn and Sörensen in 1938 (Ref. 4). The first synthesis of (3RS,3'RS)-astaxanthin (1) (Fig. 2) was

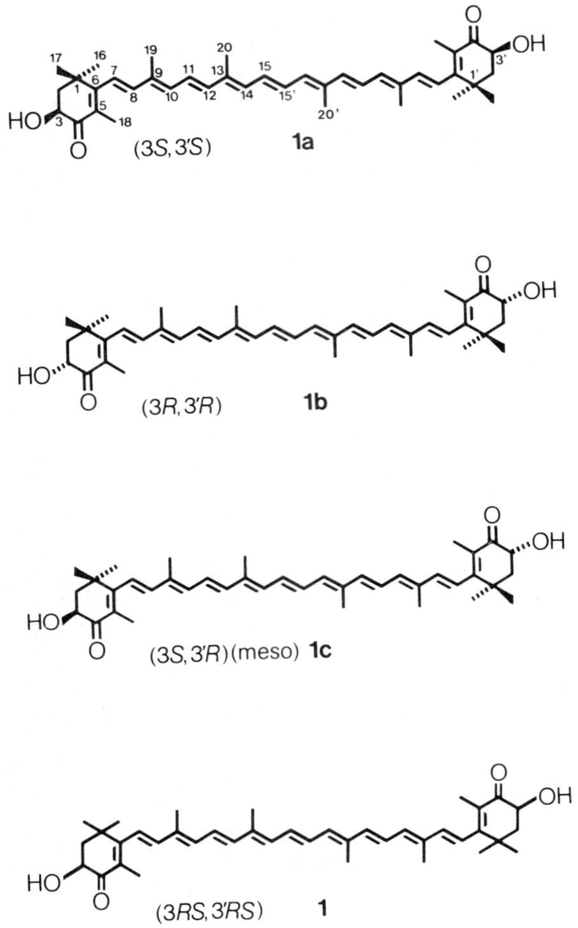

Fig. 2. Optical isomers and meso-form of astaxanthin

achieved by Leftwick and Weedon (Ref. 5). In 1974, the (3S,3'S)-configuration 1a was established for astaxanthin isolated from the green alga Haematococcus pluvialis by Andrewes, Borch, Liaaen-Jensen and Snatzke (Ref. 6). By CD comparison, the configuration of astaxanthin derived from a few other sources has also been determined to be (3S,3'S) (Ref. 7). Similar results were also obtained with zeaxanthin samples from various natural sources, which all proved to have the (3R,3'R)-configuration (Ref. 8). These findings led to the general hypothesis that natural astaxanthin should possess the (3S,3'S)-configuration.

However, in 1975, Andrewes et al. (Refs. 9, 10) reported the isolation of (3R,3'R)-astaxanthin (1b) from the yeast Phaffia rhodozyma. This unexpected result raised the question of the occurrence of enantiomeric and meso-astaxanthin in nature.

PROGRESS IN THE TOTAL SYNTHESIS OF ASTAXANTHIN

Astaxanthin is an important constitutent of fish feeds. It is deposited in the flesh of salmonids to give them their characteristic colour. Since astaxanthin cannot be synthesized by salmonids, it is necessary to include this compound in the feed to obtain adequate pigmentation. Crustacean-processing wastes or the yeast Phaffia rhodozyma can be used as a source of astaxanthin in salmonid diets. However, crustacean shells have a low astaxanthin content and a high mineral content, which is reported to cause severe practical problems when these materials are used in feed formulations (Refs. 11, 12). According to Johnson et al. (Refs. 11 12), the astaxanthin of the yeast Phaffia rhodozyma is available to rainbow trout from the diet only when the cell walls have been removed by a preceding enzymatic processing of the yeast. However, a third, and, in our opinion, probably the best solution to this problem would be to supplement the feed of cultivated salmonids with well defined nature-identical synthetic astaxanthin.

Since the first synthesis of (3RS,3'RS)-astaxanthin (1) by Leftwick and Weedon (Ref. 5), the demanding goal of a partial synthesis of astaxanthin has been taken up again in an electrochemical approach by Hall, Moss, Utley and Weedon (Refs. 13, 14). Electrolysis of astacene gave astaxanthin enoltetra-acetate which could be hydrolysed to astaxanthin in a moderate overall yield.

The development of a technical synthesis of (3RS,3'RS)-astaxanthin has been the objective of Roche chemists for the last few years.

The starting point of these investigations was the first synthesis of (3S,3'S)-astaxanthin 1a by Kienzle and Mayer (Ref. 15). Therefore, we have chosen the building scheme $C_{15} + C_{10} + C_{15} = C_{40}$ (Fig. 3) considering the phosphonium

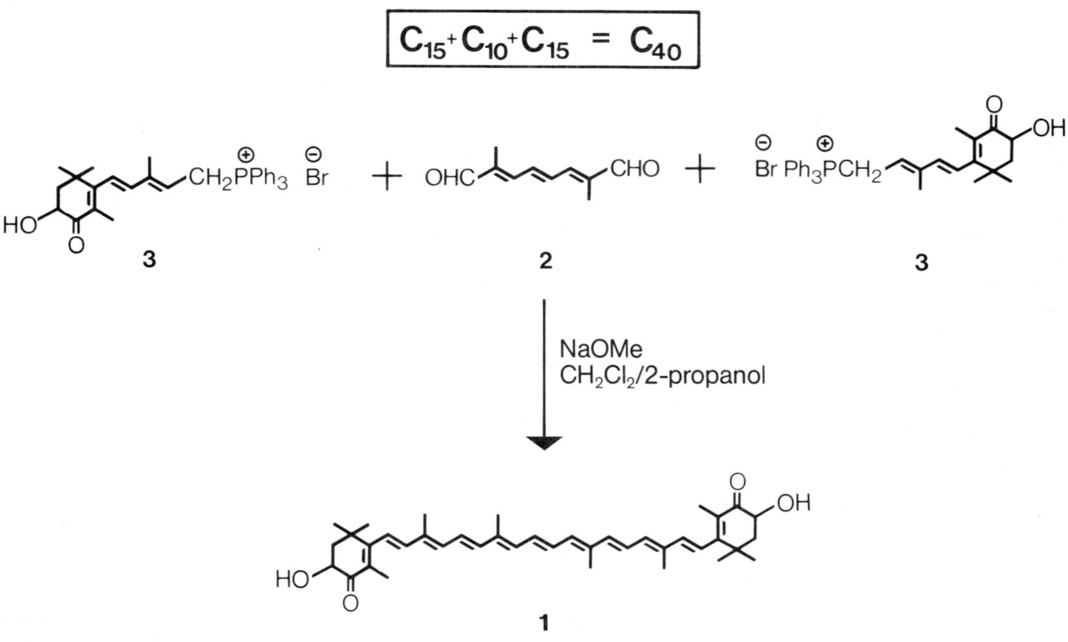

Fig. 3. Synthesis of astaxanthin

salt 3 and the C_{10}-dialdehyde 2 as most suitable building blocks. Since the C_{10}-dialdehyde is technically available, the following discussion will be focused on syntheses of the racemic and optically active unprotected C_{15}-phosphonium salts 3, 5 and 6 (Fig. 4) which were found to be superior to the protected analogues 4 and 7 (Refs. 16, 17, 18).

An efficient technical synthesis of the racemic C_{15}-phosphonium salt 3 (Fig. 5) has been developed by Widmer, Zell, Broger and their co-workers utilizing oxoisophorone 8 as a readily available starting material (Refs. 16, 17, 18). In a three-step sequence, 8 was adjusted to the oxidation level of astaxanthin to give the acetonide 11. Subsequent addition of the lithium salt of the protected acetylenic C_6-unit 12 followed by partial reduction of the resulting C_{15}-7,8-didehydro compound 13 yielded predominantly the 7,8-cis isomer 14

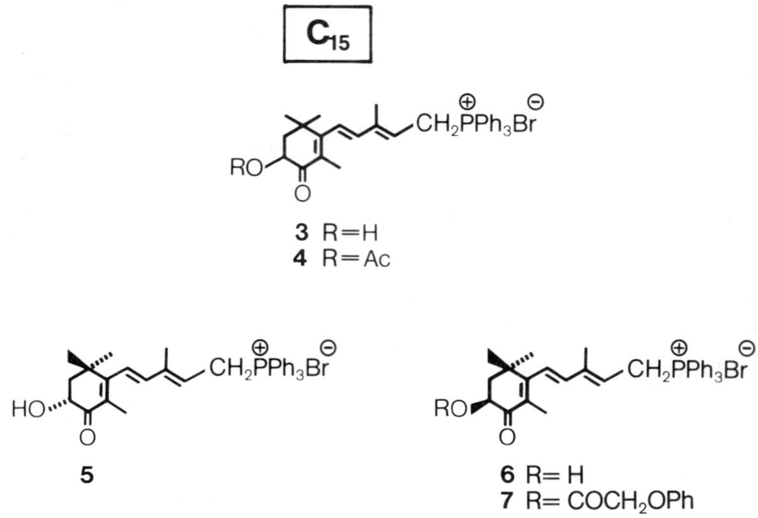

Fig. 4. C_{15}-Phosphonium salts used for the synthesis of enantiomeric-, meso- and (3RS,3'RS)-astaxanthin.

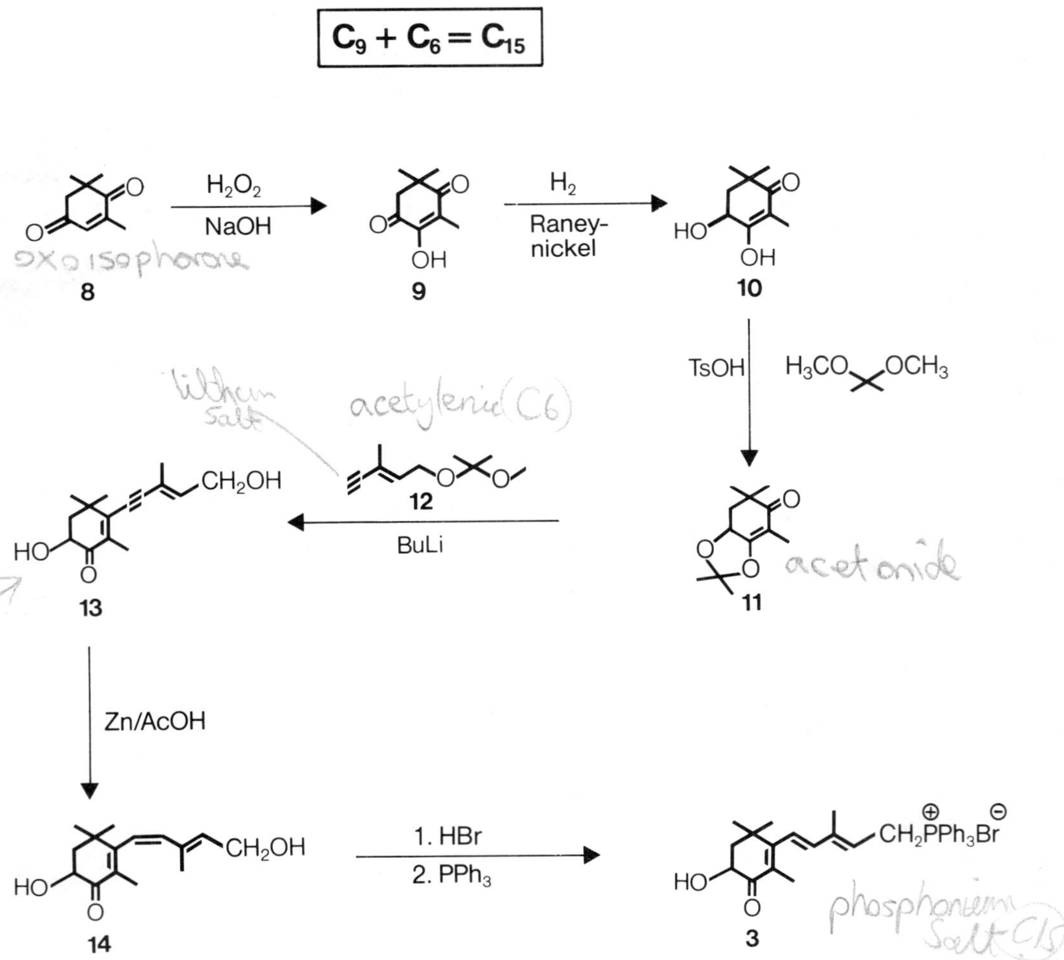

Fig. 5. Total synthesis of (3RS,3'RS)-astaxanthin from oxoisophorone.

which could be converted into the phosphonium salt 3 under simple experimental conditions. A Wittig condensation of 3 with C_{10}-dialdehyde 2 (Fig. 3) in refluxing 1,2-epoxy butane furnished (3RS,3'RS)-astaxanthin (1) of 96-98 % purity in 82.5 % yield. The whole sequence 8 → 3 → 1 has already been run on a kg scale with an overall yield of 52 % (Ref. 19).

Based on the knowledge gained in the synthesis of racemic building blocks, several new and efficient routes for the synthesis of the enantiomeric C_{15}-phosphonium bromides 5 and 6 (Fig. 6) starting from oxoisophorone derivatives

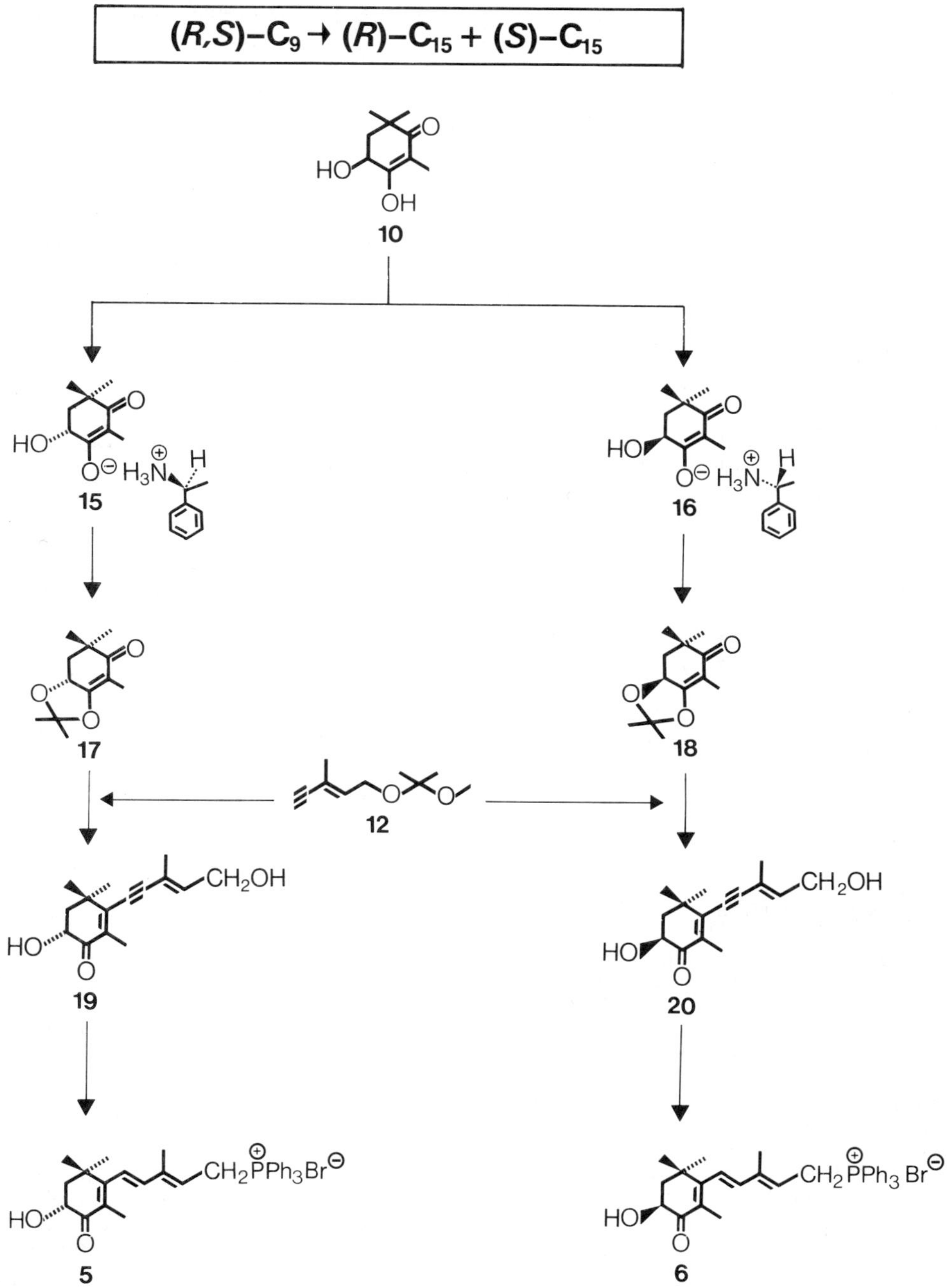

Fig. 6. Synthesis of the enantiomeric C_{15}-phosphonium salts from oxoisophorone.

have been worked out by Zell et al. (Ref. 20). As indicated in Fig. 6, partial optical resolution of the vinylogous acid 10 was realized via the crystalline salts of 10 with (S)-(-)- and (R)-(+)-1-phenylethylamine. Acidic cleavage followed by acetalization furnished the acetonides 17 and 18 only partially resolved. However, several recrystallizations from hexane yielded the optically pure acetals 17 and 18. The versatile optically active building blocks 17 and 18 were also synthesized by fermentative hydrogenation of appropriate C_9-precursors (Ref. 20). By this route, C_{15}-phosphonium salts of an optical purity of more than 99 % were obtained. These had specific rotations of + 68.8^o for 5 and -68.7^o for 6 (in ethanol).

β-Ionone (21, Fig. 7) is one of the most important intermediates in industrial

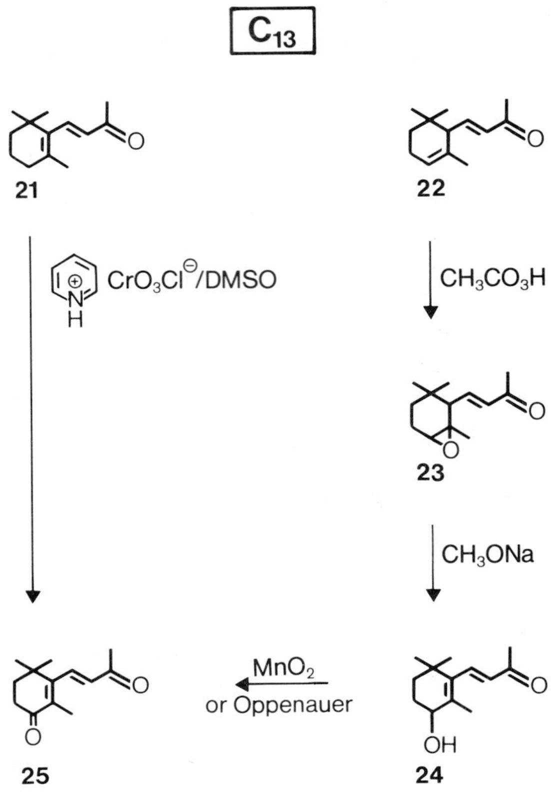

Fig. 7. Synthesis of 4-oxo-β-ionone.

syntheses of carotenoids and vitamin A (Refs. 21, 22). In an alternative route to astaxanthin (Ref. 23), we have therefore chosen β-ionone (21) as readily available starting material. As shown in Fig. 7, oxidation of β-ionone with 3 equivalents of pyridinium chlorochromate in dimethyl sulphoxide at 100° for three hours gave 4-oxo-β-ionone (25) in 50-60 % yield (Ref. 24). Alternatively, 4-hydroxy-β-ionone (24), readily prepared from α-ionone (22) according to Rosenberger (Refs. 25, 26) may be oxidized to 25 with manganese dioxide or under Oppenauer conditions (Ref. 27). The C(9)-monoacetal 27 (Fig. 8) was prepared for the specific introduction of the C(3)-oxygen functionality into the β-ionone skeleton. Treatment of 25 with 1.2 equivalents of ethyl orthoformate and 1.5 equivalents of ethylene glycol in the presence of a catalytic amount of p-toluene sulphonic acid gave a mixture of 27, 26 and 25 in the ratio of 8:1:1, from which 50 % of the desired monoacetal 27 could be isolated by crystallization from pentane at -20°. Later, we found that the diacetal 26, obtained by reaction of 25 with excess acetalization reagent, could be transformed to 96 % pure 27 in 96 % overall yield from 25 by selective hydrolysis. The monoacetal 27 proved to be a useful starting material for the synthesis of various 3,4-oxygenated xanthophylls (Refs. 24, 27, 28). Finally, racemic 3-acetoxy-4-oxo-β-ionone (28) was obtained in approx. 65 % yield by reaction of 27 with lead tetraacetate in refluxing toluene and subsequent hydrolysis of the intermediate acetal ester.

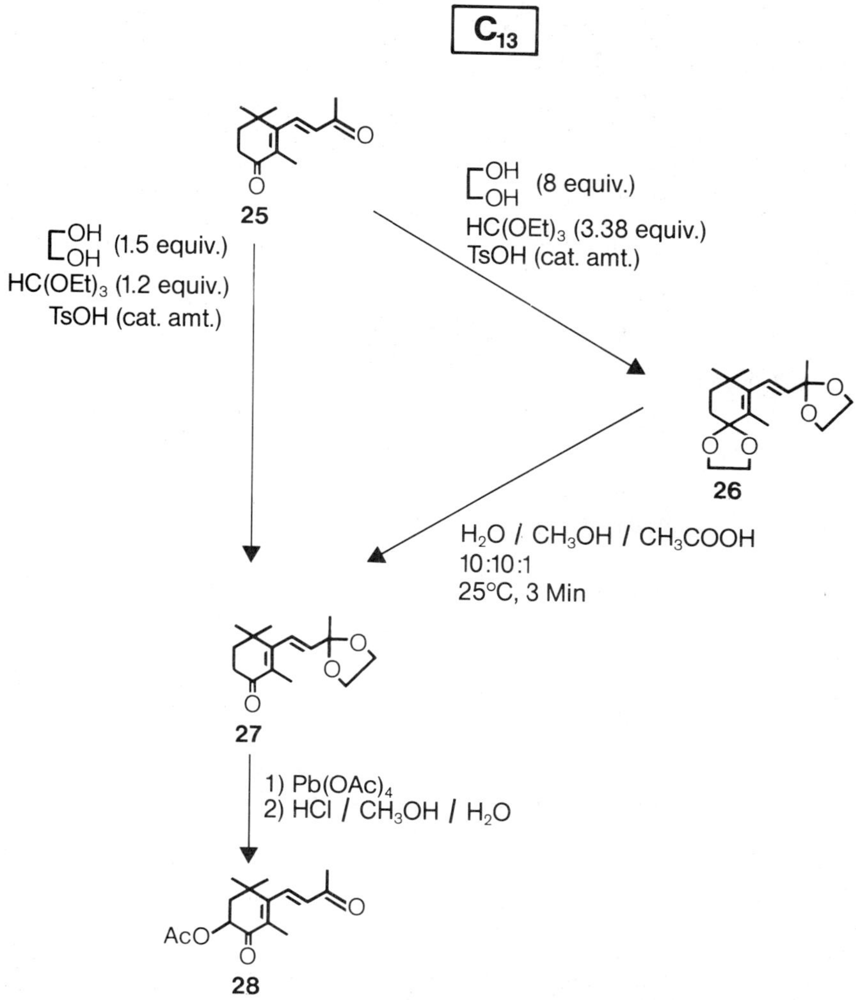

Fig. 8. Synthesis of (±)-3-acetoxy-4-oxo-β-ionone.

The transformation of 3-acetoxy-4-oxo-β-ionone (28) to the racemic C_{15}-phosphonium salt 3 (Fig. 9) required the following steps: Site-selective alkylation of 28 at C(9) with vinyl magnesium chloride in THF at -70° (Ref. 28) gave 30 as a mixture of diastereomers in more than 75 % yield. The crude product, however, contained a considerable amount of impurities which were hard to remove. Saponification of 30 with methanolic sodium hydroxide observing strict exclusion of oxygen gave the crystalline vinyl-3-hydroxy-4-oxo-β-ionol 31. The vinyl carbinol 31 was then converted into the racemic C_{15}-phosphonium salt 3 in up to 86.5 % yield under essentially the same experimental conditions as worked out for the step 14 → 3 (Fig. 5) by Widmer, Zell et al. (Refs. 16, 17). However, alkylation of 28 with lithium acetylide in THF at -70° in the presence of lithium bromide and subsequent quenching of the reaction mixture with toluene and acetic acid at -40° gave, after work-up, 84 % of the crystalline ethinyl carbinol 29. By hydrogenation in methanol over Lindlar catalyst, 29 could be converted into 30 almost quantitatively. Using this sequence, C_{15}-phosphonium salt 3 could be prepared in up to 70 % overall yield from 28.

In certain cases, site-selective alkylation of functionalized 4-oxo-β-ionone derivatives at C(9) according to the building scheme $C_{13} + C_2 = C_{15}$ may be difficult to achieve. On the other hand, functional groups can often be changed in high yield by known procedures and convenient reagents. Therefore, the readily available crystalline vinyl carbinol 31 (Fig. 10) can be consider-

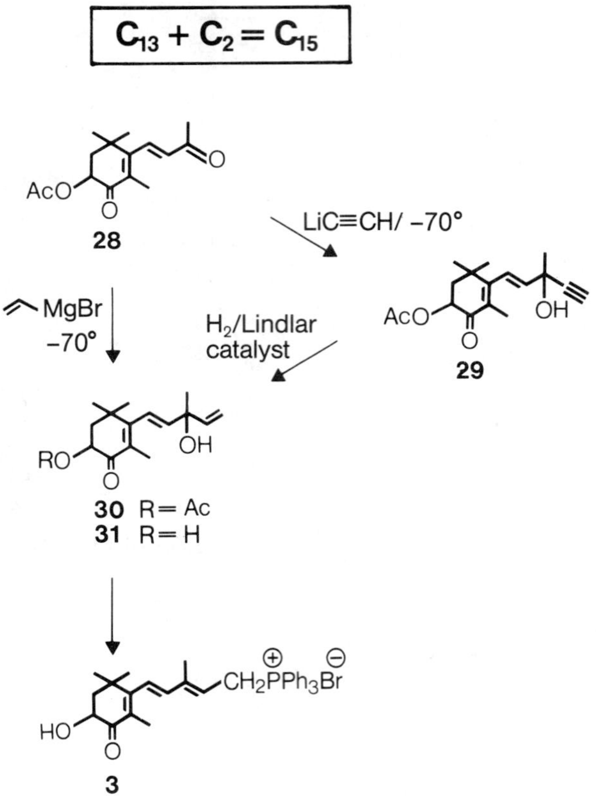

Fig. 9. Site-selective alkylation of (±)-3-acetoxy-4-oxo-ß-ionone.

ed as a common intermediate for the synthesis of 3,4-oxygenated C_{14}- and C_{15}-phosphonium salts (Ref. 27, Note a). Optical resolution of 3-acetoxy-4-oxo-ß-ionone (28) was accomplished in the following way: Esterification of the alcohol 41 with (-)-camphanic acid chloride (Note b) according to Gerlach et al. (Ref. 30) gave a mixture of diastereomeric esters 42 and 43 (Fig. 11) in more than 90 % yield. Separation into 42 (m.p. 125-126°) and 43 (m.p. 132.5-133°) was effected by fractional crystallization from ethyl acetate/hexane or diisopropyl ether or by column chromatography on silica gel. Vinylation of 42 at -70° gave a mixture of epimeric vinyl carbinols 48 in 70-75 % yield. Saponification of 48 to 50 with 1N NaOH in methanol at a temperature of -5 to 0° causes 1.5-3 % racemization, as detected by reesterification with (-)-camphanic acid chloride and HPLC analysis. Apparently, this is an inherent drawback of the saponification of the (-)-camphanates of α-hydroxy-carbonyl compounds (Refs. 23, 31). The specific rotations of the enantiomeric C_{15}-phosphonium salts obtained from this sequence were +64.4° for 5 and -63.9° for 6 (in ethanol). (3R,3'R)-Astaxanthin (1b) synthesized by this route contained 2.7 % of the meso-isomer 1c, as determined by HPLC analysis of the corresponding (-)-camphanates (Refs. 23, 32).

In a study carried out by Oritani and Yamashita (Ref. 33), a series of terpenoid secondary alcohols has been resolved microbially. Similarly, for racemic 3-acetoxy-4-oxo-ß-ionone (28), a bacillus species could be isolated from a soil sample, which hydrolyses the (R)-acetate 44 (Fig. 11) present in racemic 28 selectively to the (R)-alcohol 46 (Fig. 12). The (S)-acetate 45 remains unchanged (Ref. 23). Separation of 45 and 46 could be achieved by counter-current distribution. (S)-3-Acetoxy-4-oxo-ß-ionone (45) of approx. 97 % optical purity was obtained in 39 % yield which equals 78 % of the theoretical amount.

Note a. C_{15}-phosphonium halides of structures 33 and 34 have first been prepared by Widmer, Lukáč, Bernhard and Zell (Ref. 29) by an alternative method.

Note b. Commercially available from FLUKA AG, CH-9470 Buchs, Switzerland.

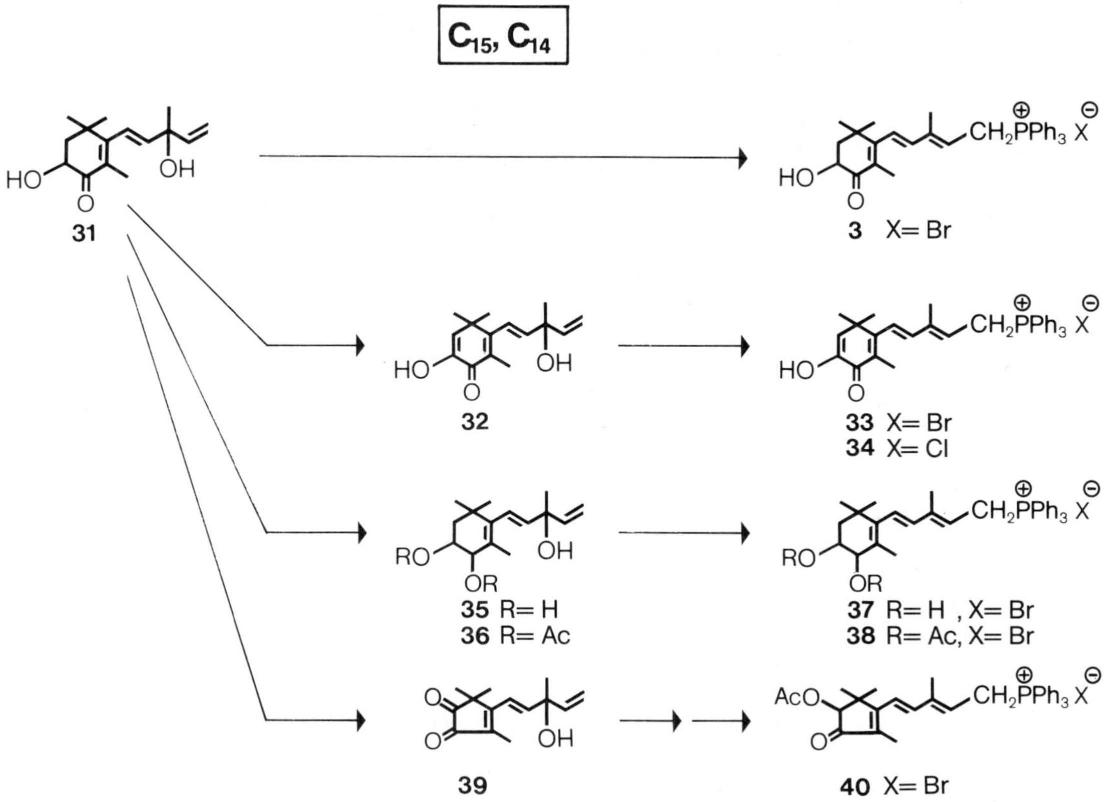

Fig. 10. Vinyl-3-hydroxy-4-oxo-ß-ionol as an intermediate for the synthesis of 3,4-oxygenated C_{15}- and C_{14}-phosphonium salts.

(R)-Acetoxy-ß-ionone (52) (Fig. 13) is an intermediate of a recently developed technical synthesis of (3R,3'R)-zeaxanthin (Refs. 34, 35). Therefore, we investigated possibilities of converting 52 into 45. Oxidation of 52 with 3 mole equivalents of pyridinium chlorochromate in dimethyl sulphoxide at 100° for 24 hours gave, after work-up and column chromatography, a 23 % yield of (S)-3-acetoxy-4-oxo-ß-ionone (45) and 26 % of unchanged starting material 52. No racemization of the product 45 could be detected (Ref. 23).

(S)-3-acetoxy-4-oxo-ß-ionone (45) prepared by one of the routes outlined in Figs. 11, 12 and 13 was alkylated site-selectively at C(9) to the carbinols 53 and 54 as described above (Fig. 9). Some differences in physical data, especially melting points, from the corresponding compounds derived from racemic 3-acetoxy-4-oxo-ß-ionone (28) were observed (Ref. 23).

ANALYSIS OF 3-HYDROXY-4-OXO CAROTENOIDS

In the light of the isolation of both enantiomers of astaxanthin from natural sources (Refs. 6, 7, 9, 10), the development of an accurate analytical method for the determination of all optical isomers of astaxanthin appeared highly desirable.

By reaction with (-)-camphanic acid chloride in pyridine according to Gerlach et al. (Ref. 30), (3RS,3'RS)-astaxanthin (1) was converted quantitatively into a mixture of diastereomers which could be separated into the esters 55a, 55b and 55c (Fig. 14) as cis/trans-mixtures by HPLC (Ref. 32), t.l.c. or even column chromatography (Ref. 31). By saponification of the separated esters 55a, 55b and 55c, all three optical isomers of astaxanthin could be obtained in yields of up to 75 % (Ref. 31). By the same procedure, (3RS)-adonirubin (3-hydroxy-ß,ß-carotene-4,4'-dione) has been resolved into its enantiomers (Ref. 31). These results demonstrate for the first time that successful resolutions may also be realized with intact C_{40}-carotenoid skeletons.

The very efficient HPLC conditions developed for the separation of the ester mixture 55a + 55b + 55c (Fig. 15) (Ref. 32) have been applied by several authors to the analysis of astaxanthin samples from various natural sources.

(R,S)-C_{13} → (R)-C_{15} + (S)-C_{15}

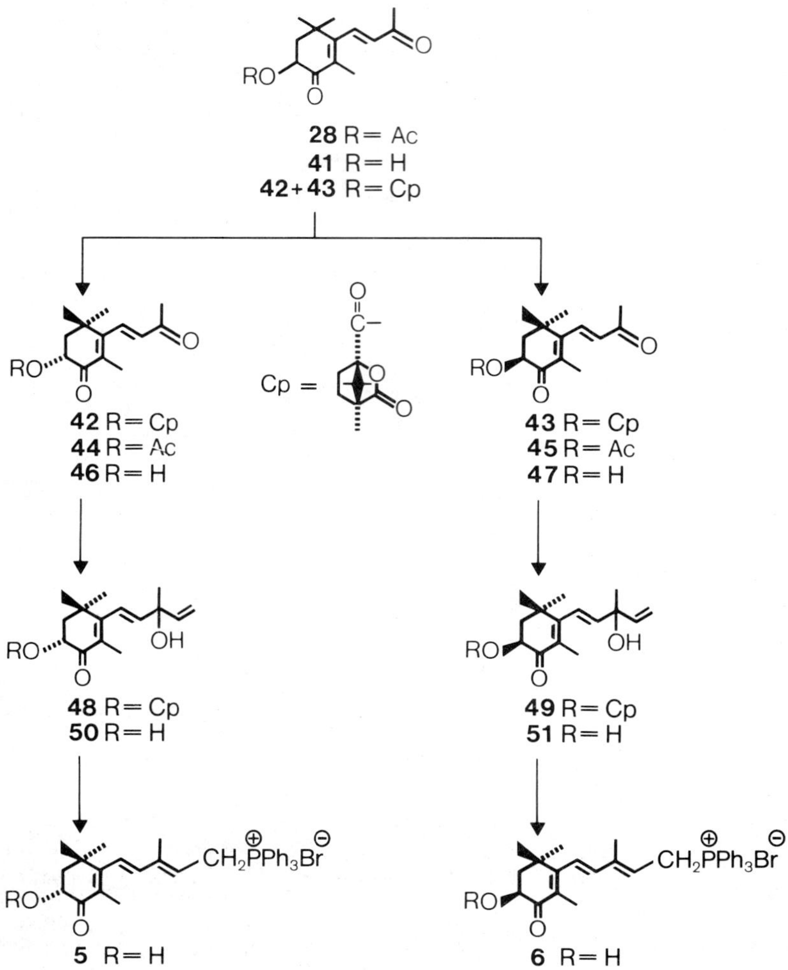

Fig. 11. Synthesis of the enantiomeric C_{15}-phosphonium salts by resolution of (±)-3-acetoxy-4-oxo-ß-ionone.

The results obtained so far are summarized in Table 1. All non-animal sources hitherto examined synthesize the pure astaxanthin isomers (3S,3'S)-1a or (3R, 3'R)-1b, whereas marine animal sources contain mixtures of all three optical isomers, including the meso form 1c.

In natural sources, astaxanthin is most frequently accompanied by minor amounts of related 3-hydroxy-4-oxo carotenoids (Refs. 2, 41-43). Moreover, xanthophylls with an α-ketol end group undergo autoxidation, especially under basic conditions, to give the corresponding diosphenols (Ref. 44). Therefore, we extended the HPLC separation technique via (-)-camphanates to some carotenoid mixtures possessing the above-mentioned end groups (Figs. 16 and 17).

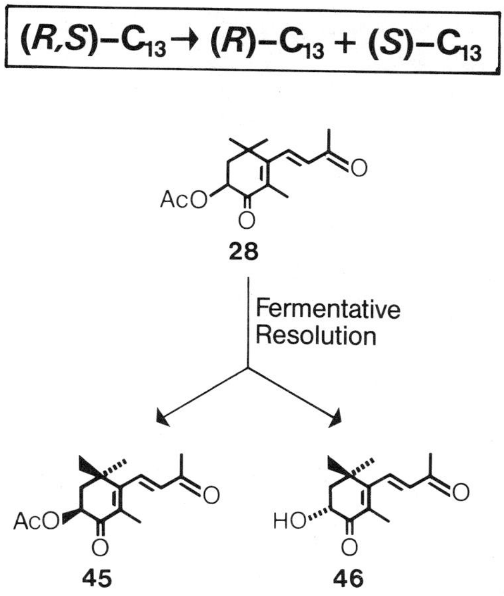

Fig. 12. Microbial resolution of (±)-3-acetoxy-4-oxo-β-ionone.

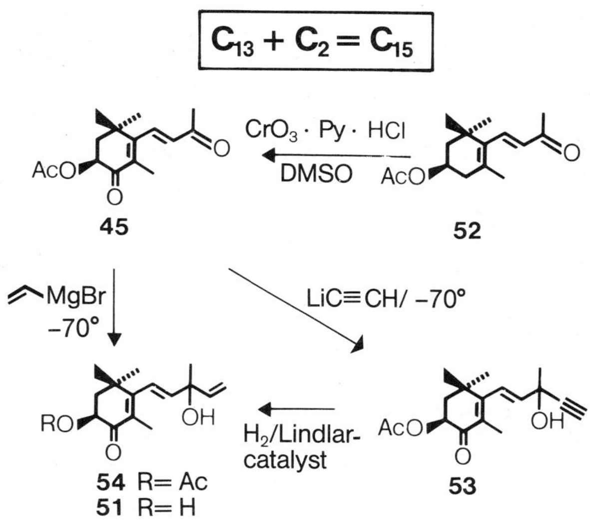

Fig. 13. Synthesis of (S)-3-acetoxy-4-oxo-β-ionone from (R)-3-acetoxy-β-ionone; site-selective alkylation of (S)-3-acetoxy-4-oxo-β-ionone.

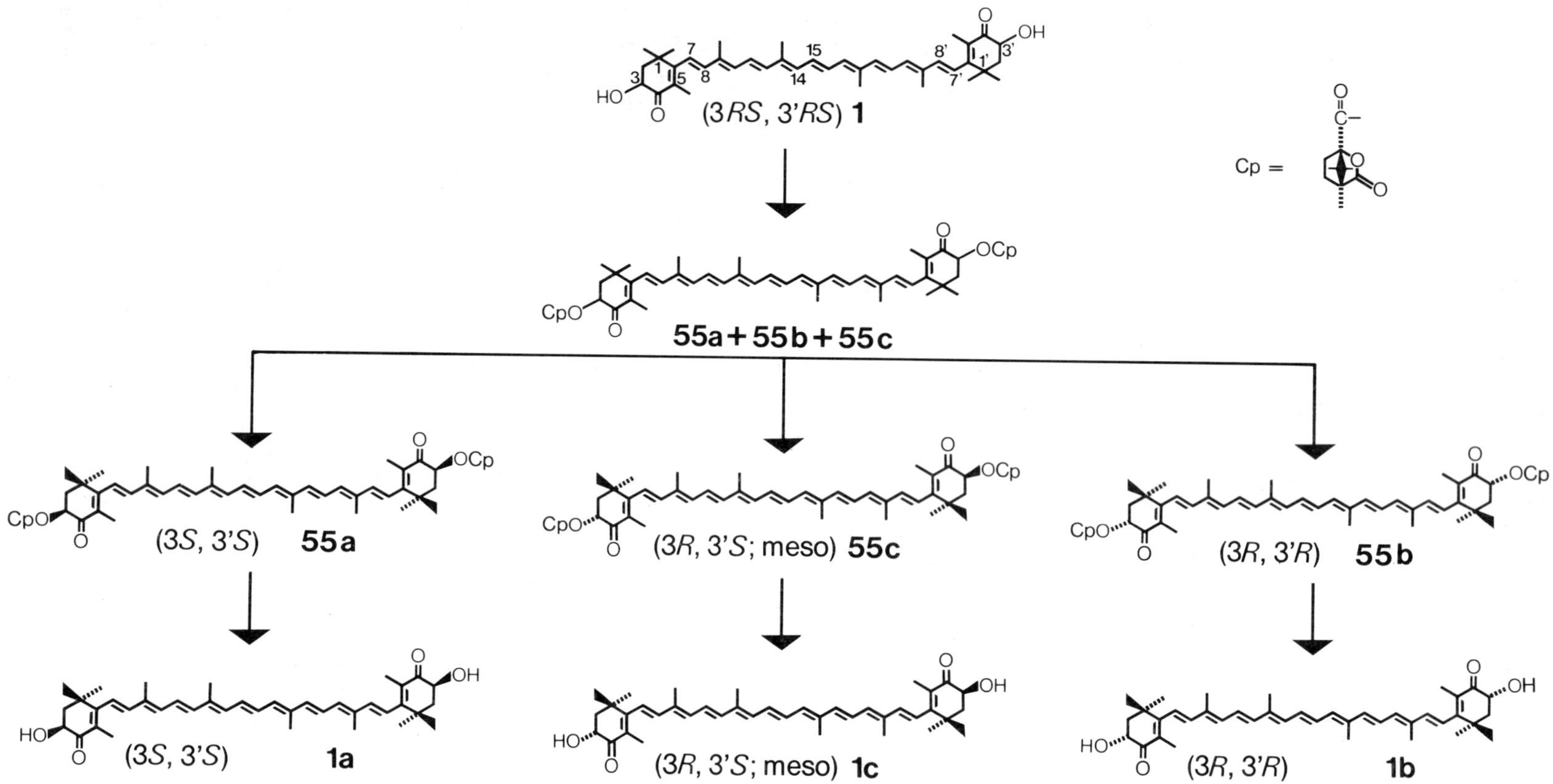

Fig. 14. Synthesis of the optical isomers and the meso-form of astaxanthin from (3RS,3'RS)-astaxanthin.

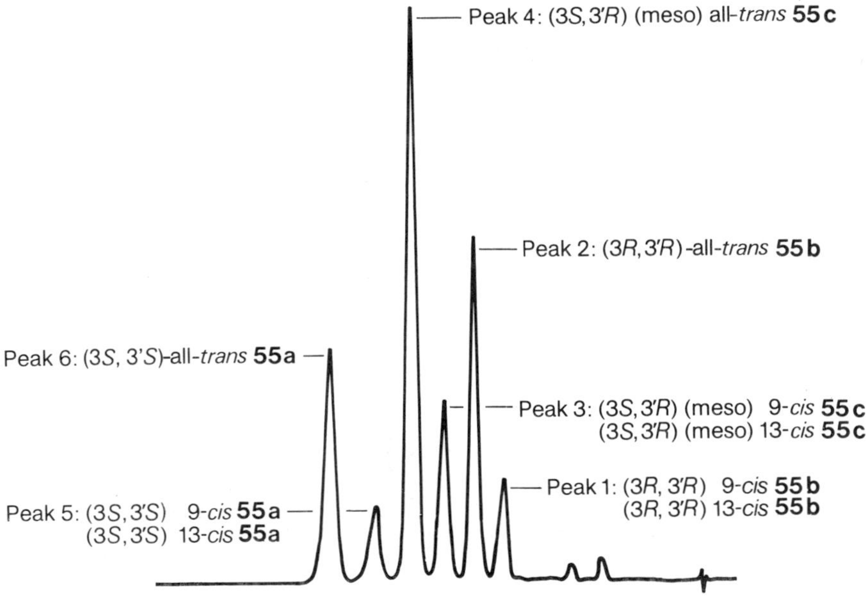

Fig. 15. HPLC separation of the (-)-camphanates of cis/trans-(3RS,3'RS)-astaxanthin.

Table 1. Occurrence of enantiomeric and meso-astaxanthin in various natural sources as determined by HPLC analysis of the corresponding (-)-camphanates (Ref. 32).

Source	1a (3S,3'S)	1b (3R,3'R)	1c (3R,3'S; meso)	Reference
Lobster eggs (Homarus gammarus)	48 % 24 %	30 % 39 %	21 % 37 %	(36)
Yeast (Phaffia rhodozyma)		>98 %		(31)
Green algae (Haematococcus pluvialis)	>99 %			(37)
Shrimps (Pandalus borealis)	25 %	23 %	52 %	(38)
Salmon (Salmo salar and oncorhynchus)	78 to 85 %	12 to 17 %	2 to 6 %	(39)
Flowers of Adonis annua	~99 %			(40)

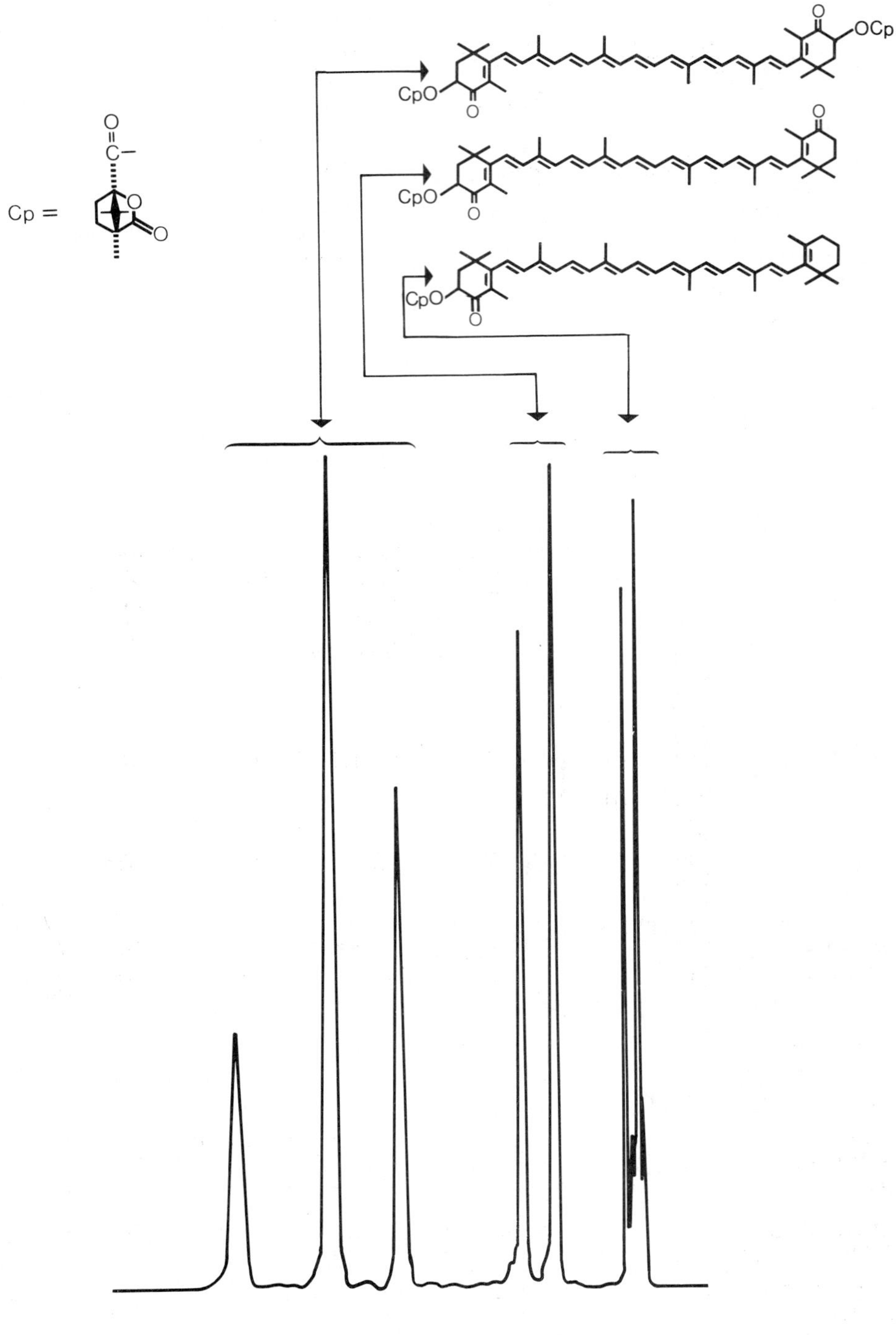

Fig. 16. HPLC separation of the (-)-camphanates of all-*trans*-(3RS,3'RS)-astaxanthin, all-*trans*-(RS)-adonirubin and *cis/trans*-(3RS)-3-hydroxy-echinenone (Ref. 31).

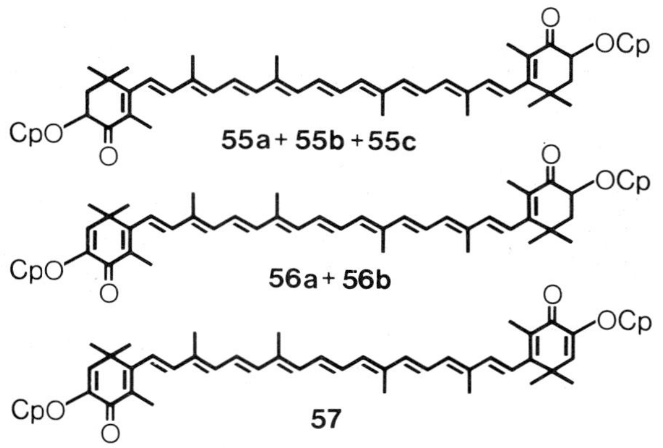

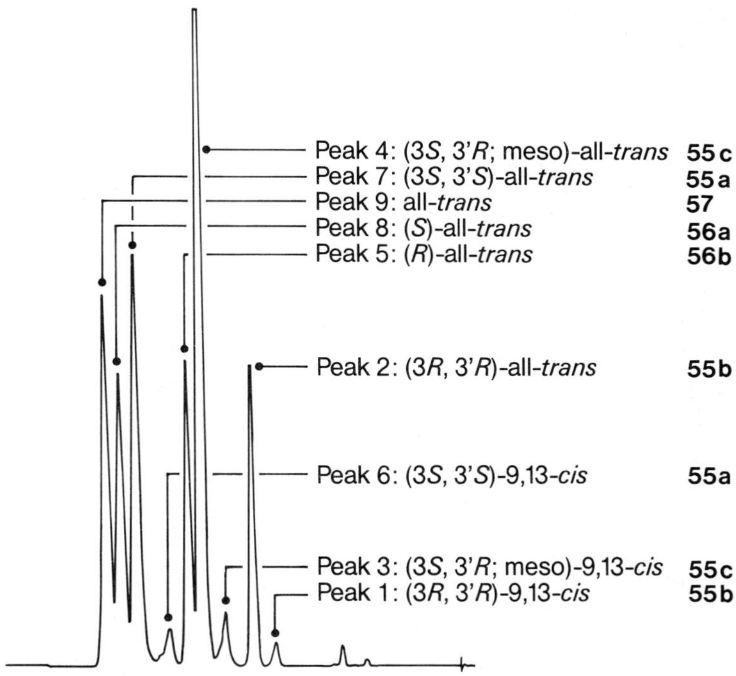

Fig. 17. HPLC separation of the (-)-camphanates of (3RS,3'RS)-astaxanthin, (3'RS)-3,3'-dihydroxy-2,3-didehydro-β,β-carotene-4,4'-dione and astacene.

SYNTHESIS OF TEDANIN, 3-HYDROXY-ECHINENONE, ADONIXANTHIN, ADONIRUBIN AND SOME RELATED XANTHOPHYLLS

Partial and total synthesis make pure carotenoids available in large quantities for structural, stereochemical and biological studies and for investigations on their suitability as supplements for food and feed. The efficiency of recently developed HPLC techniques for the identification of trace carotenoids depends on the availability of unambiguously identified reference samples. Moreover, there is always a demand for new and better methods of industrial polyene synthesis. Therefore, partial and total synthesis keep their importance and still give the synthetic organic chemist a range of unsolved problems.

Since the 1978 Madison meeting, substantial progress has been made in the field of the synthesis of unsymmetrically functionalized 3,4-oxygenated xanthophylls.

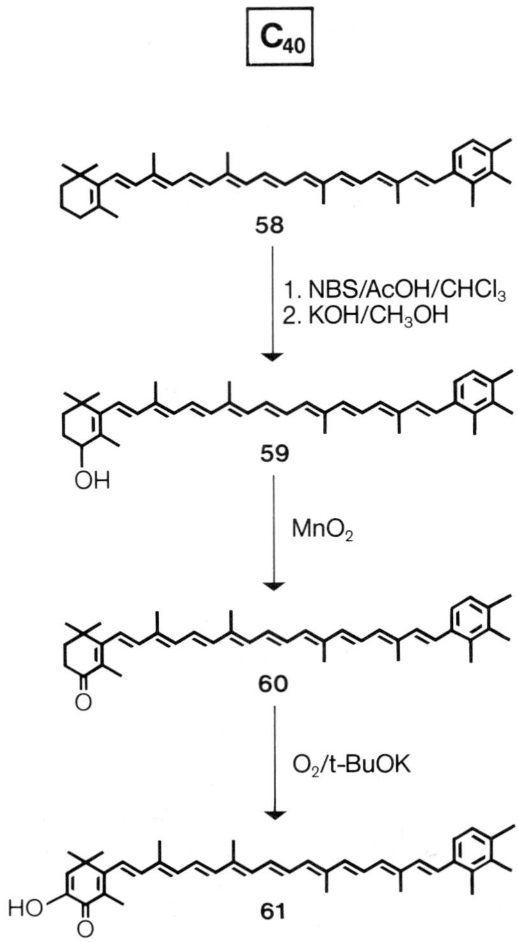

Fig. 18. Synthesis of tedanin.

Tedanin (Fig. 18: 61) was first isolated as the main carotenoid from the sea sponge Tedania digitata (O. Schmidt). Its structure has been established by Okukado (Ref. 45) on the basis of chemical and spectroscopic evidence. A total synthesis of tedanin and some related carotenoids has recently been reported with full experimental details by Yamaguchi and co-workers (Ref. 46). The synthesis of tedanin started with β,χ-carotene 58, which had previously been synthesized by Weedon and co-workers (Ref. 47) using a different building scheme. Treatment of 58 with N-bromosuccinimide and glacial acetic acid in chloroform, followed by saponification with methanolic potassium hydroxide gave the alcohol 59 in 74 % yield. Reaction of 59 with active manganese dioxide led to ketone 60 from which tedanin was obtained by oxidation with oxygen in the presence of potassium t-butoxide.

An alternative synthesis of tedanin (Fig. 19) by Yamaguchi and co-workers (Ref. 48) starts from the acetate of β-citraurin 62 which was prepared from natural zeaxanthin by a known method (Ref. 49). The C_{30}-apoaldehyde 62 was reacted with the C_{10}-phosphonium salt 63 in 1,2-epoxybutane to give a 60 % yield of 64 which could be saponified almost quantitatively to the alcohol 65. Oxidation of 65 with DMSO, TFA, pyridine and dicyclohexylcarbodiimide in benzene led to the unconjugated ketone 66 which was transformed to the enolacetate 67. Epoxidation of 67 at the 3,4-double bond could not be achieved, but by oxidation with t-butyl hydroperoxide in benzene, tedanin could be isolated in 5 % yield.

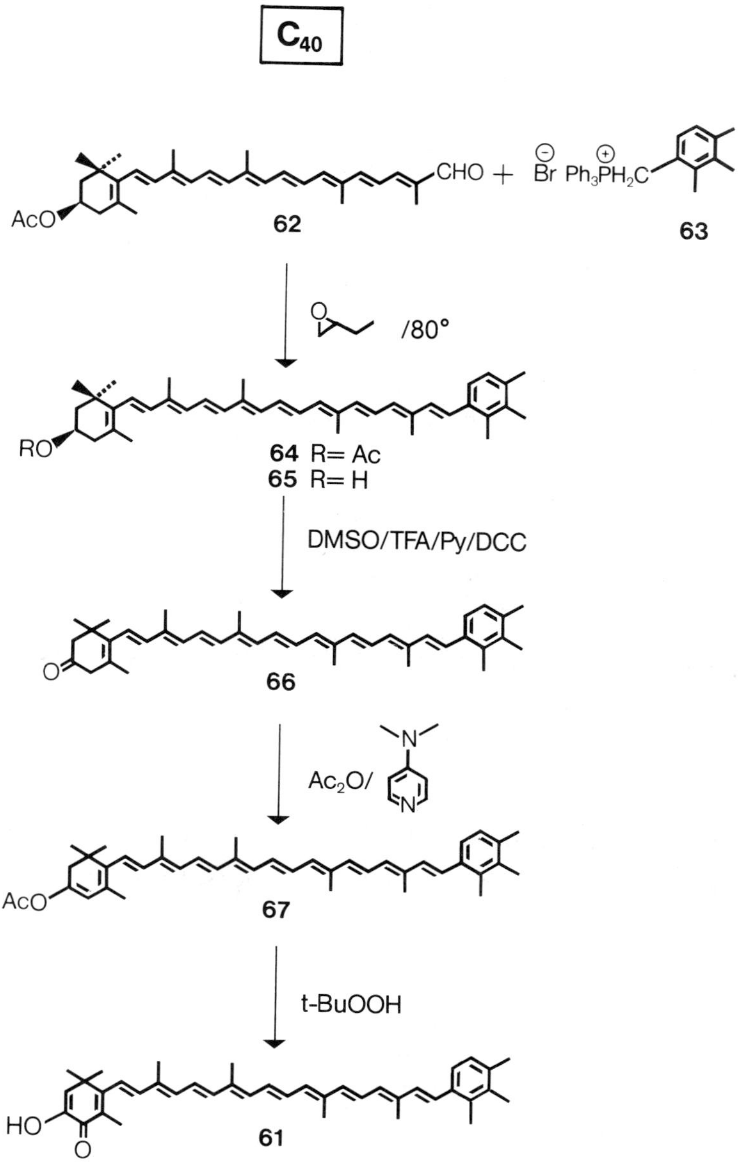

Fig. 19. Alternative synthesis of tedanin.

In 1975, the first syntheses of a series of 3,4-oxygenated xanthophylls in optically inactive form were reported by Cooper, Davis, Leftwick, Price and Weedon (Ref. 50).

With the appropriate C_{15}-phosphonium salts (Refs. 16-20, 25, 26, 35, 51) and the partially protected C_{10}-dialdehydes 68 and 69 (Fig. 20) at hand, a Roche group has recently prepared the C_{25}-apoaldehydes 70-77 (Figs. 21, 22, 23), mainly as building blocks for the synthesis of unsymmetrically functionalized xanthophylls according to the building scheme $C_{25} + C_{15} = C_{40}$ (Ref. 52). The aldehyde 70 has first been prepared by Rüegg et al. (Ref. 53) using a different scheme.

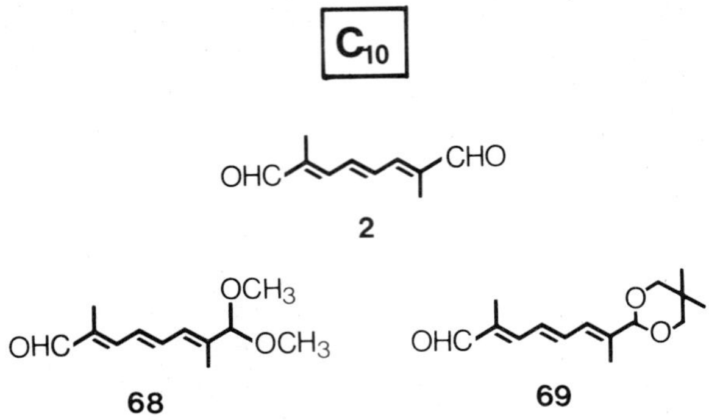

Fig. 20. C_{10}-Components used for the synthesis of unsymmetrically functionalized xanthophylls.

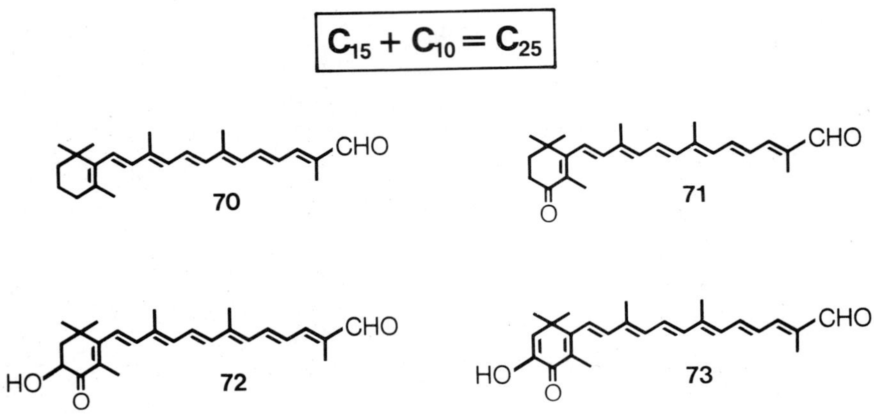

Fig. 21. Synthesis of C_{25}-apo-aldehydes.

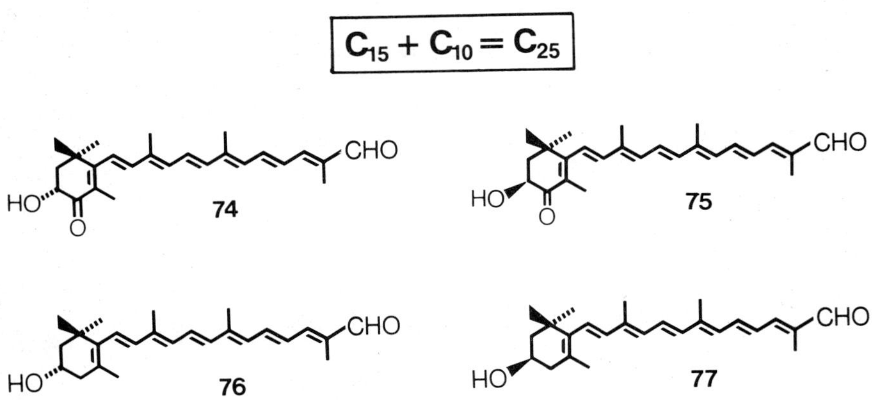

Fig. 22. Synthesis of C_{25}-apo-aldehydes.

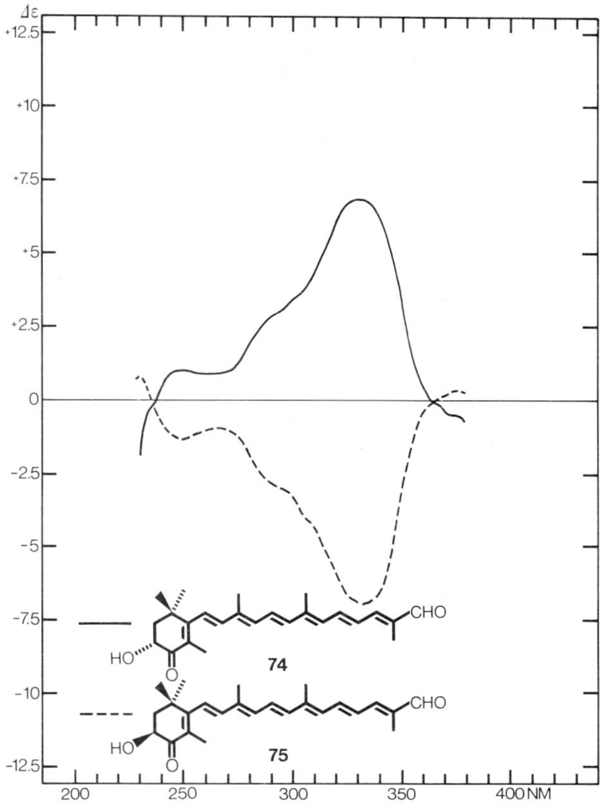

Fig. 23. CD spectra of (R)- and (S)-3-hydroxy-4-oxo-12'-apo-β-caroten-12'-al.

3-Hydroxy-β,β-caroten-4-one (3-hydroxy-echinenone) (Fig. 24) has been isolated from the yeast Phaffia rhodozyma (Ref. 41), from the green alga Sphaeroplea cambrica (Refs. 42, 54), from the flowers of Adonis annua (Ref. 55), from the spider mite Tetranychus pacificus McGregor (Ref. 56) and from crustaceans (Ref. 57). Recently, the (S)-enantiomer 80 has been isolated from a mutant strain of the bacterium Rhizobium lupini (Ref. 58). A partial synthesis starting from echinenone has been described, which gives the racemate 78 in low yield (Ref. 50).

Using refluxing 1,2-epoxybutane in the Wittig condensation of the final step, we obtained the racemate 78 (m.p. 181-183°) and both enantiomers 79 and 80 (m.p. 187-189°) in approx. 60 % yield.

3-Hydroxy-2,3-didehydro-β,β-caroten-4-one (81), usually considered as an artifact (Ref. 41), has also been prepared (m.p. 184-185°).

$C_{15} + C_{25} = C_{40}$ $C_{25} + C_{15} = C_{40}$

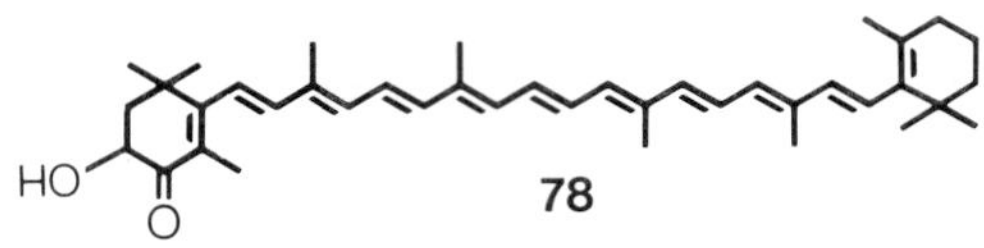

78

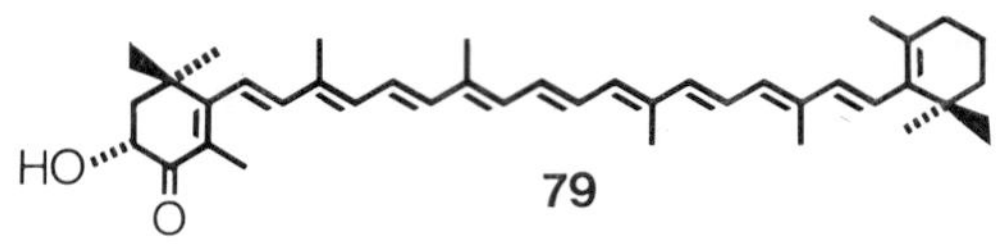

79

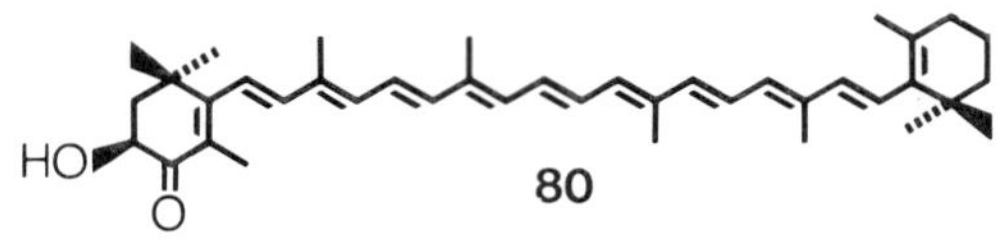

80

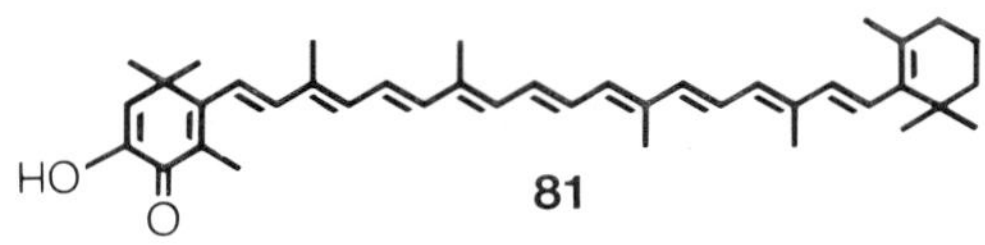

81

Fig. 24. Synthesis of 3-hydroxy-echinenones and 3-hydroxy-2,3-didehydro-β,β-caroten-4-one.

3,3'-Dihydroxy-β,β-caroten-4-one (adonixanthin, β-doradexanthin, Fig. 25) has been isolated from algae (Ref. 42), the flower of Adonis annua (Ref. 43), crustaceans (Refs. 59, 60) and from the common goldfish Carassius auratus (Ref. 61). To our knowledge, no synthesis or chiroptical data have been published. We have synthesized all four optical isomers of adonixanthin (m.p. 180-182°). In the CD spectrum, each pair of enantiomers clearly shows strong opposite Cotton effects (Fig. 26).

Recently, the temperature dependence of the CD spectra of (3S,3'R)- and (3S,3'S)-adonixanthin have been compared with those of (3R,3'R)-zeaxanthin and (3S,3'S)-astaxanthin (Ref. 62).

The corresponding enantiomeric diosphenols 86 and 87 (Fig. 27) have been obtained in approx. 40 % yield (m.p. 181-183°). The absorption value of the VIS spectrum published by Katayama et al. (Ref. 61) agreed well with our data.

$C_{15} + C_{25} = C_{40}$ $C_{25} + C_{15} = C_{40}$

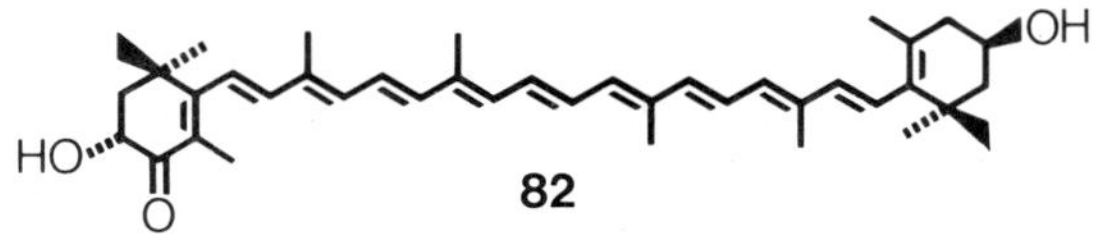

82

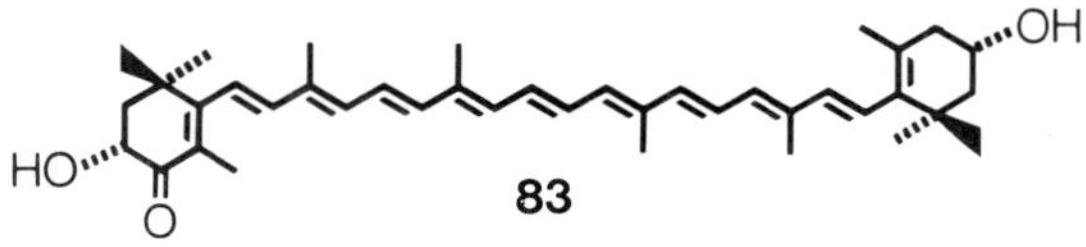

83

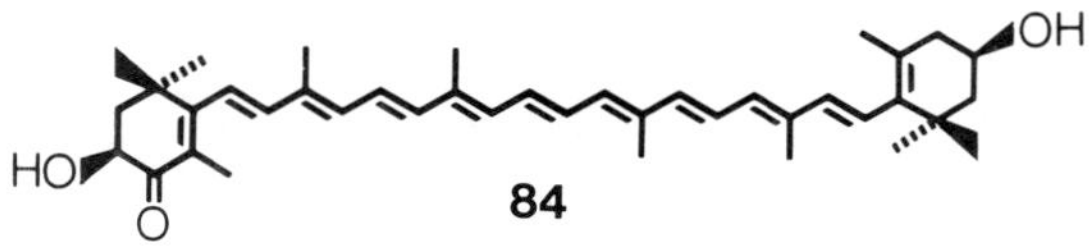

84

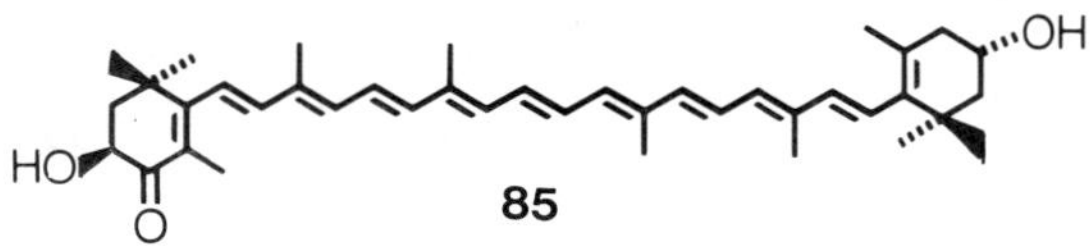

85

Fig. 25. Synthesis of (3R,3'R)-, (3R,3'S)-, (3S,3'R)- and (3S,3'S)-adonixanthin.

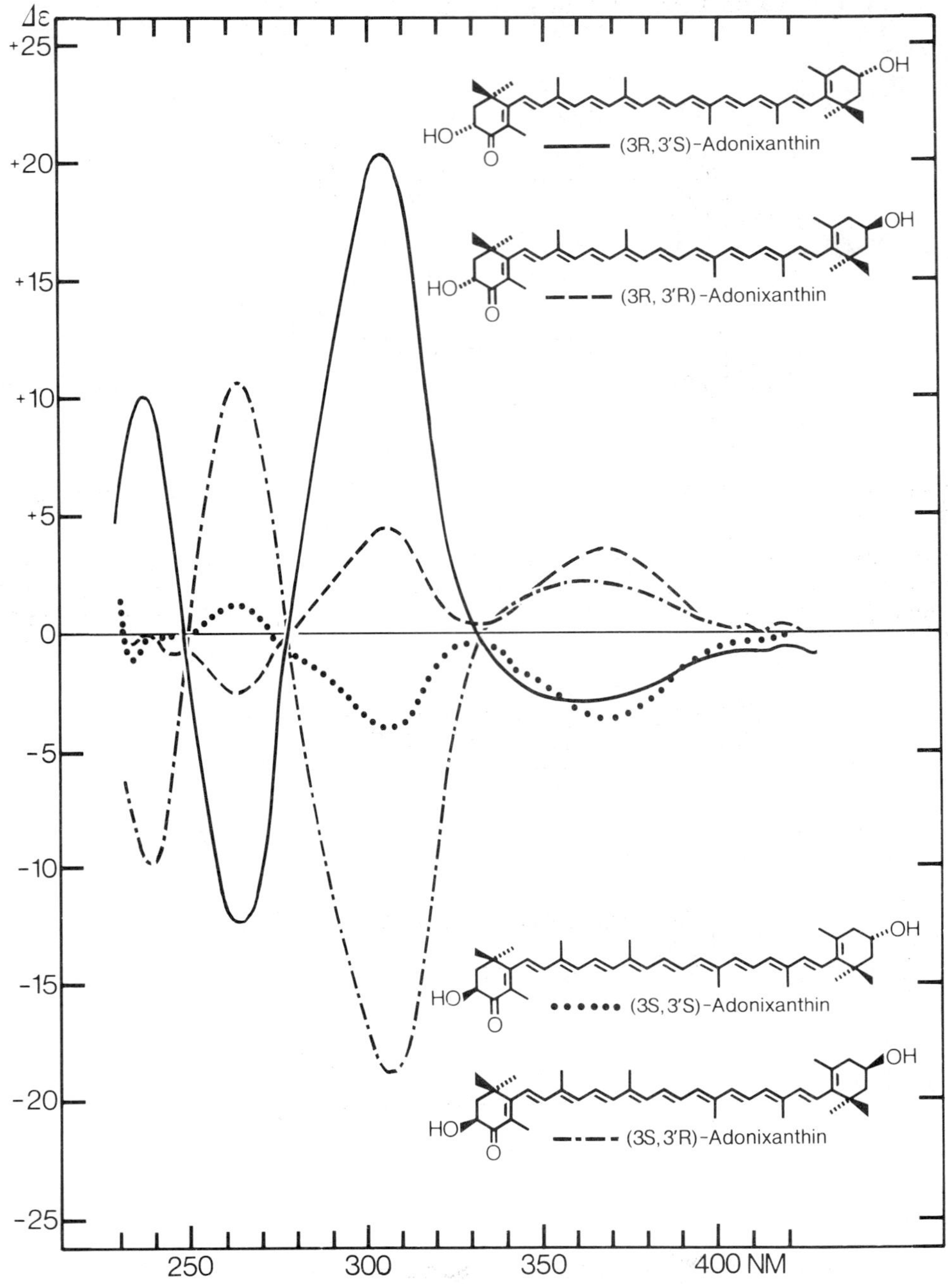

Fig. 26. CD spectra of (3R,3'R)-, (3R,3'S)-, (3S,3'R)- and (3S,3'S)-adonixanthin (dichloromethane).

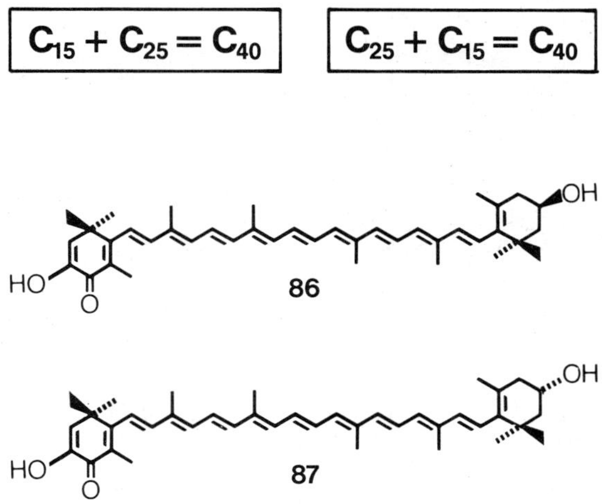

Fig. 27. Synthesis of (R)- and (S)-3,3'-dihydroxy-2,3-didehydro-β,β-caroten—4-one.

3-Hydroxy-β,β-carotene-4,4'-dione (88) (adonirubin, phoenicoxanthin)(Fig. 28) is present in the bacterium Micrococcus roseus (Ref. 63) and the yeast Phaffia rhodozyma (Ref. 41), in green algae (Ref. 42) and the flowers of Adonis annua (Ref. 55). The same pigment is also reported to occur in the hermit

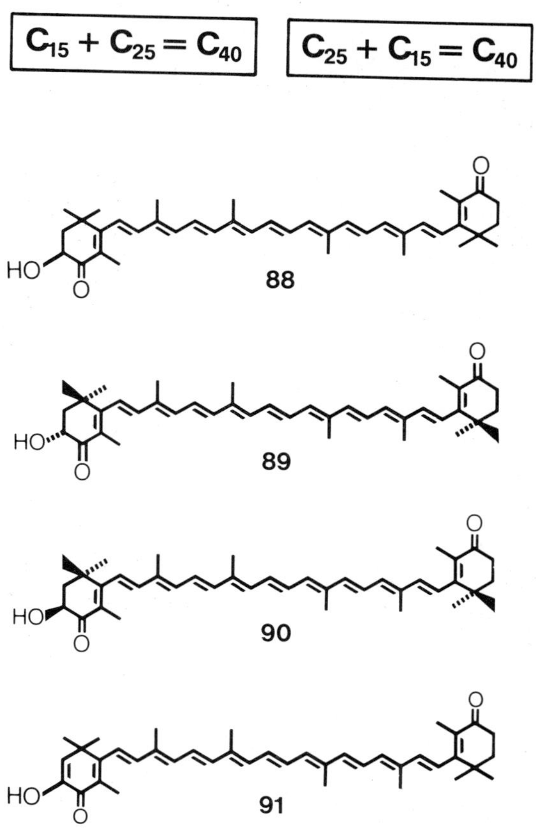

Fig. 28. Synthesis of adonirubin and phoeniconone.

$C_{15} + C_{25} = C_{40}$ $C_{25} + C_{15} = C_{40}$

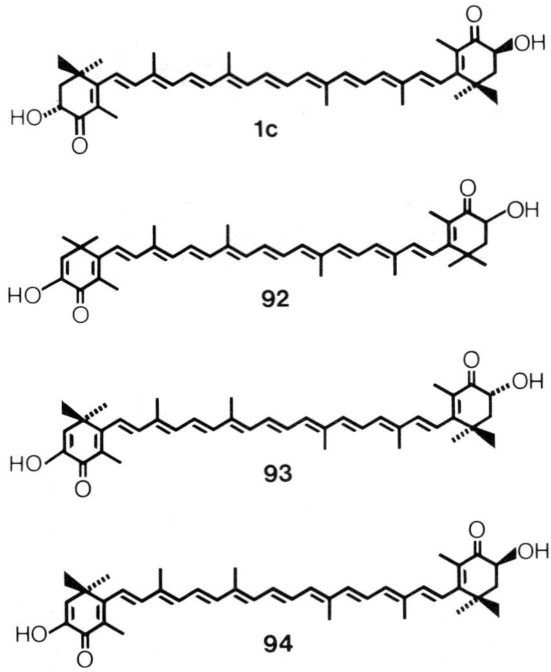

Fig. 29. Synthesis of (3R,3'S; meso)-astaxanthin and the 3,3'-dihydroxy-2,3-didehydro-ß,ß-carotene-4,4'-diones.

crab *Pagurus prideauxi* (Ref. 59), in the common goldfish *Carassius auratus* (Ref. 64) and in the plumage of birds (Ref. 65). The (S)-enantiomer 90 has been isolated from the bacterium *Rhizobium lupini* (Ref. 58). Racemic adonirubin 88 has been synthesized from canthaxanthin (Ref. 50).

We obtained the adonirubins in 55-60 % yield from the C_{25}-apoaldehyde 71 (m.p. (88): 213-215°, m.p. (89 and 90): 214-216°).

We also prepared 3-hydroxy-2,3-didehydro-ß,ß-carotene-4,4'-dione (91) (phoeniconone), which has previously been synthesized by partial oxidation of canthaxanthin (Ref. 50).

(3S,3'R; meso)-Astaxanthin 1c (Fig. 29) is a special compound in that it cannot be synthesized according to the usual symmetrical building schemes. In our hands, the scheme $C_{25} + C_{15} = C_{40}$, utilizing one of the enantiomeric C_{25}-apoaldehydes (74, 75; Fig. 22) and the appropriate C_{15}-phosphonium salt of opposite configuration (6, 5; Fig. 4) in the final Wittig condensation, proved to be very efficient. By this way, meso-astaxanthin (1c) was obtained in approx. 55 % yield.

3,3'-Dihydroxy-2,3-didehydro-ß,ß-carotene-4,4'-dione, an intermediate of the oxidation of astaxanthin to astacene, has also been prepared in the racemic (92) and optically active forms 93 and 94 (Fig. 29).

NORCAROTENOIDS

The synthesis of the enantiomeric actinioerythrols 104 and 107 (Fig. 30) and their diacetates 105 and 108 was presented at the Madison meeting (Ref. 35) and subsequently published in a short communication (Ref. 24).

By comparison of the CD spectra of the (3S,3'S)-diacetate 105 with that of actinioerythrin isolated from the sea anemone *Actinia equina*, the (3S,3'S)-configuration 106 was deduced for the natural compound. The same absolute configuration was established by Foss, Green and Rickards (Ref. 66) for actinioerythrin isolated from the sea anemone *Actinia tenebrosa* by means of oxidative degradation and comparison of one of the fragments obtained with a reference sample of known absolute configuration.

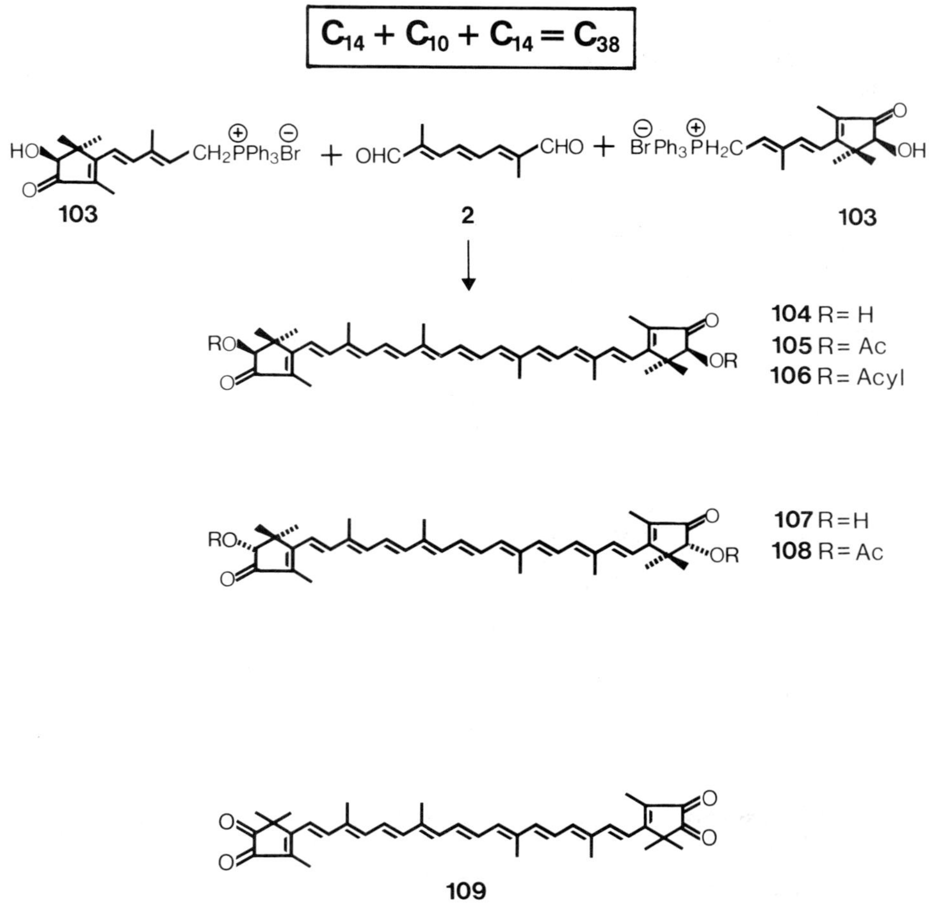

Fig. 30. Synthesis of norcarotenoids.

Although we invested some further work in the synthesis of these norcarotenoids, we have to admit that some problems have not been solved yet.

Since site-selective alkylations of 2-nor-4-oxo-β-ionone derivatives at C(9) proved to be difficult, we used the readily available C_{15}-unit vinyl-3-hydroxy-4-oxo-β-ionol (31) as starting material for the synthesis of vinyl-2-nor-3-hydroxy-4-oxo-β-ionol (101) (Figs. 10 and 31). Separation of the mixture of diastereomers 101 (= 112 + 113) was achieved by esterification at C(3) with (-)-camphanoyl chloride and separation of the ester mixture 110 + 111 by silica gel chromatography (Fig. 32). The epimeric mixtures 110 and 111 have been transformed into the optically pure C_{14}-phosphonium salts 114 and 115 using the conditions described above (Refs. 16-18).

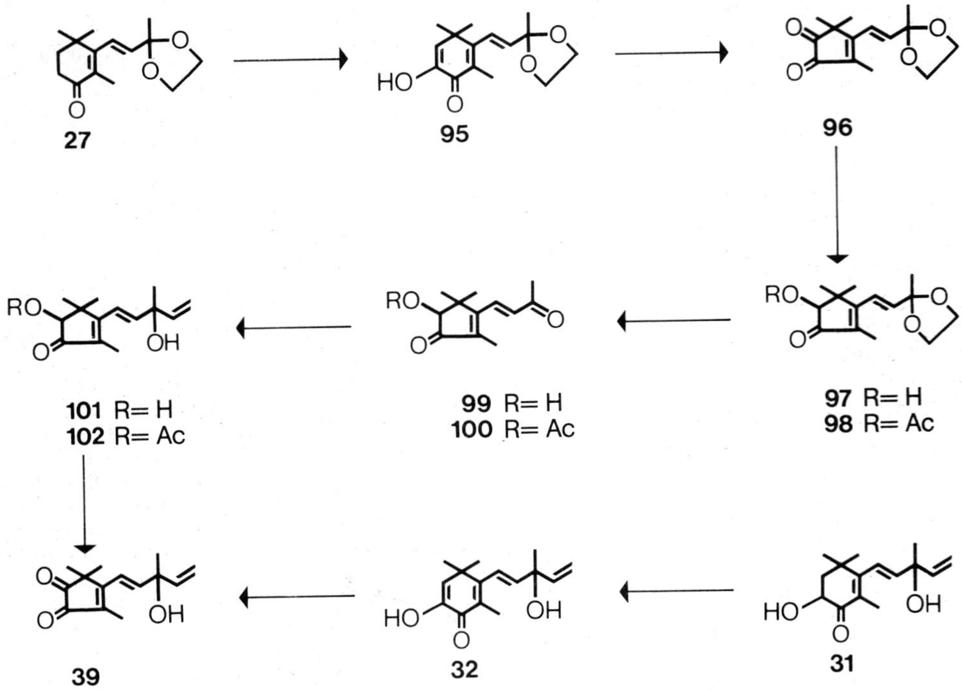

Fig. 31. Syntheses of vinyl-2-nor-3-hydroxy-4-oxo-β-ionol.

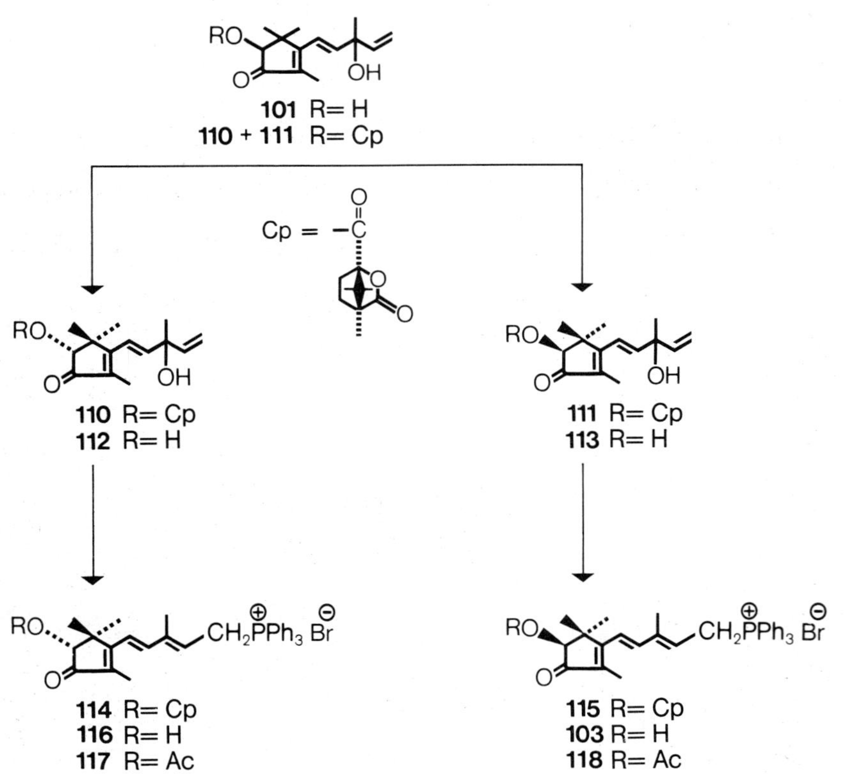

Fig. 32. Synthesis of the enantiomeric C_{14}-phosphonium salts.

Moreover, actinioerythrins were found to be much more susceptible than astaxanthin esters to racemization under basic saponification conditions. The actinioerythrols described in our paper (Ref. 24) were not completely optically pure. Unfortunately, this was only detected after publication by HPLC analysis of the corresponding di-(-)-camphanates. Nevertheless, there is fortunately no need to revise our conclusions concerning the absolute configuration of natural actinioerythrin.

Due to partial racemization, the compounds 112, 113, 116, 103, 117 and 118 could not be obtained optically pure so far.

CONCLUDING REMARKS

The foregoing discussion has shown that the search for a technical synthesis of astaxanthin has led to numerous investigations in the field of 3,4-oxygenated xanthophylls. Various methods have been presented for the synthesis of racemic and optically active 3-hydroxy-4-oxo carotenoids. A very efficient HPLC separation technique for the optical isomers of astaxanthin via the corresponding (-)-camphanates has been developed. This method has been used in studies on the natural occurrence of enantiomeric and meso-astaxanthin and may possibly further contribute to biochemical investigations. Concerning the interesting field of norcarotenoids, new routes to the synthesis of these compounds from β-ionone have been elaborated. Although technical applications of norcarotenoids are not foreseen in the near future, the very special characteristics of these compounds will certainly induce further activities in order to broaden the colour range of synthetically available carotenoids and to disclose more details of their chemical behaviour.

Acknowledgements - We should like to thank Dr. H. Mayer for stimulating advice and Dr. R. Buchecker, Prof. C.H. Eugster, Prof. S. Liaaen-Jensen, Dr. H. Pfander and Prof. B.C.L. Weedon for valuable discussions. Special thanks are due to Drs. W. Arnold, L. Chopard, G. Englert, K. Noack, W. Vetter and Mr. W. Meister for the spectral data, to Dr. R. Maurer, Mr. E. Glinz and Mr. W. Walther for the GC and HPLC analyses and to Dr. A. Dirscherl for the elemental analyses. The skilful technical assistance of Mr. K. Holzhauser, Mr. S. Jäggli, Miss K. Jakob, Mr. H. Schneider and Mr. M. Tognina is gratefully acknowledged.

REFERENCES

1. O. Straub, Key to Carotenoids: Lists of Natural Carotenoids, Birkhäuser Verlag, Basel and Stuttgart (1976).
2. B.C.L. Weedon in Carotenoids (editor O. Isler), p. 29, Birkhäuser Verlag, Basel and Stuttgart (1971).
3. S. Liaaen-Jensen in Progress in the Chemistry of Organic Natural Products 39, p. 123, Springer Verlag, Vienna and New York (1980).
4. R. Kuhn and N.A. Sörensen, Ber.Dtsch.Chem.Ges. 71, 1879 (1938).
5. A.P. Leftwick and B.C.L. Weedon, J.Chem.Soc., Chem.Commun. 49 (1967).
6. A.G. Andrewes, G. Borch, S. Liaaen-Jensen and G. Snatzke, Acta Chem.Scand., Ser.B 28, 730 (1974).
7. A. Veerman, G. Borch, R. Pedersen and S. Liaaen-Jensen, Acta Chem.Scand., Ser. B 29, 525 (1975).
8. A.J. Aasen, S. Liaaen-Jensen and G. Borch, Acta Chem.Scand. 26, 404 (1972).
9. A.G. Andrewes, M.P. Starr, H.J. Phaff and H. Hope, Fourth Int.Symp.on Carotenoids, 1975, Abstracts Contributed Papers, p. 4.
10. A.G. Andrewes and M.P. Starr, Phytochemistry 15, 1009 (1976).
11. E.A. Johnson and M.J. Lewis, J.Gen.Microbiol. 115, 173 (1979).
12. E.A. Johnson, T.C. Villa and M.J. Lewis, Aquaculture 20, 123 (1980).
13. E.A.H. Hall, G.P. Moss, J.H.P. Utley and B.C.L. Weedon, J.Chem.Soc., Chem. Commun. 387 (1978).
14. G.P. Moss, Pure Appl.Chem. 51, 507 (1979).
15. F. Kienzle and H. Mayer, Helv.Chim.Acta 51, 2609 (1978).
16. E.A. Broger, Y. Crameri, H.G.W. Leuenberger, E. Widmer and R. Zell, European Patent Application 79101400 published under Nr. 5748 (1978).
17. E. Widmer, R. Zell, T. Lukáč, M. Casadei, P. Schönholzer and E.A. Broger, Helv.Chim.Acta, in press.
18. E. Widmer, R. Zell, E.A. Broger, Y. Crameri, H.P. Wagner, J. Dinkel, M. Schlageter and T. Lukáč, Helv.Chim.Acta, in press.
19. E. Widmer, R. Zell, E.A. Broger, Y. Crameri, H.P. Wagner, J. Dinkel, M. Schlageter and T. Lukáč, Sixth Int.Symp.on Carotenoids, 1981, Abstracts Contributed Papers.
20. R. Zell, E. Widmer, T. Lukáč, H.G.W. Leuenberger, P. Schönholzer and E.A. Broger, Helv.Chim.Acta, in press.

21. A. Nürrenbach, Chemie für Labor und Betrieb 28, 171 (1977).
22. O. Isler, Pure Appl.Chem. 51, 447 (1979).
23. E. Becher, R. Albrecht, K. Bernhard, H.G.W. Leuenberger, H. Mayer, R.K. Müller, W. Schüep and H.P. Wagner, Helv.Chim.Acta, in press.
24. R.K. Müller, H. Mayer, K. Noack, J.J. Daly, J.D. Tauber and S. Liaaen-Jensen, Helv.Chim.Acta 61, 2881 (1978).
25. M. Rosenberger, DOS 2801908 (1977).
26. M. Rosenberger, P. McDougal, G. Saucy and J. Bahr, Pure Appl.Chem. 51, 871 (1979).
27. R.K. Müller, unpublished results.
28. H. Mayer and R.K. Müller, European Patent Application 79101401.2, published under Nr. 5749 (1978).
29. E. Widmer, T. Lukáč, K. Bernhard and R. Zell, Helv.Chim.Acta, in press.
30. H. Gerlach, Helv.Chim.Acta 51, 1587 (1968); H. Gerlach and W. Müller, Helv.Chim.Acta 55, 2277 (1972); H. Gerlach, K. Oertle and A. Thalmann, Helv.Chim.Acta 59, 755 (1976).
31. R.K. Müller, K. Bernhard, H. Mayer, A. Rüttimann and M. Vecchi, Helv. Chim.Acta 63, 1654 (1980).
32. M. Vecchi and R.K. Müller, HRC CC, J.High Resolut.Chromatogr.Chromatogr. Commun. 2, 195 (1975).
33. T. Oritani and K. Yamashita, Agric.Biol.Chem. 37, 1697 (1973); idem, ibid., 37, 1923 (1973); idem, ibid., 38, 1961 (1974); idem, ibid., 38, 1965 (1974); idem, ibid. 39, 89 (1975).
34. H.G.W. Leuenberger, W. Boguth, E. Widmer and R. Zell, Helv.Chim.Acta 59, 1832 (1976).
35. H. Mayer, Pure Appl.Chem. 51, 535 (1979).
36. H. Rønneberg, B. Renstrøm, K. Aareskjold, S. Liaaen-Jensen, M. Vecchi, F.J. Leuenberger, R.K. Müller and H. Mayer, Helv.Chim.Acta 63, 711 (1980).
37. B. Renstrøm, G. Borch, O. Skulberg and S. Liaaen-Jensen, Phytochemistry, in press.
38. B. Renstrøm, G. Borch and S. Liaaen-Jensen, Comp.Biochem.Physiol. 69B, 621 (1981).
39. K. Schiedt, F.J. Leuenberger and M. Vecchi, Helv.Chim.Acta 64, 449 (1981).
40. B. Renstrøm, H. Berger and S. Liaaen-Jensen, Biochem.Syst.Ecol., in press.
41. A.G. Andrewes, H.J. Phaff and M.P. Starr, Phytochemistry 15, 1003 (1976).
42. H. Kleinig, Z.Naturforschg. 22b, 977 (1967).
43. K. Egger and H. Kleinig, Phytochemistry 6, 437 (1967).
44. S. Liaaen-Jensen in Carotenoids (editor O. Isler), p. 61, Birkhäuser Verlag, Basel and Stuttgart (1971).
45. N. Okukado, Bull.Chem.Soc.Jpn, 48, 1061 (1975).
46. M. Yasuhara, K. Inanaga, T. Kumae, H.R. Brahmana, N. Okukado and M. Yamaguchi, Bull.Chem.Soc.Jpn. 53, 1629 (1980).
47. R.D.G. Cooper, J.B. Davis and B.C.L. Weedon, J.Chem.Soc. 5637 (1963).
48. A. Shimada, Y. Ezaki, J. Inanaga, T. Katsuki and M. Yamaguchi, Tetrahedron Lett. 22, 773 (1981).
49. P. Karrer, A. Rüegger and U. Solmssen, Helv.Chim.Acta 21, 448 (1938).
50. R.D.G. Cooper, J.B. Davis, A.P. Leftwick, C. Price and B.C.L. Weedon, J.Chem.Soc. Perkin I, 2195 (1975).
51. A. Rüttimann and H. Mayer, Helv.Chim.Acta 63, 1456 (1980).
52. K. Bernhard, G. Englert, H. Mayer, R.K. Müller, A. Rüttimann, M. Vecchi, E. Widmer and R. Zell, Helv.Chim.Acta, in press.
53. R. Rüegg, M. Montavon, G. Ryser, G. Saucy, U. Schwieter and O. Isler, Helv.Chim.Acta 42, 854 (1959).
54. H. Kleinig and K. Egger, Phytochemistry 6, 611 (1967).
55. K. Egger, Phytochemistry 4, 609 (1965).
56. A. Veerman, Comp.Biochem.Physiol. 42B, 329 (1972).
57. B.M. Gilchrist, Comp.Biochem.Physiol. 24, 123 (1968).
58. P. Beyer, H. Kleinig, G. Englert, W. Meister and K. Noack, Helv.Chim.Acta 62, 2551 (1979).
59. R. Castillo, R. Lenel and G. Nègre-Sadargues, Comp.Biochem.Physiol 66B, 483 (1980).
60. T. Matsuno, T. Watanabe and N. Seiichi, Bull.Jpn.Soc.Sci.Fish. 40, 619 (1974).
61. T. Katayama, H. Yokoyama and C.O. Chichester, Int.J.Biochem. 1, 438 (1970).
62. K. Noack, Helv.Chim.Acta, in press.
63. G E. Ungers and J.J. Cooney, J.Bacteriol. 96, 234 (1968).
64. M. Hata and M. Hata, Int.J.Biochem. 2, 11 (1971).
65. D.L. Fox and T.S. Hopkins, Comp.Biochem.Physiol. 17, 841 (1966); idem, ibid., 19, 267 (1966).
66. P.S. Foss, P.J. Green and R.W. Rickards, Aust.J.Chem. 31, 1981 (1978).

SYNTHESIS OF OPTICALLY ACTIVE CAROTENOIDS WITH ε-END GROUPS

H. Mayer

Department of Vitamin and Nutritional Research, F. Hoffmann-La Roche & Co., Ltd., CH-4002 Basle, Switzerland.

Abstract - Some recent advances in the synthesis of optically active carotenoids with ε-end groups are presented.

Methods for the preparation of appropriate optically active building units are discussed. Some previously unpublished work is described. This includes first syntheses of the following compounds: 1. Lutein group: (3R,3'R,6'R)-, (3S,3'S,6'S)-, (3R,3'S,6'S)- and (3S,3'R,6'R)-lutein, (3R,6'S)-3'-O-didehydrolutein (zeaxanthin metabolite). 2. Fritschiellaxanthin monoacetate. 3. Tunaxanthin group: Lactucaxanthin, (3S,6S,3'S,6'S)-tunaxanthin, chiriquixanthin A, chiriquixanthin B, (3S, 6S,3'R,6'S)- and (3R,6S,3'R,6'S)-tunaxanthin (ent.-chiriquixanthin A and B), (3R, 6R,3'S,6'S)-(meso)- and (3S,6R,3'R,6'S)-(meso)-tunaxanthin, (3R,6R,3'R,6'S)/(3S,6S, 3'S,6'R) (rac.)-tunaxanthin, and (6S,6'S)-3,3'-O-tetradehydro-tunaxanthin (zeaxanthin metabolite).

Chiroptical properties, NMR and HPLC analyses of some selected compounds are discussed.

INTRODUCTION

Carotenoids possessing ε-end groups form a major class of natural pigments (Refs. 1 & 2) which have always posed a special challenge to the organic chemist.

Much effort has been devoted to the definite establishment of structure and stereochemistry of these compounds, yet only a few have to date been synthesized. Thus, (6'R)-β,ε-carotene (α-carotene) was the first optically active carotenoid ever synthesized in its natural form (Refs. 3-6), an achievement which can certainly be regarded as a milestone in the field. The synthesis of the (6'S)-enantiomer was also reported at that time. Shortly afterwards, the synthesis of (6R,6'R)-ε,ε-carotene (ε-carotene) and its enantiomer was completed (Refs. 4, 5 & 7). (2R,6S,2'R,6'S)-2,2'-Dimethyl-ε,ε-carotene and its (2R,6R,2'R,6'R)-diastereoisomer were prepared as model compounds for decaprenoxanthin (Ref. 8). Recently, the synthesis of optically inactive 2,6-trans-2',6'-trans-decaprenoxanthin was reported (Ref. 9). 3',O-Didehydrolutein and 3'-epilutein have been obtained from lutein (Ref. 10), and (5R,6R,6'R)-5,6-dihydro-β,ε-carotene-5,6-diol and (5S,6R,6'R)-5,6-epoxy-5,6-dihydro-β,ε-carotene have been synthesized from azafrinal (Ref. 11).

It is the purpose of this paper to review some advances in the synthesis of optically active carotenoids with ε-end groups recently achieved in the Roche laboratories.

DISCUSSION

The generation of racemic ε-rings by acid catalyzed cyclization of open chain compounds may be formulated without difficulties as shown in Fig. 1. In fact, some compounds, such as racemic α-ionone, have been conveniently prepared by this route in the laboratory. Enantioselective cyclizations, however, leading to (6R)- or (6S)-configurated ε-rings (Fig. 2), as found in α- and ε-carotene, are much more difficult to achieve and have not yet been realized by chemical synthesis.

The introduction of a substituent, e.g. a hydroxyl group, into position 3 of the ε-ring complicates the situation even further (Fig. 2). By this operation, a total of four isomeric 3-hydroxy ε-end groups is obtained which may be classified as either trans or cis with respect to the relative stereochemistry at positions 3 and 6. This convenient designation will be used throughout the present discussion.

Carotenoids bearing one or two of these end groups include lutein, 3'-epilutein, the chiriquixanthins and the tunaxanthins.

Obviously, nature has solved the problem of synthesizing optically active ε-end groups in a very elegant way, however, the mechanism of the stereo- and regioselective cyclization reaction is not as simple as shown in Fig. 1. In this connection, various stereochemical aspects of the biological carotene cyclization have recently been discussed in detail (Refs. 12 & 13).

The laboratory chemist has to rely on arduous though well established methods to reach his objective. Therefore, we have decided to pursue a synthetic approach which has often proved

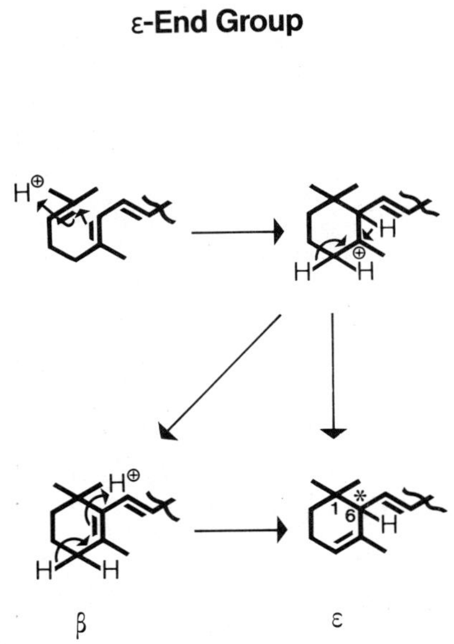

Fig. 1. Formal synthesis of ε-end groups

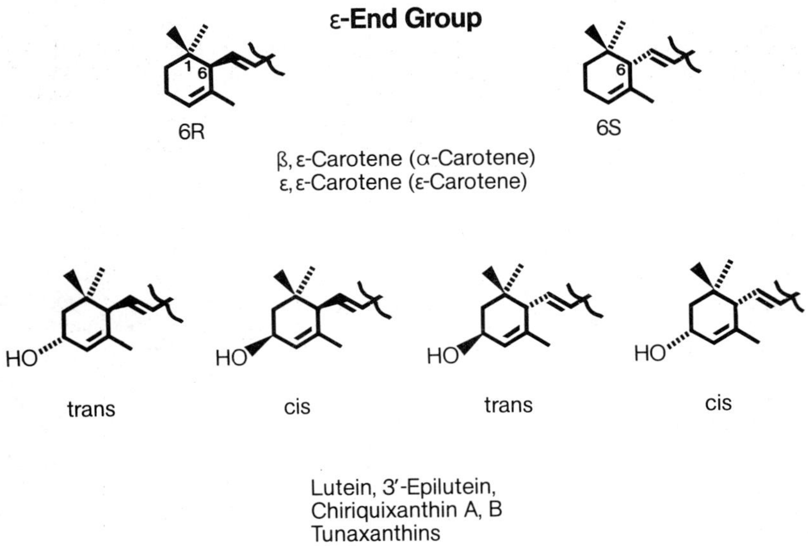

Fig. 2. Trans- and cis-3-hydroxylated ε-end groups

to be quite successful, namely to utilize small optically active building units which already possess the desired absolute configuration present in the target molecule (Refs. 13 & 14).

Lutein group

Our first goal was to develop a practical synthesis of natural (3R,3'R,6'R)-lutein to make this pigment readily available for testing as a food and feed colorant as well as for metabolic studies. Furthermore, we anticipated that a successful synthesis would also provide us with the necessary building units and know-how for the preparation of other lutein diastereomers which have not yet been detected in nature.

Lutein is very widely distributed in many algae and higher plants (Ref. 1).

The molecule possesses three chiral centres at C-3, C-3' and C-6' making possible four pairs of enantiomers (Fig. 3).

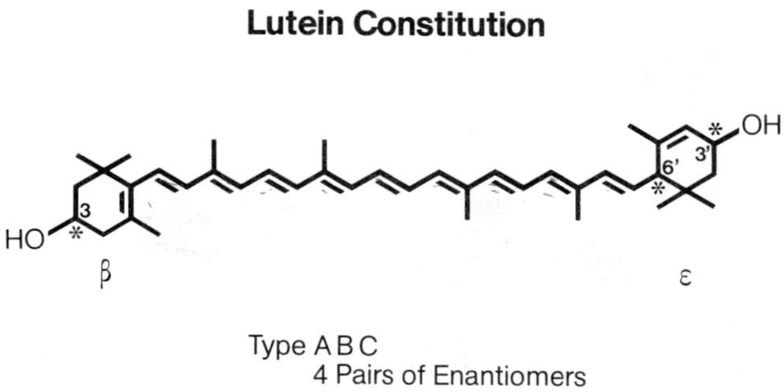

Fig. 3. Lutein constitution

The natural pigment was shown to possess the (3R,3'R,6'R)-configuration (Refs. 15-20) (Fig. 4).

Recently, the first total synthesis of optically inactive lutein and its 3'-epimer has been reported (Ref. 20).

We have chosen the building scheme $C_{15} + C_{10} + C_{15} = C_{40}$ considering the two C_{15}-phosphonium salts 1 and 2 and the readily available C_{10}-dialdehyde 3 as most suitable building units (Fig. 4) (Ref. 21). Wittig salt 1, a useful building unit for (3R,3'R)-zeaxanthin and related compounds (Ref. 14), was selected for the introduction of chirality into position 3 of the β-end group. However, the preparation of the trans-ε-ring, possessing the required (3'R,6'R)-chirality, proved to be a much more difficult task.

In order to solve this problem, we employed the acetoxy ketone 6 (Fig. 5) as key intermediate which was readily prepared from the enantiomeric hydroxy ketone 4 in the following way: Reaction of the latter compound with mesyl chloride first gave the corresponding mesylate 5 which, on treatment with tetrabutylammonium acetate, was converted into 6 with complete inversion of configuration. The introduction of the second chiral centre was achieved by diastereoselective epoxidation of the protected hydroxy ketone 7 with the sulfurylide 8 yielding the crystalline allylic epoxide 9. This was readily transformed into the protected hydroxy-α-cyclocitral 10. Subsequent chain lengthening by a Horner reaction gave the nitrile 11 which, on treatment with methyl lithium, was converted into the beautifully crystalline C_{13}-hydroxy ketone 12 in excellent optical yield.

The Wittig salts 15 and 16 were prepared as shown in Fig. 6: Vinylation of 12 gave a mixture of epimeric vinyl carbinols 13. These were smoothly transformed into the acetoxy bromide 14 by acetylation followed by reaction of the intermediate secondary acetates with hydrobromic acid. In this case, acetylation proved to be very important. Without acetylation, only destruction of 13 was observed. Subsequent treatment of 14 with triphenyl phosphine afforded the phosphonium bromide 15 which was immediately converted into the corresponding crystalline chloride 16 by treatment with aqueous sodium chloride.

The synthesis of the C_{40}-carbon skeleton was achieved according to the scheme $C_{25} + C_{15} = C_{40}$ (Fig. 7). Wittig salt 1 was first reacted with 3 to give the C_{25}-apo-compound 17 which was then condensed with 16. The reaction was carried out in a two-phase system, namely CH_2Cl_2/aqueous KOH as the base, furnishing (3R,3'R,6'R)-lutein which proved to be identical in every respect with the natural product.

The knowledge gained in the synthesis of (3R,3'R,6'R)-lutein could also be applied to the preparation of some other lutein diastereoisomers (Fig.8). Thus, utilizing the components 18

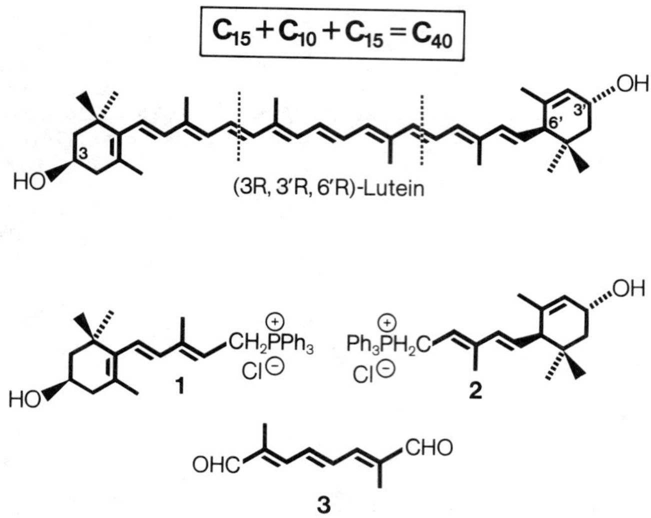

Fig. 4. Synthetic concept for (3R,3'R,6'R)-lutein

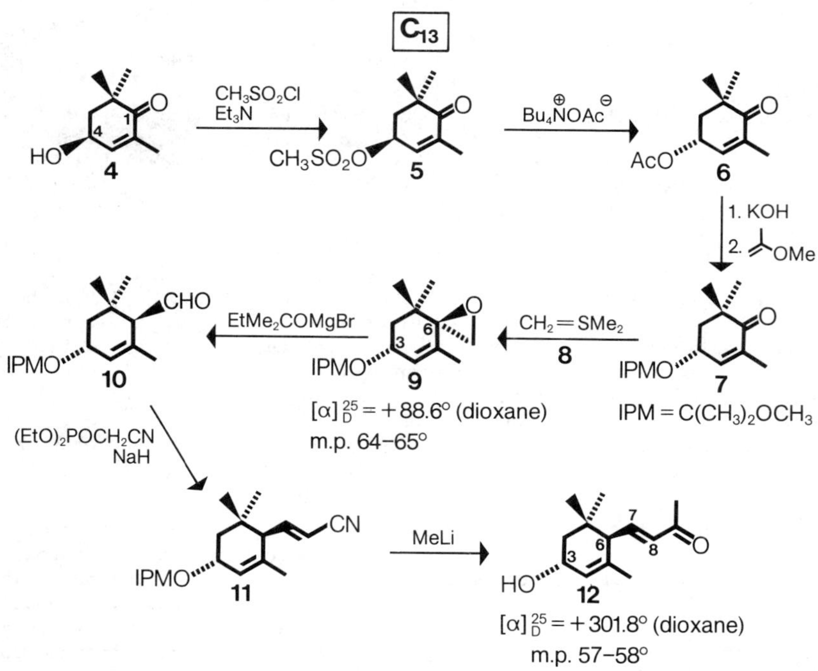

H. Mayer and A. Rüttimann, Helv. Chim. Acta 63, 1451 (1980)

Fig. 5. Synthesis of (4R)-4-acetoxy-2,6,6-trimethyl-2-cyclohexen-1-one and (3R,6R)-3-hydroxy-α-ionone

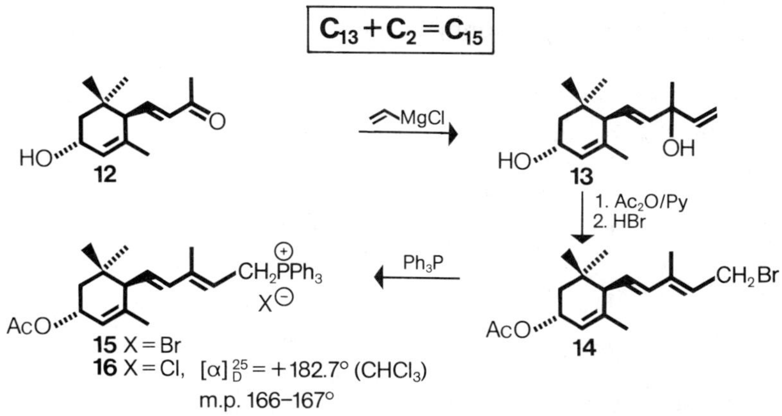

H. Mayer and A. Rüttimann, Helv. Chim. Acta 63, 1451 (1980)

Fig. 6. Synthesis of the C_{15}-Wittig salts

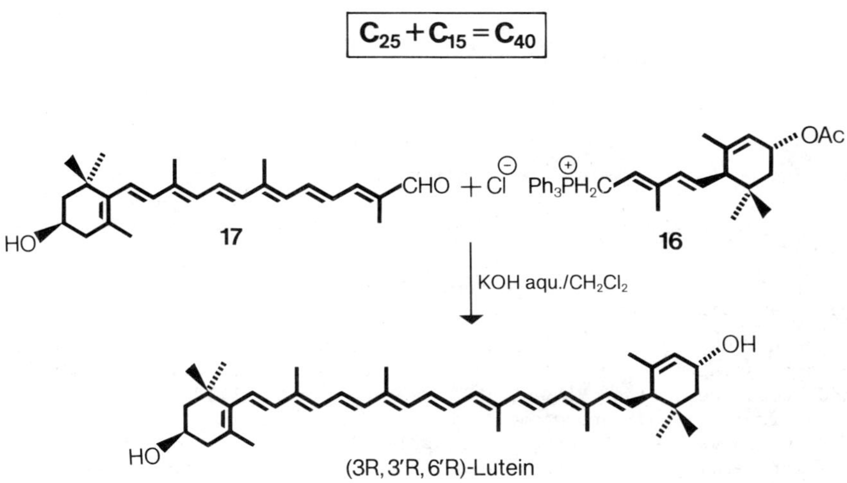

H. Mayer and A. Rüttimann, Helv. Chim. Acta 63, 1451 (1980)

Fig. 7. Synthesis of (3R,3'R,6'R)-lutein

Lutein Diastereoisomers

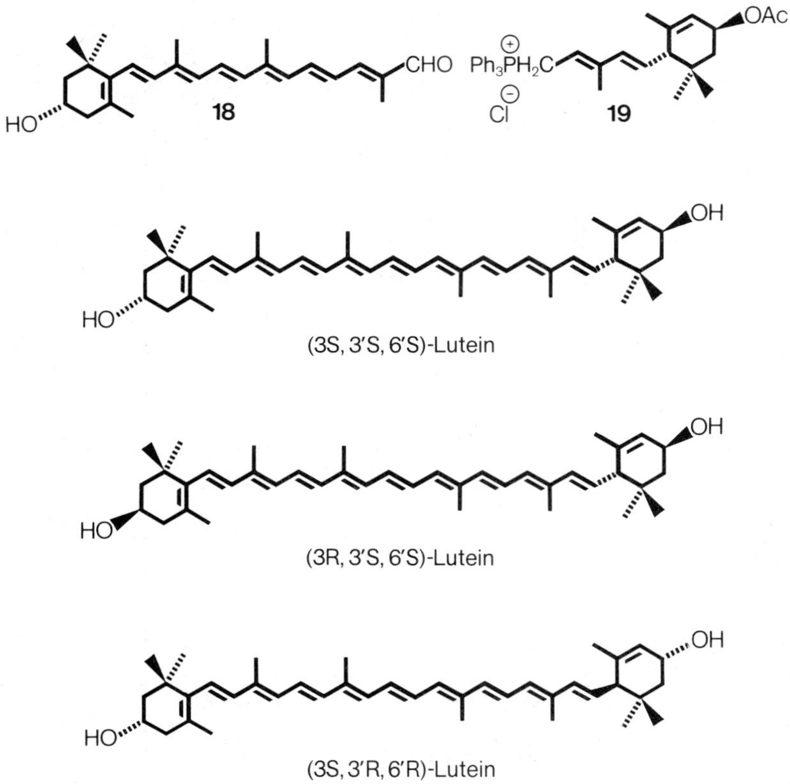

Fig. 8. Synthesis of lutein diastereoisomers

(Ref. 22) and 19 , (3S,3'S,6'S)-, (3R,3'S,6'S)- and (3S,3'R,6'R)-lutein have been synthesized in an analogous way.

The CD spectra of the four synthetic luteins are compiled in Fig. 9 clearly showing the various enantiomeric and diastereomeric relationships.

With the aid of modern techniques, research on carotenoid metabolism has become increasingly attractive. Here, the synthetic chemist can contribute by providing well defined compounds for structural and stereochemical studies. Thus, a metabolite of (3R,3'R)-zeaxanthin has recently been isolated from egg yolk and shown to be identical with the C_{40}-hydroxy ketone 20 (Fig. 10) (Ref. 23) which was readily obtained by selective Oppenauer oxidation of (3R,3'S, 6'S)-lutein. It is interesting to note that this metabolite was found to possess the (6'S)-configuration in contrast to 3'-O-didehydrolutein (Fig. 10) which has recently been isolated and fully characterized from egg yolk as possible metabolite of lutein (Ref. 24).

The CD spectra of 20 and 3'-O-didehydrolutein, obtained by Oppenauer oxidation of (3R,3'R, 6'R)-lutein, clearly show strong opposite Cotton effects at 276 and 270 nm, respectively (Fig. 11).

Fritschiellaxanthin

A new carotenoid, called fritschiellaxanthin, with an interesting combination of the astaxanthin and lutein ε-end groups, has recently been isolated and fully characterized from the green alga Fritschiella tuberosa (Ref. 10). With the necessary building units at hand, we have tried to synthesize this carotenoid according to the scheme $C_{25} + C_{15} = C_{40}$ (Fig. 12). Thus, Wittig reaction of the apo-aldehyde 21 (Ref. 14) with 16 afforded fritschiellaxanthin monoacetate whose spectral data were in complete agreement with the structure shown. However, preparation of the free pigment could not yet be achieved. Although controlled conditions for hydrolysis were applied, oxidation of the astaxanthin end group could not be prevented.

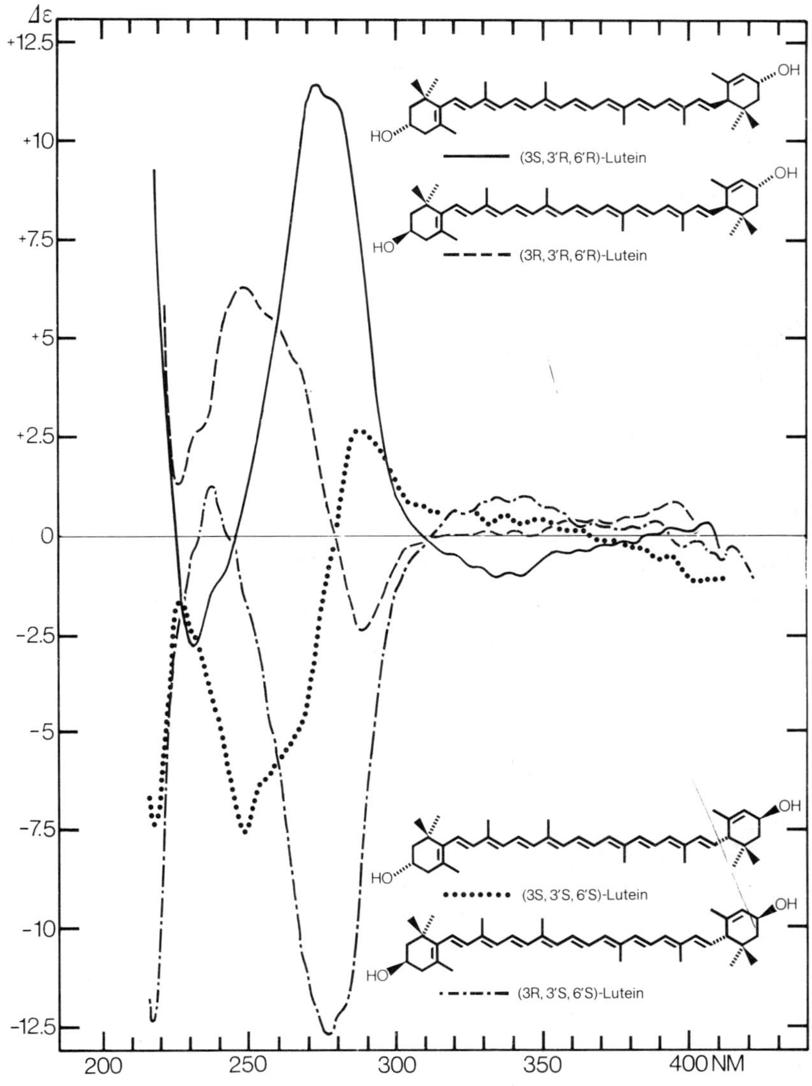

Fig. 9. CD spectra of (3R,3'R,6'R)-, (3S,3'S,6'S)-, (3R,3'S,6'S)- and (3S,3'R,6'R)-lutein (dioxane)

Tunaxanthin group

Tunaxanthin was first isolated in 1957 from bluefin tuna, Thunnus orientalis (Ref. 25) and was later found to be a common carotenoid in various other marine fishes. Structural studies suggested an ε,ε-carotene-3,3'-diol constitution for the pigment (Ref. 26) (Fig. 13) but no further support on structure and stereochemistry had been published at that time. In 1976, the first total synthesis of optically inactive 3,6-cis-3',6'-cis- and 3,6-trans-3'6'-trans-tunaxanthin was reported (Ref. 27). On the basis of NMR and TLC comparison with natural tunaxanthin, the 3,6-trans-3',6'-trans-configuration was suggested for the latter compound, but its absolute configuration was not established.

Careful consideration of the tunaxanthin structure reveals the presence of four chiral centres of type ABBA at C-3, C-6, C-3' and C-6' making possible a total of ten diastereoisomers (Ref. 28): Two pairs of enantiomers with C_2 symmetry and two pairs of enantiomers with C_1 symmetry and two optically inactive meso forms with $S_2(C_i)$ symmetry.

Today, structural elucidation and unequivocal identification of stereoisomeric carotenoids of

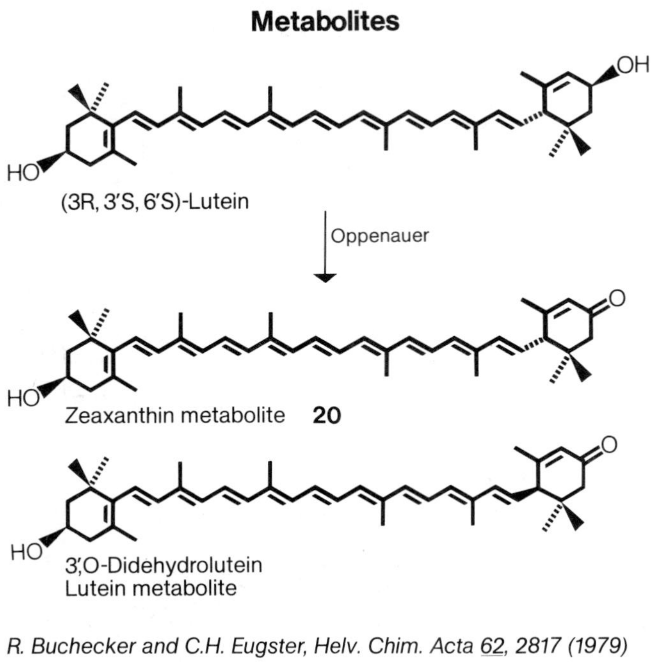

Fig. 10. Synthesis of zeaxanthin and lutein metabolite

the tunaxanthin type can be carried out on a µg scale on the basis of combined TLC, UV/VIS, NMR and CD evidence. Thus, six chiral isomers with the ε,ε-carotene-3,3'-diol constitution have recently been isolated and fully characterized from various natural sources composing what was previously known only by the single name of tunaxanthin. These include the chiriquixanthins A and B (Fig. 15) from a Costa Rican frog, Atelopus chiriquiensis (Ref. 29) and three additional isomers from various fishes, namely (3S,6S,3'R,6'S)-tunaxanthin (ent.-chiriquixanthin A) (Fig. 16) from Amanenses modestes, Thunnus thynnus, Seriola quinqueradiata (Ref. 30) and Oxyjulis californica (Ref. 28), as well as (3R,6S,3'R,6'S)-tunaxanthin (ent.-chiriquixanthin B) (Fig. 16) and (3S,6S,3'S,6'S)-tunaxanthin (ent.-lactucaxanthin) (Fig. 14) from Oxyjulis californica (Ref. 28). Very recently, a sixth chiral isomer, called lactucaxanthin (Fig. 14), has been isolated from Lactuca sativa (green lettuce) (Ref. 31).

At the outset of our synthetic activities, we were well aware of the complexity of the problem but, fortunately, the knowledge gained with lutein could also be applied to the tunaxanthin series.

Since symmetrical compounds are easier to make, our first goal was the synthesis of lactucaxanthin possessing two identical trans-ε-rings (Fig. 14). Thus, reaction of the C_{15}-Wittig chloride 16 with the C_{10}-dialdehyde 3 readily gave the desired compound whose physicochemical properties were in complete agreement with the published data (Ref. 31).

Its enantiomer, (3S,6S,3'S,6'S)-tunaxanthin, was obtained in an analogous way utilizing the corresponding enantiomeric C_{15}-phosphonium salt (Fig. 14).

Subsequent Oppenauer oxidation of lactucaxanthin afforded the diketone 22 (Fig. 15) with complete retention of configuration at C-6 and C-6'. This compound proved to be an ideal precursor for the preparation of the chiriquixanthins A and B (Fig. 15). Thus, dibal reduction of 22 gave a mixture of the two chiriquixanthins together with some lactucaxanthin which could be readily separated by preparative TLC. In this case, advantage has been taken of the two asymmetric centres at C-6 and C-6' in 22 to generate the desired trans-cis- and cis-cis-geometry, respectively.

Starting from the enantiomeric (6S,6'S)-diketone 23 (Fig. 16), the corresponding enantiomeric chiriquixanthins have been prepared in an analogous way (Fig. 16).

In this connection, it is interesting to note that diketone 23 has recently been identified as a second metabolite of (3R,3'R)-zeaxanthin in egg yolk (Ref. 23).

The described reaction sequences can be conveniently controlled by HPLC. Fig. 17 shows that excellent separation of diketone 22, lactucaxanthin and the chiriquixanthins was achieved

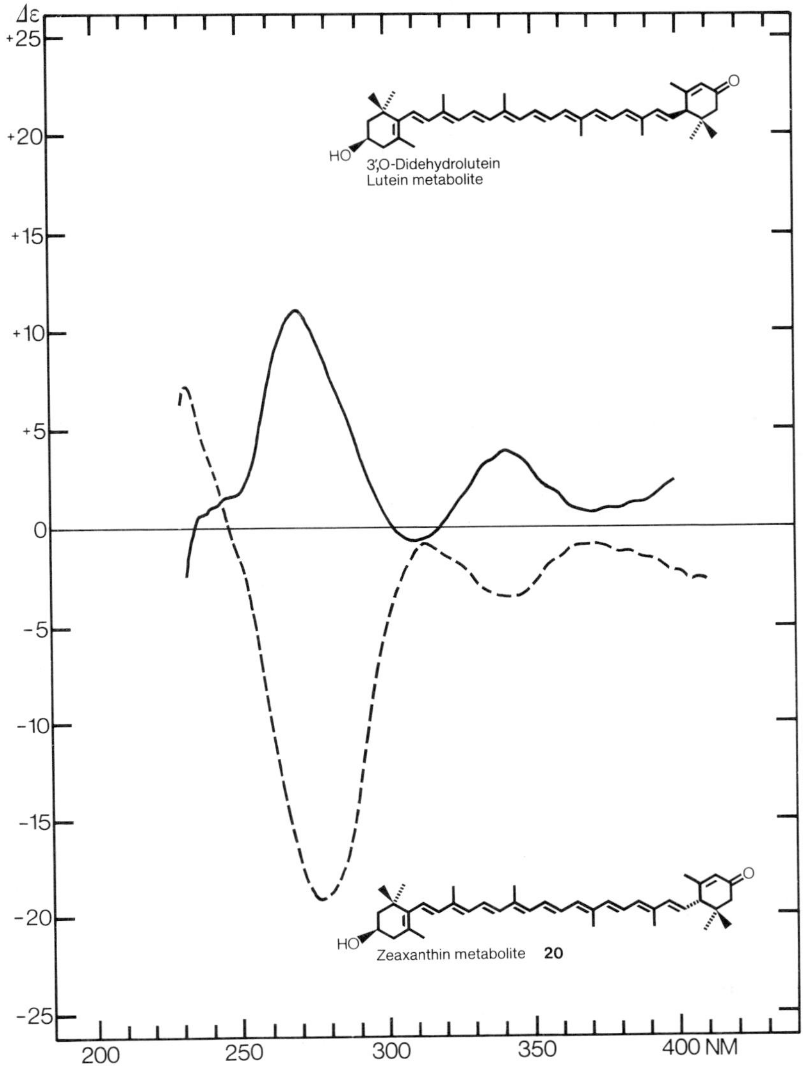

Fig. 11. CD spectra of the zeaxanthin and lutein metabolite (dioxane)

using a Spherisorb S 5-CN column with n-hexane/25 % CH_2Cl_2/0.1 % CH_3OH/0.1 % ethyl diisopropylamine as the mobile phase.

The CD spectra of the four chiriquixanthins are recorded in Fig. 18. They confirm the postulated (6R,6'R)-chirality for the natural chiriquixanthins A and B (Refs. 28 & 29) and also clearly demonstrate that the observed Cotton effects are nearly exclusively determined by the chirality at C-6 and C-6', as has already been stated earlier by several authors (Refs. 18, 28, 31-34).

The trans- and cis-configuration of the ε-rings is readily deduced from the chemical shifts of the ^{1}H-NMR signals of the 1,1-dimethyl groups (Refs. 18, 28-31). Thus, lactucaxanthin shows two methyl singlets at 0.849 and 0.998 ppm (Fig. 19), whereas for chiriquixanthin B these singlets appear at 0.852 and 0.943 ppm. As expected, chiriquixanthin A shows three signals at 0.850, 0.943 and 0.998 ppm confirming the trans-cis-configuration for the latter compound. We prefer the H-C-6 and H-C-6' doublets for clear differentiation. In this case, lactucaxanthin and chiriquixanthin B show one doublet each at 2.407 and 2.160 ppm, respectively, whereas with chiriquixanthin A two doublets are obtained at 2.405 and 2.160 ppm (Fig. 19).

The synthesis of (3R,6R,3'S,6'S)-(meso)-tunaxanthin with two enantiomeric trans-ε-rings (Fig. 20) was accomplished without major difficulties. However, special care had to be taken to prevent the generation of optical activity in the final product.

$C_{25} + C_{15} = C_{40}$

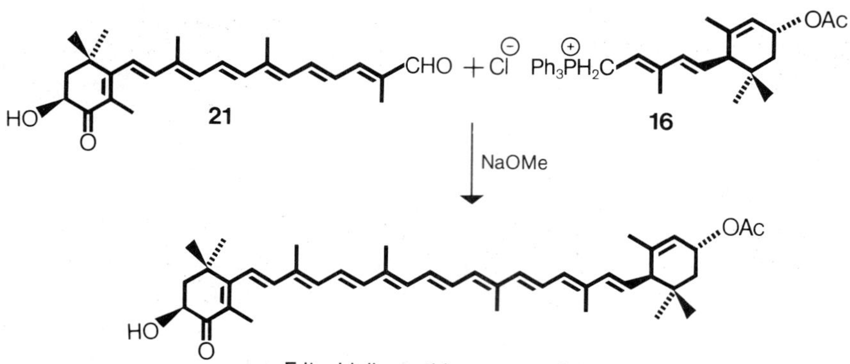

Fritschiellaxanthin monoacetate

Isolation, Stereochemistry: *R. Buchecker, C.H. Eugster and A. Weber, Helv. Chim. Acta 61, 1962 (1978)*

Fig. 12. Synthesis of fritschiellaxanthin monoacetate

Tunaxanthin Constitution

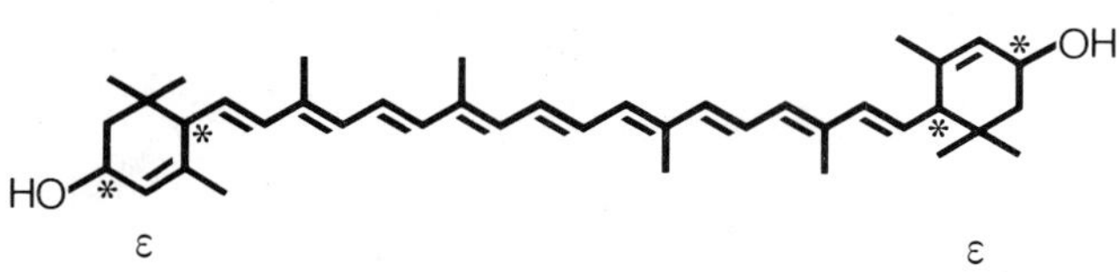

Type A B B A
2 Pairs of Enantiomers (C_2-Symmetry)
2 Pairs of Enantiomers (C_1-Symmetry)
2 Meso Forms (S_2-Symmetry)

Fig. 13. Tunaxanthin constitution

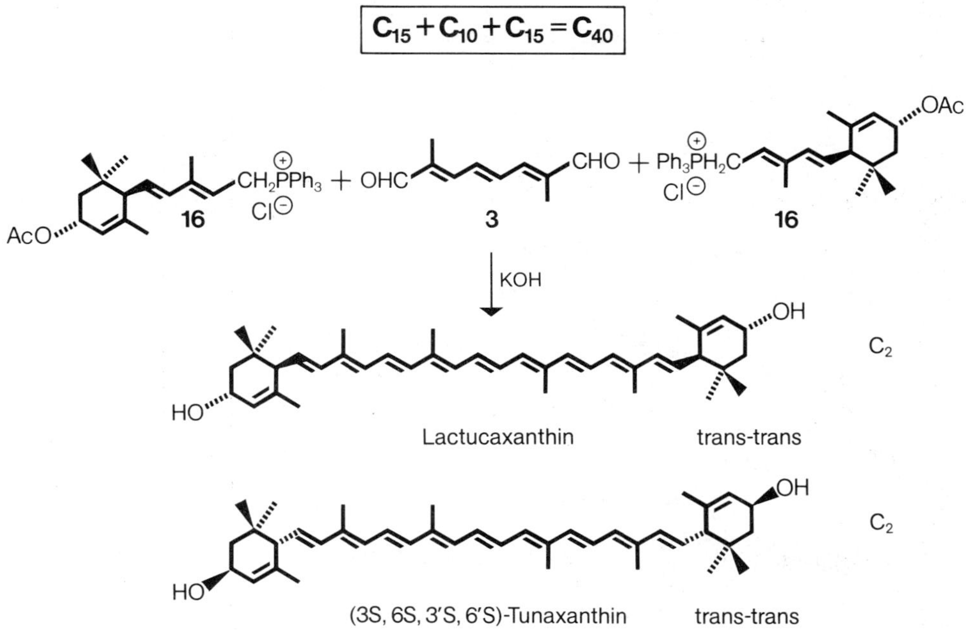

Fig. 14. Synthesis of lactucaxanthin and (3S,6S,3'S,6'S)-tunaxanthin

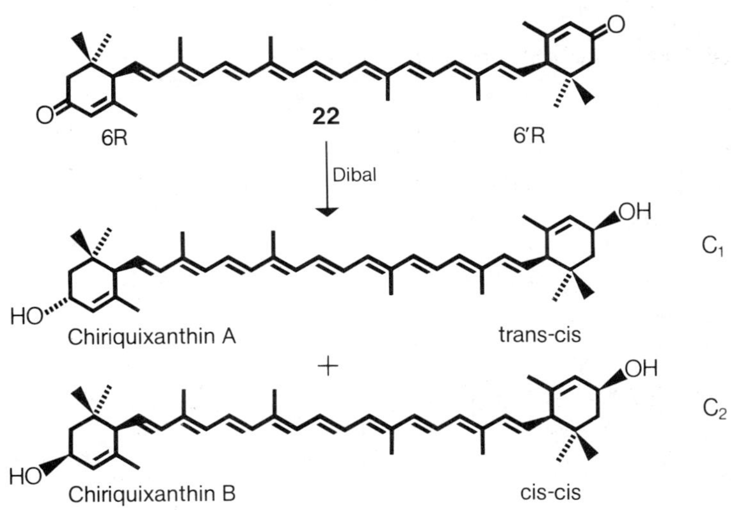

Fig. 15. Synthesis of chiriquixanthins A and B

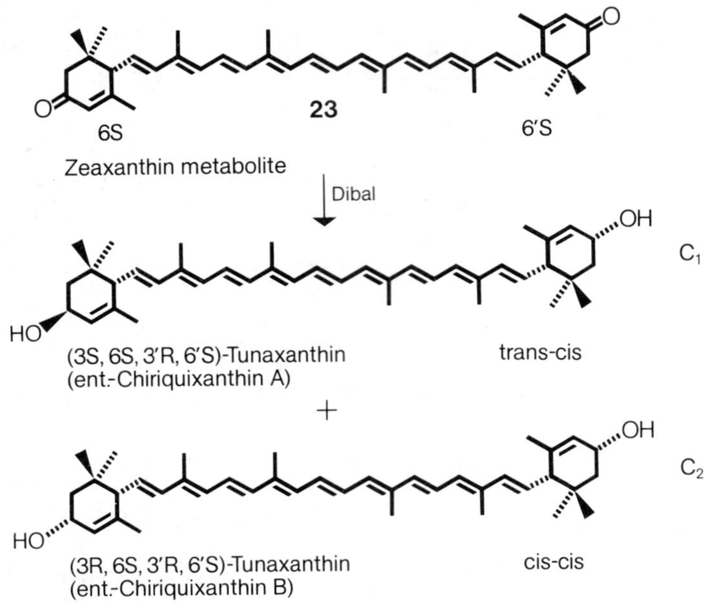

Fig. 16. Synthesis of ent.-chiriquixanthins A and B

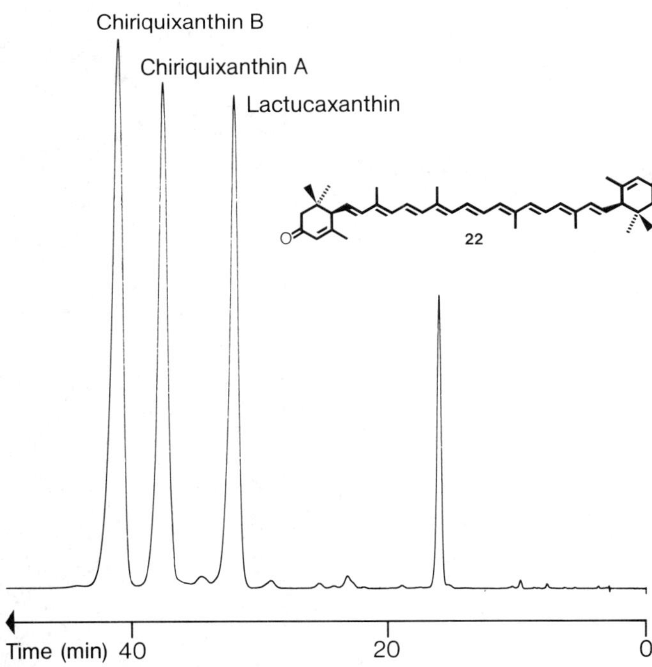

Fig. 17. HPLC of diketone 22 , lactucaxanthin and the chiriquixanthins A and B

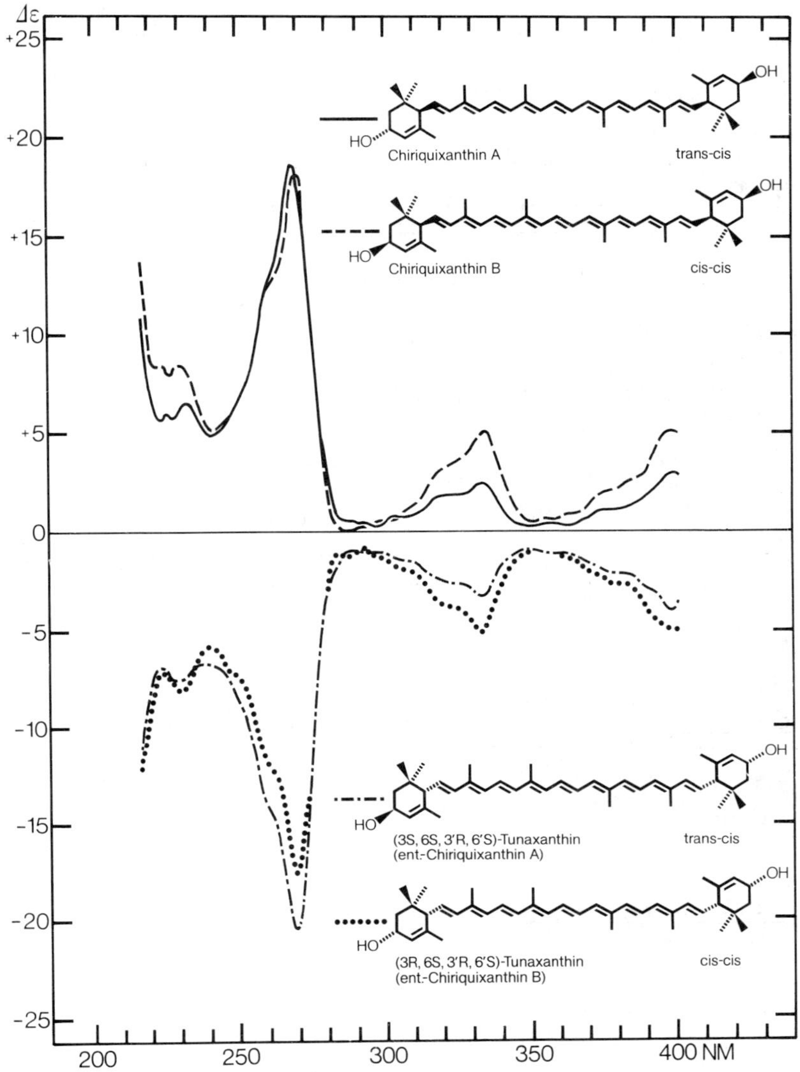

Fig. 18. CD spectra of chiriquixanthins A and B and enantiomers

This was achieved by condensation of the C_{15}-Wittig salt 16 with the C_{10}-dialdehyde 3 to give the C_{25}-apo-aldehyde 24 which was then reacted with the enantiomeric Wittig salt 19. As expected, the CD spectrum of the product showed no optical activity.

The second meso-compound, namely (3S,6R,3'R,6'S)-tunaxanthin possessing two enantiomeric cis-ε-rings (Fig. 21) was prepared starting from the (6R,6'S)-(meso)-configurated diketone 25 (Fig. 21) which was readily obtained from (3R,6R,3'S,6'S)-(meso)-tunaxanthin (Fig. 20) by Oppenauer oxidation. Thus, dibal reduction of 25 gave a mixture of the desired meso-compound and racemic trans-cis-tunaxanthin possessing the configuration shown. The meso-compound was purified by preparative TLC, but no resolution of the racemate was tried.

Concluding remarks

The foregoing discussion has shown that the synthesis of optically active carotenoids possessing ε-end groups represents a challenge. Various methods have been presented for the preparation of some more important members of this fascinating class of natural pigments. Today, even more complex structures with three and four chiral centres, such as the carotenoids of the lutein and tunaxanthin groups, can be synthesized without major difficulties. It has also become apparent, however, that the synthetic chemist has to rely more and more on modern physical techniques, such as HPLC, NMR, CD and X-ray crystallographic analysis. In the absence of X-ray analyses of intact carotenoids, synthesis provides compounds with defined absolute configurations for the confirmation of configurational assignments of the natural pig-

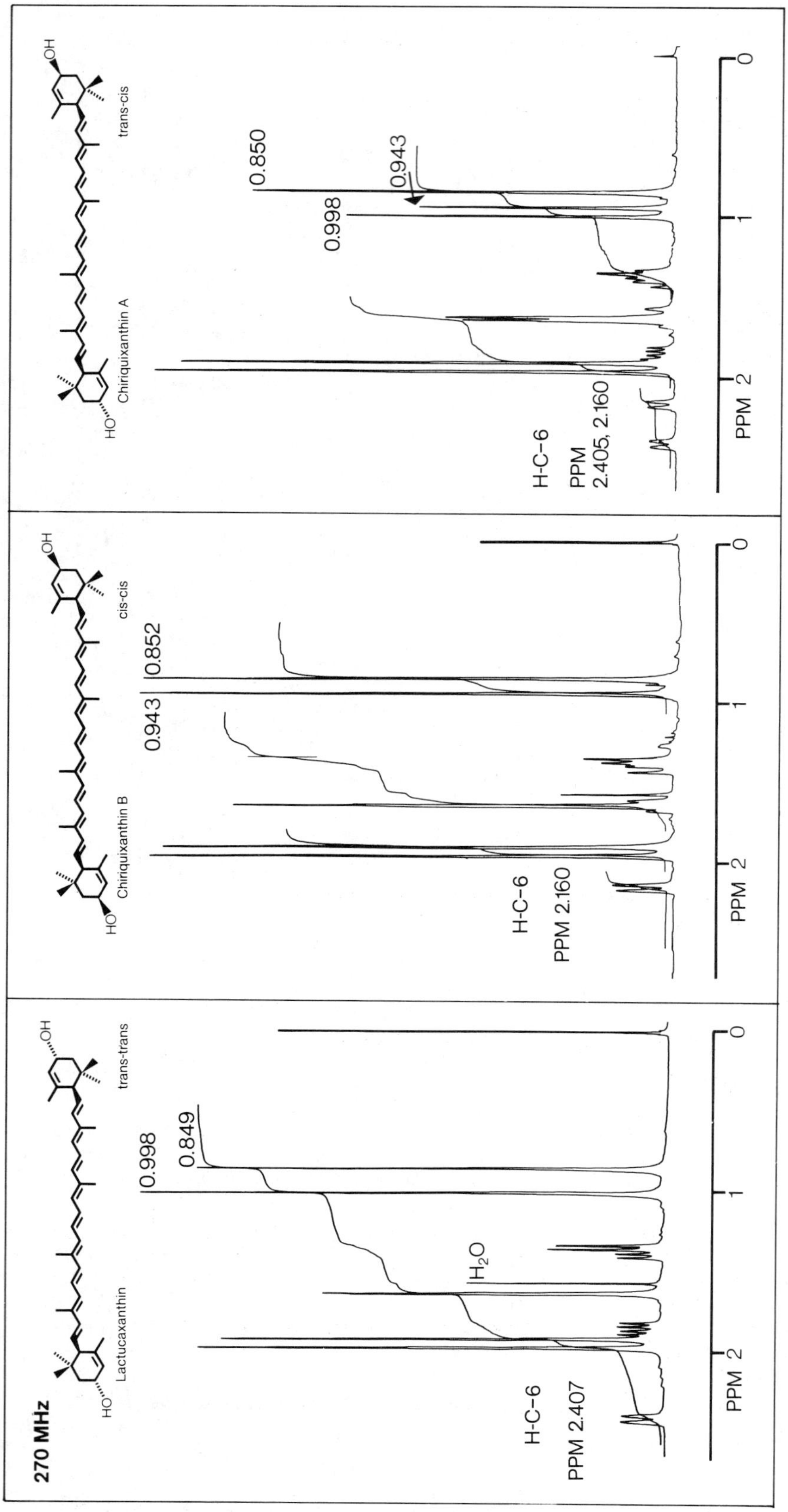

Fig. 19. 270 MHz NMR spectra of lactucaxanthin, chiriquixanthin B and chiriquixanthin A ($CDCl_3$)

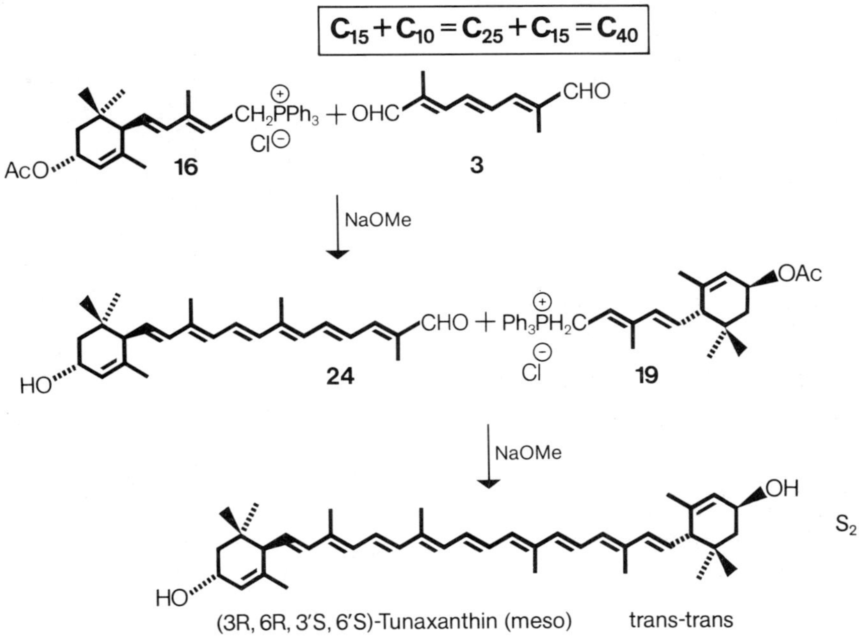

Fig. 20. Synthesis of (3R,6R,3'S,6'S)-(meso)-tunaxanthin

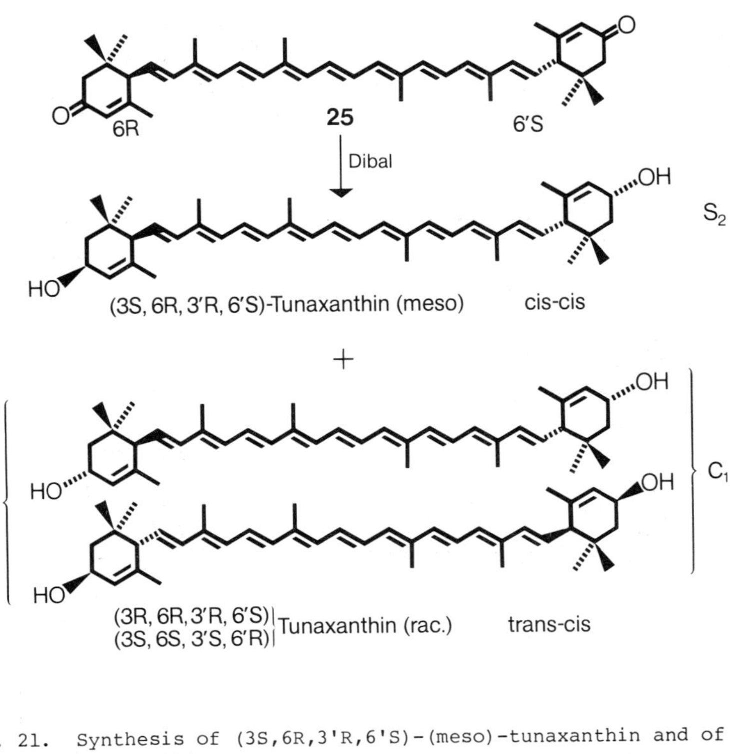

Fig. 21. Synthesis of (3S,6R,3'R,6'S)-(meso)-tunaxanthin and of racemic trans-cis-tunaxanthin

ments. Moreover, synthesis may assist the biochemist in his metabolic studies. Thus, two synthetic intermediates of the series have been shown to be interesting metabolites of (3R,3'R)-zeaxanthin, a finding which may shed some light on the biological interconversion of β- into ε-end groups.

Acknowledgements - The work described would not have been possible without the collaboration of the following scientists of the Roche group: Dr. A. Rüttimann (synthesis of key intermediates for natural lutein), Drs. R.K. Müller and K. Bernhard (synthesis of (3S)-C_{25}-apo-astaxanthinal), Dr. G. Englert, Dr. W. Arnold and Mr. W. Grunauer (NMR), Dr. W. Vetter and Mr. W. Meister (MS), Dr. L. Chopard (IR), Dr. K. Noack (CD), Dr. M. Vecchi and Mr. E. Glinz (HPLC), Dr. J.J. Daly (X-ray) and Dr. A. Dirscherl (microanalysis). Thanks are due to Mrs. K. Schiedt for providing a sample of natural lutein. Also the excellent technical assistance of Mr. K. Holzhauser and Mr. J.-M. Zielinski is gratefully acknowledged. Further, I should like to thank Prof. S. Liaaen-Jensen, Prof. C.H. Eugster and Dr. R. Buchecker for stimulating discussions and advice.

REFERENCES

1. O. Isler, Carotenoids, Birkhäuser Verlag, Basel and Stuttgart (1971).
2. O. Straub, Key to Carotenoids: Lists of Natural Carotenoids, Birkhäuser Verlag, Basel and Stuttgart (1976).
3. Ch. Tscharner, C.H. Eugster and P. Karrer, Helv.Chim.Acta 40, 1676 (1957).
4. R. Buchecker, R. Egli, H. Regel-Wild, Ch. Tscharner, C.H. Eugster, G. Uhde and G. Ohloff, Helv.Chim.Acta 52, 1729 (1969).
5. C.H. Eugster, R. Buchecker, Ch. Tscharner, G. Uhde and G. Ohloff, Helv.Chim.Acta 56, 2548 (1973).
6. L. Bartlett, W. Klyne, W.P. Mose, P.M. Scopes, G. Galasko, A.K. Mallams, B.C.L. Weedon, J. Szabolcs and G. Tóth, J.Chem.Soc. C, 2527 (1969).
7. Ch. Tscharner, C.H. Eugster and P. Karrer, Helv.Chim.Acta 41, 32 (1958).
8. A.G. Andrewes, G. Borch and S. Liaaen-Jensen, Acta Chem.Scand. B 30, 214 (1976).
9. A.K. Chopra, B.P.S. Khambay, A. Madden, G.P. Moss and B.C.L. Weedon, Chem.Commun. 357 (1977).
10. R. Buchecker, C.H. Eugster and A. Weber, Helv.Chim.Acta 61, 1962 (1978).
11. W. Eschenmoser, P. Uebelhart and C.H. Eugster, Helv.Chim.Acta 62, 2534 (1979).
12. C.H. Eugster, Pure Appl.Chem. 51, 463 (1979).
13. S. Liaaen-Jensen, Fortschr.Chem.Org.Naturstoffe 39, 123 (1980).
14. H. Mayer, Pure Appl.Chem. 51, 535 (1979).
15. C.H. Eugster, Angew.Chem. 1970, 259.
16. R. Buchecker, P. Hamm and C.H. Eugster, Chimia 25, 192 (1971).
17. R. Buchecker, P. Hamm and C.H. Eugster, Chimia 26, 134 (1972).
18. R. Buchecker, P. Hamm and C.H. Eugster, Helv.Chim.Acta 57, 631 (1974).
19. A.G. Andrewes, G. Borch and S. Liaaen-Jensen, Acta Chem.Scand. B 28, 139 (1974).
20. B.C.L. Weedon, Pure Appl.Chem. 47, 168 (1976).
21. H. Mayer and A. Rüttimann, Helv.Chim.Acta 63, 1451 (1980).
22. A. Rüttimann and H. Mayer, Helv.Chim.Acta 63, 1456 (1980).
23. K. Schiedt, Abstr.Sixth Internat.Symp.Carotenoids, 1981.
24. R. Buchecker and C.H. Eugster, Helv.Chim.Acta 62, 2817 (1979).
25. S. Hirao, J. Yamada and R. Kikuchi, Bull.Tokai Reg.Fish.Res.Lab. 16, 53 (1957).
26. G.F. Crozier and D.W. Wilkie, Comp.Biochem.Physiol. 18, 801 (1966).
27. B.C.L. Weedon, Pure Appl.Chem. 47, 167 (1976).
28. A. Bingham, D.W. Wilkie and H.S. Mosher, Comp.Biochem.Physiol. 62B, 489 (1979).
29. A. Bingham, H.S. Mosher and A.G. Andrewes, Chem.Commun. 96 (1977).
30. H. Rønneberg, G. Borch, S. Liaaen-Jensen, H. Matsutaka and T. Matsuno, Acta Chem.Scand. B 32, 621 (1978).
31. D. Siefermann-Harms, S. Hertzberg, G. Borch and S. Liaaen-Jensen, Phytochemistry 20, 85 (1981).
32. A.G. Andrewes, S. Liaaen-Jensen and O. Weeks, Acta Chem.Scand. B 29, 884 (1975).
33. A.G. Andrewes, G. Borch and S. Liaaen-Jensen, Acta Chem.Scand. B 30, 1703 (1976).
34. S. Hertzberg, G. Borch and S. Liaaen-Jensen, Acta Chem.Scand. B 33, 42 (1979).

SYNTHESIS AND STEREOCHEMISTRY OF RED PEPPER CAROTENOIDS

A. Rüttimann

Department of Vitamin and Nutritional Research, F. Hoffmann-La Roche & Co. Ltd., CH-4002 Basle, Switzerland.

Abstract - The synthesis of (3S,5R,3'S,5'R)-capsorubin, (3R,3'S,5'R)-capsanthin and (3S,5R)-cryptocapsin, the unique pigments of the red pepper fruit *Capsicum annuum*, starting from natural (+)-camphor, is reported. An alternative route to these interesting pigments, possessing five membered K-end groups, is described utilizing (3R)-3-hydroxy-β-cyclocitral - an intermediate in the technical synthesis of (3R,3'R)-zeaxanthin - as readily available starting material.

Oxidation of the above-mentioned red pepper carotenoids to (5R,5'R)-capsorubone, (3R,5'R)-capsanthone and (5R)-cryptocapsone respectively, is performed using the Oppenauer method.

The use of red pepper carotenoids as food pigmenters is discussed.

INTRODUCTION: OCCURRENCE AND HISTORY

Nature relies on a variety of compounds for pigmentation of living organisms: chlorophylls, anthocyanins, porphyrins and carotenoids, which are the most widespread, occurring in both the animal and plant kingdoms, and appear to have the most varied functions (Ref. 1). A wide variety of foods owe their colour mainly to carotenoids, which appear to be synthesized *de novo* only by higher plants, mosses, etc. The chloroplasts present in green unripe fruits, in most cases, gradually change on ripening into chromoplasts, enzymes are either newly synthesized or derepressed, while carotenoid synthesis, often of novel pigments, is enormously stimulated (Ref. 2). Typical examples are tomatoes and red peppers.

The beautiful colour of the red paprika, a variety of *Capsicum annuum* has attracted scientists for a long time. As early as 1927, a deep red pigment, called capsanthin, was first isolated from this red pepper fruit in crystalline form (Ref. 3). Subsequently, two further crystalline pigments with this unusual end group were isolated from the same source: capsorubin (Ref. 4) and in smaller amounts cryptocapsin (Refs. 5 & 6) (Fig. 1).

These three carotenoids, which belong to the unique pigments of red peppers (*Capsicum annuum*) (Refs. 6-12) are only rarely found in other sources. Pigments with this characteristic cyclopentanol end-group could be further identified in the anthers and petals of various lilies (Refs. 13 & 14), in *Berberis* fruits (Ref. 15), in the fruit peel of *Enzephalartos villosus Lehm* (Ref. 16) and in the anthers of several *Aesculus* genus (Refs. 17-19), where also the oxidized pigments capsorubone, capsanthone and cryptocapsone could be found (Fig. 2).

The structural formulae of capsanthin and capsorubin have been the subject of considerable controversy for decades (Refs. 20-32). The clue to the structure of this novel end-group was only found at the beginning of the sixties (Refs. 33-35): Oxidation of the five-membered end-groups of capsanthin and capsorubin by the Oppenauer method yielded cyclopentanone rings, which could easily be detected using IR- and ^{1}H-NMR-techniques. By correlation with (+)-camphor the (5R,5'R)-configuration was established (Refs. 32, 36 & 37). The *trans*-stereochemistry of the hydroxy group at the five-membered ring to the polyene chain was demonstrated by lactonization experiments on a degradation product (Refs. 35 & 38).

SYNTHESIS OF FIVE-MEMBERED RED PEPPER CAROTENOIDS

A) Optically inactive forms

Unequivocal proof of the structure of these new paprika pigments with the K-end-group was provided by the total synthesis of the *trans*- and *cis*-form of optically inactive capsorubin (Ref. 39) (Fig. 3).

Autoxidation of the keto acid 1 gave the α-diketone 2 which was converted into the five-membered keto acid 3 . Reduction and treatment with methyl lithium gave a mixture of *trans*- and *cis*-hydroxy ketones. The *trans*-hydroxy ketone 4 was condensed with crocetindial 5 to give optically inactive capsorubin. Unlike the *cis*-isomer, this compound was identical in

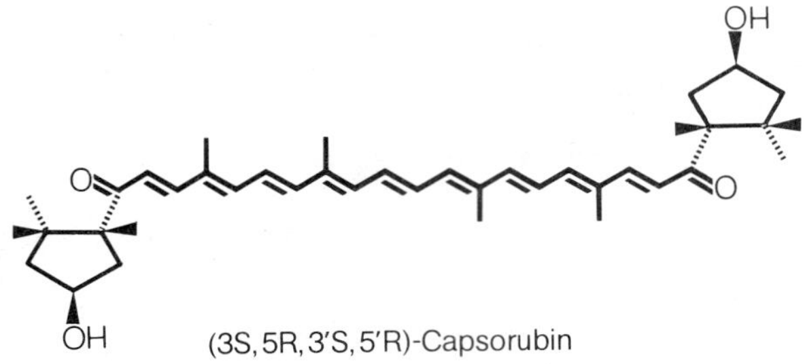

(3S, 5R, 3'S, 5'R)-Capsorubin

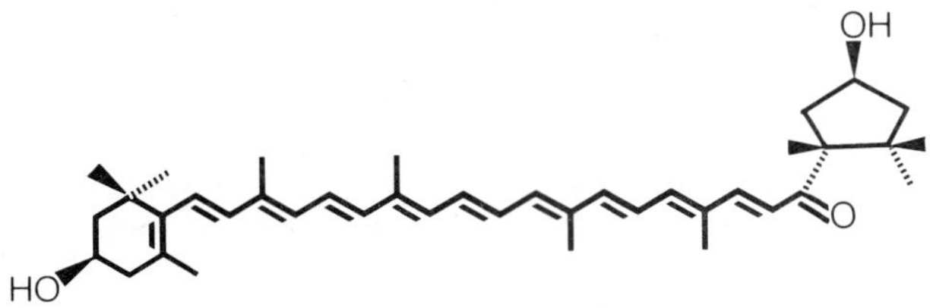

(3R, 3'S, 5'R)-Capsanthin

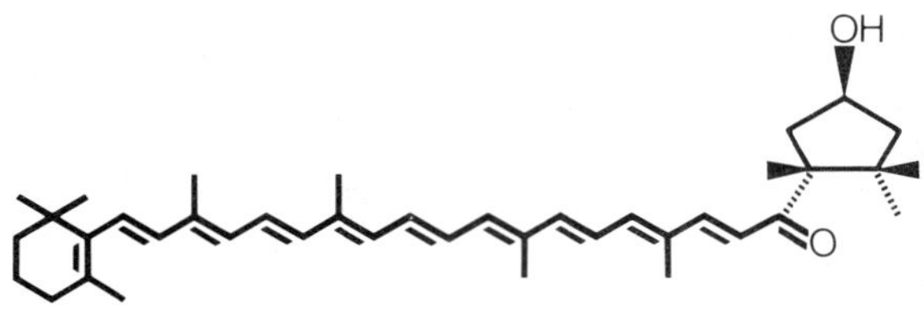

(3S, 5R)-Cryptocapsin

Fig. 1. Main carotenoids of the red paprika Capsicum annuum with cyclopentanol end-groups.

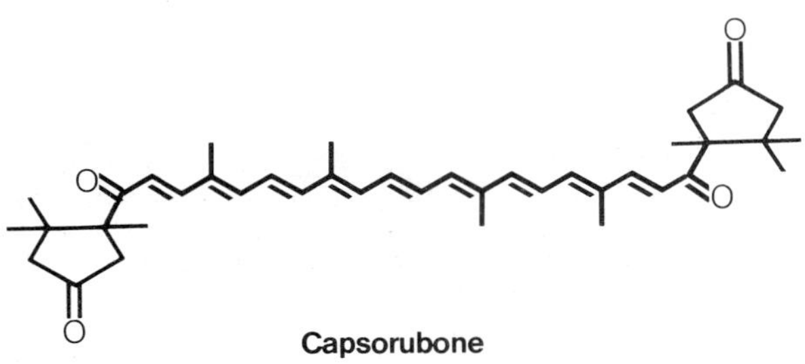

Capsorubone

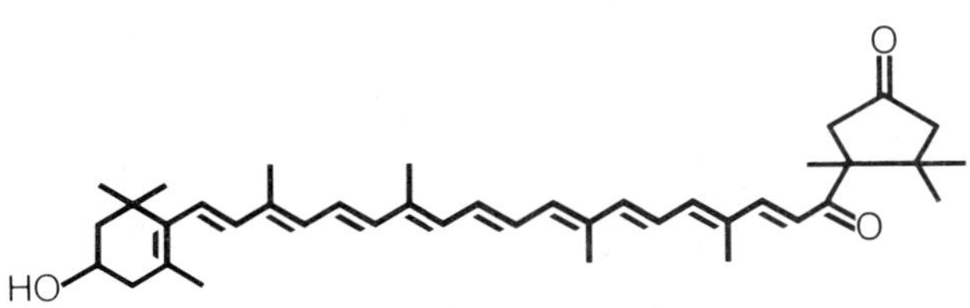

Capsanthone

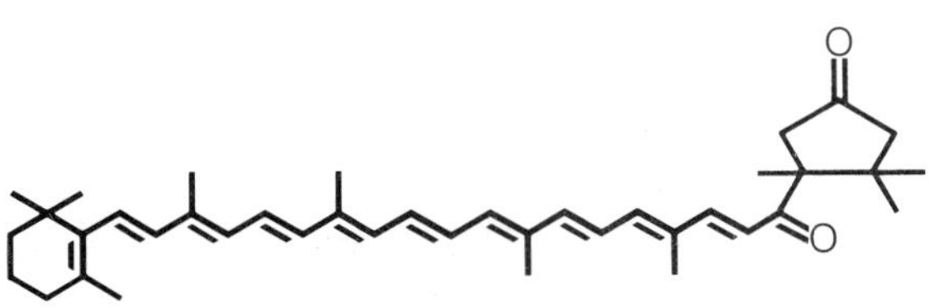

Cryptocapsone

Fig. 2. Carotenoids with cyclopentanone end-groups.

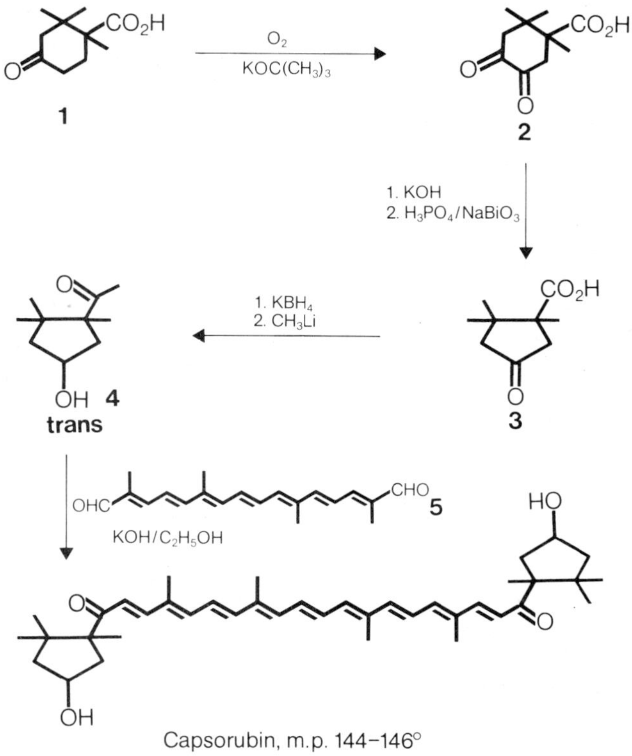

Fig. 3. Total synthesis of optically inactive capsorubin.

thin-layer chromatography, IR-, UV- and ^{1}H-NMR-spectra with the natural compound. Optically inactive capsanthin and cryptocapsin were subsequently synthesized using the same racemic end-group and compared with the naturally occurring compounds (Refs. 40-42).

B) Optically active forms

1. Synthesis of C_{10}-end-groups

From (+)-camphor

The first total synthesis of nature-identical (3S,5R,3'S,5'R)-capsorubin starting from (+)-camphor was announced in 1973 by Weedon (Ref. 43). By the same school, a new improved synthesis of this unusual pigment was reported some years later (Refs. 44 & 45) using the same starting material (Figs. 4 & 5).

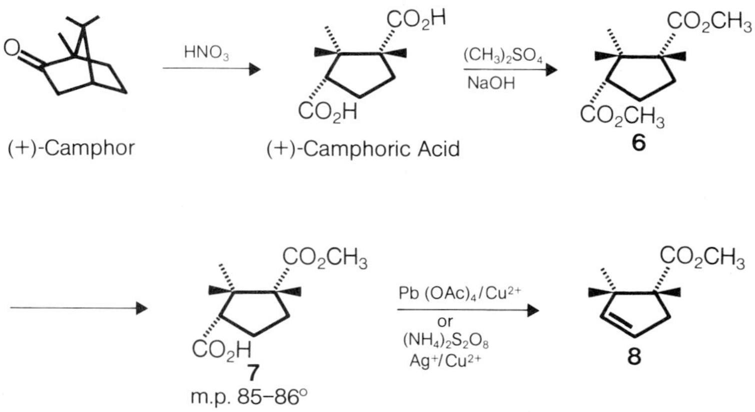

Fig. 4. Synthesis of (R)-1,1,5-trimethyl-2-cyclopentene-5-methylcarboxylate (8).

D-(+)-Camphor, which is obtained technically from the oil of the camphor tree Cinnamomum camphora using steam distillation techniques, is oxidized with nitric acid to give (+)-camphoric acid as the main product (Ref. 46). Esterification of the diacid with dimethyl sulfate and subsequent saponification of the less hindered ester of 6 with one equivalent of sodium hydroxide yielded the crystalline monoacid 7 . In a copper and silver salt catalyzed oxidative decarboxylation reaction, using lead tetraacetate or ammonium persulfate as oxidizing agent, the pure unsaturated ester 8 was obtained in high yield after distillation (Ref. 47).

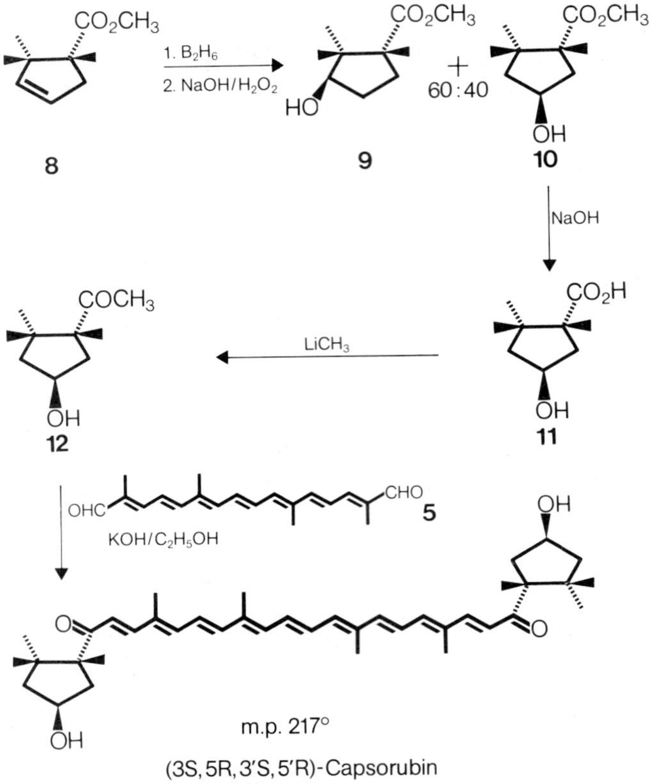

Fig. 5. Total synthesis of (3S,5R,3'S,5'R)-capsorubin (Weedon synthesis).

Introduction of the hydroxy group at the double bond of 8 was accomplished using H.C. Brown's hydroboration method (Ref. 48). Thus, treatment of 8 with diborane gave, after oxidative work-up, a mixture of isomeric hydroxy esters 9 and 10 , unfortunately with the undesired 9 as the predominant compound. Ester 10 was then hydrolyzed to the hydroxy acid 11 , which was treated with excess methyl lithium to give ketone 12 . By an aldol condensation, crocetindial 5 was reacted with this *trans*-methyl ketone 12 to give crystalline (3S,5R,3'S,5'R)-capsorubin, possessing the correct natural configuration.

The crucial step in this synthesis is obviously the introduction of the hydroxyl group in 8 . By using various sterically hindered borane derivatives, we tried to achieve a regio- and diastereoselective introduction of the hydroxy function at C-3 (Fig. 6). Thus, treatment

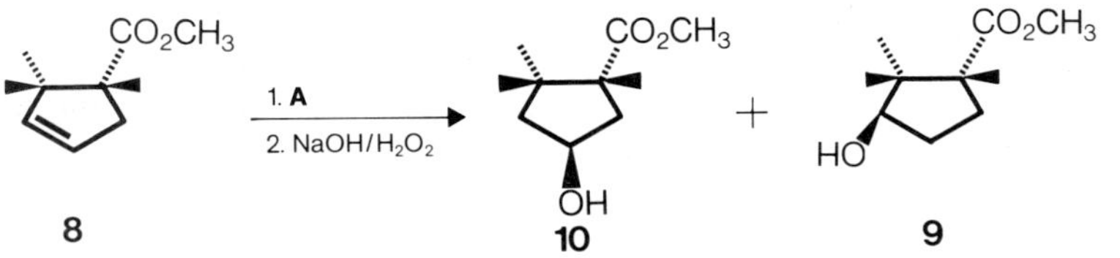

$[\alpha]_D^{25} = +105°$ (C_2H_5OH) $[\alpha]_D^{25} = +2.7°$ (C_2H_5OH) $[\alpha]_D^{25} = -29.5°$ (C_2H_5OH)

Borane Derivative (**A**)	GC-Yield (**10**+**9**)	Ratio 10:9	
		10	**9**
Borane Dimethylsulfide Complex	80%	37%	63%
Thexylborane	73%	43%	57%
Disiamylborane	60%	43%	57%
Dicyclohexylborane	16%	44%	56%
(−)-Diisopinocampheylborane	84%	25%	75%
(+)-Diisopinocampheylborane	87%	57%	43%

Fig. 6. Hydroboration of (R)-1,1,5-trimethyl-2-cyclopentene-5-methylcarboxylate (8).

of the unsaturated ester 8 with a number of known boranes listed in Fig. 6, followed by an oxidative work-up, yielded the two isomeric hydroxy esters 9 and 10 in different ratios. The corresponding cis-isomers could never be detected. (+)-Diisopinocampheylborane ((+)-$(IPC)_2BH$), derived from cheap natural (-)-α-pinene, proved to be the most selective reagent. It is interesting to note that, in this case, the two enantiomeric reagents (+)- and (-)-diisopinocampheylborane attack the double bond of the chiral substrate - not unexpectedly - in a quite different way.

To improve further the obtained ratio of 9 : 10 = 43:57, another suitable substrate for this hydroboration reaction with even more favourable sterical requirements was synthesized (Fig. 7). Thus, the five-membered ester 8 was saponified to the acid 13, which was treated with two equivalents methyl lithium to afford the volatile methyl ketone 14. A subsequent

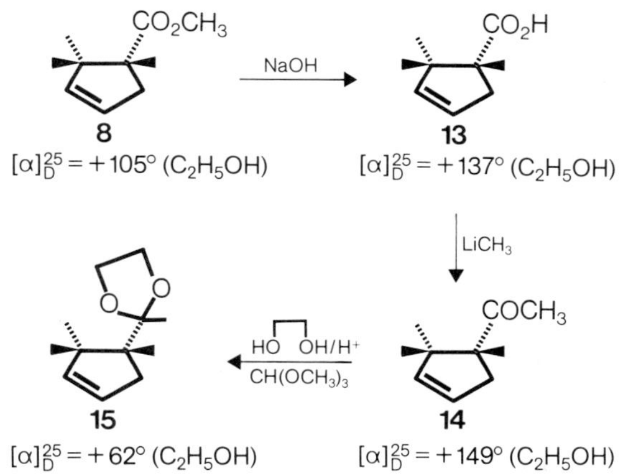

Fig. 7. Synthesis of the unsaturated ketal 15 .

acid-catalyzed ketalization with glycol yielded the desired substrate 15 in about 75 % overall yield. This compound turned out to be, indeed, a good substrate for hydroboration. A similar treatment of 15 with several boranes yielded in most cases three isomeric hydroxy ketones in various ratios (Fig. 8). This time also, a cis-isomer could be detected. Again the (+)-$(IPC)_2BH$ proved to be the reagent of choice. The desired hydroxy-ketone 12 was formed as the main product, besides only one minor isomer, which could be easily separated by chromatography.

Another highly convenient and mild procedure for the hydration of a carbon-carbon double bond was found some time ago in the oxomercuration-demercuration sequence (Ref. 49). This transformation usually proceeds without rearrangements and sometimes amazingly high regioselectivity is observed (Ref. 50). Treatment of the ketal 15 with mercuric acetate in aqueous tetrahydrofurane, followed by a reduction of the mercurial intermediate with alkaline sodium borohydride, provided, after removal of the protecting group, the two epimeric hydroxy-ketones 12 and 16 in a ratio of 85:15. (Fig. 9). The desired trans-compound 12 , which was formed as the main product, could easily be obtained pure after column chromatography. The mercury, which was obtained after work-up in metallic form, could be recovered in quantitative yield.

From (3R)-3-hydroxy-ß-cyclocitral

The paprika pigments capsanthin and capsorubin are believed to be formed in nature from zeaxanthin as first proposed in 1955 (Refs. 5, 6, 8 & 14). Now, there is strong evidence that they are both produced from zeaxanthin through the epoxides antheraxanthin and violaxanthin, respectively (Fig. 10). The key transformation to give the ketonic pigments presumably involves a pinacolic rearrangement of the epoxides, or of a closely related derivative (Ref. 51). Recently, an in vitro conversion of violaxanthin into capsorubin by a chromoplast enriched fraction prepared from semi-ripened red pepper fruits could be performed for the first time (Ref. 52).

The same type of reaction, which nature uses for this ring contraction, was utilized as the key step in an alternative approach to the C_{10}-building unit 12.

(3R)-3-Hydroxy-ß-cyclocitral (20) (Refs. 53-55), an intermediate in the technical synthesis of (3R,3'R)-zeaxanthin, proved to be a suitable starting material (Fig. 11). Reduction of the aldehyde 21 , obtained after protection of the hydroxyl function in 20 with dihydropyrane, could be carried out with sodium borohydride or lithium aluminium hydride to give the alcohol 22 . Further reduction of the alcohol to the hydrocarbon level was effected using a method developed by Corey et al. (Ref. 56): Activation of the unprotected hydroxyl group was attain-

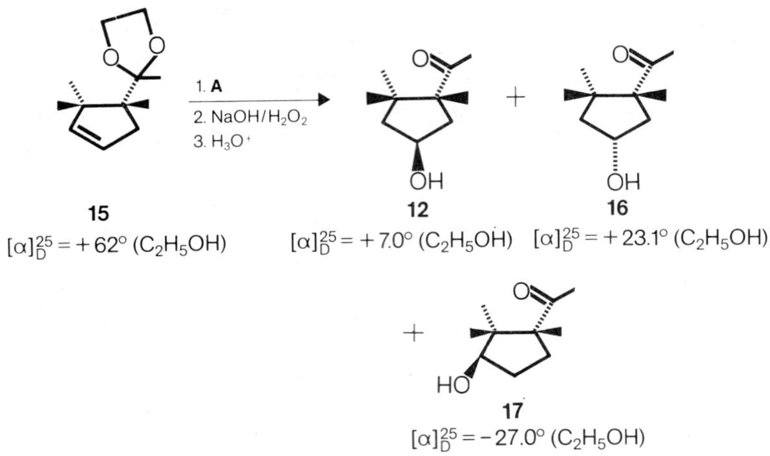

Borane Derivative (**A**)	GC-Yield (**12**+**16**+**17**)	Ratio **12**:**16**:**17**		
		12	**16**	**17**
Diborane	59%	48%	11%	41%
Thexylborane	50%	69%	4%	27%
Disiamylborane	84%	73%	5%	22%
Dicyclohexylborane	24%	63%	10%	27%
9-BBN	17%	71%	29%	–
(−)-Diisopinocampheylborane	95%	50%	9%	41%
(+)-Diisopinocampheylborane	79%	82%	–	18%

Fig. 8. Hydroboration of the unsaturated ketal 15 .

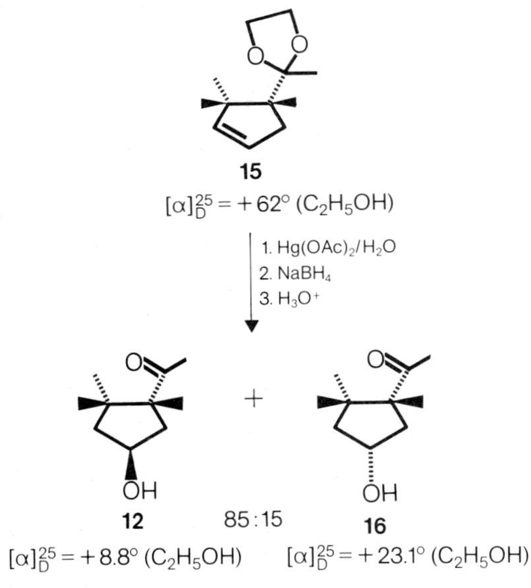

Fig. 9. Oxomercuration-demercuration of ketal 15 .

ed by treatment with the pyridine-sulfur trioxide complex. Without isolation of the intermediate sulfate monoester, a reduction with lithium aluminium hydride was performed to yield, after an acidic work-up, the alcohol 23 as a nicely crystalline compound. A subsequent epoxidation of the acetate 24 with m-chloroperbenzoic acid afforded a 2:1 mixture of isomeric epoxides 25a and 26a , which were separated by column chromatography (Fig. 12). The stereochemistry of the epoxide ring could readily be deduced from the IR-spectra of the epoxy-alcohols 25b and 26b , obtained by a simple hydrolysis of the corresponding acetates. In dilution experiments, a clear intramolecular hydrogen bonding of the hydroxy group with the epoxide ring in 25b could be observed. For this reason, a cis-configuration was assigned to this isomer (Ref. 57).

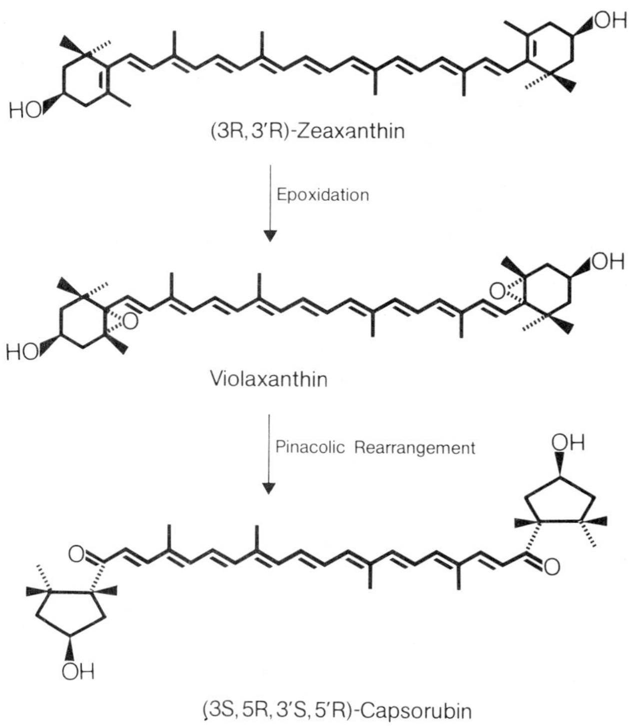

Fig. 10. Biosynthesis of (3S,5R,3'S,5'R)-capsorubin.

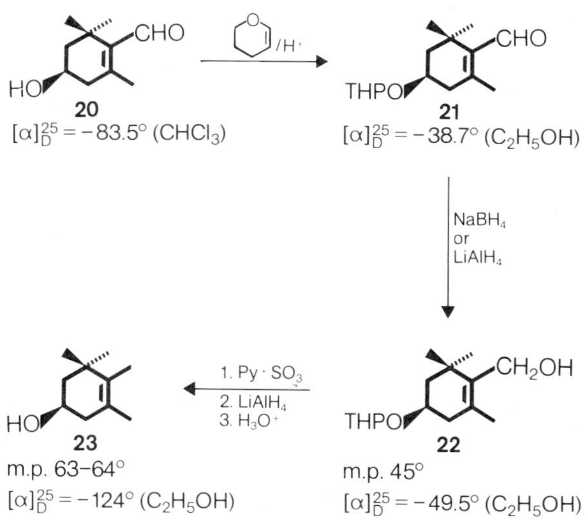

Fig. 11. Synthesis of (3R)-3-hydroxy-1,1,5,6-tetramethyl-5-cyclohexene.

The transformation of these epoxides to the five-membered methyl ketones 12 and 27 respectively, was performed using a pinacolic rearrangement (Fig. 13). A ring contraction of the trans-epoxide 26a with boron trifluoride as catalyst showed that, in up to 70 % yield, the methyl ketone 12 was formed as a single main product. The corresponding cis-epimer 27 was produced only in negligible amounts. A possible intermediate is shown in Fig. 13, arising from "axial" opening of the epoxide 26a and generation of the positive charge at C-6. A subsequent migration of a ring carbon yielded the trans-hydroxy-ketone 12 . This high stereoselectivity supports earlier findings that "axial" cleavage of tetrasubstituted epoxides with boron trifluoride is preferred over the "equatorial" cleavage by a small energy difference (Refs. 58 & 59).

A similar treatment of the cis-epoxide 25a with boron trifluoride etherate yielded, after hydrolysis, the cis-hydroxy-ketone 27 , with very high stereoselectivity. Again an intermediate, deriving from an "axial" opening of the epoxide is assumed as illustrated in Fig. 14.

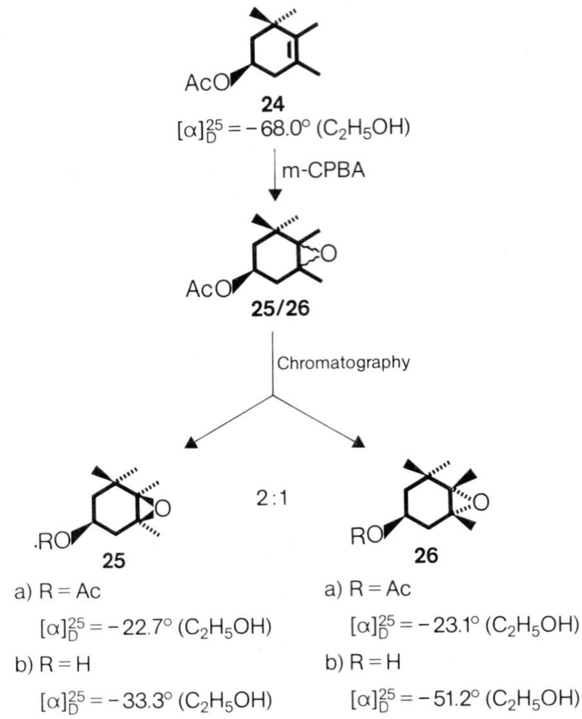

Fig. 12. Synthesis of the isomeric epoxides 25 and 26 .

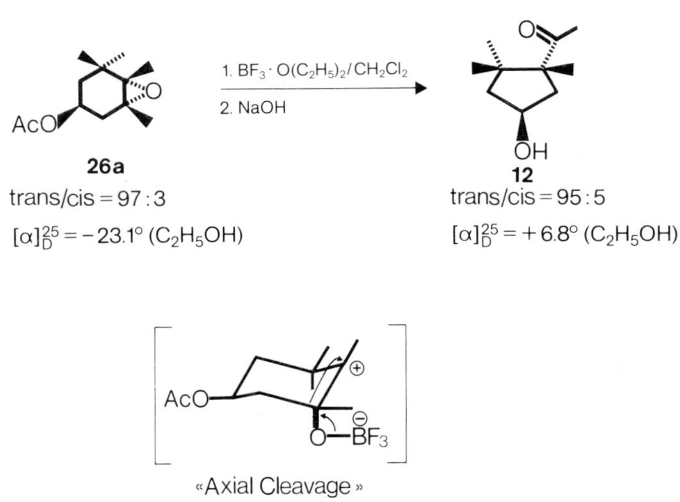

Fig. 13. Pinacolic rearrangement of the trans-epoxide 26a .

Stereochemistry of C_{10}-hydroxy ketones

The stereochemistry of the important C_{10}-building unit 12 has already been deduced earlier by correlation with the trans-hydroxy acid 11 , obtained by degradation of natural capsorubin and capsanthin (Refs. 34, 43-45). By the application of ^{1}H-NMR-spectroscopy, the position and configuration of the hydroxy group in 12 , 16 and 17 could be confirmed by considering the chemical shifts of the methyl groups and the coupling constants of the ring protons (Ref. 35).

Oxidation of the hydroxy-ketone 12 with pyridinium chlorochromate afforded in high yield the crystalline diketone 18 (Fig. 15). The same compound with identical melting point and optical rotation was obtained starting from compound 16 . Thus, the epimeric relationship of 16 and 12 could be demonstrated unequivocally. An isomeric diketone 19 with completely different physicochemical and chiroptical properties was obtained after a similar oxidation of compound 17 .

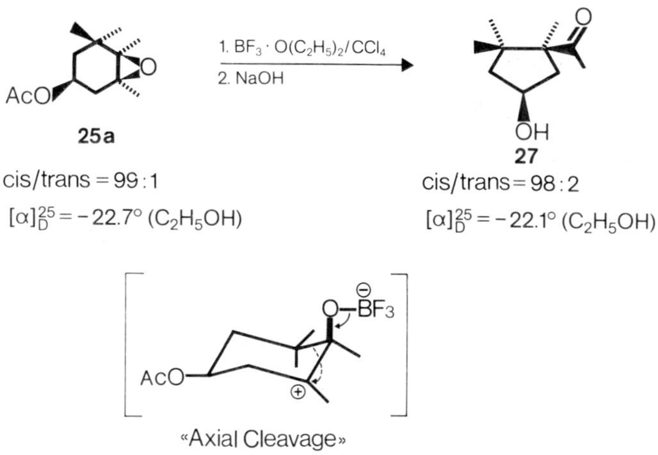

Fig. 14. Pinacolic rearrangement of the <u>cis</u>-epoxide <u>25a</u> .

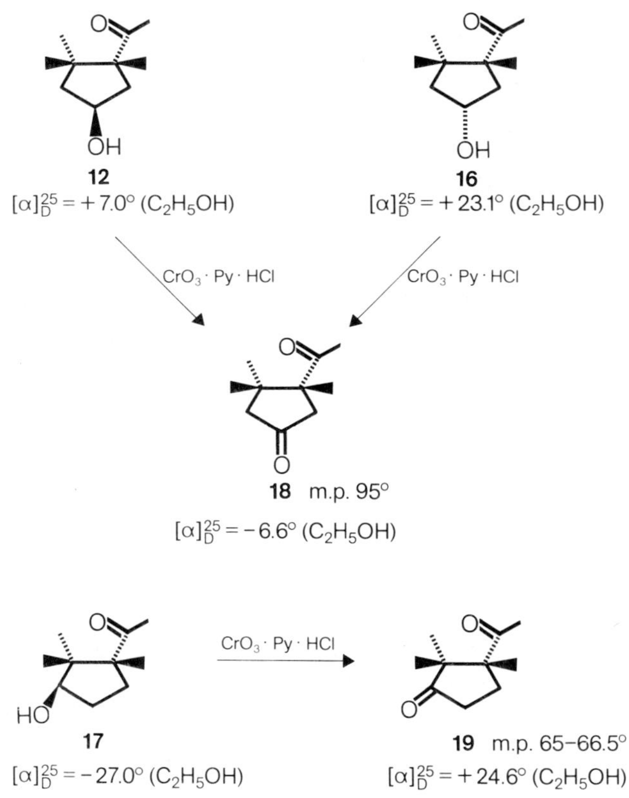

Fig. 15. Oxidation of C_{10}-hydroxy-ketones <u>12</u> , <u>16</u> and <u>17</u> .

2. <u>Synthesis of C_{40}-compounds</u>

(3S,5R,3'S,5'R)-Capsorubin, (3R,3'S,5'R)-capsanthin and (3S,5R)-cryptocapsin are unique red pepper carotenoids by virtue of the presence of a chiral acylcyclopentanol end-group. According to the building principle $C_{10} + C_{20} + C_{10} = C_{40}$ and $C_{30} + C_{10} = C_{40}$, first successfully employed by the Weedon team (Refs. 39-45) in the racemic and later also in the optically active series, all of the following carotenoids were synthesized.

By an aldol condensation, a simple and efficient coupling method, crocetindial (<u>5</u>) was reacted with a small excess of methyl ketone <u>12</u> to give nicely crystalline (3S,5R,3'S,5'R)-capsorubin, possessing the correct natural configuration at all four chiral centres (Fig. 16). The most effective base proved to be sodium hydride in toluene-tetrahydrofurane as solvent. At RT, the deep red C_{40}-compound, identical in every respect with the pigment from the red paprika, was thus smoothly formed in a few hours. From a technical point of view, it is worth

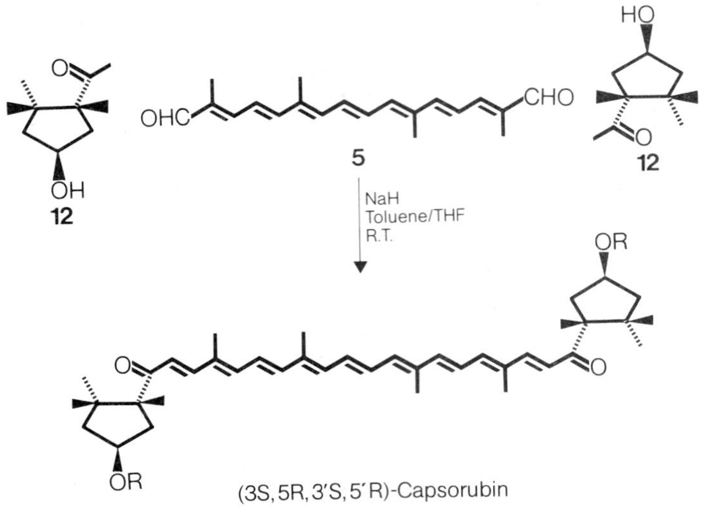

(3S,5R,3'S,5'R)-Capsorubin
R = H: m.p.: 218.5°
R = Ac: m.p.: 179–180°

Fig. 16. Synthesis of (3S,5R,3'S,5'R)-capsorubin.

noting that, in this case, no troublesome triphenylphosphine oxide is produced as a by-product but only harmless sodium hydroxide which can be neutralized by acid.

In the course of our investigation, the two isomeric xanthophylls (3R,5R,3'R,5'R)-epicapsorubin and (2R,5R,2'R,5'R)-isocapsorubin have been synthesized in a similar way, utilizing the appropriate C_{10}-end-groups <u>16</u> and <u>17</u>, respectively (Fig. 17).

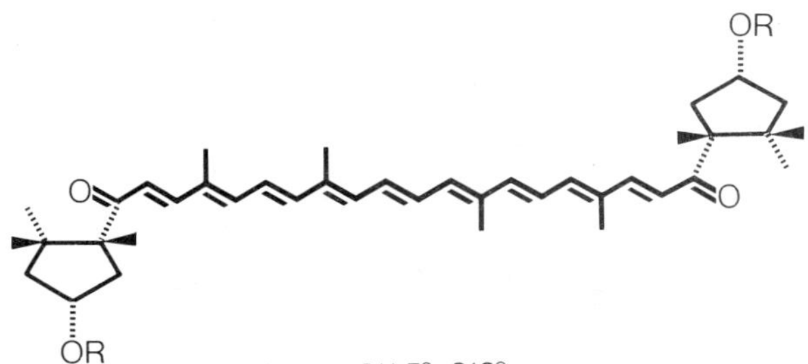

R = H, m.p.: 211.5°–212°
R = Ac, m.p.: 214°
(3R,5R,3'R,5'R)-Epicapsorubin

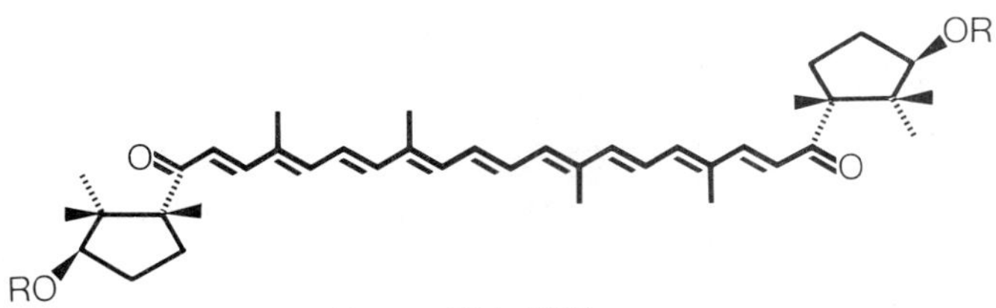

R = H, m.p.: 204–206°
R = Ac, m.p.: 183–184°
(2R,5R,2'R,5'R)-Isocapsorubin

Fig. 17. Synthesis of (3R,5R,3'R,5'R)-epicapsorubin and (2R,5R,2'R,5'R)-isocapsorubin.

(3R,3'S,5'R)-Capsanthin, a pigment with two different chiral end-groups, was prepared employing the same type of reaction (Fig. 18): Condensation of the C_{30}-apo-compound <u>29</u> with the cyclic component <u>12</u> in the usual way yielded the desired, crystalline all-<u>trans</u>-C_{40}-skeleton, which proved to be identical with natural capsanthin of established configuration. (3R)-

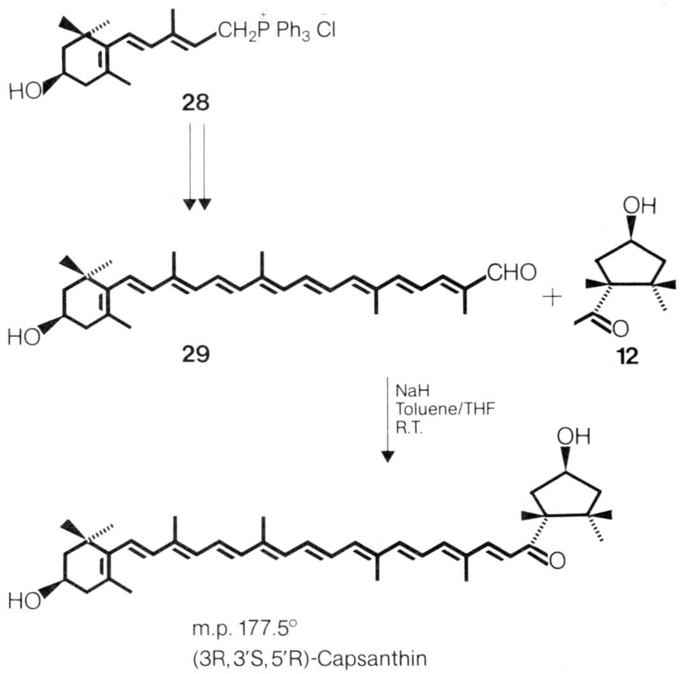

Fig. 18. Synthesis of (3R,3'S,5'R)-capsanthin.

β-Citraurin (29), also a natural product (Ref. 60), was synthesized according to known procedures (Refs. 61 & 62) from the C_{15}-phosphonium salt 28 (Refs. 53, 54 & 62), an intermediate in the technical synthesis of (3R,3'R)-zeaxanthin.

According to the same building principle $C_{30} + C_{10} = C_{40}$ (3S,5R)-cryptocapsin, a minor constituent of the red pepper fruit, was obtained as nice red crystals by a similar condensation of β-apo-8'-carotenal (30) (Ref. 63) with the cyclic ketone 12 (Fig. 19).

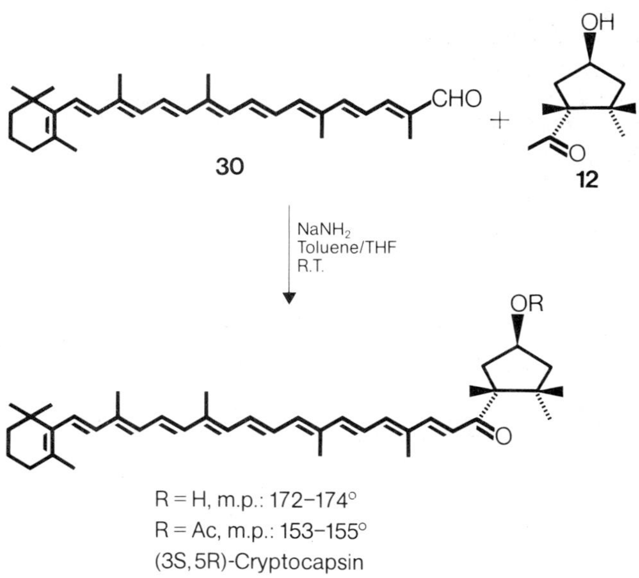

Fig. 19. Synthesis of (3S,5R)-cryptocapsin.

3) Oppenauer oxidations

In the course of our investigations we oxidized the five-membered end-groups of our synthetic C_{40}-compounds to the corresponding cyclopentanones in order to study the physical and physicochemical properties of these rarely occurring natural pigments of unknown stereochemistry (Refs. 17-19). This Oppenauer oxidation, first successfully applied by Weedon and Karrer in 1960 (Refs. 30 & 33), proved still to be the method of choice. In a clean reaction (3S,5R,

3'S,5'R)-capsorubin was oxidized to the crystalline (5R,5'R)-capsorubone using acetone and aluminium tert.-butoxide as catalyst (Fig. 20). As expected, the same compound was obtained

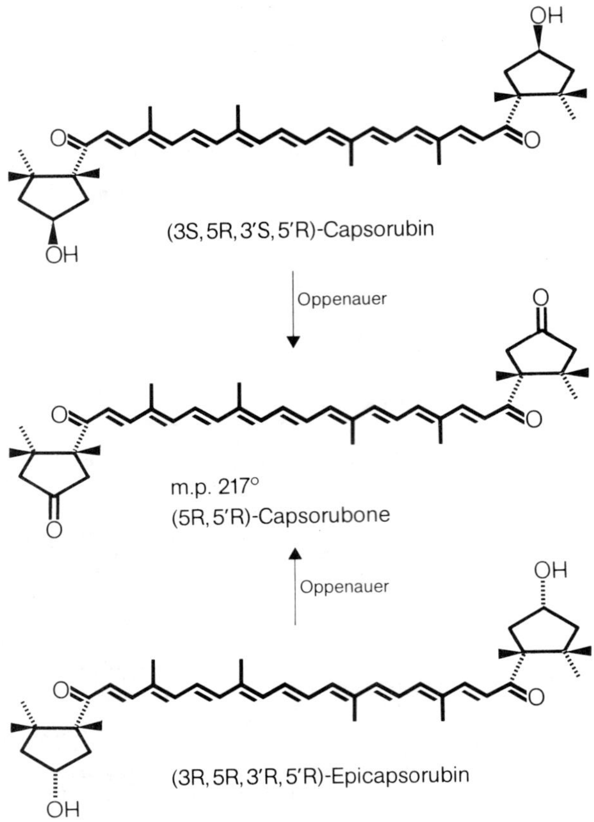

Fig. 20. Synthesis of (5R,5'R)-capsorubone.

starting from (3R,5R,3'R,5'R)-epicapsorubin.

In a similar way, (3R,3'S,5'R)-capsanthin and (3S,5R)-cryptocapsin were smoothly transformed into the desired crystalline pigments (3R,5'R)-capsanthone (Refs. 30, 33 & 34) (Fig. 21) and (5R)-cryptocapsone, respectively (Ref. 41) (Fig. 22). It is interesting to note that in (3R, 3'S,5'R)-capsanthin, the hydroxy group at the five-membered ring could be selectively oxidized, leaving the secondary (3R)-hydroxy group at the cyclohexene ring untouched.

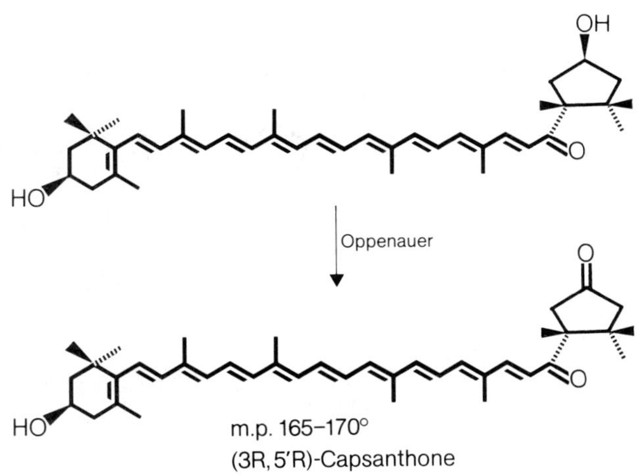

Fig. 21. Synthesis of (3R,5'R)-capsanthone.

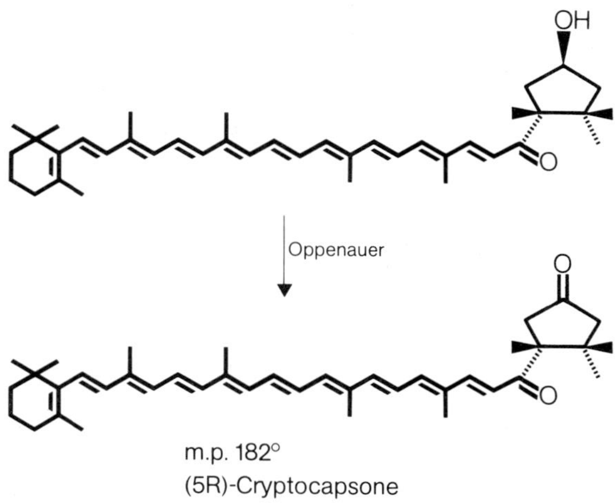

Fig. 22. Synthesis of (5R)-cryptocapsone.

4) Optical and chiroptical properties

The lovely colour of the red pepper fruits is primarily caused by the red xanthophylls capsanthin and capsorubin, which comprise together approximately 40 % of the total carotenoid composition. The UV-main absorption of these two red pigments lies at 470 nm (in hexane), similar to canthaxanthin and astaxanthin with UV-maxima at 466 and 472 nm (in hexane), respectively.

It is interesting to note that there is a remarkable difference in the absorption spectra of one of the three isomeric capsorubins, synthesized in the course of our investigation (Fig. 23).

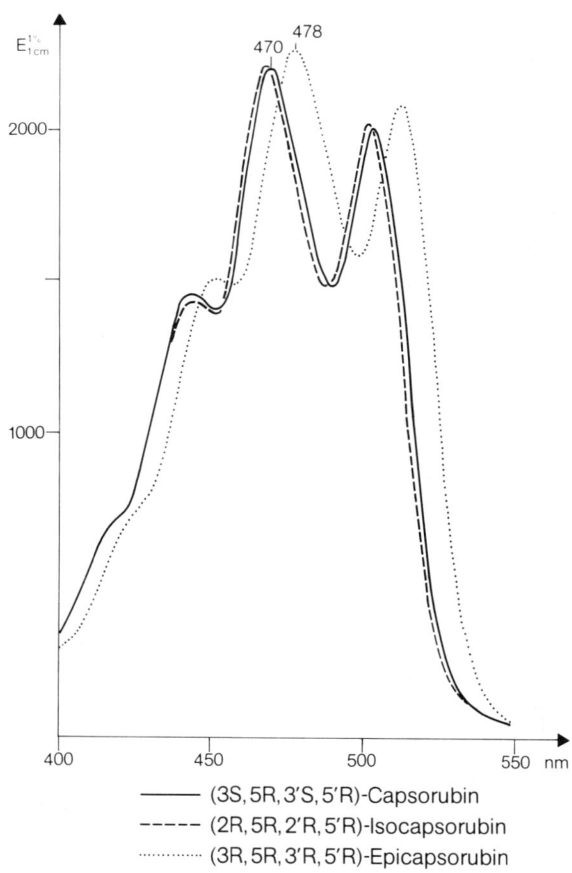

Fig. 23. UV-spectra of three capsorubin isomers.

(3R,5R,3'R,5'R)-Epicapsorubin, whose hydroxy group is cis relative to the polyene chain, has its main absorption maximum 8 nm higher than that of the two isomers with trans-stereochemistry. This causes a difference in the red colour which can easily be detected by the human eye. We assume that an interaction of the hydroxy group with the chromophore is responsible for this phenomenon.

A comparison of the CD-spectra of the same three isomeric C_{40}-compounds: (3S,5R,3'S,5'R)-capsorubin, (3R,5R,3'R,5'R)-epicapsorubin and (2R,5R,2'R,5'R)-isocapsorubin, shows clearly that the shape of the curves is, apart from small intensity differences, nearly identical (Fig. 24).

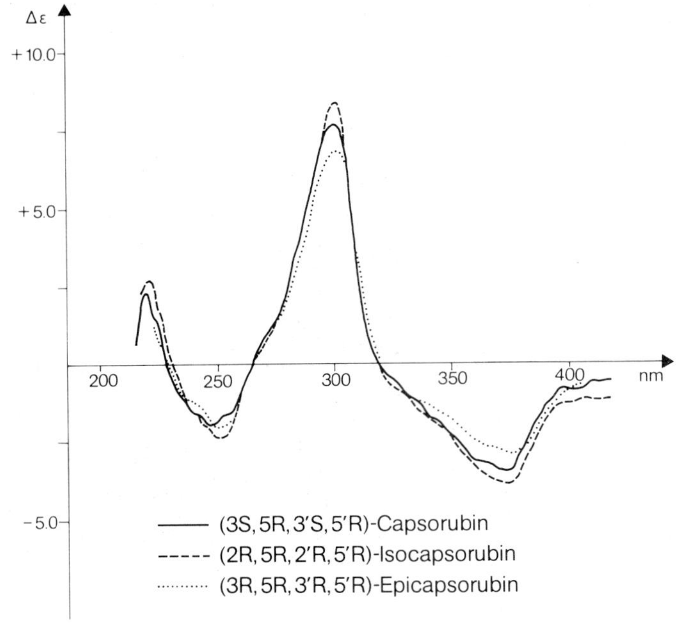

Fig. 24. CD-spectra of three capsorubin isomers.

Position and configuration of the hydroxy group at the five-membered ring have obviously only little influence on the CD-curve. The main influence is exerted by the asymmetric centre at C-5.

RED PEPPER CAROTENOIDS AS FOOD PIGMENTERS

From the earliest recorded times, man has been greatly interested in the secrets of nature's colouring matters, and searching for methods to duplicate them. Carrot extracts, palm oil extracts, annatto extracts and oleoresin of paprika, the oil extract of the red paprika *Capsicum annuum* have been used for generations as food additives (Refs. 64 & 65). The deep red extract of paprika, whose main pigments are mostly esters of capsanthin and capsorubin, finds growing technological applications. It is added to a variety of food products, such as salad dressings, sauces, soups, cheese, and particularly to meat products, including sausages, where it is legally allowed as a spice. The colour thus imparted to a product can range from a deep crimson red to a pale pinkish-yellow, depending on the concentrations used.

The advent of pure synthetic carotenoids has increased interest in colouring foods with these compounds because of obvious advantages of working with well controlled, reproducible nature-identical colour sources.

Acknowledgements: In conclusion, I should like to thank Dr. H. Mayer, Prof. S. Liaaen-Jensen, Prof. B.C.L. Weedon and Dr. H. Pfander for stimulating discussions and advice. Special thanks are due to Drs. W. Arnold, L. Chopard, G. Englert, K. Noack, W. Vetter and Mr. W. Meister for their help in the interpretation of spectral data, to Dr. M. Vecchi, Dr. R. Maurer and Mr. E. Glinz for the GC and HPLC analyses and to Dr. A. Dirscherl for the numerous chemical analyses.

The skilful technical assistance of Mr. L. Binggeli and Mr. J.M. Zielinski is gratefully acknowledged.

REFERENCES

1. B.C.L. Weedon, in Carotenoids (editor O. Isler), p. 29, Birkhäuser Verlag, Basel and Stuttgart (1971).
2. T.W. Goodwin, Food Chemistry 5, 3 (1980).
3. L. Zechmeister and L. v. Cholnoky, Liebigs Ann.Chem. 454, 54 (1927).
4. L. Zechmeister and L. v. Cholnoky, Liebigs Ann.Chem. 509, 269 (1934).
5. L. v. Cholnoky, K. Györgyfy, E. Nagy and M. Panczel, Acta Chim.Acad.Sci.Hung. 6, 143 (1955).
6. L. v. Cholnoky, K. Györgyfy, E. Nagy and M. Panczel, Nature 178, 410 (1956).
7. A.L. Curl, J.Agr.Food Chem. 10, 504 (1962).
8. B.H. Davies, S. Matthews and J.T.O. Kirk, Phytochemistry 9, 797 (1970).
9. T. Philip and F.J. Francis, J.Food Science 36, 823 (1971).
10. T. Philip, W.W. Nawar and F.J. Francis, J.Food Science 36, 98 (1971).
11. K. Langer, Separation of Carotenoids using HPLC, Ph.D. theses at the Friedrich Alexander University, Erlangen-Nürnberg 1976 (in German).
12. B. Camara and R. Monéger, Phytochemistry 17, 91 (1978).
13. P. Karrer and A. Oswald, Helv.Chim.Acta 13, 1303 (1935).
14. L.R.G. Valadon and R.S. Mummery, Z.Pflanzenphysiologie 82, 407 (1977).
15. M. Bubicz and Z. Wierzchowski, Bull.Acad.Pol.Sci. 8, 323 (1960).
16. P. Karrer and S. Ramasvamy, Helv.Chim.Acta 34, 2159 (1951).
17. G. Neamtu, G. Illyes and C. Bodea, Stud.Cercet.Biochim. 12, 77 (1969).
18. G. Neamtu and C. Bodea, Stud.Cercet.Biochim. 16, 35 (1973).
19. a) G. Neamtu and C. Bodea, Stud.Cercet.Biochim. 17, 41 (1974);
    b) G. Neamtu, G. Illyes and C. Bodea, Stud.Cercet.Biochim. 12, 77 (1969).
20. L. Zechmeister and L. v. Cholnoky, Liebigs Ann.Chem. 454, 70 (1927).
21. P. Karrer, A. Helfenstein, H. Wehrli, B. Pieper and R. Morf, Helv.Chim.Acta 14, 614 (1931).
22. L. Zechmeister and L. v. Cholnoky, Liebigs Ann.Chem. 516, 30 (1935).
23. P. Karrer and H. Hübner, Helv.Chim.Acta 19, 474 (1936).
24. L. Zechmeister and L. v. Cholnoky, Liebigs Ann.Chem. 543, 248 (1940).
25. R. Entschel, C.H. Eugster and P. Karrer, Helv.Chim.Acta 29, 1263 (1956).
26. L. v. Cholnoky, D. Szabo and J. Szabolcs, Liebigs Ann.Chem. 606, 194 (1957).
27. C.K. Warren and B.C.L. Weedon, J.Chem.Soc. 3972 (1958).
28. L. v. Cholnoky and J. Szabolcs, Acta Chim.Acad.Sci.Hung. 22, 117 (1960).
29. L. v. Cholnoky and J. Szabolcs, Experientia 43, 483 (1960).
30. R. Entschel and P. Karrer, Helv.Chim.Acta 43, 89 (1960).
31. H. Faigle and P. Karrer, Helv.Chim.Acta 44, 1257 (1961).
32. H. Faigle and P. Karrer, Helv.Chim.Acta 44, 1904 (1961).
33. M.S. Barber, L.M. Jackman, C.K. Warren and B.C.L. Weedon, Proc.Chem.Soc. 19 (1960).
34. M.S. Barber, L.M. Jackman, C.K. Warren and B.C.L. Weedon, J.Chem.Soc. 4019 (1961).
35. J.W. Faigle, H. Müller, W. von Philipsborn and P. Karrer, Helv.Chim.Acta 47, 741 (1964).
36. K. Freudenberg and W. Lwowski, Liebigs Ann.Chem. 587, 213 (1954); 594, 76 (1955).
37. F.H. Allen and D. Rogers, Chem.Commun. 837 (1966).
38. B.C.L. Weedon, in Carotenoids (editor O. Isler), p. 292, Birkhäuser Verlag, Basel and Stuttgart (1971).
39. R.D.G. Cooper, L.M. Jackman and B.C.L. Weedon, Proc.Chem.Soc. 215 (1962).
40. B.C.L. Weedon and C.K. Warren, Brit. Patent 924,255 (1963).
41. L. v. Cholnoky, J. Szabolcs, R.D.G. Cooper and B.C.L. Weedon, Tetrahedron Letters 1257 (1963).
42. B.C.L. Weedon, Pure Appl.Chem. 14, 265 (1967).
43. B.C.L. Weedon, Pure Appl.Chem. 35, 113 (1973).
44. A.K. Chopra, G.P. Moss and B.C.L. Weedon, Chem.Commun. 467 (1977).
45. A.K. Chopra, Ph.D. thesis, Queen Mary College, University of London (1976).
46. P. Heisel, I.G., DRP. 765525 (1940); Lech-Chemie Gersthofen, DBP. 879097 (1941).
47. J. Goldman, N. Jacobsen and K. Torssell, Acta Chem.Scand. B28, 492 (1974).
48. H.C. Brown, N.R. Ayyangar and G. Zweifel, J.Amer.Chem.Soc. 86, 397 (1964); J.Amer.Chem. Soc. 86, 1071 (1964).
49. H.C. Brown and P.J. Geoghegan, Jr., J.Org.Chem. 35, 1844 (1970).
50. H.C. Brown and P.J. Geoghegan, Jr., J.Org.Chem. 37, 1937 (1972).
51. B. Camara, FEBS Letters 118 (2), 315 (1980).
52. B. Camara, Bioch.Bioph.Res. C 93, 113 (1980).
53. H. Mayer, Pure Appl.Chem. 51, 535 (1979).
54. R.K. Müller, K. Bernhard, F. Kienzle, H. Mayer and A. Rüttimann, Food Chem. 5, 15 (1980).
55. A. Rüttimann and H. Mayer, Helv.Chim.Acta 63, 1456 (1980).
56. E.J. Corey and K. Achiwa, J.Org.Chem. 34, 3667 (1969).
57. R. Bonnett, A.K. Mallams, A.A. Spark, J.L. Tee, A. McCormick and B.C.L. Weedon, J.Chem. Soc. C, 429 (1969).
58. M.P. Hartshorn and D.N. Kirk, Tetrahedron 21, 1547 (1965).
59. M.S. Hadley and T.G. Halsall, J.Chem.Soc. Perkin I, 1334 (1974).
60. H. Pfander, M. Hadorn, A. Lachenmeier and G. Englert, Helv.Chim.Acta 63, 716 (1980).
61. H. Pfander, Pure Appl.Chem. 51, 565 (1979).
62. H. Pfander, A. Lachenmeier and M. Hadorn, Helv.Chim.Acta 63, 1377 (1980).

63. R. Rüegg, H. Lindlar, M. Montavon, G. Saucy, S.F. Schaeren, U. Schwieter and O. Isler, Helv.Chim.Acta 42, 847 (1959).
64. B. Borenstein and R.H. Bunnell, Advances in Food Res. 15, 195 (1966).
65. J.C. Bauernfeind, J.Agric.and Food Chem. 20, 456 (1972).

STEREOCONTROLLED SYNTHESIS OF POLYENE ISOPRENOIDS

Gerald Pattenden

Department of Chemistry, The University, Nottingham, NG7 2RD, England.

Abstract—The applications of cis-α,β-unsaturated aldehydes and cis-α,β-unsaturated phosphoranylides in the Wittig synthesis of cis-polyene isoprenoids, culminating in a total synthesis of natural methylbixin (25), are reviewed.

The potential for the Horner-Wittig reaction in the stereo-controlled synthesis of conjugated polyene isoprenoids is investigated. It is shown that the cis- and trans-phosphine oxides (31) and (32) react with cis- and trans- citrals, in single steps leading to the corresponding isomeric pentaenes (11) showing complete preservation of the cis- and trans-geometries in the starting materials. Although the single step reactions leading to (11) proceed in low overall yields (10-20%), the olefinations occur with > 98% trans-stereoselectivity. Isolation of the intermediate β-hydroxyphosphine oxides (e.g. 35) followed by treatment with sodium hydride in dimethyl-formamide, demonstrates that this feature of the reactions is associated largely with the remarkably slow rates of elimination from the erythro-intermediates in comparison with the threo-intermediates.

Condensation between (31) and the aldehyde (18) leads to the cis-6-ester (37) (34%). After conversion of (37) into the tetraenal (40), reaction with the farnesyl phosphine oxide (41), followed by separation of the erythro-β-hydroxyphosphine oxide intermediate (42), and treatment with sodium hydride in dimethylformamide leads to the di-cis-octaene (43). The octaene (43) shows closely similar spectral data to those found in natural di-cis-phytofluene (4) isolated from fruit of the Tangerine tomato. In a similar manner, reaction between the cis-phosphine oxide (31) and the dialdehyde (44) produces the di-cis-nonaene (48) which has the same chromophore as that found in di-cis-ζ-carotene (5) from Tangerine tomato fruits.

Although the overwhelming majority of natural carotenoids show an all-trans configuration about their polyene chains, a small proportion have been found to contain one or more cis double bonds, and there is reason to believe that cis-trans isomerisation plays an important part in general carotenoid biosynthesis and perhaps in some of their biological functions (Ref 1).

Bixin (1), the principal pigment in seeds of *Bixa orellana*, was the first carotenoid in which geometrical isomerism was encountered (Ref 2). Other natural cis-carotenoids of relatively long standing are central cis-phytoene (2) from tomatoes and carrots (Ref 3), and gazaniaxanthin (3) the major pigment in flowers of *Gazania rigens* (Ref 4). Taking pride of place amongst natural cis-carotenoids however is 'prolycopene' found in fruits of the Tangerine tomato, and also in certain berries and flowers. First isolated in 1941, its stereochemistry was investigated extensively by Zechmeister and his co-workers during the ensuing two decades (Refs 1 and 5). Recent applications of n.m.r. spectroscopy have now established that this intriguing pigment has the tetra-cis-lycopene structure (7) (Refs 6 and 7). Furthermore, its congeners phytoene, phytofluene, ζ-carotene and neurosporene have the poly-cis-structures (2), (4), (5) and (6) respectively (Ref 7).

The range of cis-carotenoids has been greatly extended by stereomutation studies (Refs 1 and 8), and a number of cis-compounds have been obtained by partial catalytic hydrogenation of acetylenic intermediates prepared during the

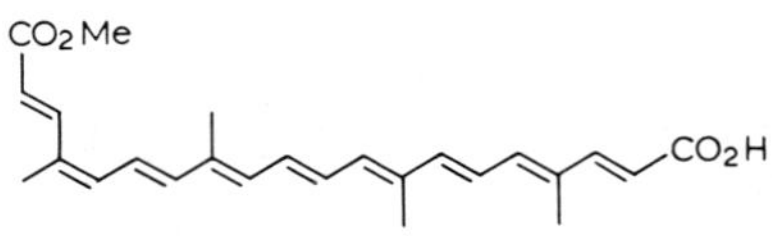

(1)

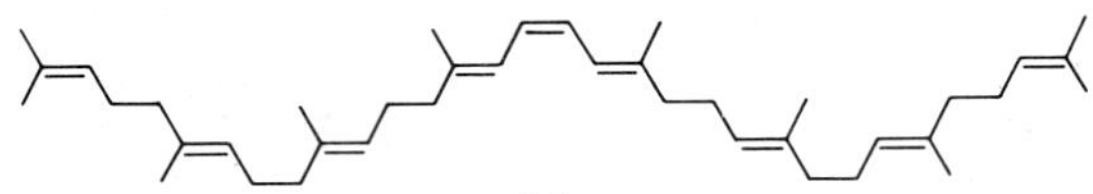

(2)

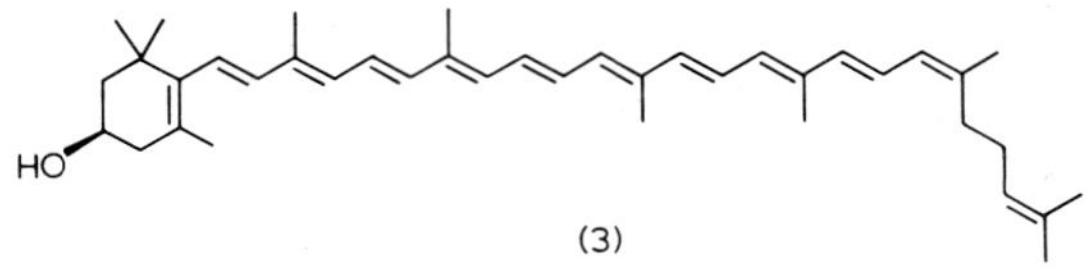

(3)

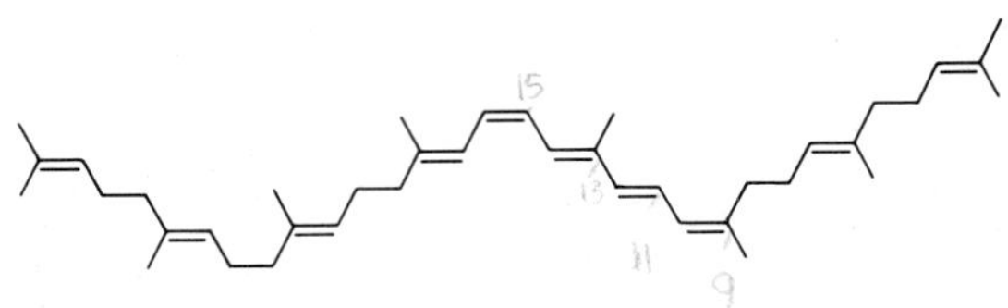

(4)

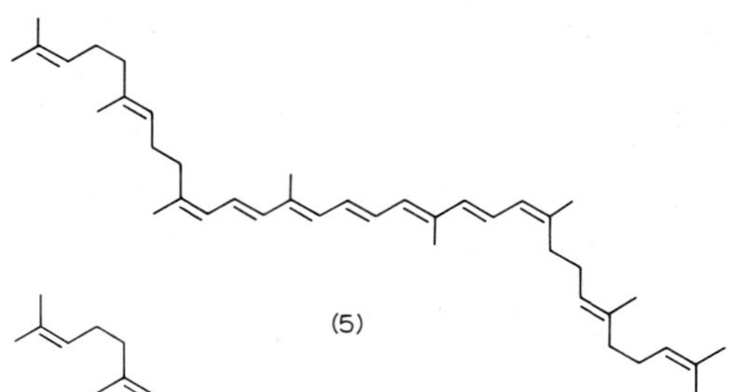

(5)

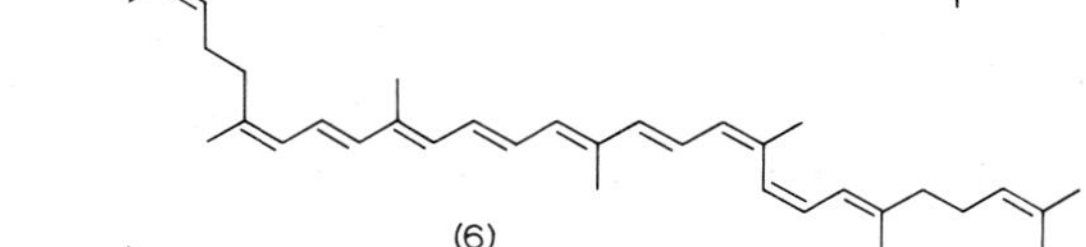

(6)

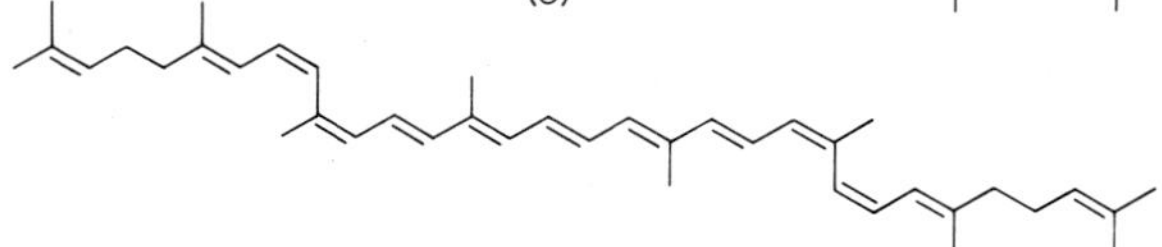

(7)

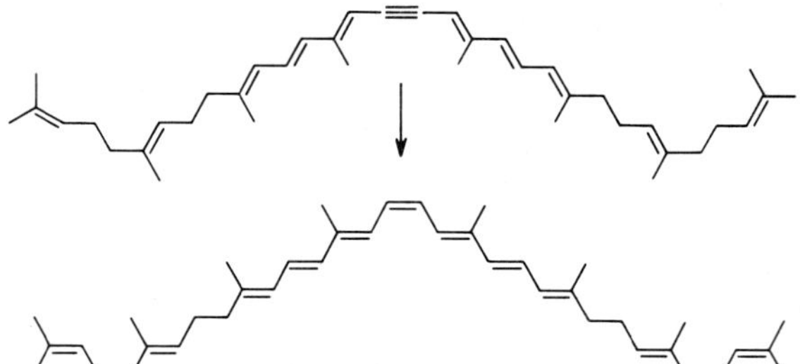

(8)

all-*trans* ζ-carotene

total synthesis of carotenoids e.g. central-cis ζ-carotene (8) (Ref 3).

The recent advances in the application of ^{13}C n.m.r. spectroscopy as a stereochemical probe amongst polyenes has greatly facilitated the determination of configuration of a number of cis-carotenoids (Refs 9 and 10). Apart from the obvious uses of acetylenic intermediates, mentioned above, progress in the development of controlled synthesis of carotenoid polyene chains with one or more cis-double bonds (whether disubstituted or trisubstituted) has however, been disappointingly slow.

In spite of the well known sensitivity of carotenoids to a wide range of conditions, the elaboration of their (all-trans) polyene chains is now relatively easy to accomplish by the well established acetylenic techniques, vinyl ether synthesis, and most important, Wittig-type reactions. Any proposed synthesis of a cis-carotenoid has to take into account this known sensitivity in addition to the established propensity with which cis-carotenoids undergo stereomutation to trans- and to other isomeric compounds. The elaboration of cis-carotenoids is therefore a daunting problem to the synthetic chemist.

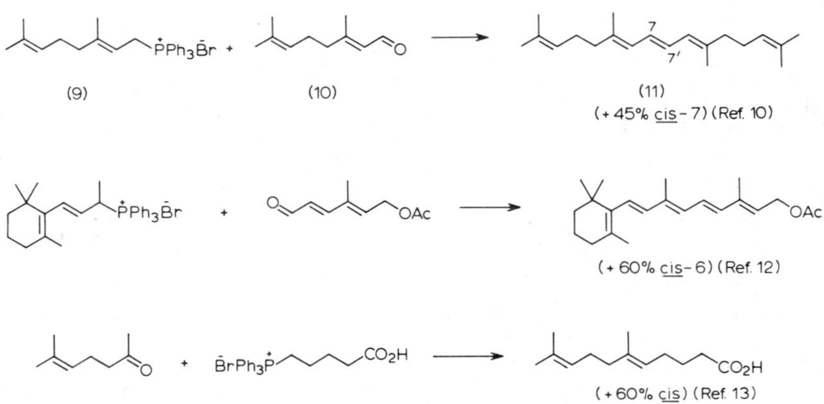

Scheme 1

The Wittig reaction has been a cornerstone in preparative polyene chemistry for almost two decades, and it is perhaps not too surprising that many of the major developments in the controlled synthesis of cis-polyene isoprenoids have attempted to use this reaction, or a variant thereof, as a key stage. Although the preparativeversatilityof the Wittig reaction is beyond question, its stereochemical course is often less predictable, and frequently leads to mixtures of cis and trans-geometrical isomers about the newly introduced double bond (Ref 11). This feature of the reaction has provoked considerable discussion regarding its general mechanism, and also much experimental work directed towards controlling the stereochemical outcome of the reaction. Indeed, a range of conditions are now available for the production of largely cis- or trans-disubstituted monoenes by the Wittig process. Sadly, these conditions seldom work when applied to the synthesis of disubstituted double bonds in conjugated polyene-isoprenoids e.g. the geranyl salt (9) and trans-citral (10) produce a mixture (ca. 1:1) of cis- and trans-isomers about the C-7, C-7' double bond in the pentaene product (11), and all attempts to synthesise trisubstituted double bonds in polyenes by the Wittig process lead to mixtures of geometrical isomers (see Scheme 1).

Much more success in the controlled synthesis of cis-polyene isoprenoids has been obtained with the use of cis-α,β-unsaturated aldehydes and cis-α,β-unsaturated ylides in the Wittig reaction. Some of the first studies of this possibility were made with cis-citral (12) which was shown to react with methyl and geranyl phosphonium salts leading to polyenes with complete preservation of the cis-geometry in the starting citral (Ref 14). In the case of the geranyl salt (9), the olefination produced a 1:1 mixture of cis- and trans- isomers about the C-7, C-7' double bond and time-consuming chromatography on silver nitrate impregnated silica gel was necessary to resolve the isomers (13) and (14). Use of the neryl phosphonium salt (15) and of cis- and trans-citral allowed us to synthesise all six geometrical isomers of the pentaene (11) including the tri-cis-isomer (16) (Ref 10). This work, along with that of

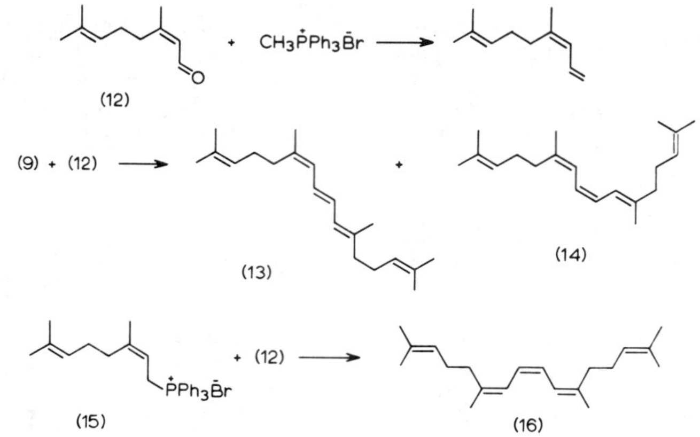

others (Ref 15) was used to assign the stereochemistry of natural *cis*- (15,15') phytoene from tomatoes. The spectroscopic data recorded for the isomeric pentaenes also suggested that the *trans*, *trans*, *cis*-configuration previously assigned to a phytoene from *Rhodospirillum rubrum* could be *cis*, *trans*, *cis* instead.

A significant breakthrough in the synthesis of carotenoids containing *cis*-trisubstituted double bonds was made with the discovery of the use of the hydroxybutenolide (17) in Wittig olefin synthesis. With a series of phosphoranylides, of 'medium' reactivity, the hydroxybutenolide led to polyene acids with complete preservation of the *cis*-geometry about the trisubstituted double bond in (17) (Scheme 2) (Ref 14 and 16). The olefinations themselves were not stereoselective, and interestingly produced a high proportion of the *cis*-olefin. Use of the hydroxybutenolide (17) and the corresponding *trans*-aldehyde (18) in Wittig reactions with geranyl and neryl phosphonium salts provide convenient syntheses of all eight geometrical isomers of the triene system in (19) (Ref 17).

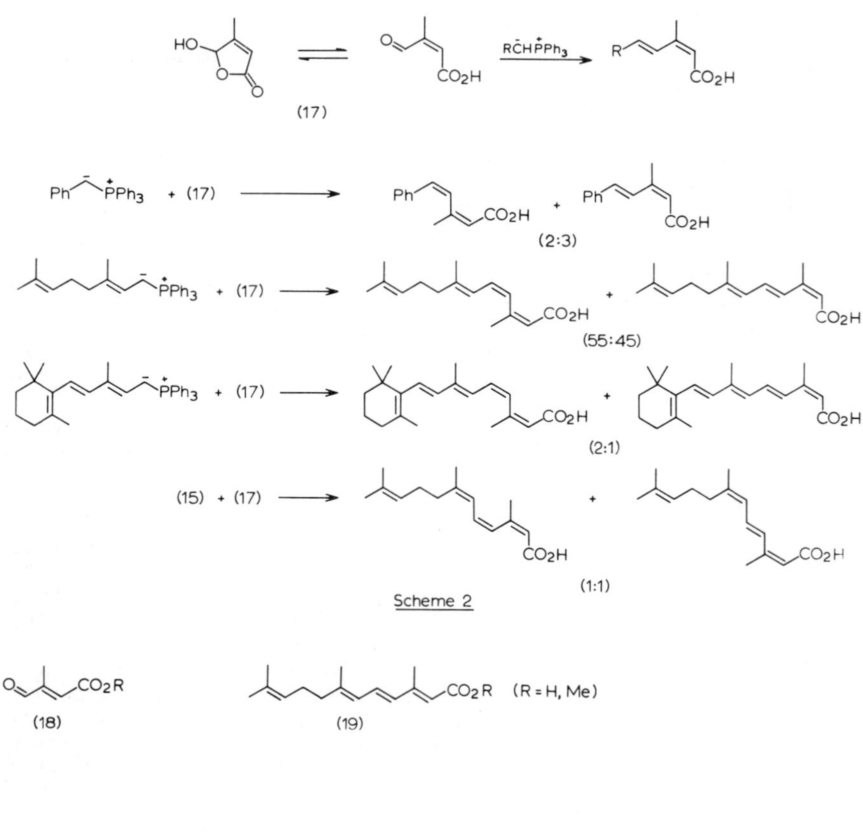

Scheme 2

Reaction between the hydroxybutenolide (17) and the stable phosphorane (20) or the phosphonate ester carbanion (21) has been shown to lead to high yields of the cis-dienoic acid (22) resulting from exclusive trans-olefination (Ref 14). This dienoic acid (22) was then used as a central intermediate in our synthesis of natural methylbixin (25) (Ref 18). Thus, conversion of the acid into the corresponding acid chloride, and reduction of the latter with lithium tri-t-butoxyaluminium hydride yielded the cis-aldehyde (23) with complete preservation of stereochemistry. Reaction between the aldehyde (23) and the C_{17}-phosphonium salt (24) then gave natural methylbixin (25) as the major product.

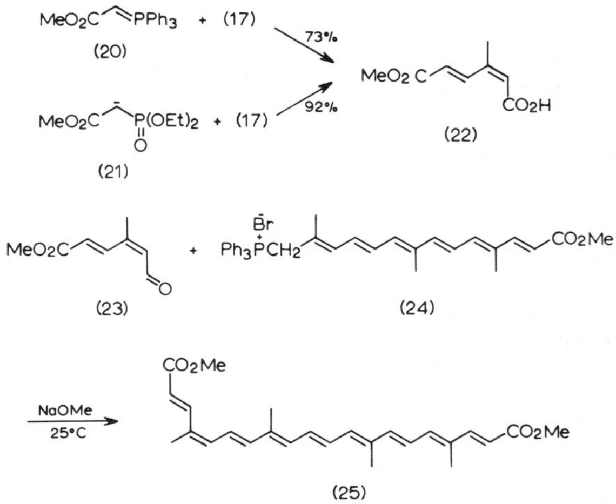

Further examples which highlight the use of cis-α,β-unsaturated aldehydes and phosphoranylides in the Wittig synthesis of cis-carotenoids are the synthesis of 13-cis-β-carotene (27) from the cis-pentaenal (26) (Ref 19) the synthesis of 9,9'-di-cis-alloxanthin (29) from the cis-salt (28) and the C_{10}-trienedial (44) (Ref 20) and the use of neryl salt (15) in the formation of 5-cis-lycopene (30) and of (±)-gazaniaxanthin (3) (Ref 17).

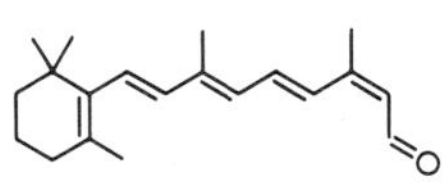

(26)

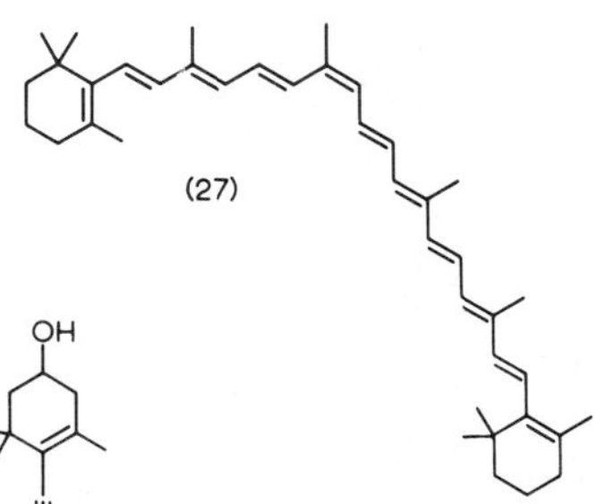

(27)

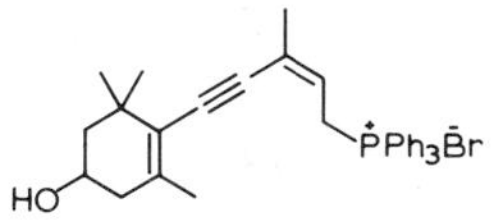

(28)

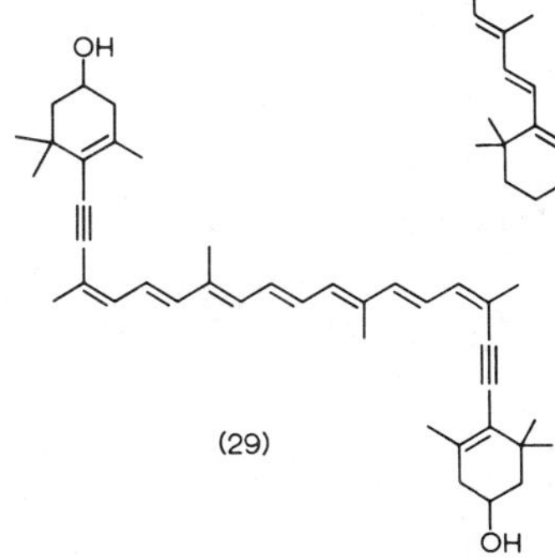

(29)

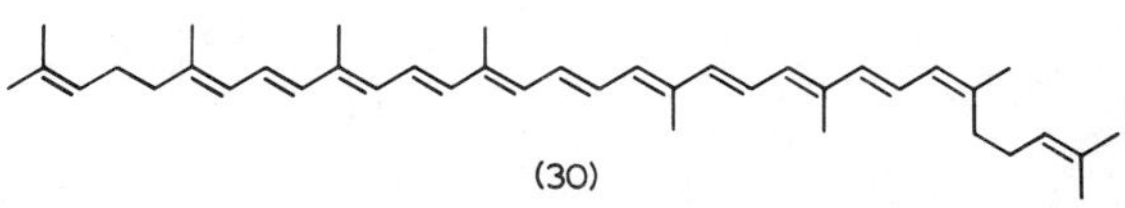

(30)

It is important to stress that although the above methodology of using cis-α, β-unsaturated aldehydes and phosphoranylides provides a useful entry to cis-polyene isoprenoids, the Wittig olefinations themselves almost invariably produce mixtures of cis- and trans- isomers about the newly introduced double bonds. Time consuming chromatography and/or fractional crystallisation, which are frequently accompanied by stereomutation and equilibration of the isomeric polyenes, is then essential to separate the pure geometrical isomers. This feature of the Wittig synthesis of carotenoids raises its ugly head time and time again, and emphasises the need for an alternative to the Wittig reaction for the controlled synthesis of isomeric conjugated polyenes. At the same time however, any new method must incorporate all the desirable practical advantages of the Wittig reaction when handling polyenes (low temperature, mild base conditions, inert atmosphere, diffuse light) if it is to compete in any way.

Some four years after Wittig and Schöllkopf published their now celebrated paper describing the Wittig reaction (Ref 21) Horner and his co-workers (Ref 22) outlined the use of the corresponding diphenylphosphine oxide carbanion intermediate, as an alternative to triphenylphosphoranylide, in the synthesis of alkenes. Today this reaction has been dubbed the Horner variant of the Wittig reaction and more generally the Horner-Wittig reaction. Although sporadic reports of the use of phosphine oxide anions in alkene synthesis appeared in the literature during the ensuing fifteen years (Ref 23) it is not until recently that attention has been given to the Horner-Wittig reaction as an alternative to the Wittig process in the synthesis of isomeric alkenes (Ref 24). Our contemporaneous investigations of poly-cis carotenoids found in fruits of the Tangerine tomato (Ref 7), and the associated difficulties in assigning their stereochemistries due to the dearth of suitable model poly-cis compounds led us to explore the potential for the Horner-Wittig reaction in the polyene area (Ref 25 and 26).

We began these studies with an investigation of the use of the cis- and trans-phosphine oxides (31) and (32) in the synthesis of stereoisomers of the pentaene (11) by reaction with cis- and trans- citral. The phosphine oxides (31) and (32) were produced from nerol and geraniol respectively, following conversion to the corresponding allylic chlorides, reaction with diphenylphosphide, and oxidation of the resulting tertiary phosphines with hydrogen peroxide. They were clearly distinguished by mixed m.p. and n.m.r. data.

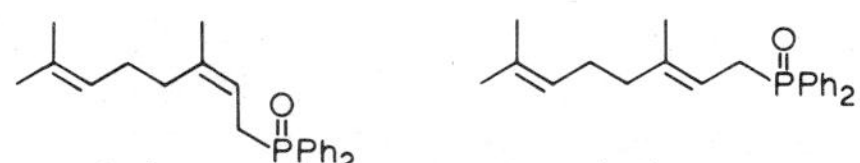

(31) (32)

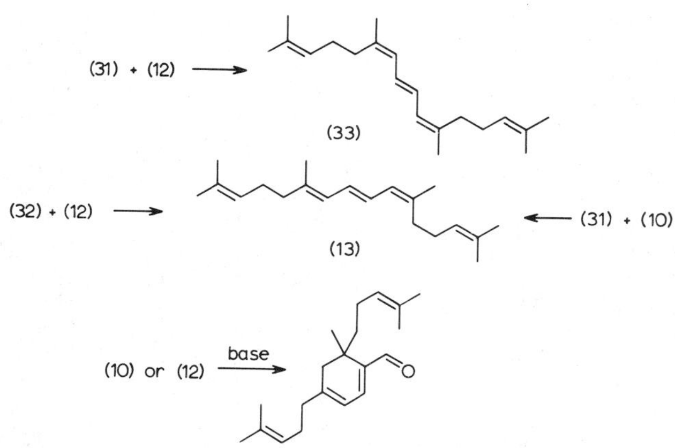

Metallation of the individual phosphine oxides at -78° using n-butyl lithium, followed by reaction with cis- or trans-citral and warming to 25°, led to the corresponding isomeric pentaenes showing complete preservation of the cis or trans-geometries in the starting materials, and with > 98% trans-olefination. Thus, the phosphine oxide (31) and cis-citral led to (33), whilst the phosphine oxide (32) and cis-citral, or the phosphine oxide (31) and trans-citral both produced (13). These results are to be contrasted with those obtained with the corresponding cis and trans-phosphonium salts (i.e. 9 and 15) which gave rise to the corresponding cis-olefination products (cis:trans ca. 1:1) concurrently.

The most disappointing feature of the Horner-Wittig syntheses of the isomeric pentaenes (11) was the low yields recorded (10-20%) in comparison with those obtained in the corresponding Wittig reactions (ca. 70%). In addition, using the single step conditions described, from each reaction we recovered up to 50% of the starting phosphine oxide, and upwards of 15% of the cyclohexadiene by-product (34) produced from self-condensation of citral (Ref 27). A wide range of alternative reaction conditions were investigated in order to optimise the yields in these reactions, but in those instances where we were able to increase yields (≯ 50%), we also observed extensive stereomutation about the double bonds of the starting phosphine oxides.

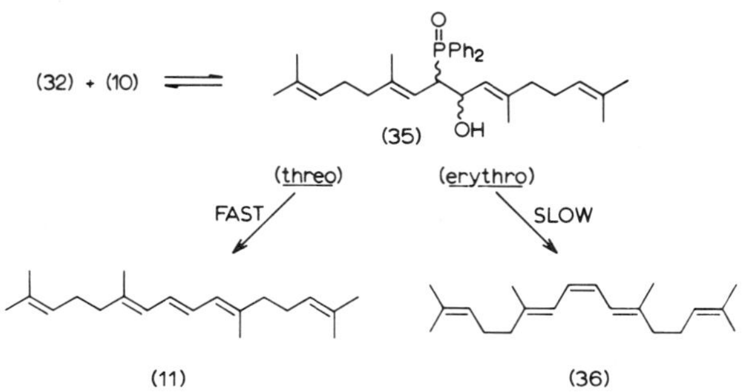

Scheme 3

Further experiments, designed to examine other features which might control the yield and stereochemical outcome of the olefinations, established that the isolation of only trans-olefination products in the single step reactions was associated entirely with the much slower rates of β-elimination from the erythro-β-hydroxyphosphine oxide intermediates produced in the reactions. This feature was substantiated when the threo- and erythro-intermediates (e.g. 35) were separated from reactions quenched after short periods of time at -60° and the individual intermediates treated in a separate step with sodium hydride in dimethylformamide (Ref 28). Thus, the trans-phosphine oxide (32) and trans-citral, at -60°, produced a 1:1 mixture of threo- and erythro-β-hydroxyphosphine oxide intermediates (35) in a combined yield of 73%. Treatment of the purified threo-intermediate with sodium hydride in dimethylformamide then led to the all-trans-pentaene (11) in 70% yield within 0.5 h., whereas the corresponding erythro-β-hydroxyphosphine oxide intermediate, under the same conditions in the same period of time, gave only a 18% yield of the trans-cis-trans-triene (36) [contaminated with ca. 10% of the all-trans-triene (11)], the major product being the trans-phosphine oxide (32) (Scheme 3). In a similar manner, this two stage procedure, using cis-phosphine oxide (31) and trans-citral, produced (75%) a 3:2 mixture of the corresponding threo- and erythro-β-hydroxyphosphine oxide intermediates; subsequent treatment of the threo-intermediate then gave the cis-trans-trans-pentaene (13) in 74% yield.

The above data go some way to explaining the low yields and exclusive trans-olefinations observed in the single step syntheses of the isomeric pentaenes (11): (i) formation of the β-hydroxyphosphine oxide anion intermediates is fast and reversible; this is clear from the observed accumulation of (34), and the observed isomerisation of the starting phosphine oxide with time, (ii) syn-elimination from the threo-diphenylphosphine oxide anion intermediate is energetically favoured over the erythro-intermediates, and it is this 'kinetic' effect which accounts for the observed (apparent) trans-stereoselectivity, rather than any other effect.

Having established the use of the single step Horner-Wittig reaction in the synthesis of *trans*-disubstituted double bonds set within a conjugated polyene isoprenoid system, we turned our attention to longer functionalised polyenes (e.g., 37, 45) required for elaboration to the di-*cis* pentaene and heptaene chromophores present in phytofluene (4) and ζ-carotene (5) respectively, found in fruit of the Tangerine tomato.

Thus, metallation of the *cis*-phosphine oxide (31) followed by reaction with the *trans*-ester (18,R=Me) led, in a single step, to the *trans*-2,*trans*-4, *cis*-6-tetraenoate (37) in 34% yield. In a similar manner, Horner-Wittig reactions between (31) and the hydroxybutenolide (17), and between (17) and the *trans*-phosphine oxide (32) produced the corresponding *cis*-2,*trans*-4, *cis*-6-(38) and *cis*-2,*trans*-4,*trans*-6 (39) tetraenoic acids respectively. The exclusive *trans*-olefinations observed in these single-step reactions were obtained at the expense of low overall yields (≯ 34%). It is recalled that the corresponding Wittig reactions, using both (9) and (15), produced the acids (38) and (39) and the ester (37) in higher overall yields (∿ 75%), but upwards of 40% *cis*-olefinations were observed concurrently.

(31) + (18) ⟶

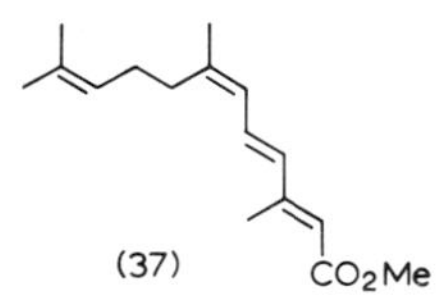

(37)

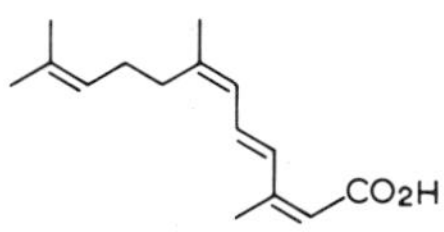

(38)

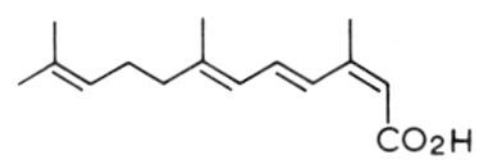

(39)

Conversion of the *trans*-2,*trans*-4,*cis*-6-ester (37) into the tetraenal (40), followed by Horner-Wittig reaction with farnesyl phosphine oxide (41), and treatment of the purified *erythro*-β-hydroxyphosphine oxide (42) with sodium hydride in dimethylformamide led to the di-*cis*-octaene (43) which showed closely similar spectral data to those found in natural di-*cis*-phytofluene (4) from Tangerine tomato fruits (Ref 7).

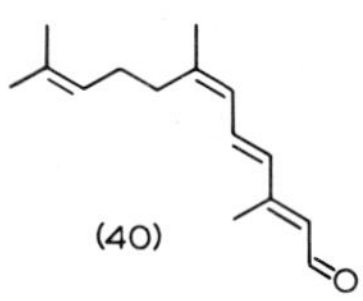

(40)

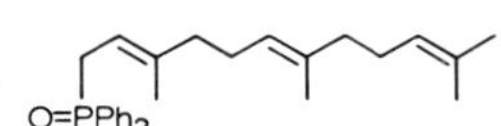

(41)

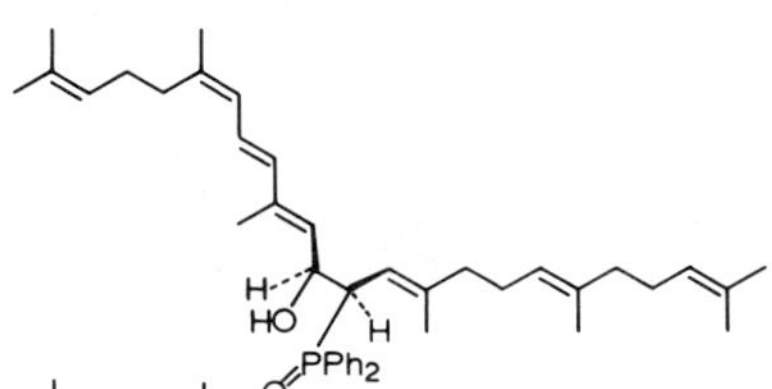

(42)

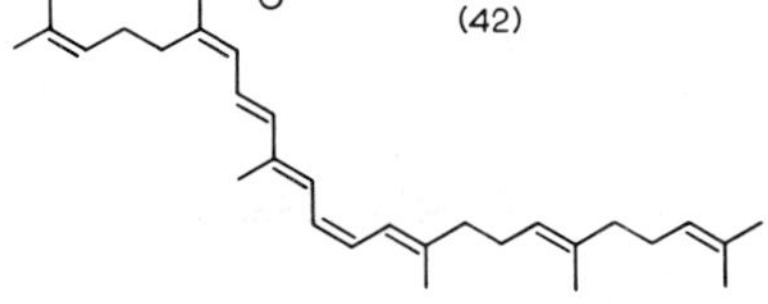

(43)

Although the Horner-Wittig syntheses of the hexaenal (45) and the nonaene (47), from (31) and the dialdehyde (44), proceeded in reasonable yield and with almost complete *trans*-olefination, they were accompanied by isomers resulting from stereomutation (20-30%) about the double bond in the starting phosphine oxide. Thus, condensation between two mole equivalents of the *cis*-phosphine oxide (31) and the dialdehyde (44), led (33%) to the *cis*-10-hexaenal (45) accompanied by *ca* 30% of the all-*trans*-isomer (46). Similarly, reaction between the all-*trans*-hexaenal (46) and (31) produced (70%) the *cis*-nonaene (47) contaminated with *ca* 25% of the all-*trans*-nonaene. Interestingly, the Horner-Wittig reaction between (44) and 4 mole equivalents of the *cis*-phosphine oxide (31), led in one step to the di-*cis*-nonaene (48) in 86% yield; once again however, the condensation was accompanied by stereomutation about the double bond in (31). The C_{40}-prenylogue of (48) [i.e. di-*cis*-ζ-carotene (5)] has been found along with (4) in Tangerine tomato fruits.

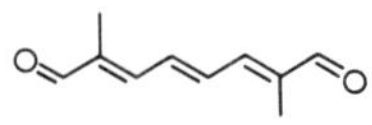

(44)

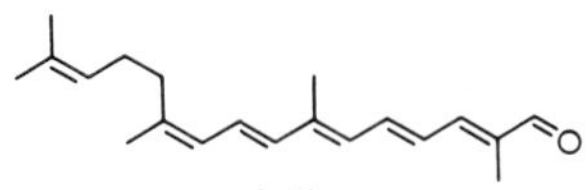

(45)

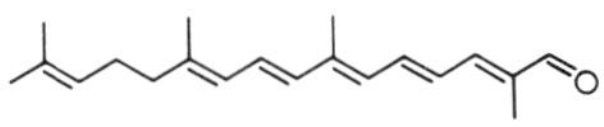

(46)

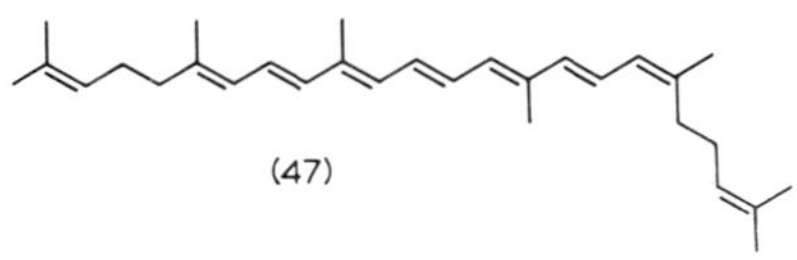

(47)

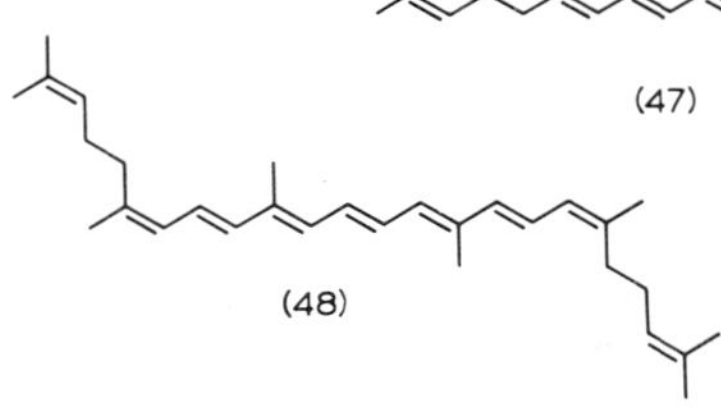

(48)

The present results, and the synthesis of the di-*cis*-polyene (43) in particular, fully demonstrate the scope of the Horner-Wittig reaction in the controlled synthesis of *trans*- and *cis*-disubstituted double bonds set within a conjugated polyene isoprenoid framework. Although overall yields in the *single step* Horner-Wittig reactions are not always high, this feature has to be offset against the almost exclusive *trans*-olefinations observed in all the cases studied; concurrent stereomutation about the double bonds of α,β-unsaturated phosphine oxides can present problems. An added bonus associated with the Horner-Wittig reaction over the Wittig reaction is the possibility of isolation of the intermediate β-hydroxyphosphine oxides (≡ 'betaines'). Subsequent elimination from the separated *erythro*-intermediates then permits the synthesis of *cis*-disubstituted double bonds [(see synthesis of (43)], thus avoiding the tedious chromatography often necessary in the purification of *cis*- and *trans*- isomers produced from the corresponding Wittig reactions.

Acknowledgements - I am grateful to Linda Carey (née Barlow) and John M. Clough for their dedicated and enthusiastic collaboration in much of the work I have described. It is also a pleasure to acknowledge a scientific debt to Professor B.C.L. Weedon, who introduced me to this area of research.

References

1. See 'Carotenoids', ed. O. Isler, Birkhäuser, Basel, (1971), and L. Zechmeister, 'cis-trans-Isomeric Carotenoids, Vitamin A and Arylpolyenes Springer-Verlag, (1962).
2. J. Herzig and F. Faltis, Justus Liebigs Ann. Chem. 431, 40 (1923); M.S. Barber, A. Hardisson, L.M. Jackman and B.C.L. Weedon, J. Chem. Soc. 1625 (1961).
3. J.B. Davis, L.M. Jackman, P.T. Siddons, and B.C.L. Weedon, J. Chem. Soc. (C). 2154 (1966).
4. B.O. Brown and B.C.L. Weedon, J. Chem. Soc., Chem. Commun. 382 (1968).
5. L. Zechmeister, A.L. LeRosen, F.W. Went and L. Pauling, Proc. Nat. Acad. Sci. U.S.A. 27, 468 (1941); A.L. LeRosen and L. Zechmeister, J. Am. Chem. Soc. 64, 1075 (1942).
6. G. Englert, B.O. Brown, G.P. Moss, B.C.L. Weedon, G. Britton, T.W. Goodwin, K.L. Simpson and R.J.H. Williams, J. Chem. Soc., Chem. Commun. 545 (1979).
7. J.M. Clough and G. Pattenden, J. Chem. Soc., Chem. Commun. 616 (1979).
8. For a recent illustration see: G. Englert and M. Vecchi, Helv. Chim. Acta 63, 1711 (1980).
9. G. Englert, Helv. Chim. Acta. 58, 2367 (1975); G.P. Moss, Pure Appl. Chem. 47, 97 (1976); M. Baranyai, J. Szabolcs, G. Toth and L. Radics, Tetrahedron 32, 867 (1976).
10. L. Barlow and G. Pattenden, J. Chem. Soc., Perkin Trans I, 1029 (1976).
11. See I. Gosney and A.G. Rowley in 'Organophosphorus Reagents in Organic Synthesis', ed. J.I.G. Cadogan, Academic Press (1979).
12. H. Pommer, Angew Chem. 72, 811 (1960).
13. J.J. Plattner, U.T. Bhalerao and H. Rapoport, J. Amer. Chem. Soc., 91, 4933 (1969), idem, ibid. 92, 3429 (1970).
14. G. Pattenden and B.C.L. Weedon, J. Chem. Soc. (C). 1984 (1968).
15. N. Khan, D.E. Loeber, T.P. Toube and B.C.L. Weedon, J. Chem. Soc., Perkin Trans I, 1457 (1975).
16. G. Pattenden and B.C.L. Weedon, J. Chem. Soc. (C) 1997 (1968).
17. L. Carey (née Barlow) Ph.D. Thesis, University of Nottingham, 1976.
18. G. Pattenden, J.E. Way and B.C.L. Weedon, J. Chem. Soc. (C). 235 (1970).
19. J.D. Surmatis, U.S. Pat. 3,367, 985 (1968); Chem. Abs., 68, 114786 (1968).
20. B.C.L. Weedon, Rev. Pure Appl. Chem. (Australia), 20, 51 (1970) cf. G.P. Moss, Pure and Applied Chem., 51, 507 (1979).
21. G. Wittig and U. Schöllkopf, Chem. Ber. 87, 1318 (1954).
22. L. Horner, H. Hoffman and H.G. Wippel, Chem. Ber. 91, 61 (1958).
23. L. Horner, Fortschr. Chem. Forsch, 7, 1 (1966); B.J. Walker in 'Organophosphorus Reagents in Organic Synthesis' ed. J.I.G. Cadogan, Academic Press, (1979).
24. see B. Lythgoe, T.A. Moran, M.E.N. Nambudiry and S. Ruston, J. Chem. Soc., Perkin. Trans I, 2386 (1976); A.H. Davidson and S. Warren, ibid., 639 (1976); M. Schlosser and H.B. Tuong, Chimia (Switz), 30, 197 (1976).
25. J.M. Clough and G. Pattenden, Tetrahedron Lett. 4159 (1978).
26. J.M. Clough and G. Pattenden, Tetrahedron Lett. 5043 (1979).
27. A.F. Thomas and R. Guntz-Dubini, Helv. Chim. Acta 59, 2261 (1976).
28. cf. A.J. Bridges and G.H. Whitham, J. Chem. Soc., Chem. Commun. 142 (1974).

ELECTROCHEMICAL REACTIONS APPLIED TO POLYENES AND CAROTENOIDS

James H.P. Utley

Department of Chemistry, Queen Mary College, Mile End Road, London E1 4NS, UK

Abstract - The selectivity and mildness of chemical conditions associated with electrochemical reductions have been exploited for syntheses and transformations of polyenes and carotenoids. Suitable cathodic reactions include: hydrogenation and cleavage; pinacolisations modified by chromium(III); the reductive coupling of polyenylphosphonium salts; and the synthesis of polyenes by Wittig reactions induced by electrogenerated base.

INTRODUCTION

Carotenoids and polyenes are notoriously sensitive to severe chemical conditions and much of the art of synthesis in this area is concerned with the development of mild methods which avoid over-oxidation, over-reduction, acid or base catalysed rearrangement or general degradation. In this context electrochemical methods may have much to offer. The key step is electron transfer, and control of current and potential can give selectivity in oxidation and reduction reactions. Because the rate of electron transfer is dependent on potential, rather than temperature, difficult redox reactions may be conducted under otherwise mild conditions.

The range of reactive intermediates accessible electrochemically is displayed in Scheme 1 and their chemical behaviour is remarkably similar to that of the same species formed homogeneously. One important consequence of heterogeneous generation is that, because high local concentrations of intermediates are formed, dimerisation reactions are often favoured. In suitable aprotic solvents an electroactive range of +3.0 to -3.0 V is achievable and this may be equated with a possible modification of the energy of activation for electron transfer by *ca*. 290 kJ mol^{-1}. In practical terms solvated electrons may be generated at the cathodic limit and carbon-carbon and carbon-hydrogen bonds cleaved oxidatively at the anodic limit.

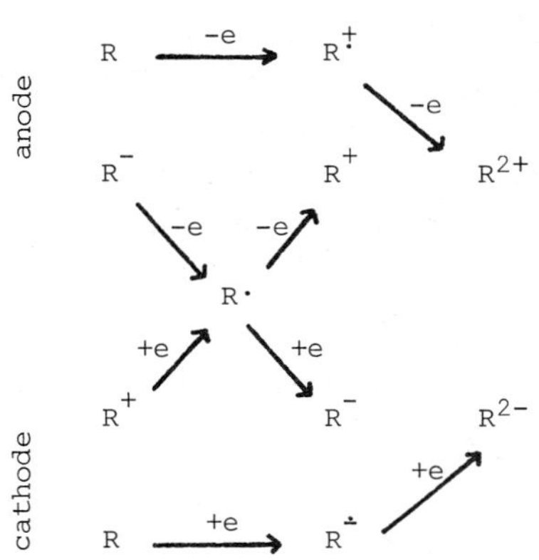

radical-cations

carbocations

carbanions

radical-anions

Scheme 1. Organic reactive intermediates produced at electrodes.

The examples of electrosynthesis described in this paper are intended to illustrate, in the context of polyene chemistry: (1) selective cathodic hydrogenation and cleavage; (2) cathodic hydrodimerisation; and, (3) the convenient cathodic generation of bases.

CATHODIC HYDROGENATION AND CLEAVAGE

Canthaxanthin is smoothly reduced (Ref. 1) in a 2 F mol^{-1} reaction and in the presence of acetic anhydride gives a good yield of the retro-diacetate (1). Hydrolysis, separately or *in situ*, provides overall an indirect and highly selective method of hydrogenation (Scheme 2). Mild conditions are maintained throughout and it is therefore possible to carry out the

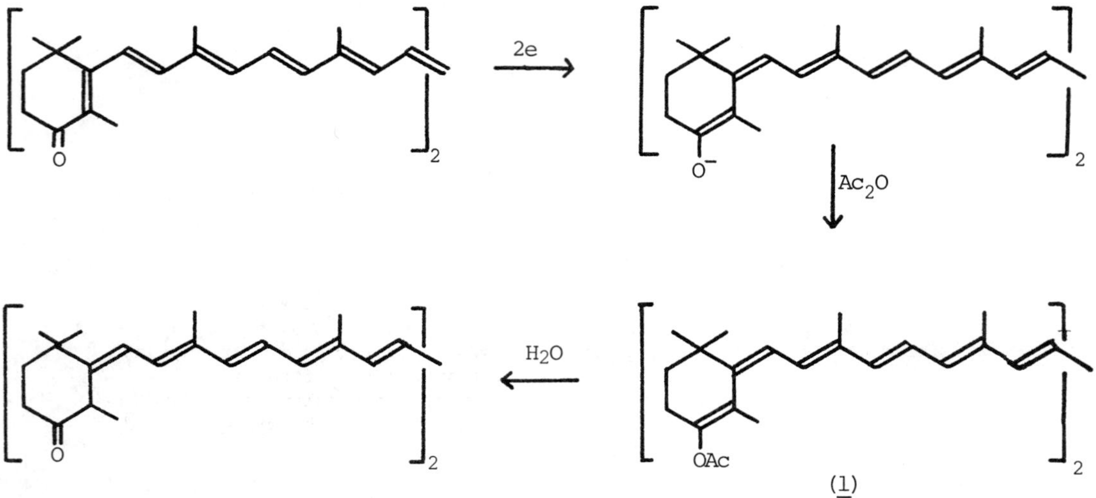

Scheme 2. Cathodic acylation and hydrogenation of Canthaxanthin

reaction under kinetic control; the major product is the relatively unstable 5,5'-dihydro-canthaxanthin. The same reaction has been applied to other polyene carbonyl compounds, e.g. crocetindial and 4-keto-β-ionone (Ref. 2); in each case high yields of retro-diacetates are formed. The hydrolysis (and hence hydrogenation) products are very sensitive to air-oxidation but the diacetate formed from 4-keto-β-ionone undergoes stepwise hydrolysis firstly to the monoacetate (2) and then to (3).

(2) (3)

The conditions for electrolysis, and valuable clues to mechanism, are provided by cyclic voltammetry. The mechanism outlined in Scheme 2 is based soundly on cyclic voltammetric experiments. For several acetates cyclic voltammetry indicates that they undergo irreversible reduction at relatively modest potentials (Table 1). Preparative scale

TABLE 1. Cyclic voltammetric data[a] for benzylic and polyene acetates

Compound	$-E_p$/V *vs.* Ag-AgI
p-$MeO_2C.C_6H_4.CH_2OAc$	1.58
E-Ph(AcO)C:C(OAc)Ph (7)	1.54
Vitamin A acetate	1.32
Zeaxanthin diacetate	1.00
Isozeaxanthin diacetate	0.87; 1.07; 1.54
Crustaxanthin tetraacetate (6)	0.67
(β-Carotene	1.08; 1.50)

a. N,N-Dimethylformamide - Hg drop cathode - scan rate 0.1 or 0.3 Vs^{-1}

electrolysis reveals that the irreversible chemical reaction following electron transfer is loss of acetate ion (Scheme 3). The fact that this can be achieved under chemically mild conditions is the basis of simple and efficient syntheses (Ref. 3) of axerophtene (4) and 3,4,3',4'-tetradehydro-β-carotene (5) from, respectively, vitamin A acetate and crustaxanthin tetraacetate (6). Cathodic reduction of vicinal diacetates results more often than not in elimination of both acetate groups. The mechanism is undoubtedly stepwise, e.g. by the choice of sufficiently protic conditions one acetate only is removed from stilbene dioldiacetate (7) (Ref. 4), yet it did not prove possible to halt the reduction of crustaxanthin tetraacetate at the zeaxanthin diacetate stage.

$$RCH_2OAc \xrightarrow{e} [RCH_2OAc]^{\cdot -} \xrightarrow{-OAc^-} [RCH_2^{\cdot}] \xrightarrow[H^+]{e} RCH_3$$

Scheme 3. Cleavage of acetates

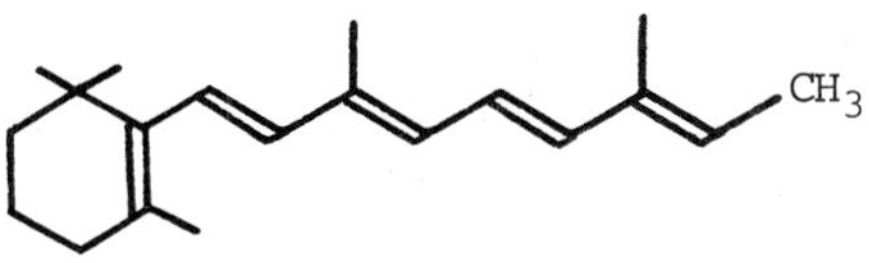

(4)

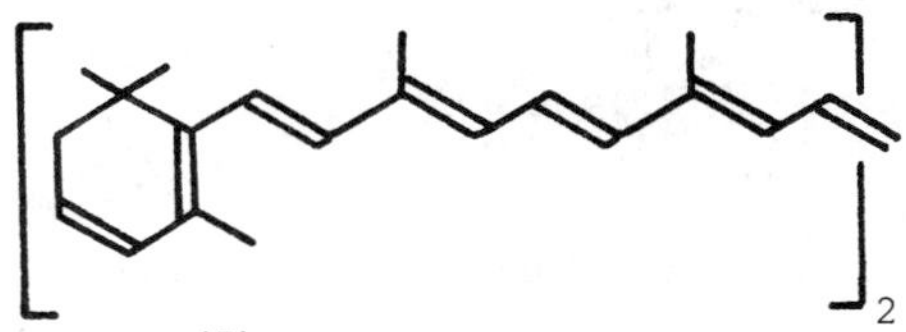

(5)

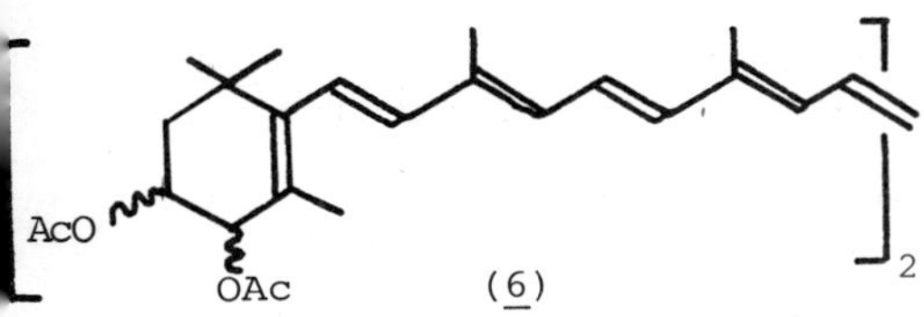

(6)

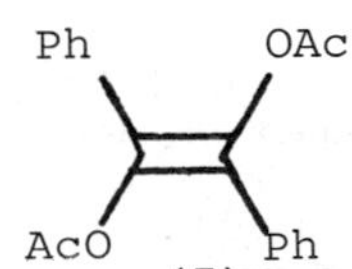

(7)

A strategy for the electrosynthesis of carotenoids is given in Scheme 4; the dimerisation reaction will be discussed below but the point of immediate interest is that reductive cleavage is involved in the final step. It is not always convenient or easy to convert allylic hydroxyls into good anionic leaving groups such as acetate. Consequently conditions under which hydroxyl might be persuaded to depart from radical-anions were sought. The

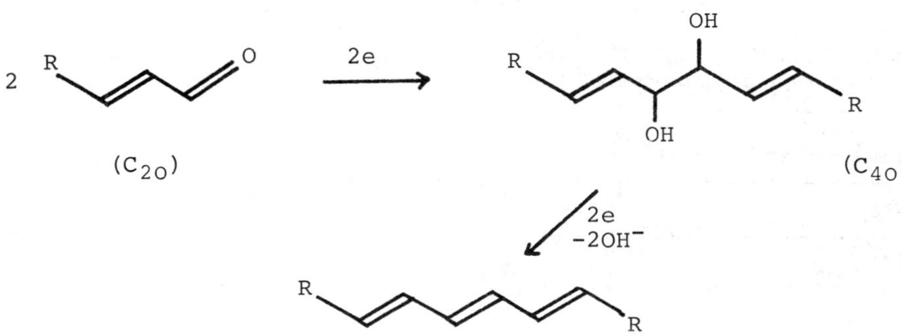

Scheme 4. A strategy for electrosynthesis of carotenoids

methyl ester of abscisic acid would seem to be ideal for such a study; the hydroxyl is activated towards cathodic cleavage both by the cyclic enone system and by the unsaturated ester function. This interpretation is supported by the low reduction potential in N,N-dimethylformamide ($E_p = -1.38$ V *vs.* Ag/AgI) of the ester. Controlled potential electrolysis, however, resulted in the formation of the bicyclic ester (8) and cyclic voltammetric experiments on model compounds strongly suggest that reaction proceeds according to Scheme 5. The hydroxyl group in the abscisic acid ester exercises the important function of inhibiting conjugation between the flanking unsaturated systems (Ref. 5).

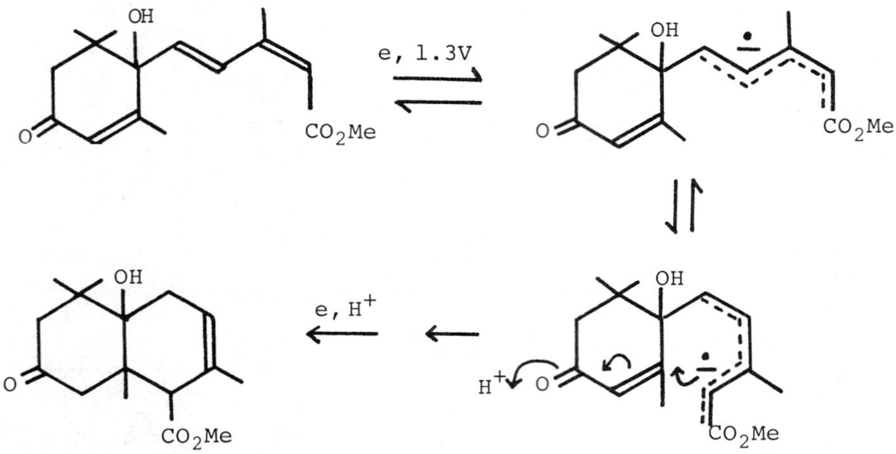

Scheme 5. Cathodic cyclisation of methyl abscisate

CATHODIC HYDRODIMERISATION

Cathodic pinacolisation has been extensively studied and its successful application often depends upon the correct choice of a protic electrolyte. Strongly acidic conditions are ruled out for polyenes and carotenoids and attempts to use the electrochemical method have been dominated by the need to "neutralise" the radical-anions, and hence encourage dimerisation, without using destructive chemical conditions. In the important case of the hydrodimerisation of retinal a simple and apparently effective method is to use diethylmalonate as a proton donor (Ref. 6).

Following an earlier interest in the pinacolisation of α- and β-ionone and of retinal (Ref. 7) we have explored the role of chromium(III) in modifying these reactions. The usefulness of chromium(III) salts in promoting pinacolisation is illustrated by the results given in Table 2 (Ref. 8); as a point of comparison it should be noted that the cathodic pinacolisation of benzophenone has previously only been achieved using strong aqueous mineral acid as solvent. The mechanism of the reaction in the presence of chromium(III) has been thoroughly investigated (Ref. 8) and the key step is electron transfer to a complex of the carbonyl compound with chromium(III); the polarisation of the carbonyl group which this causes is the reason why the chromium(III) modified pinacolisations occur at such conveniently low potentials.

TABLE 2. Pinacolisation[a] modified by chromium(III)

Carbonyl compound	$-E_{red.}$/V *vs.* Ag-AgI	Yield of pinacol (%)
Ph_2CO	1.00	70
PhCHO	0.90	51
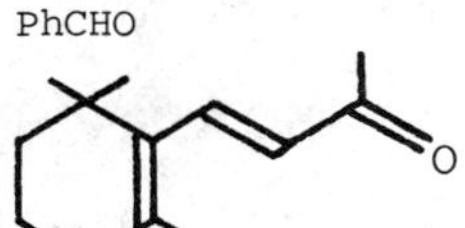	0.95	75
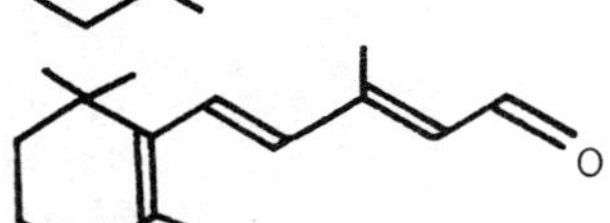	0.80	60
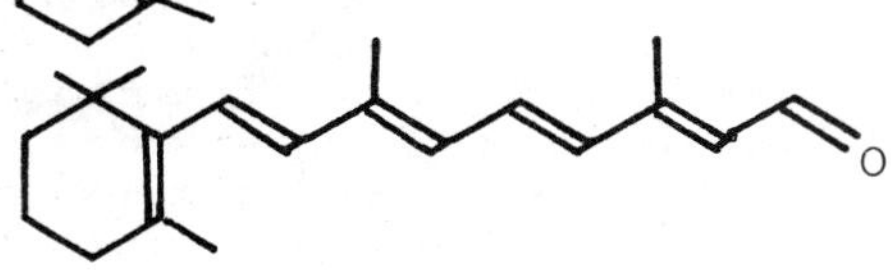	0.80	25

a. N,N-Dimethylformamide-$NaClO_4$ (0.15 mol dm^{-3}), Hg cathode, divided cell, $CrCl_3.6H_2O$ (*ca.* 10^{-2} mol dm^{-3}), carbonyl compound (*ca.* 10^{-2} mol dm^{-3}).

Existing chemical methods for the reductive cleavage and elimination of vicinal hydroxyl groups are inadequate for the final conversion of pinacol into polyene as envisaged in Scheme 4. For instance, retinal may be converted into the corresponding pinacol in acceptable yield and yet the final conversion into β-carotene gave only 3% yield using the conventional reagent (PI_3-CS_2-pyridine). A promising electrochemical method has now been developed (Ref. 9) which is based on the low potential cathodic fragmentation of oxalates. Good results have been obtained for simple vicinal diols (Table 3) and an important improvement on earlier cathodic methods is that the olefinic products are unreactive at the low potentials required for oxalate reduction. This method has yet to be applied to a polyene pinacol.

TABLE 3. The cathodic reduction[a] of oxalates

Oxalate	$-E_{red}$/V (*vs.* Ag-AgI)	Products (%)	
meso-HOCH(Ph)CH(Ph)$O_2C.CO_2Et$	1.30	*meso*-HO.CH(Ph)CH(Ph).OH	(31)
		HO.CH(Ph)CH_2Ph	(11)
		trans-PhCH:CHPh	(23)
meso-$EtO_2C.CO_2CH$(Ph)CH(Ph)$O_2C.CO_2Et$	1.20	*trans*-PhCH:CHPh	(80)
(±)-$EtO_2C.CO_2CH$(Ph)CH(Ph)$O_2C.CO_2Et$	1.20	*trans*-PhCH:CHPh	(75)
meso-$PhO_2C.CO_2CH$(Ph)CH(Ph)$O_2C.CO_2Ph$	1.10	*trans*-PhCH:CHPh	(45)
		meso-HO.CH(Ph)CH(Ph).OH	(22)

a. Divided cell, Hg cathode, N,N-dimethylformamide - Bu_4NClO_4 (0.1 mol dm^{-3})

Polyene-substituted phosphonium salts are well characterised and readily accessible intermediates for polyene synthesis. The electroreduction of 'onium salts has also been the subject of much mechanistic study and as one of the competing reactions following electron transfer is known to be dimerisation the cathodic dimerisation of polyene-substituted phosphonium salts is obviously worth exploring (Scheme 6). Systematic study reveals that optimum conditions for coupling involve the use of aluminium cathodes (Ref. 10). The method

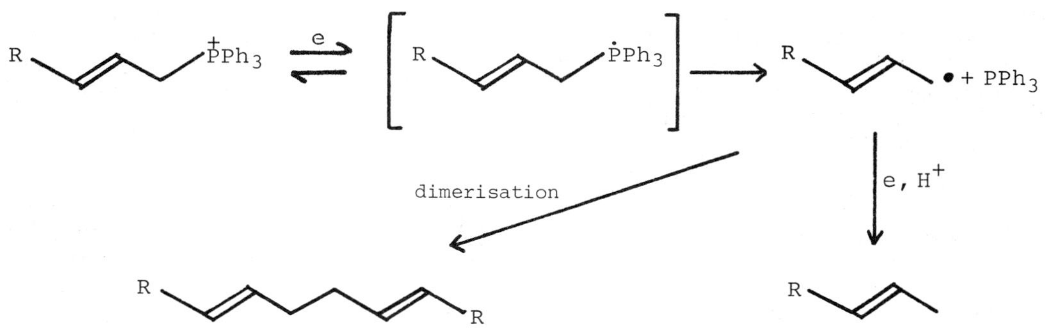

Scheme 6. Cathodic cleavage of phosphonium salts.

was explored using benzyl-, allyl-, cinnamyl-, and polyenylphosphonium salts; representative results are included in Table 4. It will be seen that moderately efficient coupling is obtained and the yields must be judged against the paucity of alternative routes to these particular products. The cells used are undivided ones of simple construction, the electrodes (aluminium) are cheap, and the reaction is best run at constant current rather than at constant potential.

TABLE 4. Cathodic coupling[a] of phosphonium salts

Phosphonium salt	Coupling product
$PhCH_2\overset{+}{P}Ph_3\overset{-}{NO_3}$	$PhCH_2CH_2Ph$ (56%)
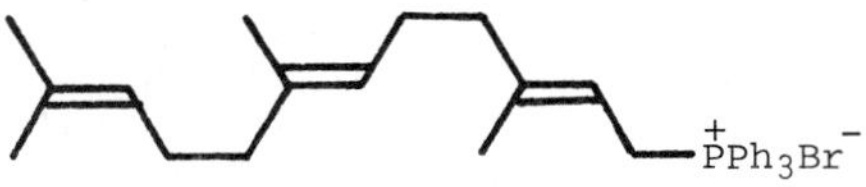	— [b]
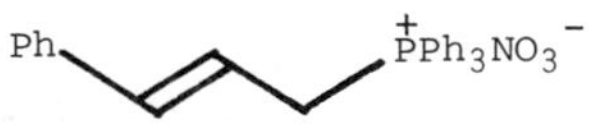	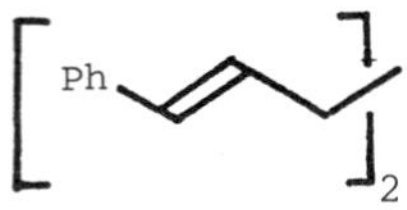 (15%) 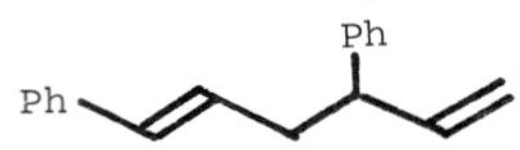 (13%)
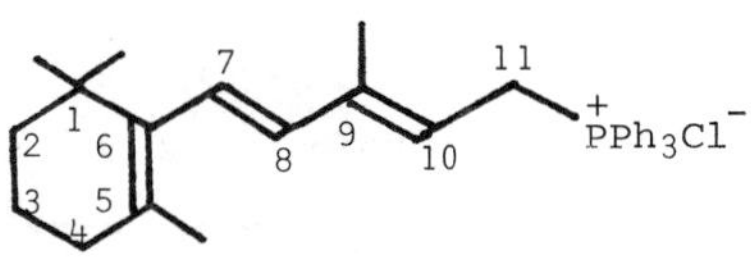 (9)	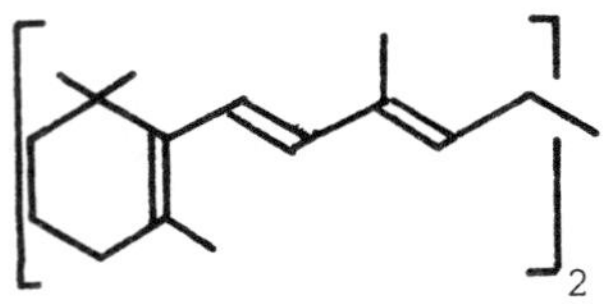 (11%) 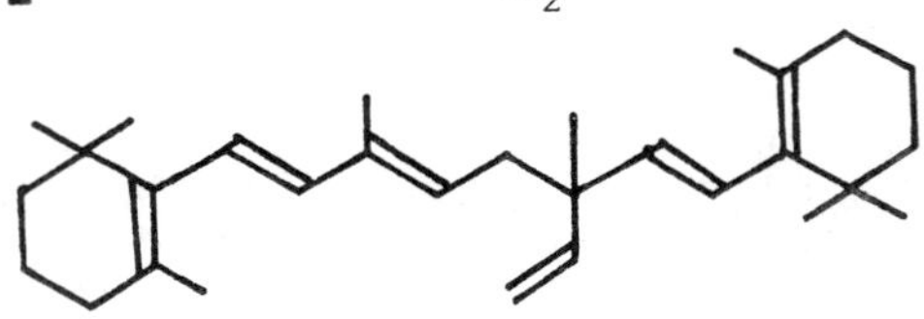 (6%)

a. Al cathode, N,N-dimethylformamide, 2.5 F mol^{-1}, *ca.* 0.25 A cm^{-2}

b. Major product, α-farnesene (32%)

Coupling from the C_{15} polyenylphosphonium salt (9) is interesting in that *trans*-isomers only are formed and the dimer resulting from symmetrical coupling at C-9 is absent. This is analogous to the result of the experiments involving the cinnamylphosphonium salt; the product of symmetrical coupling is in this case a known compound which would undoubtedly have survived the reaction conditions. For the C_{15} system products involving coupling at C-5 and C-7 are also absent, presumably as a consequence of the steric hindrance which also limits and directs the cathodic pinacolisation of polyene carbonyl compounds.

THE CATHODIC GENERATION OF BASES FOR USE IN THE WITTIG REACTION

The coupling reactions described above proceed with the consumption of 1 F mol^{-1} and under the forcing conditions (high current density) used for preparative electrolysis the dimerisation of radicals competes well with further reduction to the corresponding carbanions, i.e. 2 F mol^{-1} reduction (see Scheme 6). Cyclic voltammetry, in dry N,N-dimethylformamide, reveals, however, that an alternative 1 F mol^{-1} process may operate for benzyl-, allyl-, cinnamyl-, and polyenylphosphonium salts. Reduction peaks, additional to those of the starting materials and the products of hydrogenolysis, have been identified as being associated with the corresponding ylids (Ref. 11). The mechanism of ylid formation in these circumstances is that given in Scheme 7. The ease of formation of the ylids, and their evident stability, suggested that preparative use might be made of polyenyl-substituted ylids formed *via* bases cathodically generated from added reducible compounds (pro-bases). The effectiveness of such bases in generating ylids by *in situ* reaction with phosphonium salts can be monitored by cyclic voltammetry. Cyclic voltammetry can also be used to select combinations of pro-base, phosphonium salt, and carbonyl compound

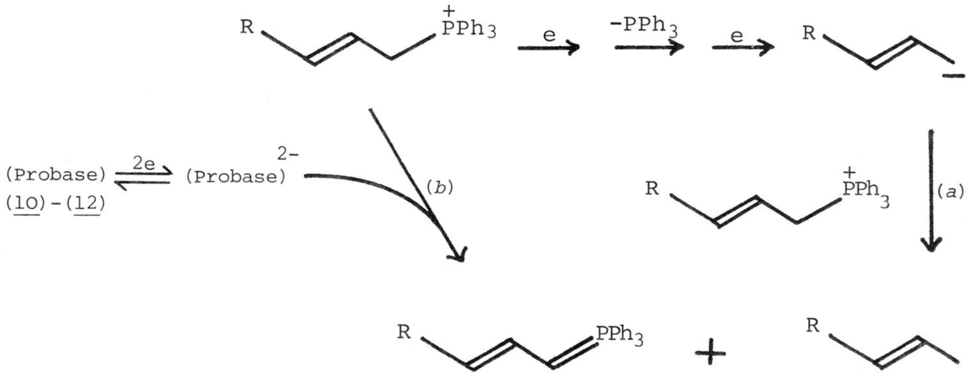

Scheme 7. Cathodic formation of ylids; (*a*) intermolecularly (*b*) *via* external, electrogenerated, base.

in which it is the pro-base which is the more easily reduced. These ideas are illustrated by Fig. 1 in which the effect of added phosphonium salt on the cyclic voltammogram of 9-fluorenyl-1,1-dicyanomethylene (10), (a pro-base), are clearly seen; the ylid formed by reduction at -0.95 V (*vs*. Ag/AgI) is itself reduced at $E_p = -1.93$ V. The two reduction peaks of (10) correspond to formation of firstly the radical-anion and then the dianion. It is the dianion which acts as base and the effect of proton donation from added phosphonium salt is to quench the reversible formation of dianion (Fig. 1). Similar behaviour is found for the pro-bases (11) and (12).

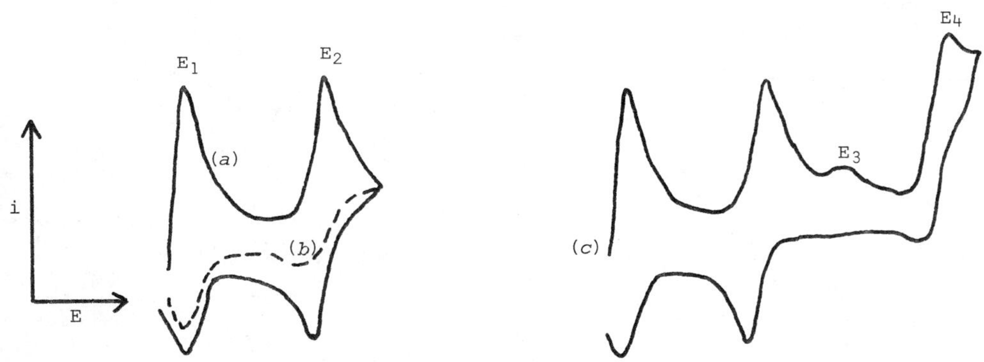

Conditions: DMF-Bu_4NI, vitreous C cathode; 0.3 V s^{-1}

Curves: (*a*) probase (10), scan reversal at -1.1 V (*vs*. Ag/AgI); (*b*) (10) + PhCH:$CHCH_2\overset{+}{P}Ph_3$, reversal at -1.1 V; (*c*) as (*b*) but reversal at -2.1 V.

Peak potentials: E_1, -0.11 V (1e reduction of (10)); E_2, -0.90 V (1e reduction of $(10)^{\dot{-}}$); E_3, -1.28 V (reduction of PhCH:$CHCH_2\overset{+}{P}Ph_3$); E_4, -1.93 V (reduction of ylid).

Figure 1. Cyclic voltammetry of (10) and PhCH:$CHCH_2\overset{+}{P}Ph_3$

The preparative application of this method of ylid formation involves conducting electrolysis, at the potential for dianion formation, in the presence of less easily reduced phosphonium salts and carbonyl compounds. The reduction potentials of the latter are, of course, easily determined by preliminary cyclic voltammetric experiments. Advantages to be expected from the method are: convenience (no special drying of the solvent is necessary); control over the rate of generation of the base (*via* concentration and current); deployment of a range of bases in one solvent system; and control over added salts.

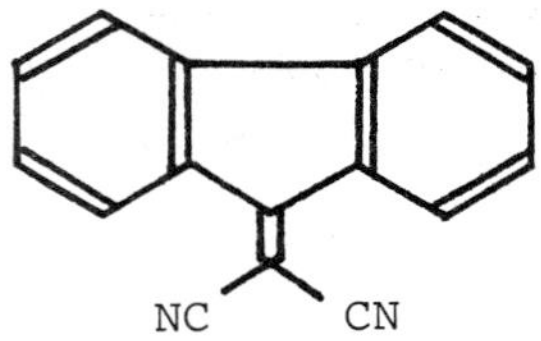

(10)

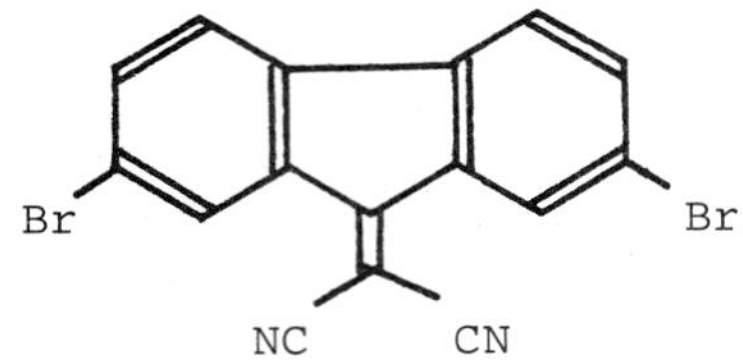

(11)

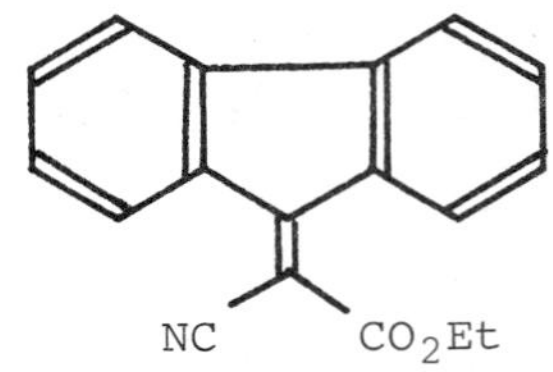

(12)

The results of preparative scale experiments of relevance to polyene synthesis are displayed in Table 5. As with many Wittig reactions the important influence of cations, both on yield and stereochemistry, can be seen. Optimum conditions are the employment of (12) as pro-base in the presence of a lithium salt. The precise control of conditions which is a feature of the electrochemical method results in good reproducibility of yields and proportions of stereoisomers. In addition the work-up procedure is simple and by controlling the extent of reduction no more than the required amount of base is generated. This offers the prospect of conveniently preparing, and isolating, relatively unstable polyenes.

TABLE 5. Wittig syntheses *via* cathodically generated[a] base in N,N-dimethylformamide

Phosphonium salt	Carbonyl compound	Pro-base[b]	Electrolyte cation ($0.1\ mol\ dm^{-3}$)	Alkene product (%); [*trans:cis*]
$PhCH_2\overset{+}{P}Ph_3$	PhCHO	(10)	Bu_4N^+	Stilbene (46); [1.56]
			Li^+	Stilbene (74); [0.69]
$PhCH_2\overset{+}{P}Ph_3$	PhCHO	(11)	Bu_4N^+	Stilbene (38); [0.92]
			Li^+	Stilbene (21); [1.00]
$PhCH_2\overset{+}{P}Ph_3$	PhCHO	(12)	Bu_4N^+	Stilbene (58); [1.00]
			Li^+	Stilbene (94); [1.17]
$PhCH_2\overset{+}{P}Ph_3$	PhCH:CHCHO	(11)	Bu_4N^+	1,4-diphenylbutadiene (34, *trans*)
$PhCH:CHCH_2\overset{+}{P}Ph_3$	PhCHO	(11)	Bu_4N^+	1,4-diphenylbutadiene (64, *trans*)
(9)[c]	(13)[d]	(10)	Li^+	Vitamin A acetate (30); [0.56]
		(12)	Li^+	Vitamin A acetate (40); [0.32][e]

a. Divided cell, Hg pool, $2\ F\ mol^{-1}$, reactants *ca.* $10^{-2}\ mol\ dm^{-3}$

b. Reduction potentials (V *vs.* Ag-AgI): (10), -0.90; (11), -0.60; (12), -0.80

c. See Table 4.

d. 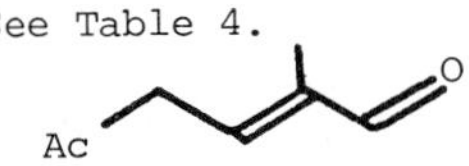 (13)

e. Corresponds to 76% 11-*cis*, 24% all-*trans*

Acknowledgement - This work was partially supported by the S.R.C. and by equipment grants from the Royal Society and the University of London Central Research Fund.

REFERENCES

1. E.A.H. Hall, G.P. Moss, J.H.P. Utley, and B.C.L. Weedon, *J. Chem. Soc., Chem. Commun.*, 586 (1976).
2. E.A.H. Hall, *Ph.D. Thesis (London University)* (1977).
3. J.G. Gourcy, M. Hodler, B. Terem, and J.H.P. Utley, *J. Chem. Soc., Chem. Commun.*, 779 (1976)
4. C. Adams, N.M. Kamkar, and J.H.P. Utley, *J. Chem. Soc., Perkin Trans. 2*, 1767 (1979).
5. B. Terem and J.H.P. Utley, *Electrochim. Acta*, 24, 1081 (1979).
6. L.A. Powell and R.M. Wightman, *J. Am. Chem. Soc.*, 101, 4412 (1979).
7. R.E. Sioda, B. Terem, J.H.P. Utley, and B.C.L. Weedon, *J. Chem. Soc., Perkin Trans. 1*, 561 (1976).
8. D.W. Sopher and J.H.P. Utley, *J. Chem. Soc., Chem. Commun.*, 1087 (1979).
9. D.W. Sopher and J.H.P. Utley, *J. Chem. Soc., Chem. Commun.*, 134 (1981).
10. J.H.P. Utley and A. Webber, *J. Chem. Soc., Perkin Trans. 1*, 1154 (1980).
11. V.L. Pardini, L. Roullier, J.H.P. Utley, and A. Webber, *J. Chem. Soc., Perkin Trans. 2*, in the press.

N.M.R. OF CAROTENOIDS

Gerhard Englert

Central Research Units, F. Hoffmann-La Roche & Co., Ltd., CH-4002 Basle (Switzerland)

Abstract - The advantages and some applications of high-field p.m.r. spectroscopy especially for the elucidation of the structures of *cis*-isomeric carotenoids are discussed. Examples are presented of the high sensitivity of modern instruments enabling p.m.r. spectra to be run from sample quantities below 1 μg and ^{13}C-n.m.r. spectra from quantities of less than 1 mg. The characteristic p.m.r. data of a great number of typical end groups are given. Some applications of the homonuclear Overhauser effect and of the two-dimensional J-resolved p.m.r. spectroscopy are presented. The potential use of ^{17}O-n.m.r. spectroscopy in the field of carotenoids is discussed.

INTRODUCTION

In recent years nuclear magnetic resonance (n.m.r.) spectroscopy has become a tool of increasing importance in the field of carotenoids. This is mainly caused by two facts. Firstly, modern instruments are now using high or very high magnetic fields of up to 140 kG (14 tesla), corresponding to p.m.r. frequencies of up to 600 MHz. With these instruments the dispersion and spectral resolution of the otherwise strongly overlapping signals typical for the spectra of carotenoids are so advantageously enhanced that such spectra can frequently be largely understood and interpreted.

A second reason for the increasing importance of n.m.r. is the fact that the increase of the magnetic field strength (together with the advent of Fourier-transform techniques) was paralleled by a significant increase in the sensitivity. As will be shown below, it is possible now to run p.m.r. spectra of carotenoids from sample quantities below 1 μg and ^{13}C-n.m.r. spectra from less than 1 mg if correspondingly longer accumulation times of up to several days can be tolerated. Together with the application of chromatographic methods such as h.p.l.c. this opened up the possibility of elucidating the structure of compounds even if they are available only in very small quantities. An important application in this respect is the elucidation of the structure of *cis*-isomeric carotenoids as will be discussed below.

A further advantage of n.m.r. can be seen in the fact that a number of powerful experimental methods has been developed for the solution of complicated structural problems. Two examples thereof, the homonuclear Overhauser technique and the newly available two-dimensional n.m.r. spectroscopy, will be treated briefly. Furthermore, the present sensitivity of ^{13}C-n.m.r. and the potential application of ^{17}O-n.m.r. in the field of carotenoids will be discussed with the aid of some typical spectra.

As is seen from this survey my contribution will not provide a review of the extended n.m.r. literature of carotenoids but I would rather like to present some recent results and applications obtained in our laboratory selected from the point of view of a spectroscopist rather than a chemist.

P.M.R. AT HIGH MAGNETIC FIELDS

The striking increase of information in a high-field p.m.r. spectrum is demonstrated in Fig. 1. Here, the 90 MHz spectrum (top) of astaxanthin is compared to the spectrum run at 400 MHz (middle and bottom). In the first spectrum the olefinic part consists of a broad hump and only from the integral can useful information be extracted, namely the approximate number of olefinic protons. In the 400 MHz spectrum, on the other hand, the enhanced dispersion by a factor of 4.4 makes possible the identification and assignment of all proton signals.

Some general remarks on the p.m.r. spectra of carotenoids should be inserted here. The assignments given here and in some later examples cannot be discussed in detail. They are based on comparison with suitable reference compounds and in most cases on corresponding decoupling experiments. It is evident from the 400 MHz spectrum in Fig. 1 that even the olefinic proton signals are frequently sufficiently separated from each other to make possible the application of this method and to find the different coupling partners.

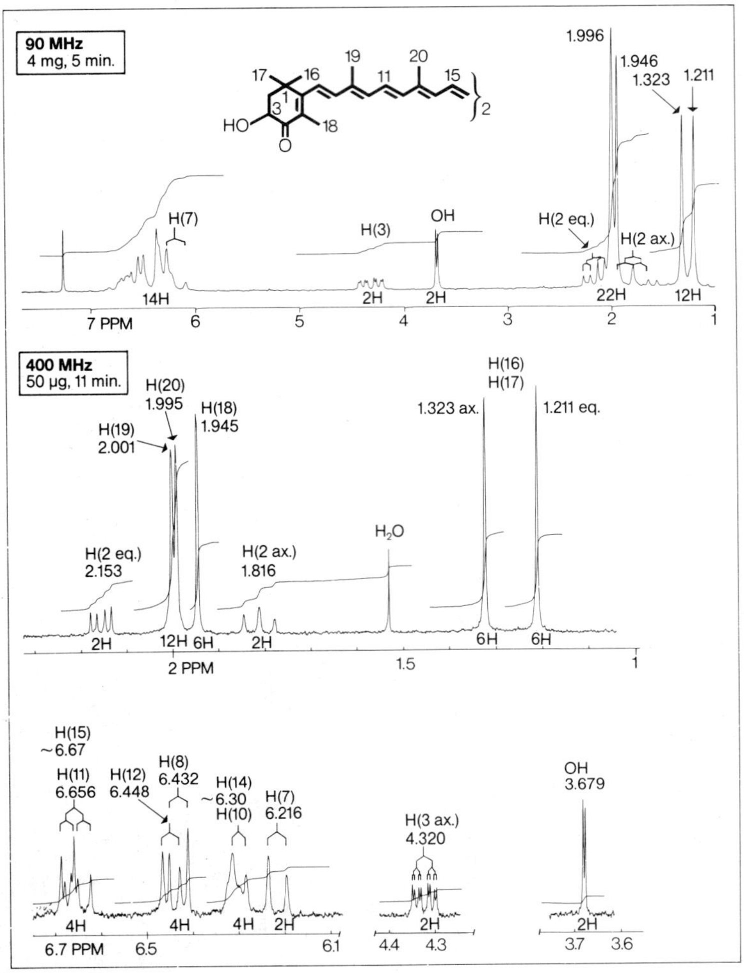

Fig. 1. F.T.-p.m.r. spectra of astaxanthin in $CDCl_3$. Top: 90 MHz, 4 mg in 0.5 ml, accumulation time 5 min. Center and bottom: 400 MHz, 50 µg in 0.16 ml, 180 pulses of 90° flip angle, 11 min.

A general feature of the spectrum of all-*trans* carotenoids such as astaxanthin is the observation that the signals of H(11) and H(15) are usually found at lowest field near 6.7 ppm, and those of H(12), H(14) and H(10) at slightly higher fields. The positions of the latter as well as those of the two doublets of H(7) and H(8) strongly depend on the type of end group.

The additional deshielding of H(11) and H(15) can be intuitively interpreted by the assumption that it is caused by the strong steric interactions with the hydrogens of the "in-chain" methyl groups. The explanation of this additional downfield shift by strong van der Waals interactions with proton internuclear distances as small as 2.2 Å can be successfully applied in the interpretation of the chemical shift differences between all-*trans* and *cis* compounds as will be seen later.

The 400 MHz spectrum in Fig. 1 also demonstrates as a first example the high sensitivity of a modern FT-instrument. It was measured in 11 minutes by application of 180 pulses of 90° flip angle from a sample quantity of only 50 µg. A reduction of the measuring time by a factor of ca. 10 without significant loss of information is clearly possible.

Since the accumulation time necessary for a desired signal-to-noise ratio is (under optimum conditions) inversely proportional to the square of the sample quantity one can predict that a sample of ca. 1 µg should be accessible in roughly 1 or 2 days of accumulation. This is indeed possible as is shown in Fig. 2. Here the two sections of the 400 MHz p.m.r. spectrum of ca. 1.5 μg of lactucaxanthin are presented measured in 13 hours. The structure of this carotenoid was very recently elucidated (Ref. 1). According to a preceding h.p.l.c. examination by Dr. M. Vecchi (Basle) the sample which was kindly provided by Prof. S. Liaaen-Jensen originally consisted of one main component the spectrum of which is shown, and two minor components presumably isomers. After the sample was identified (relative geometry) by comparison of its spectrum with that of an authentic sample (Ref. 2) the sample quantity of 1.5 μg was estimated by UV/VIS-spectroscopy from the known molar absorptivity.

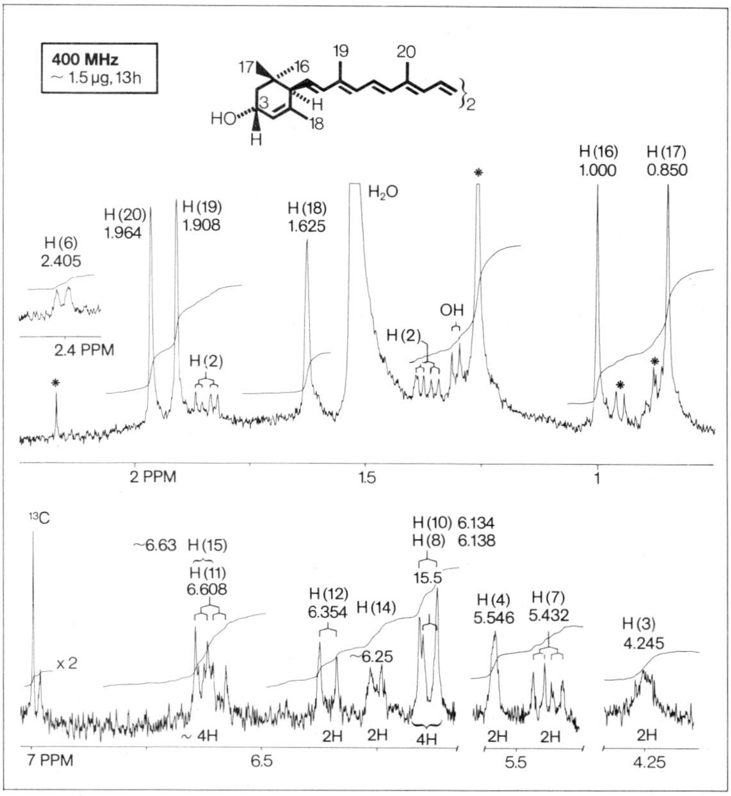

Fig. 2. 400 MHz p.m.r. spectrum of lactucaxanthin; ca. 1.5 μg in 0.12 ml $CDCl_3$ (100 % D quality); 13 hours accumulation; *impurities.

Countless difficulties and problems are encountered if one attempts to run p.m.r. spectra of such small sample quantities. Thus it is difficult to find a solvent of sufficient purity, to handle the sample preparation without the introduction of impurities, and to have a probe head and sample tubes free of background signals. Fortunately the extremely strong signal at 7.26 ppm being caused by the remaining protons of the so-called 100 % D chloroform (isotopic purity ≥ 99.96 %) is frequently outside the interesting spectral region. Thus, only the upper ^{13}C-side band with 0.55 % of the intensity of the main signal is shown at the low-field edge of the olefinic part of the spectra. The next strongest signal near 1.5 ppm is due to the extremely small water content of the solvent. Both signals can cause difficulties with the dynamic range of the instrument. A further problem is the observation that carotenoids frequently possess a considerably reduced chemical stability if dissolved as extremely small quantities.

Despite these difficulties it is possible, in principle, to reduce further the sample quantity. In Fig. 3 is shown the 400 MHz p.m.r. spectrum of 0.25 μg of canthaxanthin obtained as the result of the accumulation of 116'000 free induction decays in 116 hours. The ^{13}C-side band of the solvent is now more than 10 times as intense as the strongest peak in the olefinic range. The sample was prepared by twofold dilution of a first solution with a known quantity of canthaxanthin. All the signals are visible and the integrals are mostly accurate within ca. 20 %. I consider that this spectrum which was presumably obtained from the smallest sample quantity ever used for the recording of the p.m.r. of a carotenoid convincingly demonstrates the high sensitivity and power of modern high-field p.m.r. instruments.

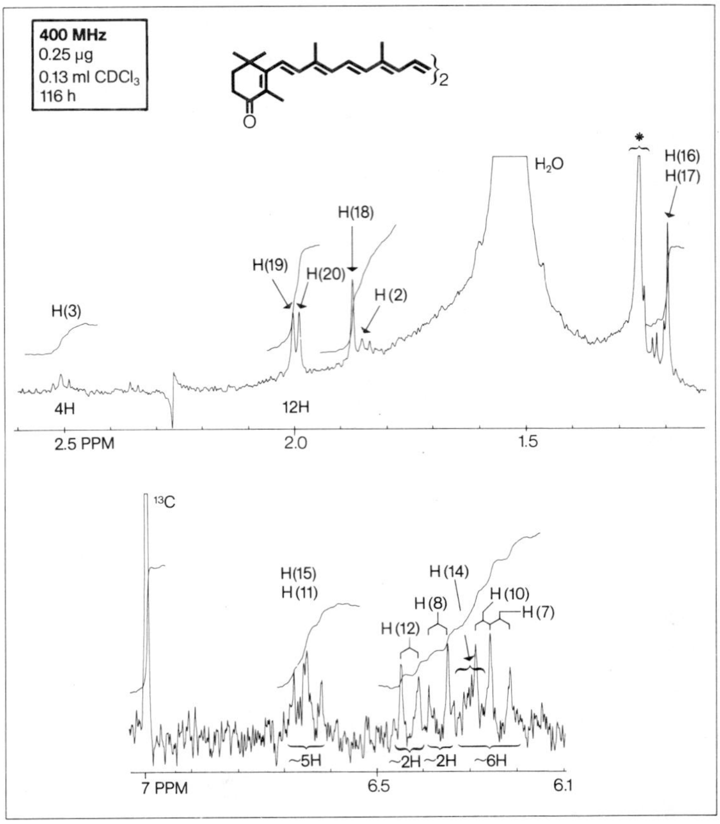

Fig. 3. 400 MHz p.m.r. spectrum of canthaxanthin; 0.25 µg in 0.13 ml $CDCl_3$ (100 % D quality); 116'000 pulses in 116 hours; * impurities.

P.M.R. DATA OF END GROUPS

The characterization of an unknown carotenoid usually begins with the identification by p.m.r. of the specific type of end group. During the last years we have compiled a collection of p.m.r. data of numerous end groups of natural and synthetic carotenoids and some examples are presented in Table 1. The chemical shifts in ppm and, in a few cases, the coupling constants in Hz, are average values taken mostly from several high-field spectra of retinoids and carotenoids. This collection of data displays an extended version of our previous one (Ref. 3) and will certainly be of great practical use for the identification of carotenoids. It is impossible here to discuss the data of Table 1 in detail. A few remarks, however, will be helpful.

Since it was found that the presence of a 9-cis configuration (in contrast to the much smaller contribution of a 13-cis configuration) may significantly influence some of the chemical shifts of the end groups these cases have been separately included in the data file. In a few cases the assignment of the α- or β- and axial or equatorial orientation of protons or methyl groups was possible based on the observed spin couplings or on homonuclear Overhauser experiments. It is thought that the chemical shifts of most end groups are reliable within ± 0.02 ppm if the side chain attached to the end group is at least a tetraene with no strongly anisotropic group at the end of the chain. The nature of the end group, on the other hand, will also influence to some extent the position of the signals of the polyene chain, albeit with decreasing magnitude along the chain. Therefore, the shifts of protons H(7), H(8), H(10) and H(19) are included in Table 1.

Table 1. Characteristic p.m.r. data of some typical end groups of natural and synthetic carotenoids (solvent $CDCl_3$).

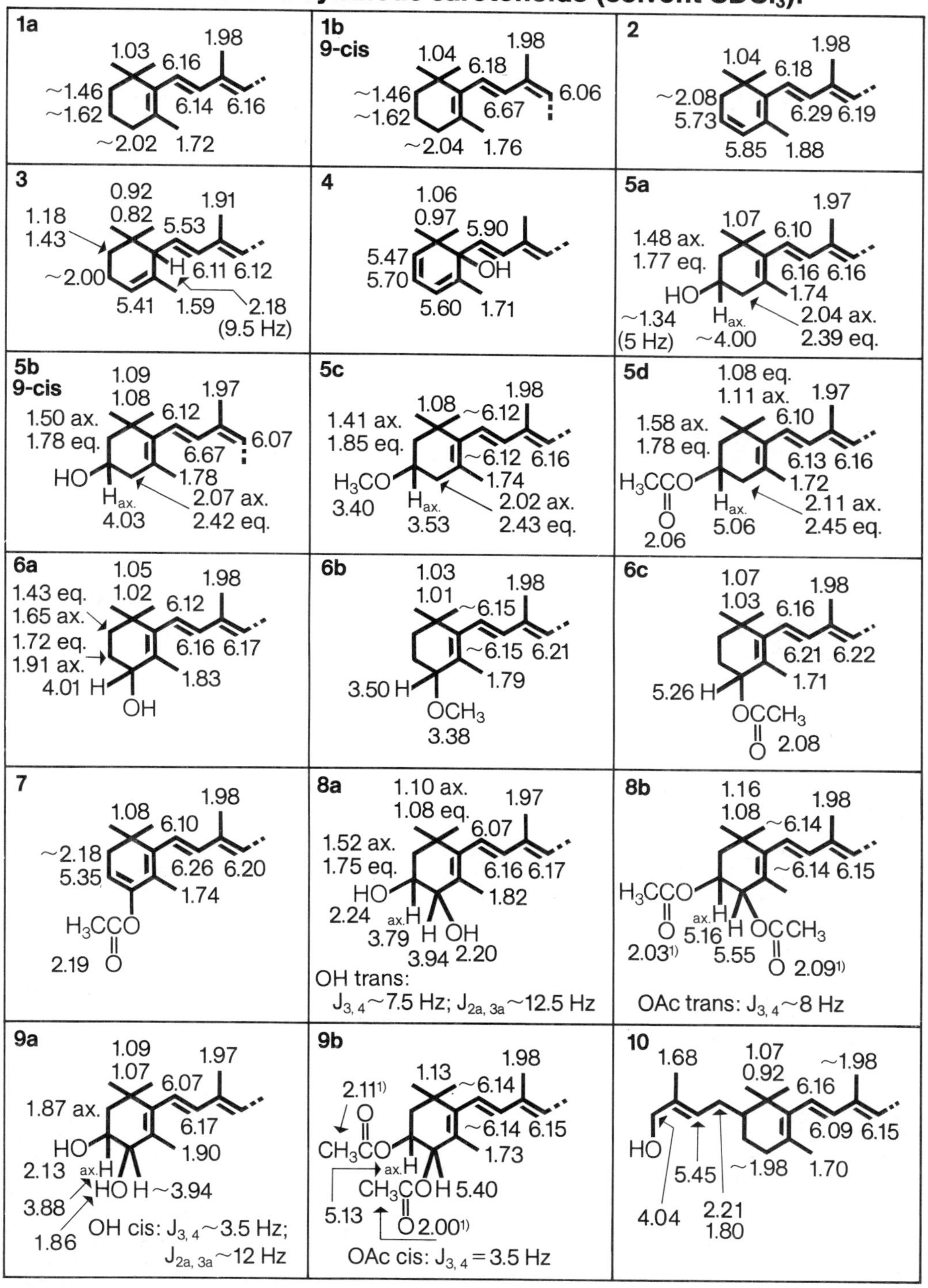

[1]Corresponding assignments may be reversed.

Table 1. Continued

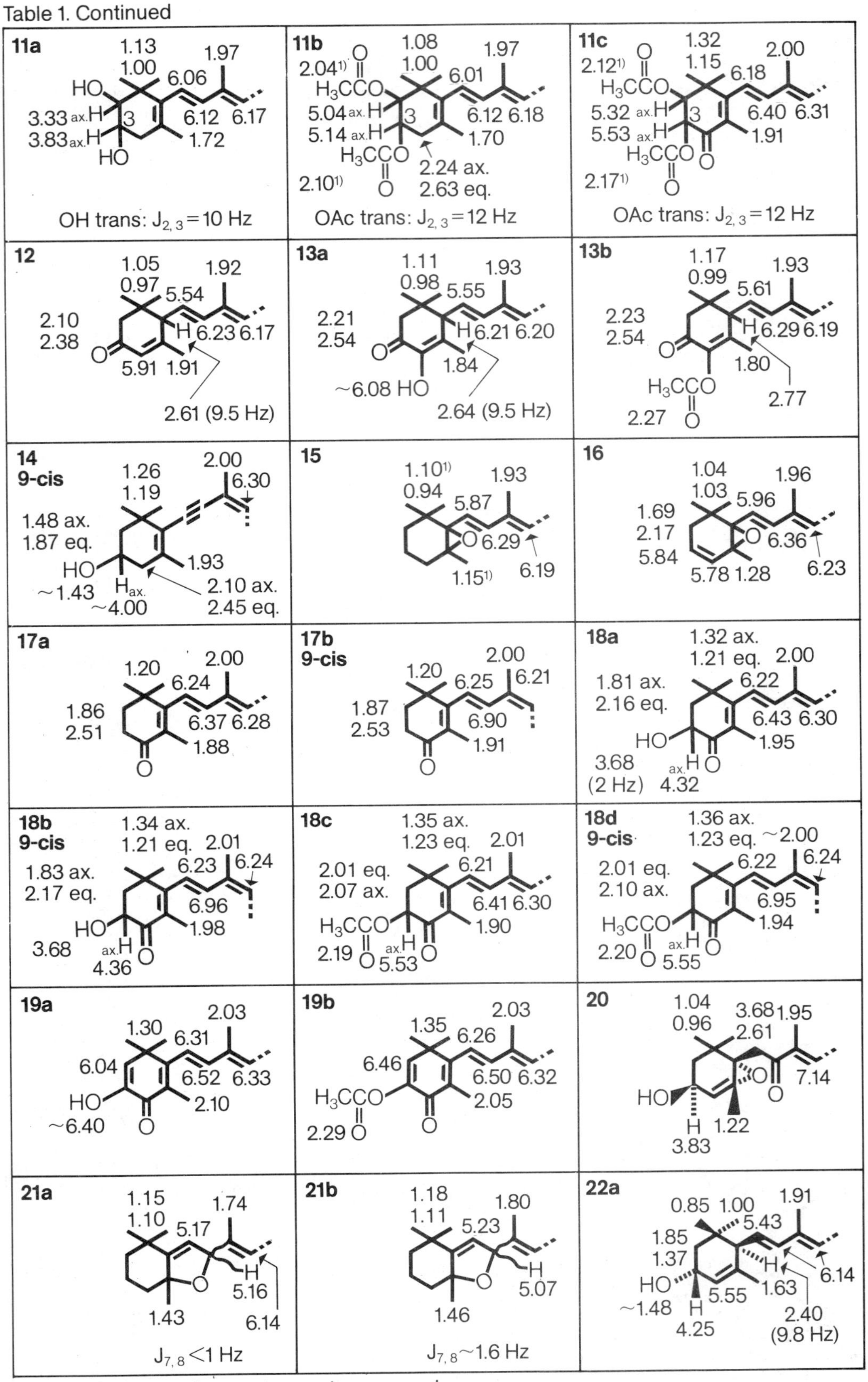

1) Corresponding assignments may be reversed.

Table 1. Continued

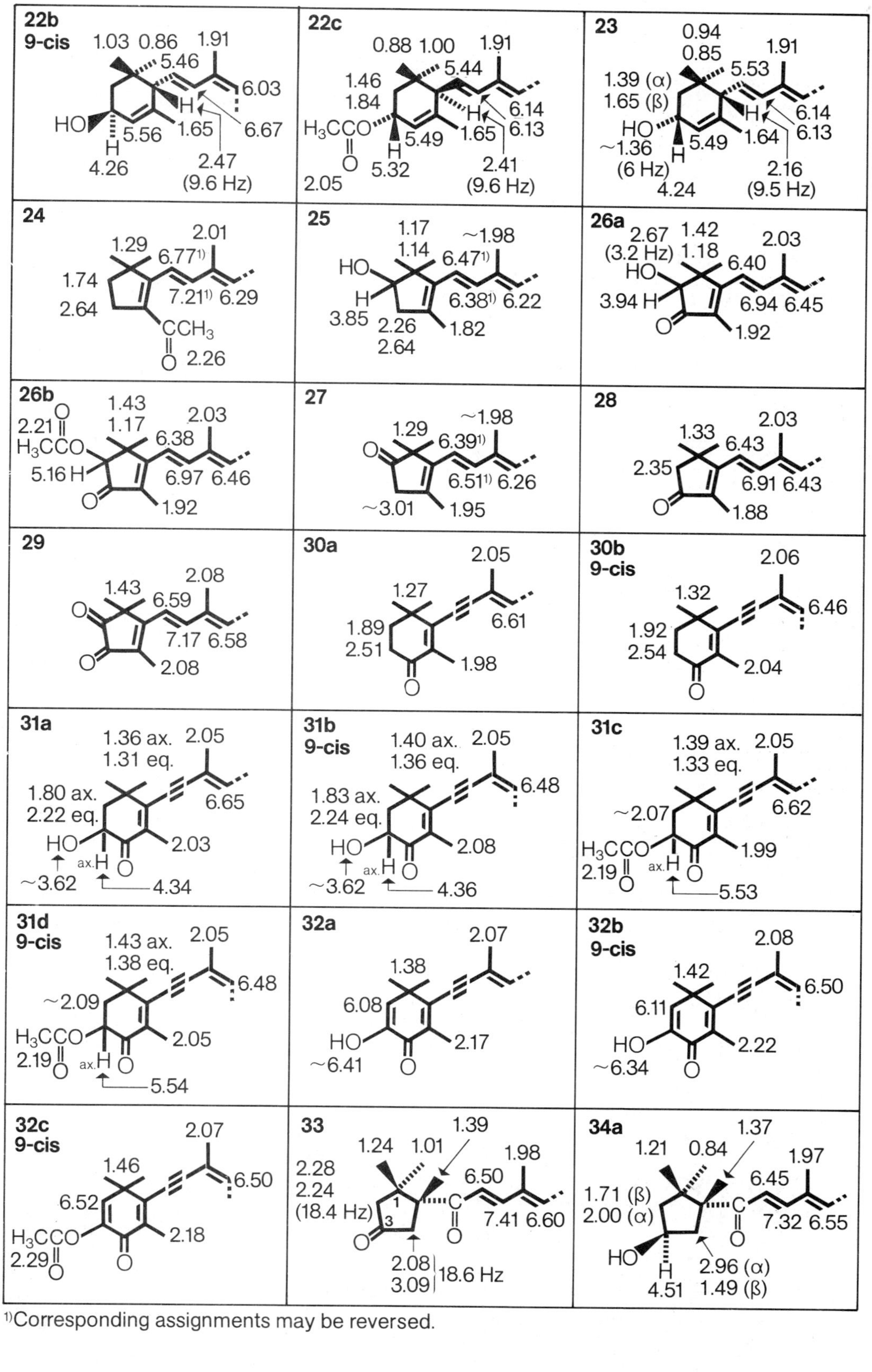

1)Corresponding assignments may be reversed.

Table 1. Continued

34b

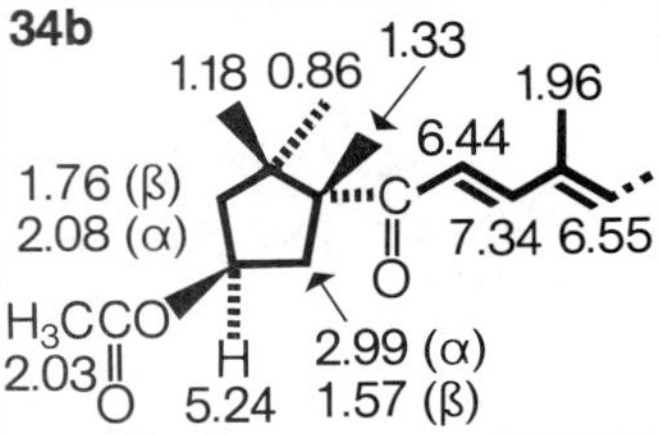

35a

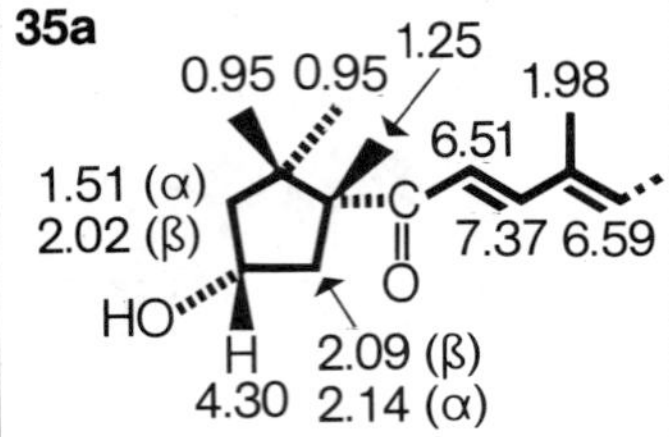

35b

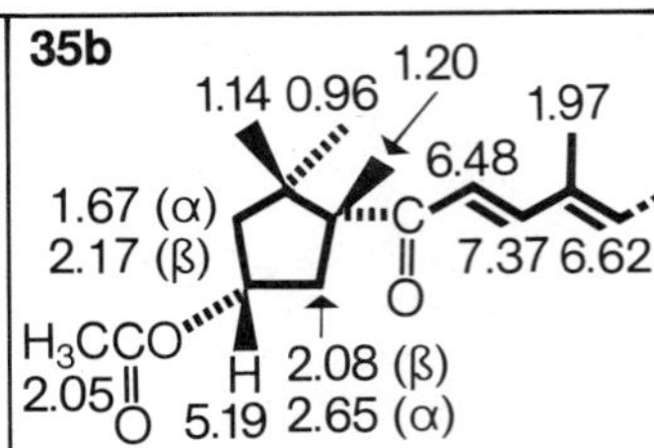

36a

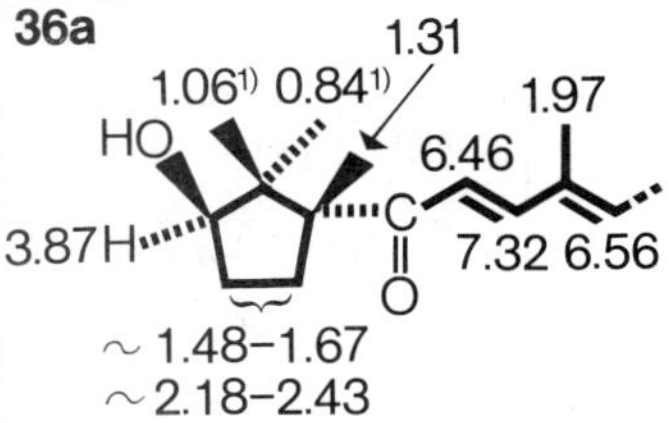

36b

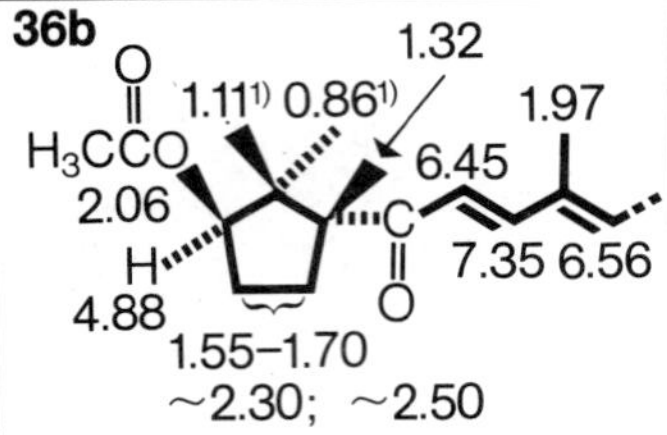

37

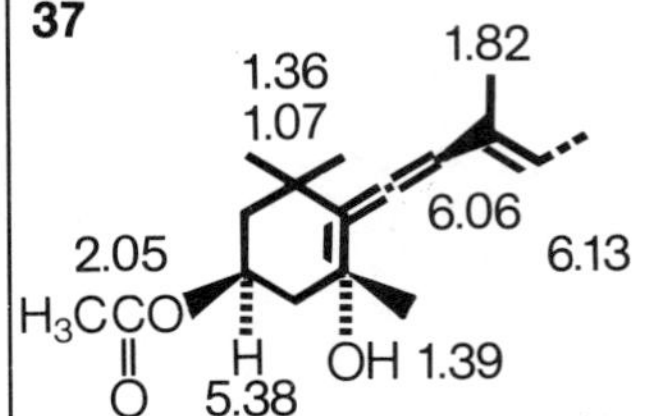

38a

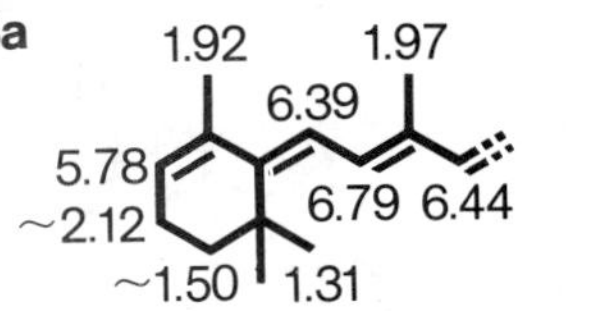

38b

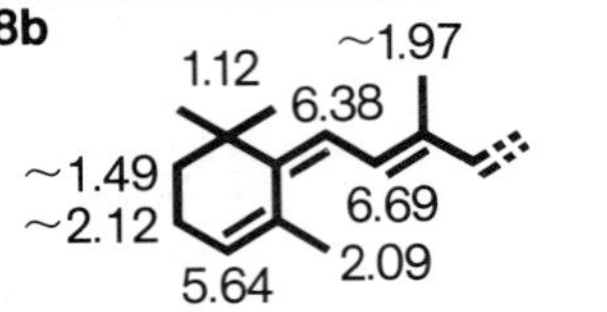

39a

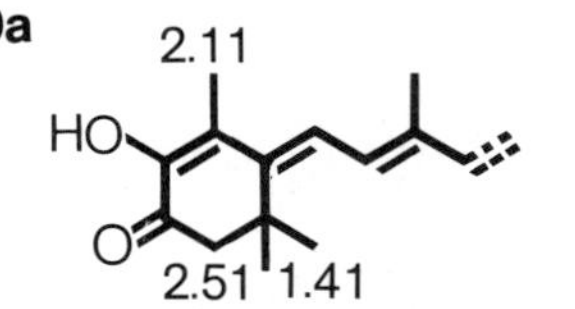

39b

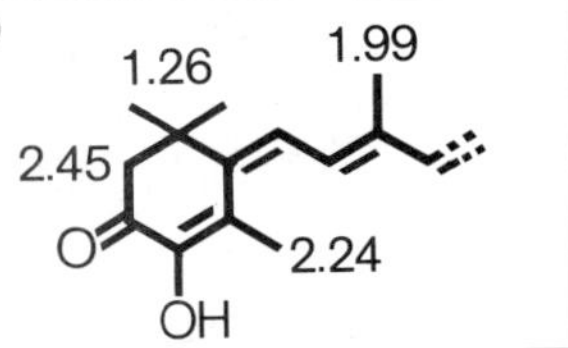

40a

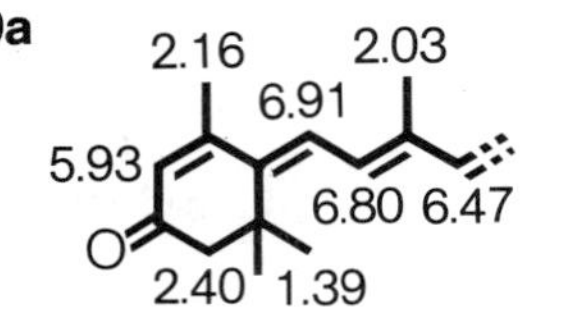

40b

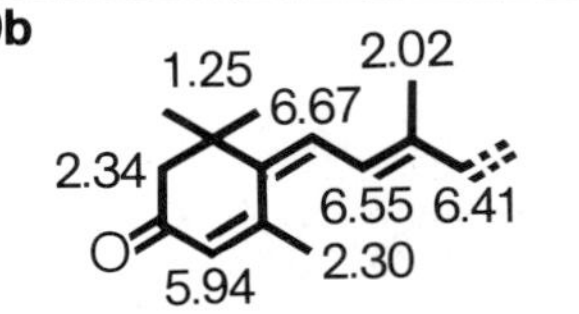

41a

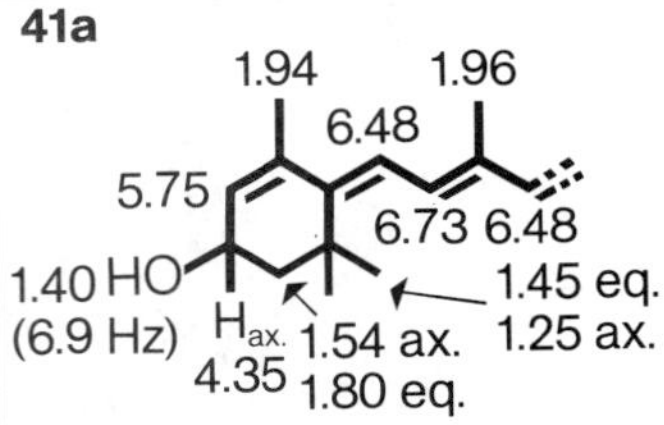

41b

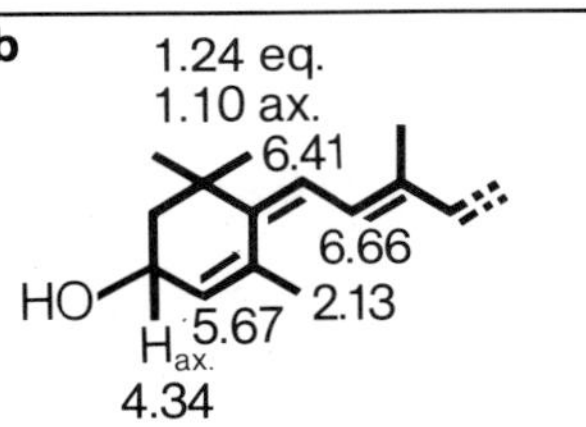

41c

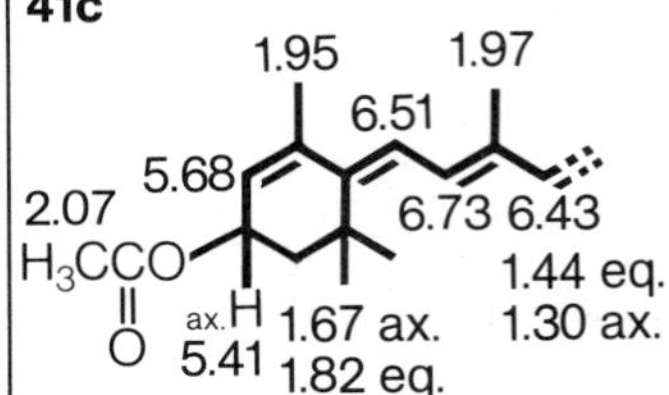

41d

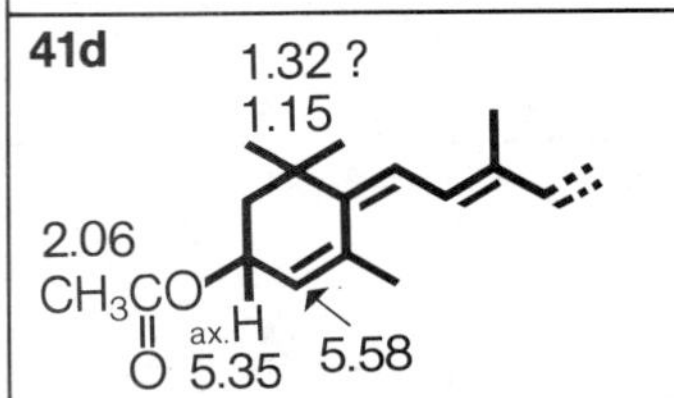

42a

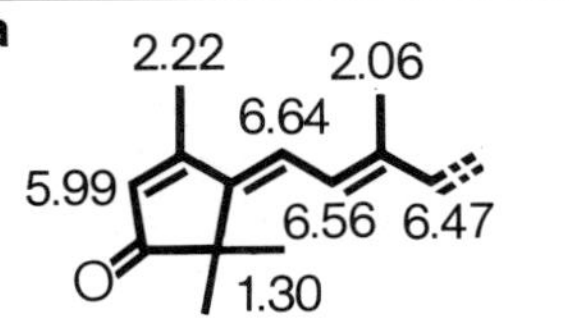

42b

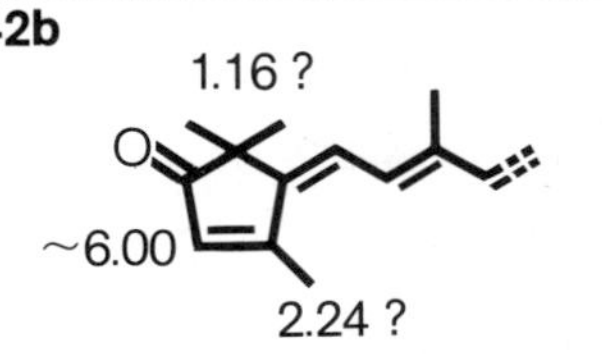

43

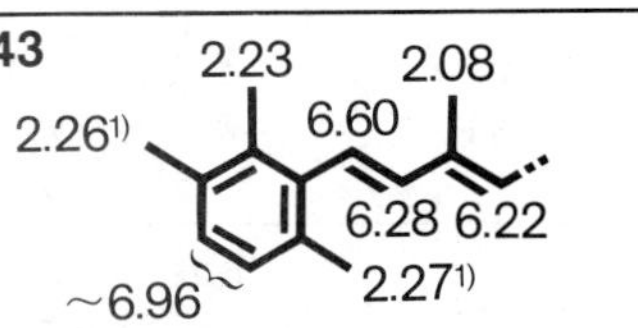

44

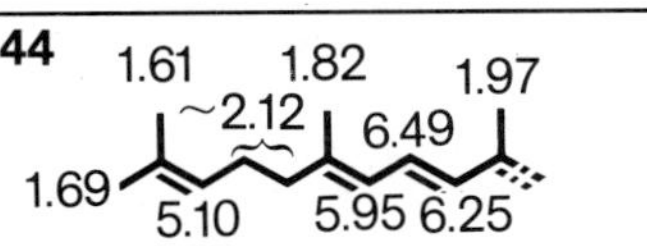

45

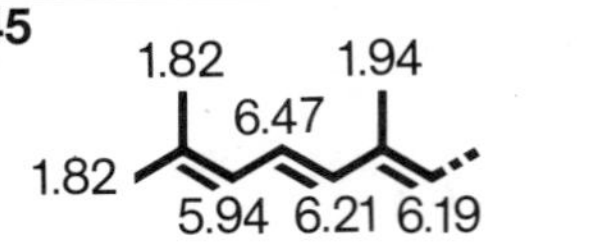

46

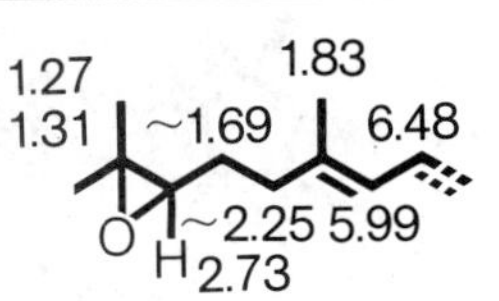

47

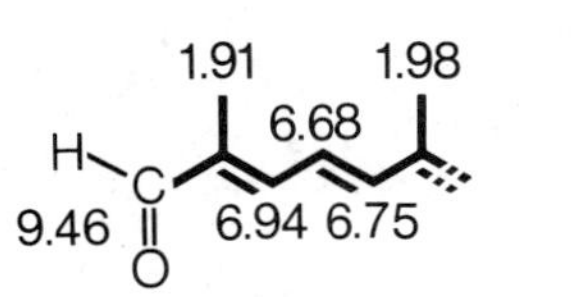

48

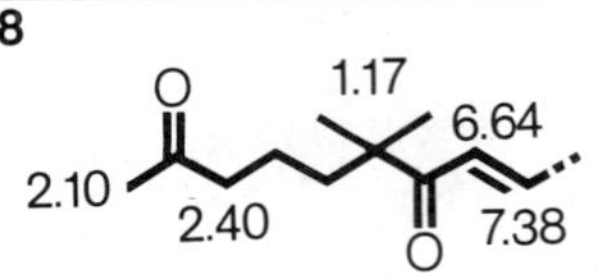

[1]Corresponding assignments may be reversed.

Some of the end groups are representatives of the class of retro carotenoids. Due to the shift of their double bonds their chemical shifts are, in general, completely different from normal carotenoids. By means of interproton Overhauser experiments the Trondheim group and I have recently proved that eschscholtzxanthin, rhodoxanthin and other related compounds, in general, possess preferentially Δ6,6'-di-trans configurations (Ref. 4). The latter have significantly different and therefore characteristic chemical shifts compared to the corresponding cis isomers which are sometimes observed as by-products. A number of such examples are given in Table 1 (see nos. 38 - 42).

In the meantime it was possible to separate completely by h.p.l.c. the three major isomers of rhodoxanthin, namely the all-trans, the 6-mono- and the 6,6'-di-cis isomers and to confirm their structures by 400 MHz p.m.r. spectroscopy including Overhauser experiments (Ref. 5). The all-trans structure of a further retro carotene, namely the 2,2'-dinor analogue of rhodoxanthin, will be proved below.

Since in many publications retro compounds can still be found presented as 6-cis it is strongly recommended that this habit should be left for those cases where the cis structure has been specifically proved by spectroscopic or other methods.

P.M.R. OF CIS ISOMERS

When a natural or synthetic carotenoid has been isolated and its end groups and the length of its polyene chain identified, a frequently encountered further task for p.m.r. is the confirmation of the all-trans or the deduction of the specific cis structure. In practice, this is in many cases hampered by the fact that cis isomers may be encountered as by-products in only very small concentrations. Therefore, the application of ^{13}C-n.m.r. is frequently excluded.

During the last few years we have successfully applied high-field p.m.r. spectroscopy to the elucidation of the structure of many cis isomeric retinoids and carotenoids. These compounds were in a few cases isolated by h.p.l.c. either as by-products of a synthesis or, in most cases, from a mixture artificially prepared by photoisomerization or refluxing in a suitable solvent (Ref. 6 & 7). In Zechmeister's monograph on cis-trans isomeric carotenoids (Ref. 8) a very comprehensive review on the preparation and isolation of numerous isomers is given, although their structural elucidation was only possible in a few simple cases due to the lack of high-field p.m.r. spectroscopy.

In Table 2 a survey is presented of some of the cis isomeric C_{40} carotenoids which were isolated so far, mostly by h.p.l.c. in quantities between 5 and 100 μg and identified by p.m.r. It is seen that the so-called unhindered cis isomers with 9-, 13- and 15-cis and combinations thereof occur relatively frequently. In contrast, the hindered cis isomers 11-cis and 9,11-di-cis were only available in the case of canthaxanthin and a number of apo-carotenoids not shown in the table. These isomers may have a reduced stability and we actually preferred to run their p.m.r. spectra at lower temperatures (between 0 and -20°).

Instead of discussing all the different spectra in detail I would rather like to present some empirical rules and figures extracted from our data which will certainly be very useful for the elucidation of related cis isomeric structures. For this purpose Fig. 4 shows a number of structural elements found in different cis isomers together with the value of the so-called isomerization shift Δ, that is the difference in ppm of the chemical shifts of the protons of the cis and trans compounds. As is seen this Δ-value is very characteristic and indicative for a given position of the cis bond in the polyene chain.

The strong downfield shift of approximately 0.5 ppm of the signals of H(8) in 9-cis, of H(10) in 11-cis, of H(12) in 13-cis compounds can again be interpreted as being at least partly caused by the newly introduced strong steric interaction with protons H(11), H(20) and H(15), respectively. Conversely, the increased shielding of the protons attached to the convex side of the molecules may be partly due to a release of some interactions.

It should be pointed out that the shifts of the "in-chain" methyl groups are, in general, very poorly indicative for the position of the cis bond and a significant shift change of ca. 0.1 ppm was observed only in the case of the two hindered cis isomers 11-cis and 9,11-di-cis Whether this result can be generalized seems, however, doubtful since in the spectrum of prolycopene which was recently identified as the 7,9,9',7'-tetra-cis isomer of lycopene (Ref. 9, 10 and 11) a corresponding downfield shift of the signal of H(19,19') of only 0.03 ppm was measured although a 7,9-di-cis configuration is intuitively expected to show similar Δ-values to the 11,13-di-cis structural unit.

A few further remarks concerning the data presented in Fig. 4 seem to be useful. If two cis bonds are present and sufficiently separated from each other, the effects of both are strictly additive as in the 9,9'-di-cis and 9,13'-di-cis isomers. In contrast, the Δ-values of a 9,13 -di-cis compound significantly deviate from additivity and this simplifies its differentiation from the 9,13'-di-*cis*.

TABLE 2. *Cis*-isomeric carotenoids identified by application of 270 MHZ or 400 MHz p.m.r. spectroscopy

Compound	Astaxanthin diacetate	Astaxanthin	Canthaxanthin	β-Carotene	Zeaxanthin	β-Cryptoxanthin	Lutein
9-*cis* 9'-*cis*	+	+	+	+	+	+	+ +
11-*cis*			+				
13-*cis* 13'-*cis*	+	+	+	+	+		+ +
15-*cis*	+	+	+	+	+	+	+
9,9'-di-*cis*	+		+	+	+		
9,11-di-*cis*			+				
9,13-di-*cis*	+	+	+	+			+
9,13'-di-*cis*	+			+			+
9,15-di-*cis*	+		+				
13,13'-di-*cis*	+		+	+			+
13,15-di-*cis*	+						
Ref.	a)	b)	c)	d)	e)	f)	g)

a) G. Englert and M. Vecchi, Helv. Chim. Acta 63, 1711 (1980).
b) G. Englert and V. Meduna, unpublished.
c) G. Englert and P. Kreienbühl, unpublished.
d) M. Vecchi and G. Englert, unpublished.
e) R. Marbet, H. Mayer and G. Englert, unpublished.
f) K. Bernhard and G. Englert, unpublished.
g) Mrs. K. Schiedt, M. Vecchi and G. Englert, unpublished.

It is clear that the reliability of the data presented in Fig. 4 heavily depends on the correctness of the assignments of the signals to the corresponding protons. That this is by no means always a trivial task is demonstrated as an example by the 400 MHz spectrum of 9-*cis* astaxanthin shown in Fig. 5. Due to the unsymmetric structure almost all the signals are doubled. In this and related cases a very simple method has proved useful when beginning the assignments. All signals of the *trans* half of the molecule can be easily identified by comparisonwith the spectrum ofthe all-*trans* compound. For the rest of the signals a few selective decoupling experiments are in general sufficient to link the remaining coupling partners. A further very powerful but time-consuming method, namely the two-dimensional J-spectroscopy, can also be helpful for the understanding of very complex spectra as will be demonstrated later.

HOMONUCLEAR OVERHAUSER EXPERIMENTS

Nuclear Overhauser (N.O.) experiments between protons are an extremely useful technique for the elucidation of the structure of stereoisomers. The N.O. effect is based on the known fact (Ref. 12) that two protons or groups of protons which are spatially sufficiently close to each other in a molecule are the main source of their mutual relaxation. This relaxation is predominantly caused by the time-dependent direct dipolar (through-space) couplings being modulated by the molecular tumbling in the liquid. Any change of the population of the spin states of either proton is partly transferred via relaxation processes to the other one. Thus, if one signal in a spectrum is saturated by the application of second radio-frequency of sufficient power this may result in a change of the population of the spin states of the neighbouring protons detected as a change of their signal intensity. For protons in molecules of small or medium size the N.O. enhancement is, in general, positive and always smaller than the theoretically predicted maximum of 50 % increase referred to the unperturbed signals. In practice, N.O. enhancements between ca. 10 and 25 % are considered as being strong effects. Since the enhancement is inversely proportional to the sixth power of the interproton distance a small increase of the distance will necessarily result in a rapid decrease of the observed effect.

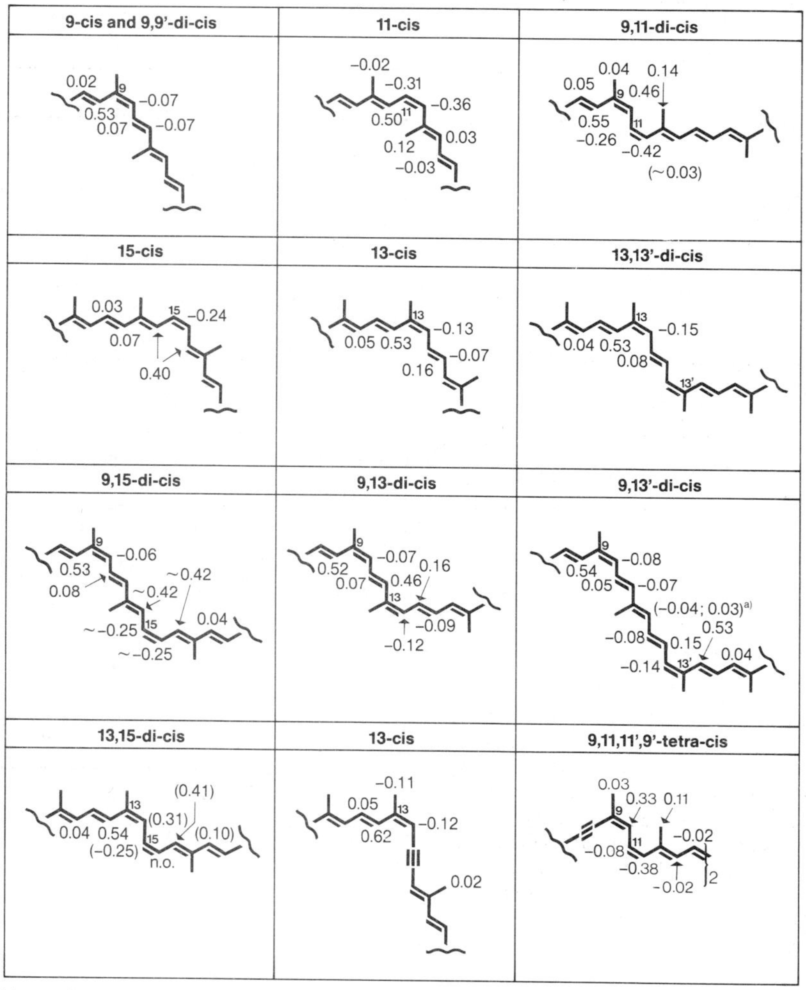

Note a): Slightly different values were obtained for the different compounds.

Fig. 4. Average values of the p.m.r. isomerization shifts $\Delta = \delta_{\underline{cis}} - \delta_{\underline{trans}}$ in ppm (solvent $CDCl_3$) for 12 different cis isomeric structures. Tentative values are given in parentheses.

By an improved experimental technique, the so-called N.O. difference spectroscopy, it is a simple routine experiment on modern FT-spectrometers to measure precisely N.O. enhancements down to ca. 1 % even in cases where the signals are strongly overlapped. This is possible since only the enhancement of the signals, that is the difference of the signal intensities with and without saturation, is directly measured. In this experiment the frequency of the decoupler is first set on the signal to be irradiated for 6 to 8 seconds. Then, after it is switched off, the excitation pulse is applied and the accumulation in the computer memory of the free induction decay (FID) is carried out as usual. The decoupler frequency is then positioned outside the spectrum (off-resonance) and, after a waiting-time, the subsequent FID is subtracted from the previous one. This procedure is automatically repeated under full computer control until the signal-to-noise of the resulting difference FID is satisfactory. After Fourier transformation the spectrum contains a strong negative signal due to the signal which was saturated in one half of the scans and some smaller, mainly positive signals, which are caused by the increase of intensity by the N.O. effect. All other signals without Overhauser enhancement are cancelled.

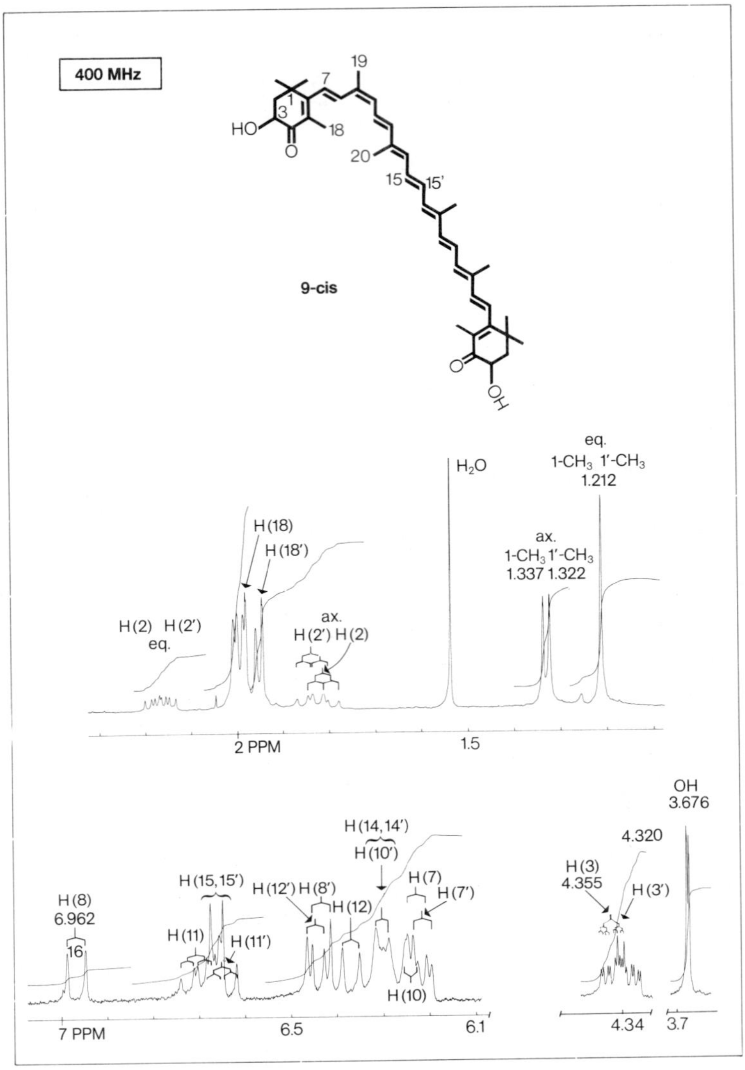

Fig. 5. 400 MHz p.m.r. spectrum of 9-cis astaxanthin; ca. 2 mg in 0.6 ml $CDCl_3$.

The magnitude of the achieved saturation and the increase of intensities by the N.O. effect can be quantitatively measured by comparison of the integrals with those of a control spectrum which was accumulated with one half the number of scans as above but with the decoupler frequency always off-resonance. The power of this method, which avoids complications due to decoupling effects, the shift of the signals due to Bloch-Siegert effects, and problems caused by signal overlapping, will be demonstrated in the following applications.

A first example is shown in Fig. 6. On the top trace is seen the olefinic part of the 400 MHz p.m.r. of 2,2'-dinor-rhodoxanthin the synthesis of which was recently described by Kienzle and Minder (Ref. 13). This compound is shown to be the all-trans compound by the following arguments: Saturation of protons H(16,17) absorbing at 1.302 ppm gives a strong enhancement of 11 % of H(8) and only weak effects at H(7) and H(4) of ca. 3 %. This proves that protons H(16,17) and H(8) are spatially close and hence that Δ6,6' are trans as depicted in the formula.

Interestingly the saturation of protons H(18) gives, besides a strong effect on H(4), only an unexpectedly weak enhancement of H(7). The strong enhancement of H(4) is explained by the fact that mainly protons H(18) are contributing to the relaxation of H(4), whereas H(7) is certainly additionally relaxed by other protons. The two experiments, however, indicate that Δ6,6' must be trans. The further two experiments with irradiation of the signals of H(19) and H(20) with enhancements of H(7) and H(11), and H(11) and the multiplet of the strongly coupled protons H(14,15,15',14') prove that Δ8, 10, 12 are trans as expected.

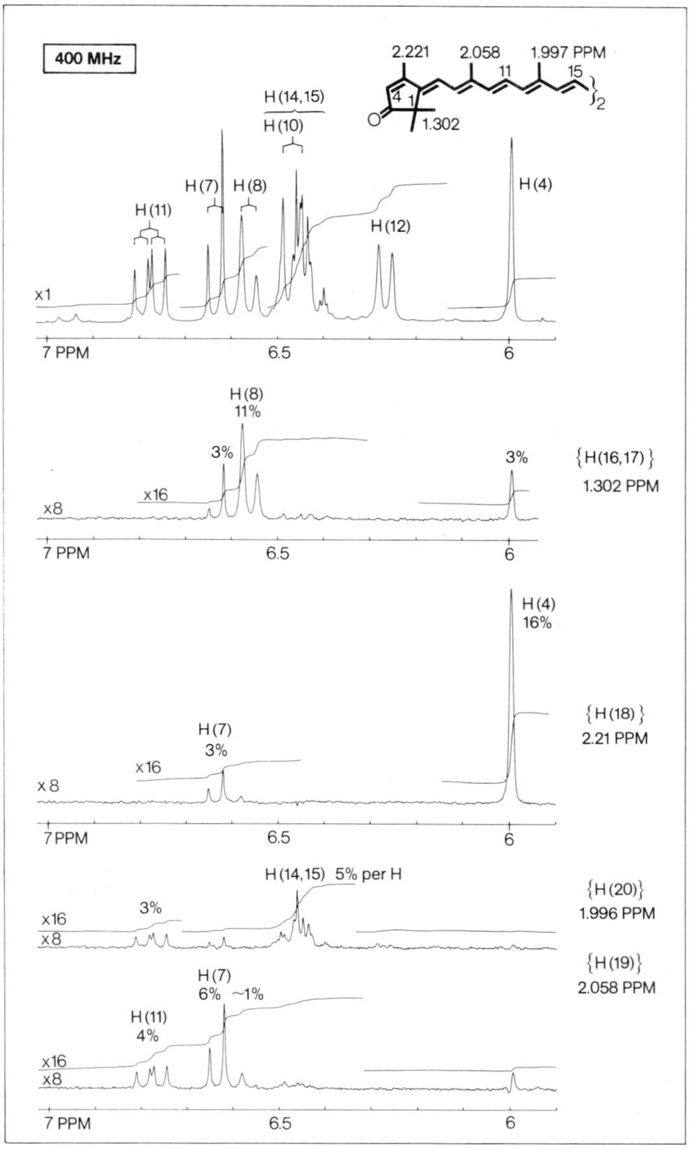

Fig. 6. Top: Olefinic part of the 400 MHz p.m.r. spectrum of 2,2'-dinor-rhodoxanthin in $CDCl_3$.
Lower traces: N.O. difference spectra obtained upon partial saturation of the signals of the different methyl protons.

It should be pointed out that in this and the following N.O. experiments it is only the relative magnitude of the enhancements which is relevant and not the absolute values. This is due to the fact that the power of the irradiation used in these experiments was, in general, smaller than that necessary to completely saturate the transition in order to avoid or reduce the saturation of neighbouring signals. Therefore, the observed N.O. enhancements may be significantly smaller than the theoretically expected values for a given interproton distance.

In Fig. 7 the 400 MHz p.m.r. spectrum is shown of all-trans 15,15'-didehydro-8'-apo-β-caroten-8'-al. Irradiation of protons H(18) results in N.O. enhancements of H(8) and H(7) with the former distinctly greater. This is in agreement with the known fact that the actual configuration is nearer to 6-s-cis than trans and hence the former is shown in the formula. Saturation of protons H(19) give N.O. effects at H(11) and H(7) proving Δ7 and Δ9 are trans. Irradiation of H(20) and H(20') gives similarly enhancements of H(11) and the multiplet of the strongly coupled H(11) and H(12').

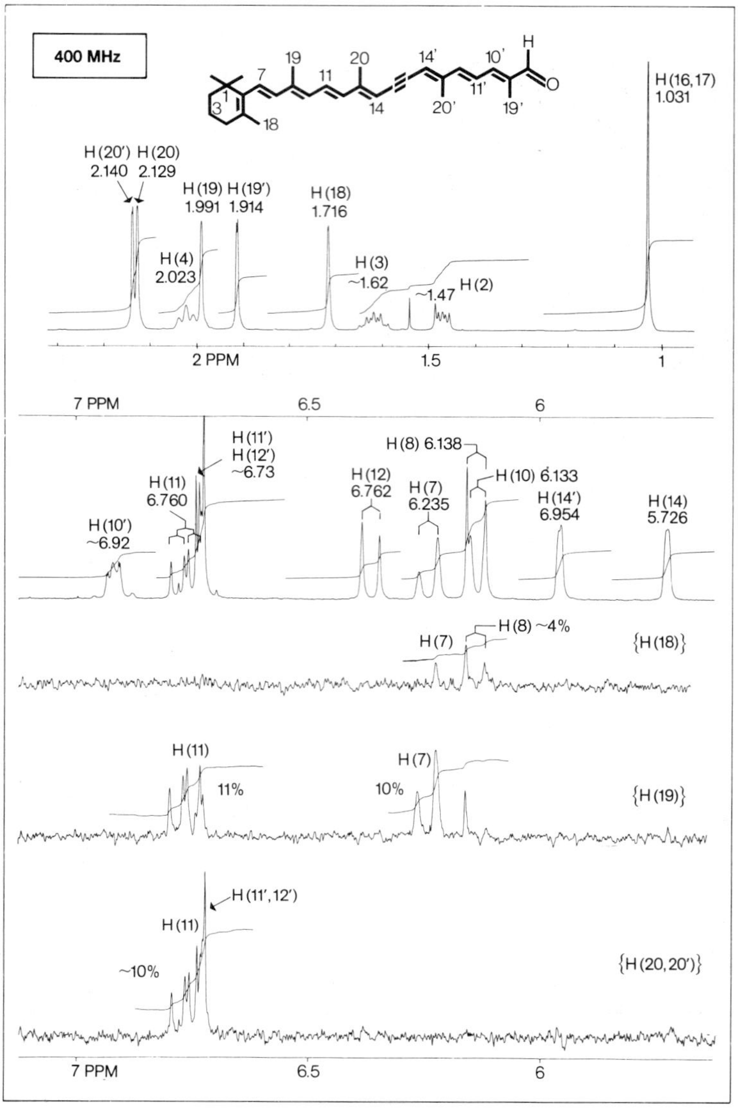

Fig. 7. 400 MHz p.m.r. spectrum and N.O. difference spectra of 15,15'-didehydro-8'-apo-β-caroten-8'-al ($CDCl_3$).

Up to now only signals of the methyl protons were saturated. In Fig. 8 it is demonstrated for the same compound that N.O. enhancements are in the same way measurable if the olefinic signals are saturated provided they are sufficiently separated from each other.

In the first experiment the signal of the aldehyde proton is saturated which then appears as a negative signal in the difference spectrum. By comparison with the control spectrum obtained with a corresponding number of scans and with the decoupler off-resonance it can be deduced from the integral that the aldehyde proton was approximately 90 % saturated. The only other signal, now with positive intensity, belongs to H(10'). This proves that both protons are spatially close to each other, i.e. that Δ9' is trans and the single bond between C(8') and C(9') prefers the s-trans configuration.

Conversely, if H(10') is saturated an even stronger enhancement of H(8') (which is practically solely relaxed by H(10')) is observed. The positive effect on H(12') is also detected. However, this signal is too close and therefore a direct saturation cannot be avoided when irradiating H(10'). The next three N.O. experiments prove that H(12) and H(14) are on the same side of the olefinic chain as well as H(14') and H(12'). Thus, the whole geometry of the olefinic chain is easily deduced.

The next three figures show N.O. difference experiments with the corresponding 9'-cis carotenal the structure of which was conclusively proven by these experiments.

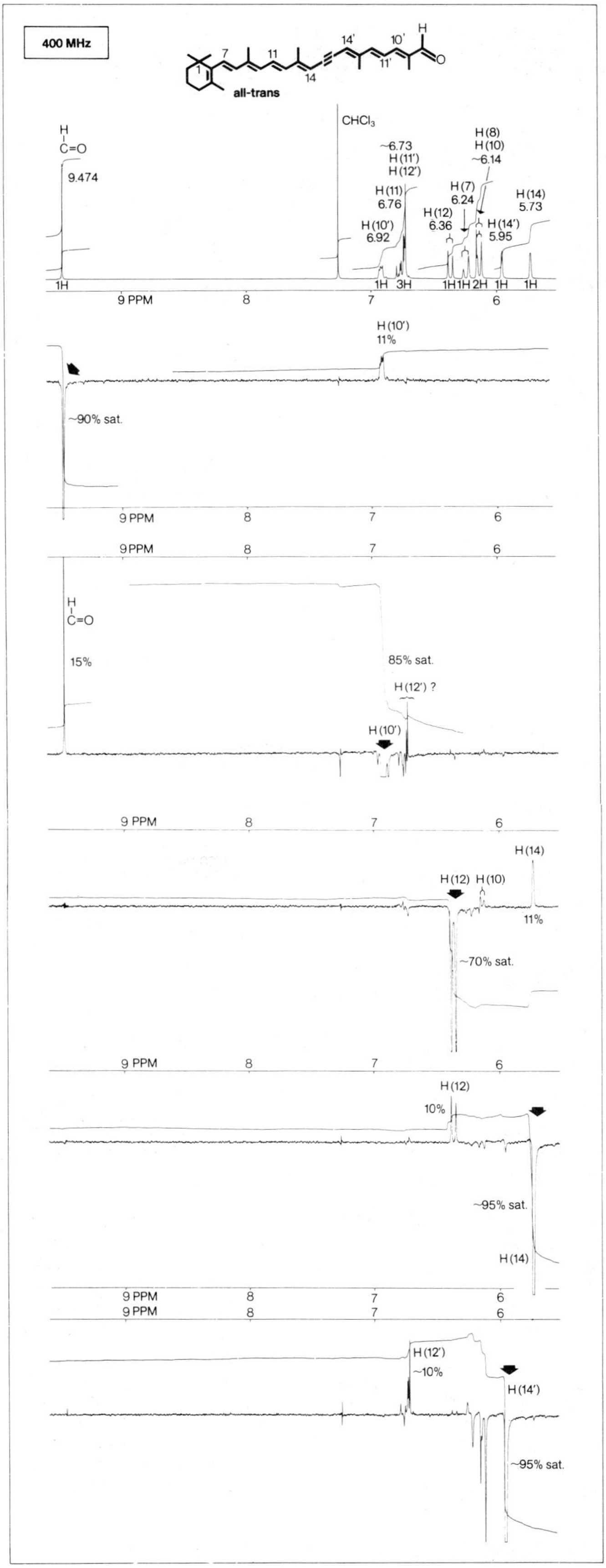

Fig. 8. 400 MHz p.m.r. spectrum and N.O. difference spectra of 15,15'-didehydro-8'-apo-β-caroten-8'-al ($CDCl_3$). The positions of the irradiation are indicated by arrows.

Fig. 9 shows the result of the saturation of the different methyl signals. The N.O. effects at H(8) upon irradiation of H(18) and at H(7) and H(8) upon irradiation of H(16,17) may again be qualitatively interpreted by the assumption that in solution the 6-s-configuration is probably nearer to 6-s-*cis* than *trans*, a result which has been confirmed in several other cases of compounds with β- end groups. From the three further experiments the last one, namely irradiation of H(19') and the N.O. enhancement of H(10') is decisive for the proof of the 9'-*cis* configuration of this compound.

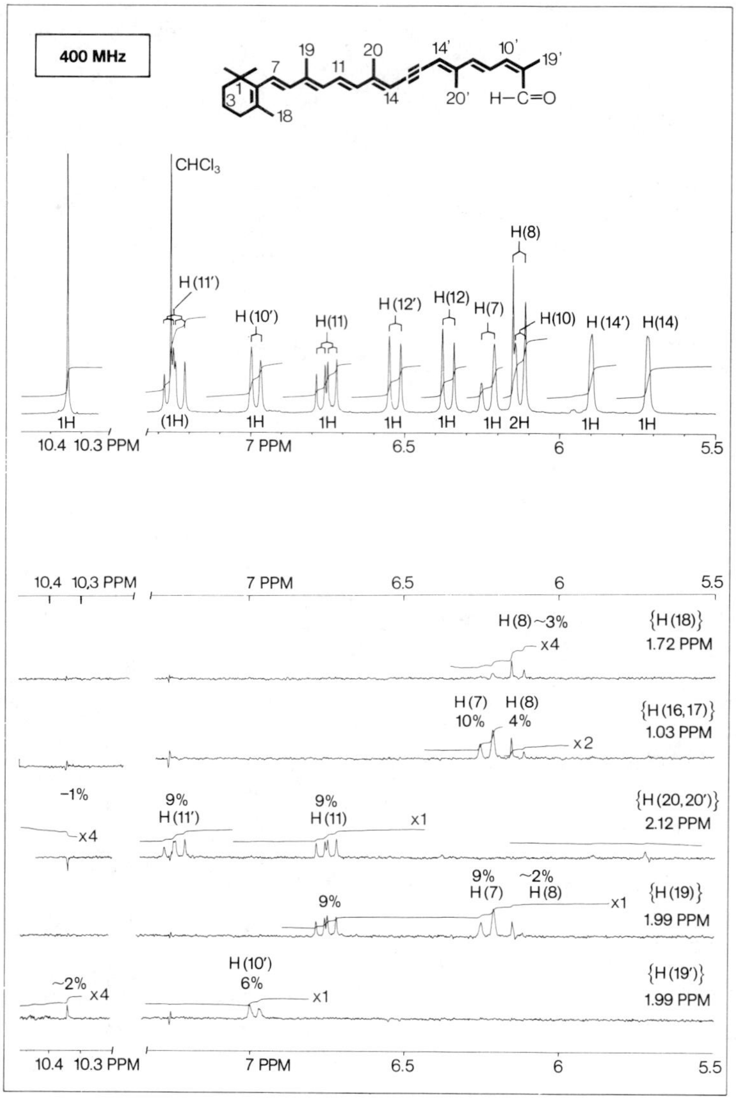

Fig. 9. 400 MHz p.m.r. spectrum (olefinic section) and N.O. difference spectra of the 9'-*cis* isomer of 15,15'-didehydro-8'-apo-β-caroten-8'-al ($CDCl_3$).

Fig. 10 shows further experiments with the same compound with irradiation of some olefinic protons. These experiments again demonstrate how one can start at one end of the molecule and derive a conclusive picture of the geometry of the olefinic chain.

In the literature it is frequently stated that N.O. enhancements of methyl signals are unobservably small due to the fact that the three protons are mainly relaxed by each other (Ref. 14). Hence, their N.O. enhancement upon irradiation of a spatially proximate olefinic proton is expected to remain very small. With the N.O. difference technique, however, it is possible to measure N.O. enhancements with sufficient sensitivity and two examples are presented in Fig. 11. Here is shown the aliphatic part of the same 9'-*cis* carotenal as before.

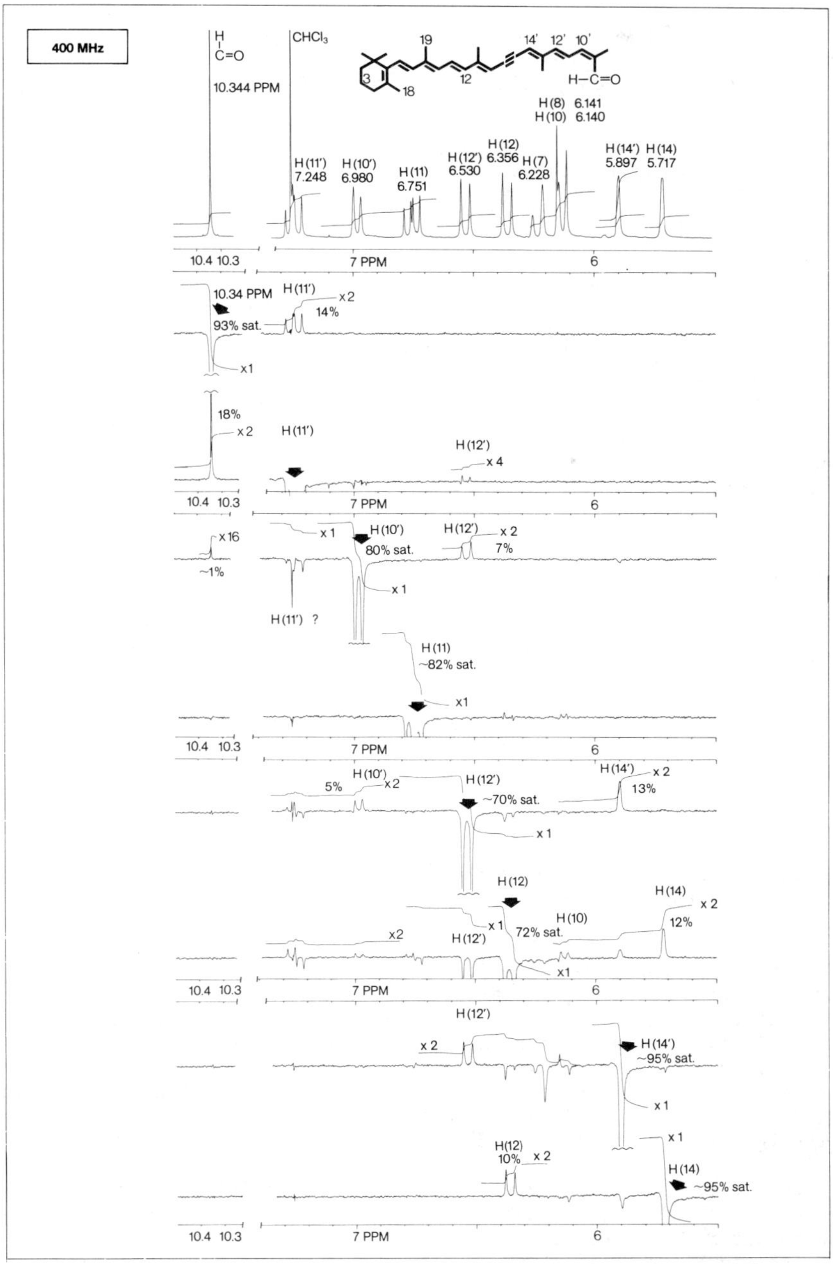

Fig. 10. 270 MHz p.m.r. spectrum (olefinic section) and N.O. difference spectra of 9'-cis 15,15'-didehydro-8'-apo-β-caroten-8'-al ($CDCl_3$).

Irradiation of the signals of H(10') and H(11') give N.O. enhancements of ca. 2 % of H(19') and of ca. 3 % of H(20'). Although these effects are small they are no doubt a positive indication of the shown molecular geometry. In addition, irradiation of H(16,17) gives a small (~ 5 %) and a very small enhancement of the neighbouring protons H(2) and H(3). In this way, the neighbouring protons of an unknown end group might be located in a complex spectrum.

In Fig. 12 is presented the 400 MHz spectrum of 2,2'-dinor-β,β-carotene-4,4'-dione (Ref. 13). Here, irradiation of H(16,17) clearly gives enhancements of H(8) and H(7) of approximately the same magnitude. Irradiation of H(18) also results in a N.O. enhancement of both protons. An obvious explanation of these results is the assumption that the actual configuration of the molecule in solution is approximately in the middle between 6-s-cis and 6-s-trans. The two further experiments, namely irradiation of the two "in-chain" methyl groups giving N.O. enhancements mainly of H(7) and H(11), and of H(11') and H(15), respectively, are in agreement with the known all-trans configuration of the olefinic chain.

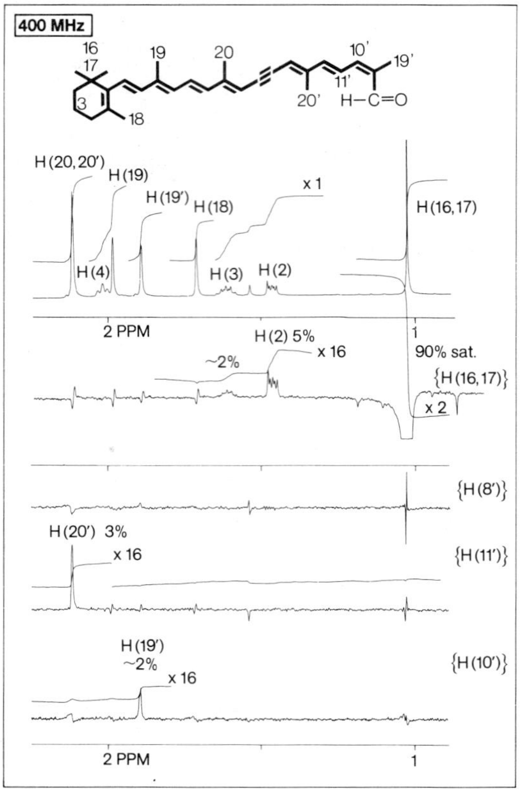

Fig. 11. 400 MHz p.m.r. spectrum (aliphatic part) and N.O. difference spectra of 9'-cis 15,15'-didehydro-8'-apo-β-caroten-8'-al ($CDCl_3$).

N.O. experiments not only can reveal the geometry of a polyene chain but can also be successfully used for the assignment of the axial and equatorial or α and β orientation of protons or methyl groups of the end groups (see Table 1). For example, in Fig. 13 the 270 MHz spectrum is shown of all-trans zeaxanthin diacetate. In contrast to zeaxanthin the diacetate has slightly differently shielded methyl groups attached to C(1). As is seen from the two N.O. experiments the methyl group absorbing at slightly lower field must be in a 1,3-diaxial relationship to H(3). That the latter is axial follows from the large coupling constants of 12 and 10 Hz to the two axial partners at C(2) and C(4).

By a series of selective decoupling experiments it was possible to unequivocally link the axial and equatorial methyl protons with the corresponding ^{13}C-signals in the ^{13}C-n.m.r. spectrum. As a result it was found that the ^{13}C-signal at 28.6 ppm corresponds to the axial methyl carbon, the signal at 30.1 ppm to the equatorially oriented methyl group. Hence, the relative position of the two types of signals in the p.m.r. and the ^{13}C-n.m.r. are interchanged.

In the course of ^{13}C-labelling studies in the biosynthesis of lycopene and its cyclisation to zeaxanthin it was found by the Liverpool group that the C(1) methyl substituents retain their individuality since enrichment of ^{13}C was only observed at the carbon giving rise to the signals at 28.8 ppm of zeaxanthin and at 28.6 ppm of the diacetate. The latter signal was unequivocally assigned in the described experiments to the axial methyl group. Concerning the biosynthetic conclusions to be drawn from these experiments I refer to Ref. 15.

These selected applications of the N.O. effect clearly demonstrate the great use and power of this technique. In the following section some examples of a relatively recent method, the so-called two-dimensional J-spectroscopy (2DJ) are presented which, to the best of my knowledge, has not yet been applied in the field of carotenoids.

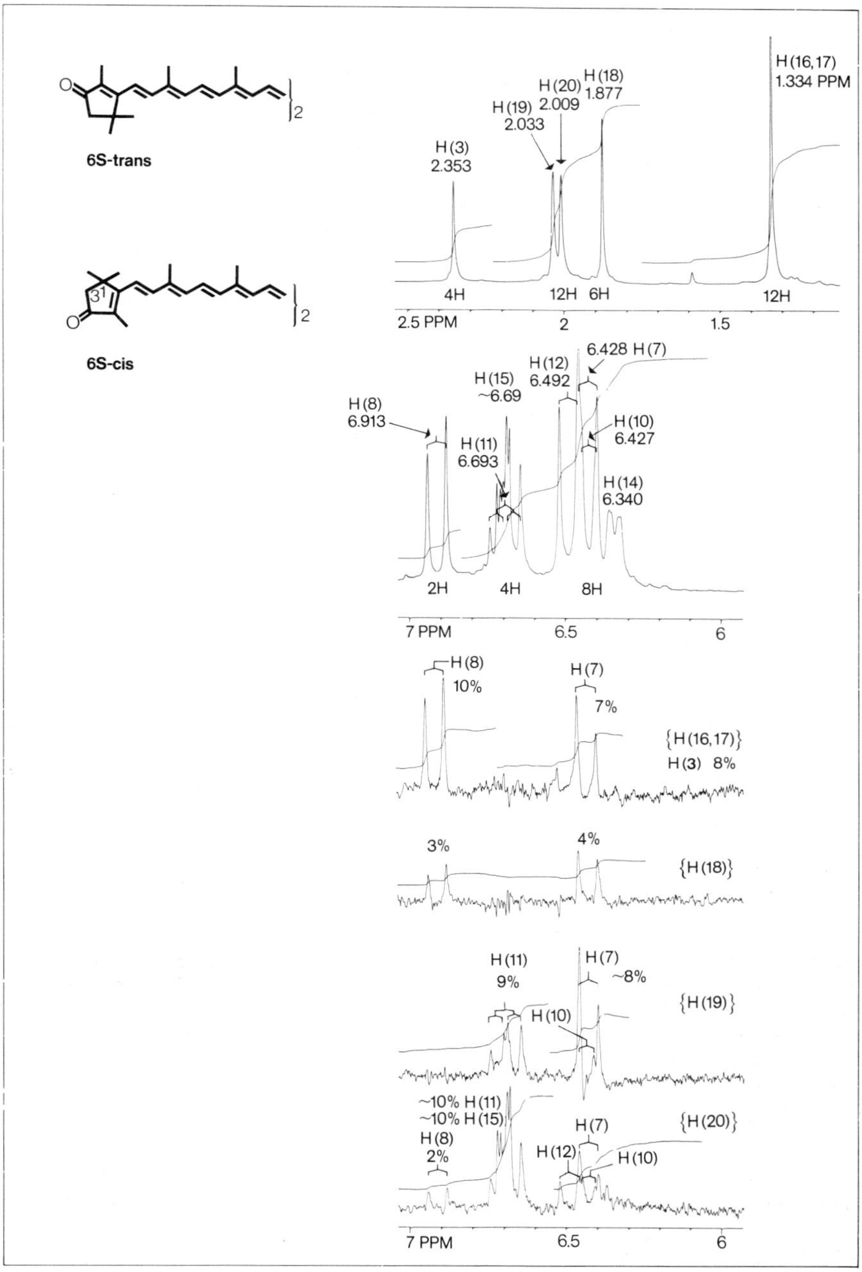

Fig. 12. 270 MHz p.m.r. spectrum and N.O. difference spectra of 2,2'-dinor-β,β-carotene-4,4-dione ($CDCl_3$).

2DJ-RESOLVED P.M.R. SPECTROSCOPY

From several different two-dimensional n.m.r. methods now available (Ref. 16 & 17) the so-called 2DJ-resolved spectroscopy (where J stands for the usual J spin-spin coupling) is probably of specific interest here since it exhibits a very elegant and effective means of separating and identifying the different multiplets of a strongly overlapping spectrum.

The principles and the experimental details of the 2DJ-spectroscopy cannot be treated here in detail. The basic experimental sequence consists of a 90° pulse at the beginning of the so-called evolution period of duration t_1. In the middle of it (at $t_1/2$) a 180° pulse is applied producing a spin-echo at the end of the evolution period. Now, the signal accumulation of duration t_2 starts. In a series of measurements t_1 is varied leading to a phase modulation of the signal at the beginning of the accumulation period. Instead of only one time variable one has now two which, after a two-dimensional Fourier transformation and some data manipulation, yield a 2DJ-spectrum. The practical aspects are seen in the following figures.

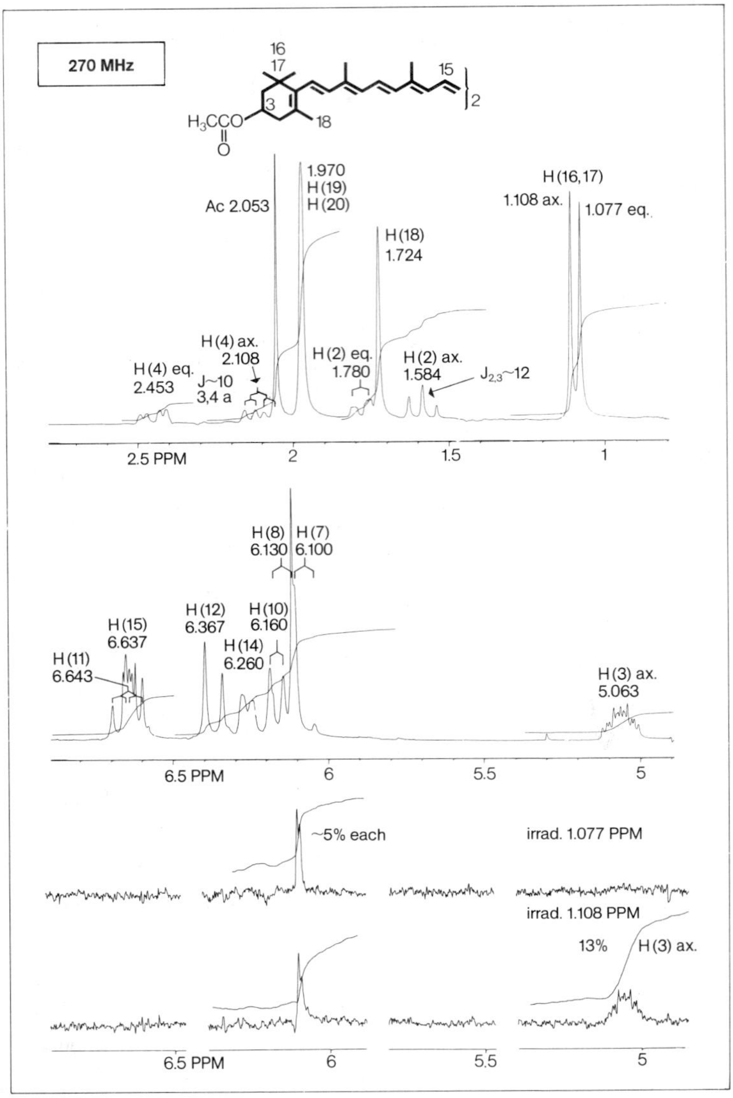

Fig. 13. 270 MHz p.m.r. spectrum of zeaxanthin diacetate in $CDCl_3$. Bottom: N.O. difference spectra upon partial saturation of the signals of the equatorial and axial methyl protons at C(1).

In a normal or one-dimensional (1D) spectrum (see top of Fig. 14) the different multiplets appearing at specific chemical shifts and with typical J-couplings are spread along the single frequency axis and are, therefore, strongly overlapping.

In a 2DJ-spectrum (see Note a), on the other hand, the chemical shift and spin coupling information are spread along two different frequency axes, the δ- and J-axes, as is seen in Fig. 14. Thus, a 2DJ-spectrum has two frequency axes and, of course, a third dimension containing the intensities. It appears as if each J-multiplet was simply rotated about its center frequency, i.e. about its chemical shift. If one looks along the J-direction every multiplet produces a single peak in this projection on the δ-axis. The peak positions correspond to the different chemical shifts.

Note a. The Bruker FTNMR2D-Program version 801010 was used for these measurements.

This δ-projection therefore looks as if all the protons were decoupled from each other, as in a broad-band homonuclear decoupled spectrum. The ideal separation of the two frequency axes is possible only for the case of weakly coupled spin systems (Ref. 18) and this ideal condition is certainly only approximated in the case of the olefinic protons of a carotenoid. This causes the appearance of some extra peaks and artifacts in the shown 2DJ-spectrum. In addition, some further signals arise from the folding of signals from outside the measured region.

A 2DJ-plot as the one seen at the bottom of Fig. 14 is actually not very informative since many of the signals are masked by other stronger ones. A much better way is to plot the different cross sections along the J-axis which are selected at those positions on the δ-axis corresponding to the maxima of the δ-projection, i.e. at the exact chemical shifts of the J-multiplets. This is shown in Fig. 15 where all these J-cross sections are shown starting at low-field with the chloroform singlet and ending-up with the multiplet of H(3) at higher field. In this way, a complex spectrum has been separated into the basic multiplets from which it is built up.

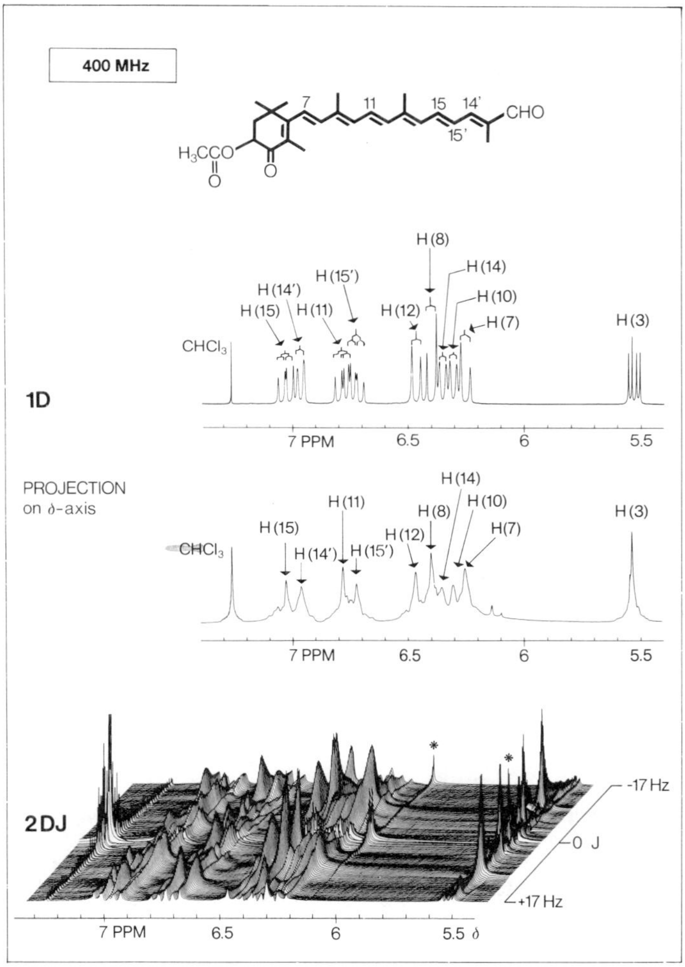

Fig. 14. Top: 400 MHz p.m.r. spectrum (olefinic section) of 3-acetoxy-4-oxo-12'-apo-β-caroten-12'-al in $CDCl_3$. Middle: Projection of the 2DJ-spectrum on the δ-axis. Bottom: 2DJ-spectrum (128 x 8192 data points, 0.27 Hz per point); * artifacts.

A further property of 2DJ-spectroscopy is seen at the doublets of protons H(14') and H(8). These signals show additional and well-resolved long-range splittings which are, in general, unobservable in a 1D experiment. The basic theory of 2DJ-spectroscopy shows that along the J-axis it is the natural line-width of the signals (as in a spin-echo experiment) which is observed provided the digital resolution can be made sufficiently high. This means that any residual field inhomogeneity will not contribute to the line-width along the J-axis, thus 2DJ-spectroscopy leads to an improved resolution.

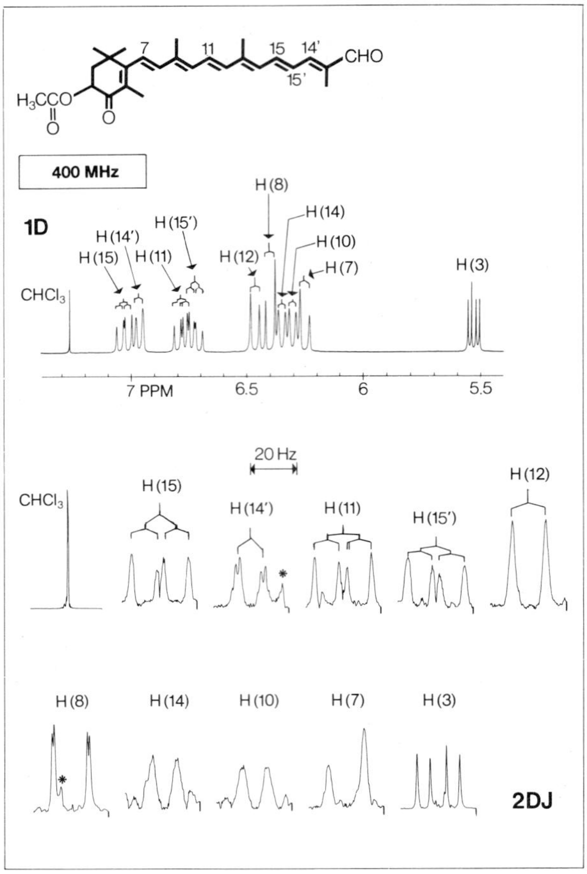

Fig. 15. Top: 400 MHz p.m.r. spectrum (olefinic section) of 3-acetoxy-4-oxo-12'-apo-β-caroten-12'-al in $CDCl_3$. Bottom: Cross sections of the 2DJ-spectrum along the J-axis taken at the peak positions of the projection on the δ-axis (middle of Fig. 14); * artifacts.

In Fig. 16 are presented the two low-field sections of the 1D-spectrum of 9-cis astaxanthin (top) and the J-cross sections, showing the multiplets which could be sorted out by the 2DJ-method. All multiplets were detected despite the relatively poor signal-to-noise ratio with the exception of the expected doublet of H(10) which, according to double resonance experiments must be hidden near 6.23 ppm.

That the quality of the separation of the δ- and J-information along the two frequency axes can be perfect if the protons are only weakly coupled is demonstrated in Fig. 17, where only the section of the 1D-spectrum is shown with the two slightly differently shielded protons H(3) and H(3') of 9-cis astaxanthin (bottom, left), together with the δ-projection with the two singlet signals and the two J-cross sections with the completely separated multiplets.

On the basis of my own limited experience with this new experimental technique I do feel that its application in specific cases of great complexity could be of great use in the field of carotenoids although a considerable amount of instrument time is necessary to perform such experiments.

HIGH-FIELD ^{13}C-N.M.R. SPECTROSCOPY

As an excellent supplement to p.m.r., ^{13}C-n.m.r. spectroscopy has become of increasing importance in the field of retinoids and carotenoids (see e.g. Ref. 19, 20 & 21). However, its application is greatly hampered by the relatively low sensitivity compared to p.m.r. Although the sensitivity of modern instruments has steadily increased over the years the sample quantity necessary for a broad-band decoupled ^{13}C-n.m.r. spectrum of good quality must still be of the order of 1 mg if excessive accumulation times are to be avoided. This means that compared to p.m.r. ca. 500 to 1000 fold larger sample quantities must be available.

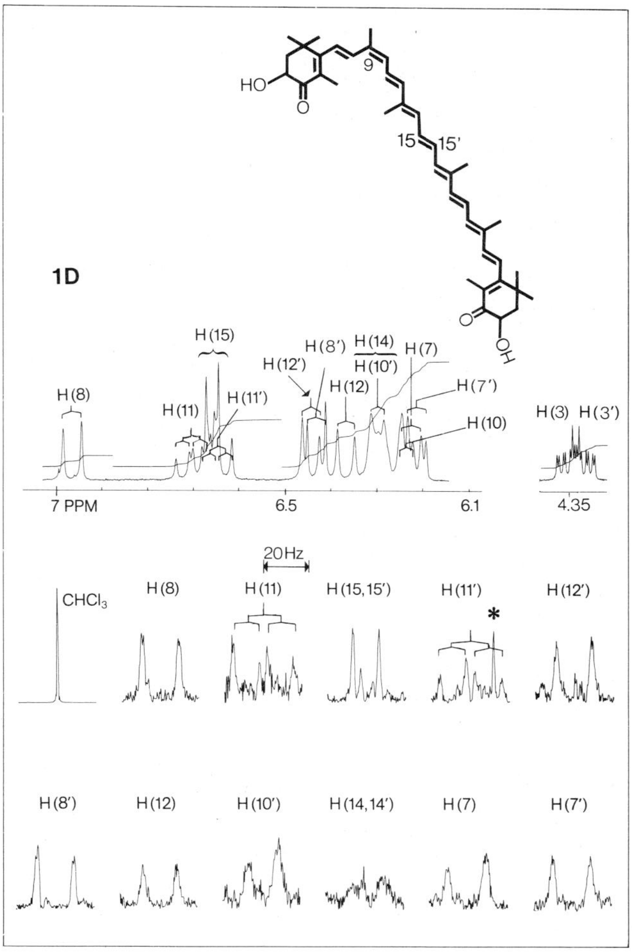

Fig. 16. Top: Low-field part of the 400 MHz p.m.r. spectrum of 9-cis astaxanthin in $CDCl_3$. Bottom: Cross sections of the 2DJ-spectrum along the J-axis taken at the peak positions of the projection of the 2DJ-spectrum on the δ-axis.

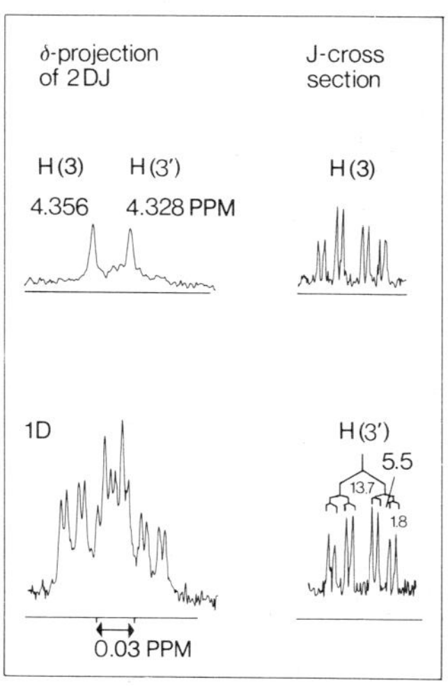

Fig. 17. Bottom left: Superimposed signals of H(3) and H(3') of 9-cis astaxanthin in the 1D spectrum. Top left: Projection of the 2DJ-spectrum on the δ-axis. Right: J-cross sections.

Fig. 18 shows two examples demonstrating the sensitivity of a modern high-field instrument operating at 100.6 MHz corresponding to a p.m.r. frequency of 400 MHz. On top is seen the ^{13}C-n.m.r. of 3 mg of cryptocapsin acetate obtained in ca. 3 hours. The lower spectrum of 1 mg of lactucaxanthin was accumulated in 12 hours (see Note a). The latter should be compared to the previously shown p.m.r. in Fig. 2 corresponding to a factor of 670 in the sample quantity necessary.

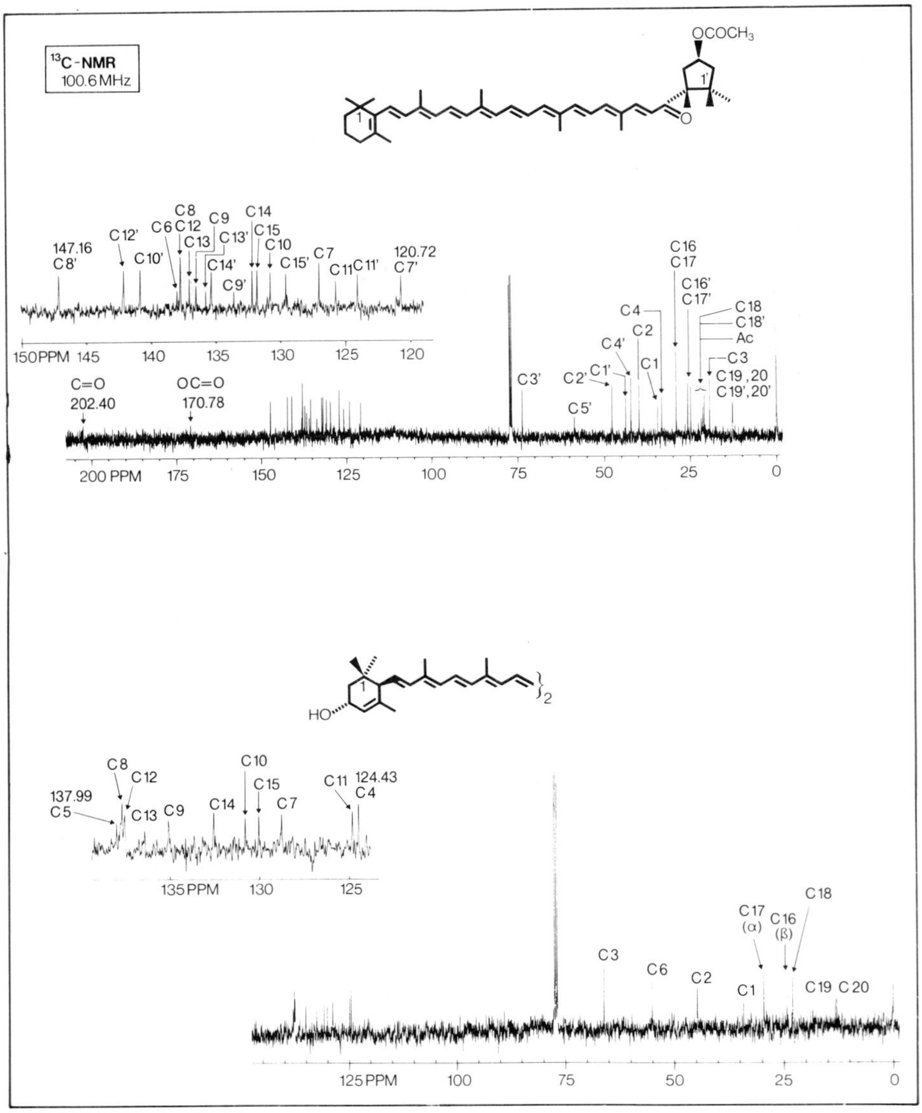

Fig. 18. ^{13}C-n.m.r. spectra at 100.6 MHz. Top: Cryptocapsin acetate, 3 mg in 0.14 ml $CDCl_3$, accumulation 3.2 h. Bottom: Lactucaxanthin, 1 mg in 0.14 ml $CDCl_3$, 12 h.

Two reasons for the reduced sensitivity of ^{13}C-n.m.r. are the low isotopic abundance of only 1.1 % and the smaller magnetic moment of the ^{13}C-nucleus. A further important drawback of quaternary carbons is the fact that their spin-lattice relaxation time T_1 can be rather long compared to protonated carbons since the former are frequently only insufficiently relaxed by the more distant protons in the molecule. A long T_1 means that the corresponding ^{13}C-signal is readily saturated. In order to avoid this, the duration of the high-frequency pulse and hence the flip angle of the nuclear magnetization must be reduced for a given repetition rate of the pulse. An additional drawback of unprotonated carbons is caused by the fact that at higher frequencies the nuclear Overhauser enhancement caused by the broad-band decoupling of the protons may be significantly reduced.

Note a. The samples were kindly provided by Drs. A. Rüttimann and H. Mayer of our Company.

These two effects are clearly visible in the spectra of Fig. 18 where the signals of all the quaternary carbons are smaller or even hardly detectable. Although this has the advantage of making possible the identification of these types of carbons it is evident that the absence of one or more signals can be crucial for the elucidation of the structure of an unknown carotenoid. In order to make sure that all quaternary carbon signals are visible it is frequently necessary to reduce the flip angle to ca. 30° and to increase the total accumulation time considerably.

The theory of spin-lattice relaxation predicts (Ref. 22) that at higher magnetic fields the dipolar contribution to the relaxation is reduced and hence T_1 should become longer. This would then mean that the gain in sensitivity at higher frequencies would be partly compensated by an increase of the T_1's.

To investigate this problem the ^{13}C-n.m.r. spin-lattice relaxation times T_1 of a number of retinoids and carotenoids were measured at 68 MHz. A representative example is presented in Fig. 19. Here, the T_1's in seconds of the different carbons of astaxanthin diacetate are given, measured at 68 MHz by the Freeman-Hill inversion recovery method.

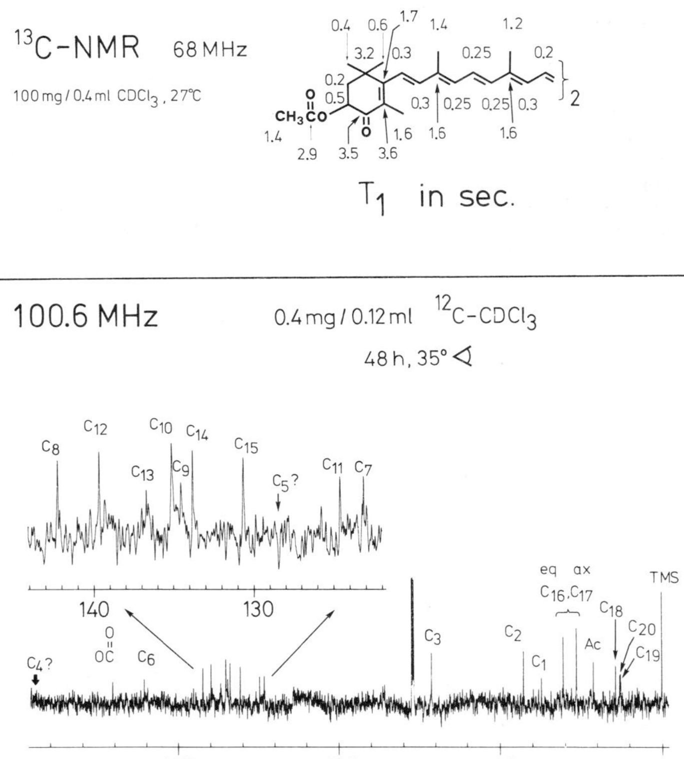

Fig. 19. Top: ^{13}C-n.m.r. spin-lattice relaxation time T_1 in sec. of astaxanthin diacetate (68 MHz). Bottom: 100.6 MHz ^{13}C-n.m.r. spectrum of 0.4 mg astaxanthin diacetate in 0.12 ml ^{12}C-$CDCl_3$, 48 h, flip angle 35°, 21°C.

It is seen that the protonated carbons have reasonably short T_1's even at this high frequency. Only the methyl carbons C(18), C(19) and C(20) possess distinctly greater T_1's reflecting their higher internal mobility compared to C(16) and C(17). Here the longer T_1 of 0.6 sec is assigned to the axial, the shorter T_1 of 0.4 sec to the equatorial methyl group. It is clear from this brief discussion that T_1-measurements can be very successfully utilized for the assignment of the signals since the different carbons can be grouped according to their expected T_1-values.

Important from the point of view of sensitivity is the observation that the longest T_1's due to C(5) and C(4) are only about 3.5 sec. A corresponding measurement at 22 MHz gave ca. 7 sec for both carbons. Therefore, the T_1's of quaternary carbons at higher magnetic fields are actually shortened by other additional relaxation mechanisms (Ref. 22). This is the reason why the situation, although worse than that found in p.m.r., is much better than originally anticipated. One should, however, keep in mind that a variation of the T_1's by a factor of up to 20 and the reduction of the nuclear Overhauser enhancement put stringent limitations on the sensitivity of ^{13}C-n.m.r. if all quaternary carbons are to be detected in a spectrum.

As a further practical example is shown in Fig. 19 the ^{13}C-n.m.r. spectrum at 100.6 MHz of astaxanthin diacetate accumulated with a pulse angle of 35° from only 0.4 mg in 48 hours. As a consequence of the relatively long T_1 the two quaternary carbons C(4) and C(5) are actually not detected and an even longer accumulation time would be needed. In general, a renunciation of the detection of the quaternary carbon signals could reduce the observation time by roughly a factor of 10.

We turn now to the possible application of a still more insensitive method, namely ^{17}O-n.m.r. spectroscopy.

POTENTIAL APPLICATION OF ^{17}O-N.M.R.

In addition to hydrogen and carbon-13 many carotenoids contain oxygen which is, in principle, accessible by n.m.r. through the isotope oxygen-17. Although the ^{17}O-n.m.r. of organic compounds has been reported for more than 20 years its routine application is strongly hampered by the low natural abundance of only 0.037 % and the strong quadrupole moment of oxygen-17. The latter has the very unfavourable effect of strongly broadening the signals by quadrupole relaxation (Ref. 23). Thus, typical line-widths which are roughly proportional to the molar volume and the viscosity of the solution, between 50 Hz and up to several kHz have been observed. The total chemical shift range for ^{17}O in diamagnetic molecules is of the order of 1000 ppm compared to ca. 250 ppm in ^{13}C-n.m.r.

In practice, the lower abundance and considerably larger line-width reduces the sensitivity of ^{17}O-n.m.r. by a factor of 1000 to 10'000 for medium molecular weights compared to ^{13}C-n.m.r. This is obvious from the two spectra of vitamin A-acetate obtained from 0.6 g dissolved in 1.5 ml $CDCl_3$ (Fig. 20). The upper ^{13}C-n.m.r. at 100.6 MHz was measured with only one pulse, the lower 54.2 MHz ^{17}O-n.m.r. of the same sample in the same probe head had to be measured by accumulation of 200'000 FID's in 4 hours. The total sweep-width was 50 kHz. As a reference the signal of H_2O is used appearing near the high-field end of the usual chemical shift range. The line-width of this medium sized molecule is already ca. 1 kHz, explaining one part of the considerable loss in sensitivity.

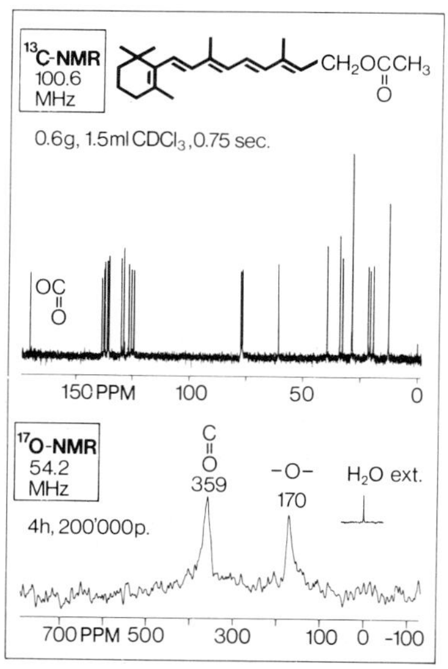

Fig. 20. 100.6 MHz ^{13}C-n.m.r. (top) and 54.2 MHz ^{17}O-n.m.r. of vitamin A-acetate (0.6 g in 1.5 ml $CDCl_3$)

In order to study the potential applicability of ^{17}O-n.m.r. in the field of carotenoids the spectra of 17 compounds were taken starting from small molecules related to some typical end groups and reaching up in the molecular size to canthaxanthin. The results are presented in Fig. 21. The accumulation times needed were between a few minutes and ca. 24 hours depending on concentration and molecular weight. The chemical shifts are given with reference to the signal of external H_2O (δ = 0). In parentheses, the observed line-widths in kHz are given in-

creasing from ca. 0.4 kHz to almost 9 kHz in the case of canthaxanthin. This large line-width significantly reduces the spectrum quality and the accuracy of the measured chemical shift. On the other hand, a clear separation of the different types of oxygen functions is possible as shown at the bottom of Fig. 21.

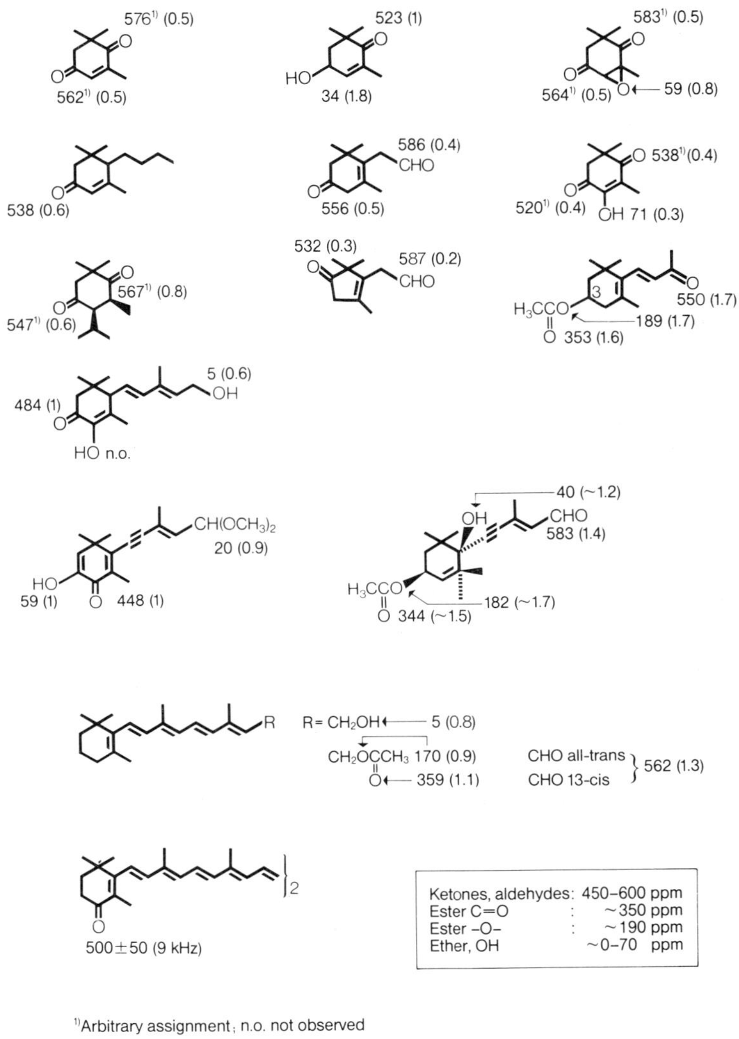

Fig. 21. Survey of some ^{17}O-n.m.r. chemical shifts, measured at 54 MHz in $CDCl_3$. External H_2O served as the reference. In parentheses are given the line-widths in kHz.

On the basis of these preliminary results one can predict that future applications of ^{17}O-n.m.r. spectroscopy to problems of carotenoid chemistry will certainly be limited to very specific cases. However, a reliable judgement must await further experiments.

Acknowledgement - I should like to express my gratitude to all my colleagues who provided the compounds the spectra of which were described. I should like to specifically mention here Drs. K. Bernhard, P. Kreienbühl, H. Mayer, R.K. Müller, A. Rüttimann and R. Zell, as well as Mrs. K. Schiedt and Mr. V. Meduna.

In addition I also gratefully mention my close co-operation with Dr. M. Vecchi and Mr. E. Glinz (h.p.l.c.) and the skilful technical assistance of Messrs. P. Casagrande and W. Grunauer who ran most of the spectra.

REFERENCES

1. D. Siefermann-Harms, S. Hertzberg, G. Borch and S. Liaaen-Jensen, Phytochem. 20, 85-88 (1981).
2. H. Mayer, Abstracts, 6th International Symp. Carotenoids, 1981.
3. W. Vetter, G. Englert, N. Rigassi and U. Schwieter, Spectroscopic Methods, Chapter IV in Carotenoids, O. Isler (Edit.), 189-266, Birkhäuser, Basle (1971).
4. A.G. Andrewes, G. Englert, G. Borch, H.H. Strain and S. Liaaen-Jensen, Phytochem. 18, 303-309 (1979).
5. G. Englert and M. Vecchi, to be published.
6. G. Englert, S. Weber and M. Klaus, Helv. Chim. Acta 61, 2697-2708 (1978).
7. G. Englert and M. Vecchi, Helv. Chim. Acta 63, 1711-1718 (1980).
8. L. Zechmeister, Cis-Trans Isomeric Carotenoids, Vitamins A and Arylpolyenes, Springer-Verlag, Wien (1962).
9. G. Englert, B.O. Brown, G.P. Moss, B.C.L. Weedon, G. Britton, T.W. Goodwin, K.L. Simpson and R.J.H. Williams, J.C.S. Chem. Comm. (1979), 546-547.
10. J.M. Clough and G. Pattenden, J.C.S. Chem. Comm. (1979), 616-619.
11. G. Englert, Helv. Chim. Acta 62, 1497-1500 (1979).
12. J.H. Noggle and R.E. Schirmer, The Nuclear Overhauser Effect, Chemical Applications, Academic Press, New York and London (1971).
13. F. Kienzle and R.E. Minder, Helv. Chim. Acta 61, 242-249 (1978).
14. R. Rowan III, P.H. Mazzocchi, C.A. Kanagy and M. Regan, J. Magn. Res. 39, 27-30 (1980).
15. G. Britton, T.W. Goodwin, W.J.S. Lockley, A.P. Mundy, N.J. Patel and G. Englert, J.C.S. Chem. Comm, 1978, 27-28.
16. R. Freeman and G.A. Morris, Bull. Magn. Res. 1, 5-26 (1980).
17. W.P. Aue, J. Karhan and R.R. Ernst, J. Chem. Phys. 64, 4226-4227 (1976).
18. G. Wider, R. Baumann, K. Nagayama, R.R. Ernst and K. Wüthrich, J. Magn. Res. 42, 73-87 (1981).
19. G. Englert, Helv. Chim. Acta 58, 2367-2390 (1975).
20. G. Moss, Pure & Appl. Chem. 47, 97-102 (1976).
21. M. Baranyai, P. Molnar and J. Szabolcs, Tetrahedron 37, 203-207 (1981).
22. F.W. Wehrli and T. Wirthlin, "Interpretation of Carbon-13 NMR Spectra", Heyden, London 1976.
23. Th.St. Amour and D. Fiat, Bull. Magn. Res. 1, 118-129 (1980).

CIRCULAR DICHROISM OF CAROTENOIDS AND ITS USE IN INVESTIGATIONS OF THEIR STRUCTURES, CONFIGURATIONS AND CONFORMATIONS

Klaus Noack

Central Research Units, F. Hoffmann-La Roche & Co., Ltd., CH-4002 Basle (Switzerland)

Abstract - A carotenoid with a β-end-ring is an intrinsically chiral chromophore by virtue of the twist about the formal single bond connecting the planar conjugated chain with the end-ring. Steric hindrance prevents the double bond in the ring from lying coplanar with the chain. Fixation of the conformation of the ring itself by an equatorial substituent at C(2) and/or C(3) gives preference to one handedness of the twist of the ring against the chain resulting in an intrinsically chiral conjugated chain.

With this model many features of the c.d. spectra of carotenoids can be understood. Three rules have been given to describe the experimental observations[4]. 1. All-*trans* and di-*cis* isomers have very similar c.d. spectra, which are approximately mirror-images of those of the mono-*cis* isomers of the same carotenoid. 2. The c.d. spectra of carotenoids with only one end-ring do not invert on *cis*-isomerization. 3. The c.d. spectra are temperature-dependent.

These rules are shown to hold for a number of *trans*, mono- and di-*cis* astaxanthin diacetates.

The limitations and possible extensions of these rules are explored with other carotenoids, including those with epoxy rings and ε-rings, such as lutein isomers and epimers and chiriquixanthin epimers and related compounds.

The conformational flexibility has implications for the use of the c.d. spectra in the determination of the absolute stereochemistry.

The c.d. spectra of 9-mono-*cis* and 9,9'-di-*cis* astaxanthin diacetates at -180°C are strongly concentration-dependent, which suggests an association of these compounds at low temperature in solution.

INTRODUCTION

Most of the naturally occurring carotenoids possess at least one asymmetric carbon and occur in nature in optically active form (i.e. Ref. 1). One can therefore expect optical rotatory dispersion (o.r.d.) and circular dichroism (c.d.) spectra to be useful tools in carotenoid research. From the o.r.d. and c.d. spectra one should, at least in principle, be able to deduce the absolute stereochemistry of these compounds. In practice there is, unfortunately, a long way to go towards this goal and we doubt that this aim will ever be realized. To understand why it is so difficult to establish the absolute stereochemistry directly from the c.d. spectrum one must try to understand what structural and conformational features influence the c.d.

Even if the absolute stereochemistry cannot be deduced from the c.d. spectrum there is a great deal of useful information which can be gained from it. Some of the important areas to which the study of those spectra has made a useful contribution are the following:
1. The most obvious use is in quantitative and qualitative analysis: The confirmation of the identity or non-identity of two compounds, the enantiomeric purity with respect to a known standard and so on. Recently, by the use of optically active shift reagents and optically active derivatives, nuclear magnetic resonance (n.m.r.) and high pressure liquid chromatography (h.p.l.c.) have also become efficient tools in the analysis of enantiomeric composition and purity of carotenoids (Ref. 2 & 3). They can in favourable cases give the enantiomeric purity without a known standard. But c.d. is generally easier and more generally applicable and all three methods complement each other. The purely analytical aspects of c.d. will not be treated further here. They are, of course, very important in the determination of the absolute stereochemistry by chemical correlations with known products.
2. From the c.d. information on spectroscopic properties and the electronic structure can be obtained in conjunction with and supplementary to the information from the absorption spec-

tra. An understanding of these properties and of the origin of the c.d. spectra is necessary if one wants to use the c.d. for the determination of the absolute configuration.

3. The determination of the absolute stereochemistry is of course the highest goal the natural product chemist hopes to attain with the help of the c.d. spectra. Often an empirical approach of close inspection of the spectra of related compounds has to be used. When conformations are unknown and when there is a lack of theoretical understanding of the origin of the c.d. an unambiguous assignment of the absolute configuration from the c.d. is not possible.

4. Finally the c.d. spectra can be used for the investigation of special properties of carotenoids. The temperature dependent c.d. allows the study of the dynamic behaviour and conformational equilibria (Ref. 4) and the energy difference between conformers. The concentration dependence may be used to detect association and aggregation in solution. Some examples will be given later in this lecture.

This lecture reviews results obtained by us recently and will give examples to illustrate many of these points as well as raising the problem posed by attempts to place the interpretation of the c.d. spectra of optically active carotenoids on a sound theoretical basis.

No attempt has been made to give a comprehensive review of the numerous other works on the c.d. spectra of carotenoids found in the literature.

SOME GENERAL RULES

Jensen has recently assembled a list of all known chiral centers in naturally occurring carotenoids (Ref. 5). From this impressive list it is clear that most carotenoids owe their optical activity to asymmetrically substituted carbon atoms at cyclic end groups. Typical examples are astaxanthin, lutein and chiriquixanthin A.

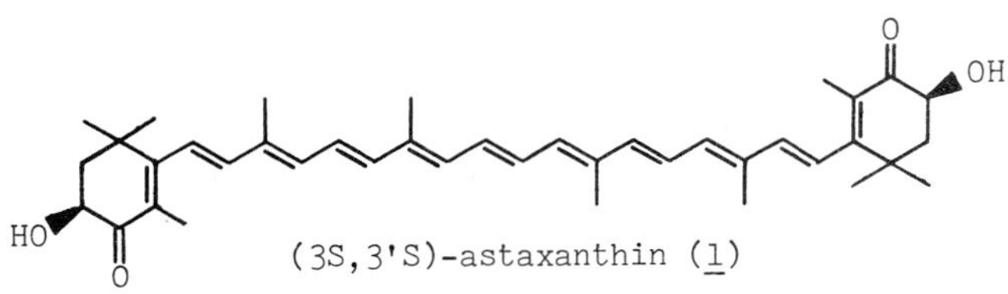

(3S,3'S)-astaxanthin (1)

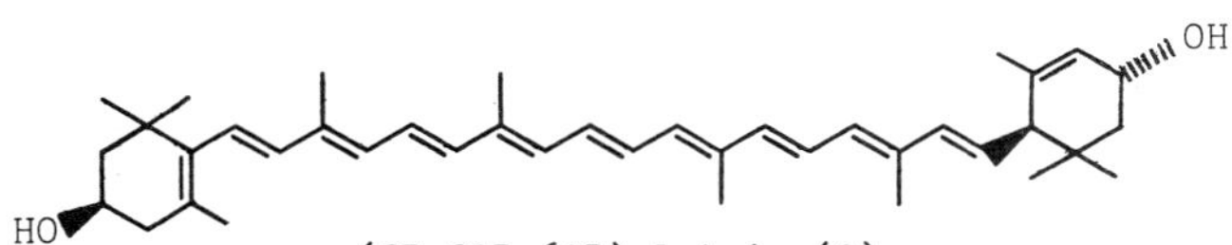

(3R,3'R,6'R)-lutein (2)

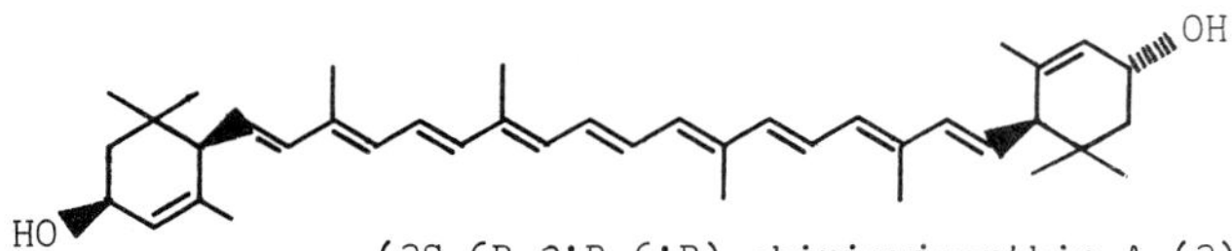

(3S,6R,3'R,6'R)-chiriquixanthin A (3)

In 1 the double bonds in both end-rings are formally conjugated to the chain, in 2 one of the end-rings is conjugated with the chain and in 3 the double bonds in both end groups are separated by two single bonds from the conjugated chain. But many other examples are known, including epoxy-rings, substituted open ends and allenic double bonds. However, in most cases the asymmetric centers are located near the ends of the conjugated chain.

The c.d. bands of the carotenoids are observed in the same wavelength region as the absorption. This implies that the whole chromophoric system is responsible for the c.d. We must therefore examine how optical activity is induced into the long almost planar chain of conjugated double bonds from one or both of its ends. The best studied and understood examples are those with at least one formally conjugated end-ring which bears one or more asymmetrically substituted carbons: the "substituted β-end-ring type". Typical examples are zeaxanthin, β-cryptoxanthin and rubixanthin and their Z-isomers.

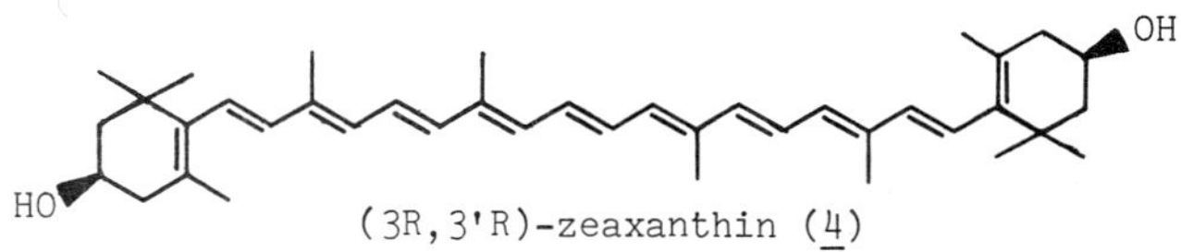
(3R,3'R)-zeaxanthin (4)

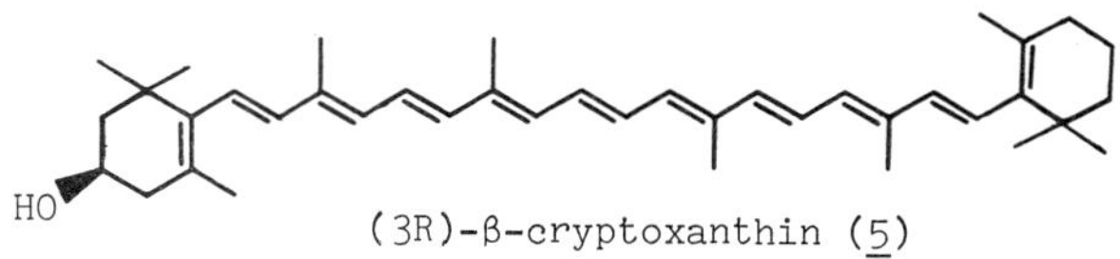
(3R)-β-cryptoxanthin (5)

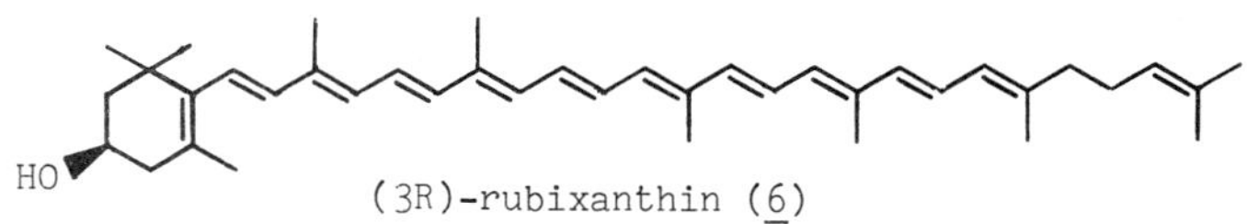
(3R)-rubixanthin (6)

We have recently shown that by a careful study of a number of compounds of this general type a good deal can be learned and understood about the optical activity of carotenoids (Ref. 4). A more theoretical study has also appeared (Ref. 6). I shall first summarize our work and then treat a number of more complicated cases we have studied recently.

Three rules were given to describe our experimental results on the "β-end-ring type" compounds:
Rule 1. The bands in the c.d. spectra of all-*trans* and di-*cis* isomers of carotenoids with two β-end-rings are opposite in sign to the mono-*cis* isomers of the same carotenoid.
Rule 2. In pairs of all-*trans* and mono-*cis* isomers of half-carotenoids or carotenoids with only one β-end-ring the c.d. spectra have the same sign.
Rule 3. The c.d. spectra of carotenoids are strongly temperature-dependent.

Similar observations on the sign inversion of all-*trans* and mono-*cis* compounds have been made by others (Ref. 7,8,9). Rule 1 holds also if only one of the two β-end-rings is asymmetrically substituted as in 5. As illustration of rule 3 may serve 4, where the Δε-values increase several fold and 1 where an inversion of sign on cooling from ambient temperature to -180°C is observed.

We have shown (Ref. 4) that these rules can be rationalized if there is a steric hindrance between the H-atoms on C(7) and on C(8) and the methyl groups on C(5) and C(1) preventing the C-atoms C(5), C(6), C(7) and C(8) from being coplanar or, in other words, preventing the coplanarity of the double bond in the ring with the conjugated chain. Thus, one or both ends of the whole conjugated system are twisted resulting in an intrinsically chiral chromophore. It can be concluded from molecular models and calculations (Ref. 21) as well as from crystal structure analysis (Ref. 22) that two distorted s-*cis* conformations of slightly different energy with the ring "up" or "down" are possible. In carotenoids without asymmetric centers one form is converted into its mirror image of identical energy by simultaneous rotation and ring inversion (as in β-carotene or the unsubstituted side of 5).

In this case one has a (racemic) mixture of rapidly interconverting chiral molecules. When there is a substituent at either C(3) and/or C(2) the two ring conformations have different energies. Since the conformation with the equatorial substituent is strongly favoured, the ring interconversion is prevented. Therefore the two twist forms around C(6) - C(7) become energetically different and hence in the equilibrium mixture one of the two forms predominates. This is why a c.d. spectrum can be observed. Since the energy difference is only small the equilibrium and hence the c.d. spectrum are temperature-dependent.

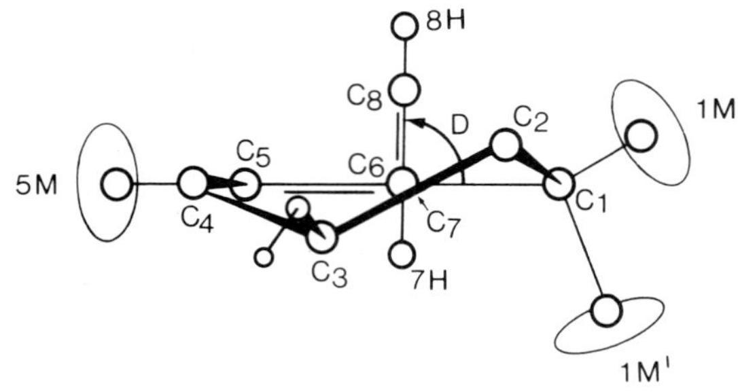

Fig. 1. 3-hydroxy β-ionone end-ring, viewed along the C(6)-C(7)-bond from one end across the ring.

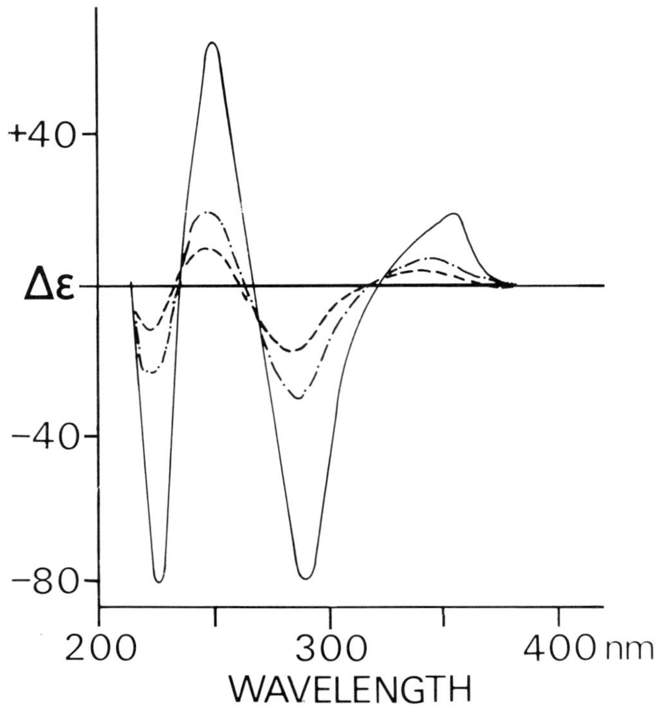

Fig. 2. C.D. spectrum of (3R,3'R)-zeaxanthin
----- +20°C, -·-·- -60°C, ——— -180°C

The model of the twisted conjugated chain gives an explanation of rule 1, namely the sign change between the all-trans, di-cis and the mono-cis isomers (Ref. 4 & 6). Figure 3 shows the twisted all-trans and 15-cis zeaxanthin, both of symmetry C_2 and of the same absolute configuration at C(3) and C(3'). The C_2-axis is tilted by 90°.

In trans-zeaxanthin it is perpendicular to and in the cis isomer it lies in the plane of the conjugated chain. The chiralities of the two are opposite. They have the same relationship to each other as twisted s-trans and s-cis butadiene (Fig. 4).

It has been shown that the c.d. spectra are expected to be of opposite sign (Ref. 10 & 11). Recently, calculations have been carried out for the whole conjugated carotenoid chain which also predicted the sign inversion on cis-isomerization (Ref. 6).

Rule 2 was derived from the c.d. of all-trans and 9-mono-cis didehydro-apo astaxanthin. A poster at this symposium by Buchecker et al. showed that, in the case of all-trans rubixanthin and 3 of its mono-cis isomers, clearly inversion of sign is observed. Rule 2, therefore, needs further definition (Ref. 23).

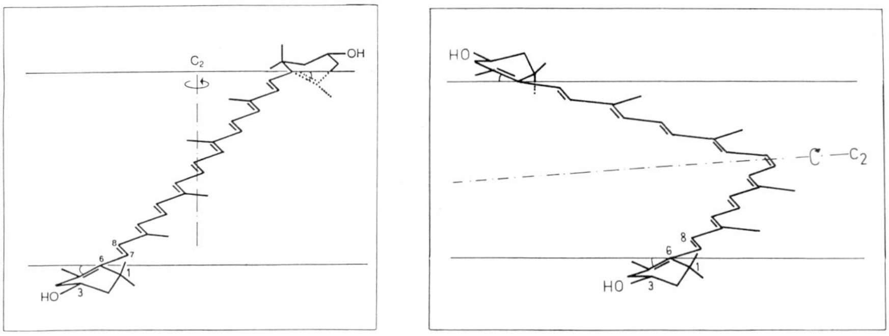

Fig. 3. Conformations of twisted trans and 15-cis (3R,3'R)-zeaxanthin.

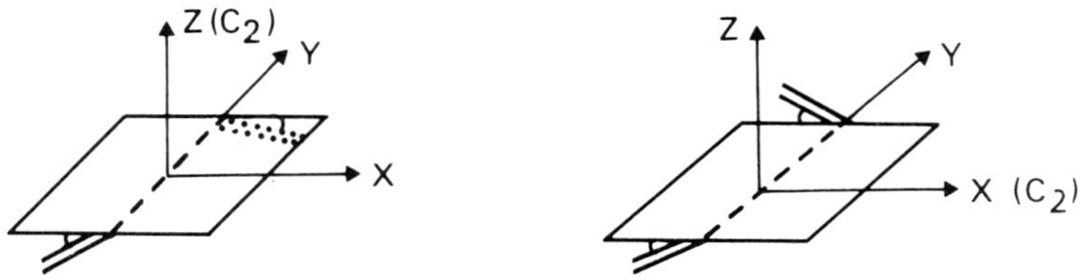

Fig. 4. Skewed s-trans and s-cis butadiene.

DETERMINATION OF THE EQUILIBRIUM CONSTANT FOR ZEAXANTHIN

Using an approach given by Moscowitz et al. (Ref. 12 & 13), it is possible to determine the free energy difference of two conformers in a dynamic equilibrium by means of the temperature dependent c.d. spectra. Briefly, the equilibrium constant can be written as

$$K = (R_a - R_o^T) / (R_o^T - R_b) \qquad (1)$$

where R_o^T is the observed rotational strength at absolute temperature T and R_a and R_b the rotational strengths of the lower energy conformer a and higher energy conformer b respectively. From the assumption of a Boltzmann distribution an equation relating R_o^T to R_a and R_b was derived.

$$R_o^T = (R_a - R_b)\,[1 + \exp(-\Delta G^o/NkT)]^{-1} + R_b \qquad (2)$$

Here N is Avogadro's number, k is Boltzmann's constant and ΔG^o the standard Gibbs free energy change for the reaction a$\rightleftharpoons$b.

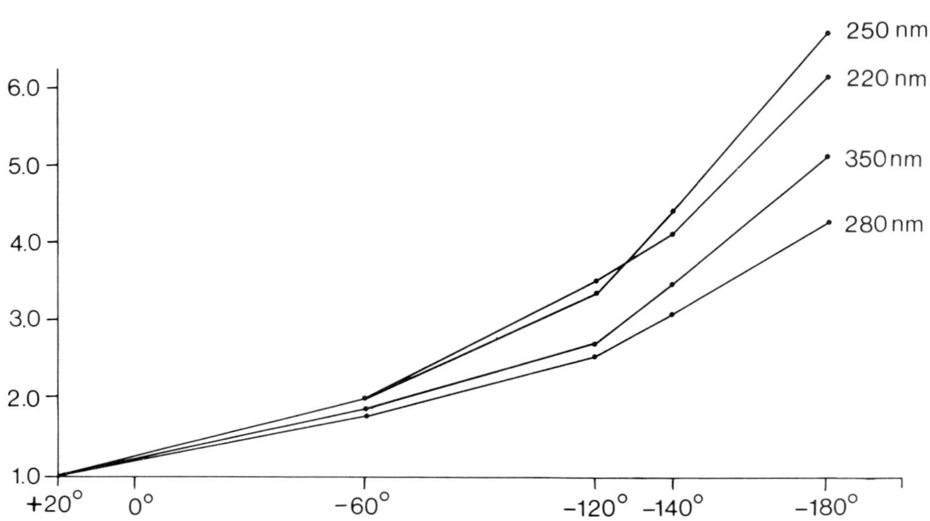

Fig. 5. Relative Δε-values of the c.d. maxima vs. temperature, referred to Δε at RT, for (3R,3'R)-zeaxanthin.

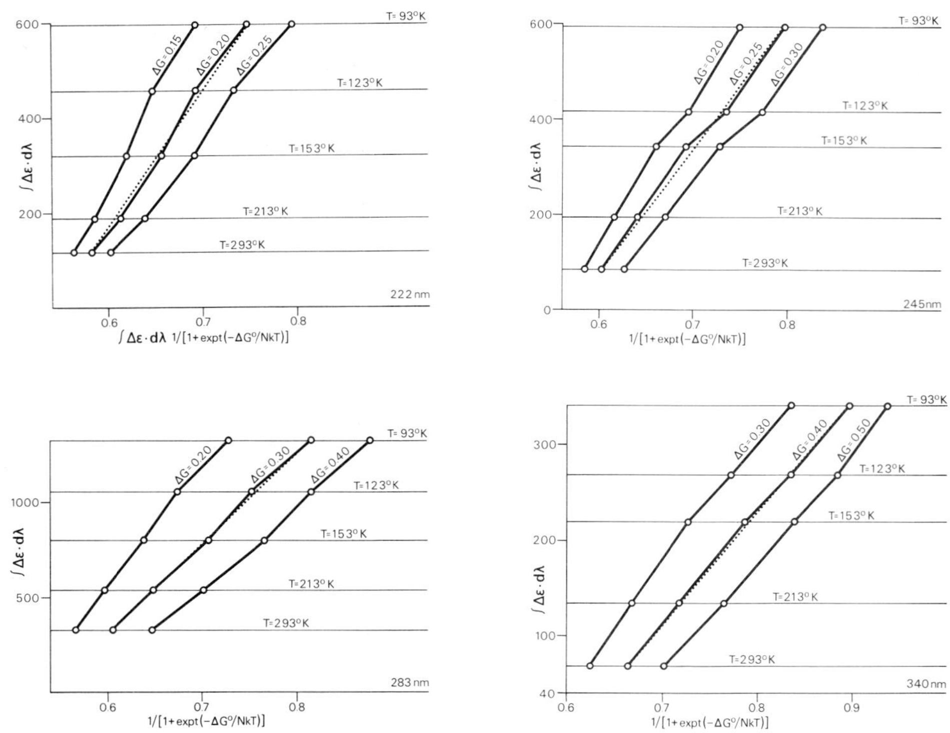

Fig. 6. Plots of eq. 2 for the 4 c.d. maxima of (3R,3'R)-zeaxanthin for 3 trial ΔG^o (kcal/mole)-values each.

It follows from eq. 1 and eq. 2 that a plot of R_o^T vs. $1/[1 + \exp(-\Delta G^o/NkT)]$ should yield a straight line for the proper value of ΔG^o. We have tried this approach on the data for zeaxanthin. Fig. 5 shows a plot of the relative Δε-maxima vs. temperature, referred to Δε at 20°C, for (3R,3'R)-zeaxanthin.

It is immediately obvious that the different bands do not vary in the same way. This is almost certainly due to partial overlap of the close lying positive and negative maxima (Fig. 2). Therefore, the ΔG^o-values determined for the different bands will also vary. One can nevertheless estimate a figure for the magnitude of the energy difference. Fig. 6 gives the plots of equation 2. The best straight line yielding the ΔG^o and two neighbouring lines are drawn. The mean ΔG^o lies somewhere between 0.2 and 0.4 kcal/Mol.

C.D. SPECTRA OF ASTAXANTHIN DIACETATE ISOMERS

We have recently extended our studies of the c.d. spectra of carotenoids to include the temperature- and also the concentration-dependence of a series of mono-*cis* and di-*cis* astaxanthin diacetates (Ref. 14). We had at our disposal the (3S,3'S)-astaxanthin diacetate and its 9-*cis*, 13-*cis*, 9,9'-di-*cis*, 9,13'-di-*cis*, 9,13-di-*cis* and 13,13'-di-*cis* isomers.

The isomers were obtained by h.p.l.c.-separation of an iodine catalyzed equilibrium mixture (Ref. 2), and the structures were determined by proton magnetic resonance (Ref. 2).

As expected, these compounds exhibit strongly temperature-dependent c.d. spectra. The signs invert on cooling, as has been observed before with all-*trans* astaxanthin itself (Ref. 4). They conform with one exception to rule 1 (opposite sign of all-*trans* and di-*cis* vs. mono-*cis* compounds). Fig. 7 - 10 give 4 typical spectra at room temperature and -180°C. The 13,13'-di-*cis* isomer shows in contrast to the other isomers, under the longest wavelength band, the opposite sign to the all-*trans* isomer. For the other bands, however, this compound also obeys the rule 1.

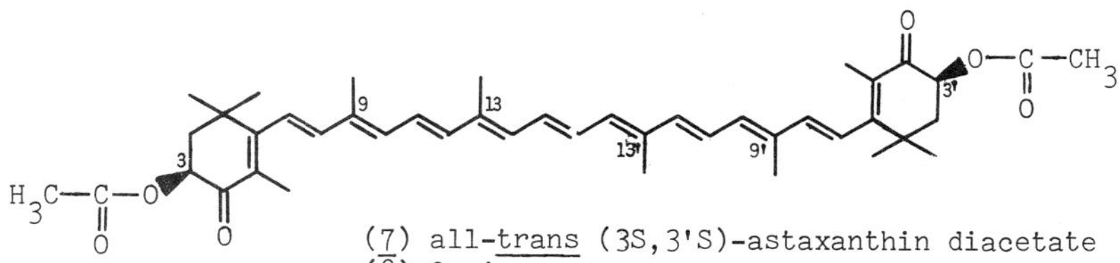

(7) all-trans (3S,3'S)-astaxanthin diacetate
(8) 9-cis
(9) 13-cis
(10) 9,9'-di-cis
(11) 9,13'-di-cis
(12) 9,13-di-cis
(13) 13,13'-di-cis

An unexpected observation has, however, been made with 9-cis and 9,9'-di-cis astaxanthin diacetate: The c.d. is not only temperature-dependent but at low temperature also depends strongly on the concentration. At the concentration normally employed (about 70 to 90 μM) and at -180°C both compounds show a surprisingly strong c.d. under the longest wavelength band. This c.d. shows distinct splitting and a change of sign across the band. The maxima and minima do not coincide with the maxima in the absorption spectra at the same temperature. Upon 10 to 30 fold dilution the maxima shift and become much weaker. They now coincide with the absorption maxima (Fig. 11).

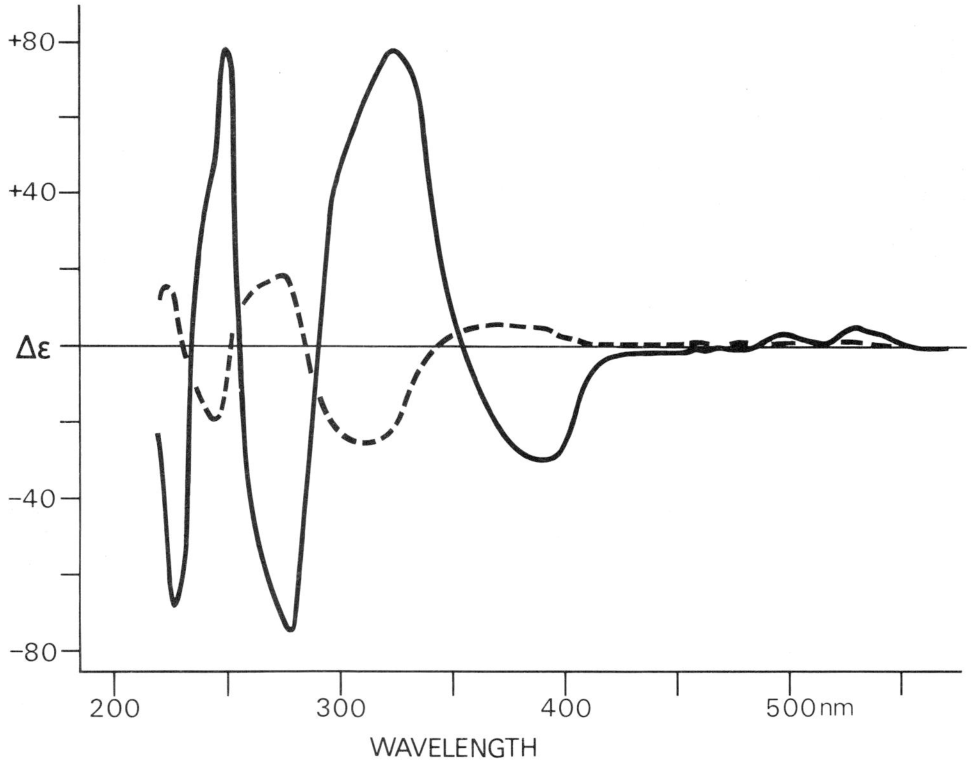

Fig. 7. C.D. spectra of (3S,3'S)-astaxanthin diacetate at RT -----, at -180°C ———.

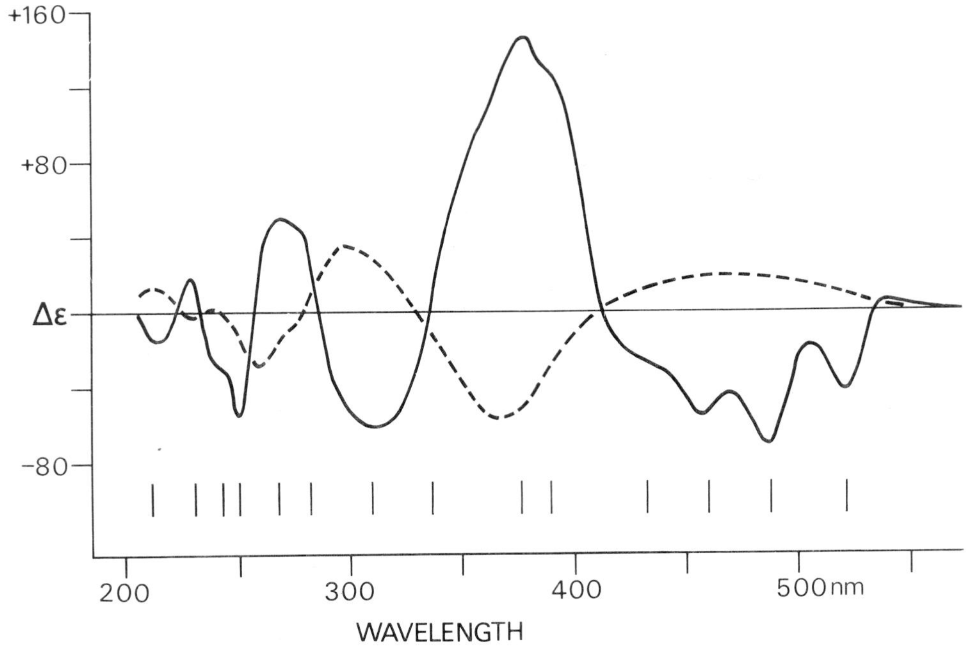

Fig. 8. C.D. spectra of (3S,3'S)-13-cis astaxanthin diacetate at RT -----, at -180°C ———, bars indicate positions of absorption maxima or shoulders at -180°C.

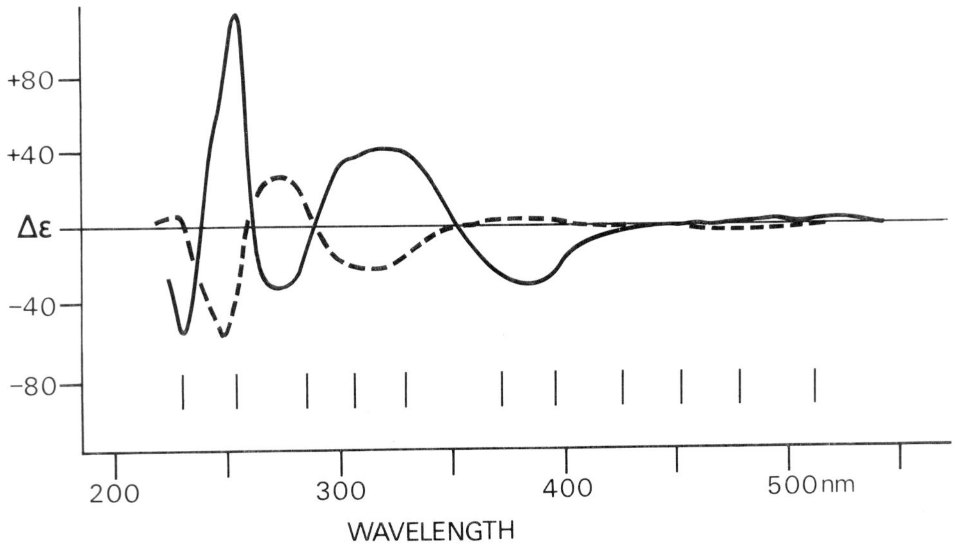

Fig. 9. C.D. spectra of (3S,3'S)-9,13-di-cis astaxanthin diacetate at RT -----, at -180°C ——— , bars indicate positions of absorption maxima or shoulders at -180°C.

This behaviour is indicative of aggregation and arises from exciton interaction between monomers (Ref. 15). Unfortunately no detailed conclusions can be drawn from the spectra at the present time without some knowledge of the number of monomers in the aggregate. The presence of a 9-cis bond seems to be necessary for this oligomerization since in the all-trans and the other mono- and di-cis isomers there is a good coincidence of the c.d. and absorption maxima and no sign change in the c.d. under the main absorption band is observed. Since the aggregation is only observed at temperatures below about -150°C, the forces which hold the aggregates together must be very weak. It does not seem to occur in 9,9'-di-*cis* zeaxanthin as indicated by the coincidence of absorption and c.d. peaks and the absence of bisignate bands in the c.d. (Ref. 4). Owing to lack of material we were unable to check whether aggregation occurs in 9,9'-di-*cis* zeaxanthin diacetate nor whether it occurs in free 9-*cis* or 9,9'-di-*cis* astaxanthin. We favour the idea that aggregation is a consequence of interaction of the polyene chains. Models show that in the all-*trans* and the mono- and di-*cis* forms except the 9-*cis* and 9,9'-di-*cis* the bulky geminal dimethyl groups prevent a close approach of the two chains. In the 9-*cis* and the 9,9'-di-*cis* forms the rings are turned away and a long stretch of the chains can approach each other closely. However, this model is admittedly conjectural at this stage.

These examples show that c.d. can help in the detection of rather subtle interactions in these compounds.

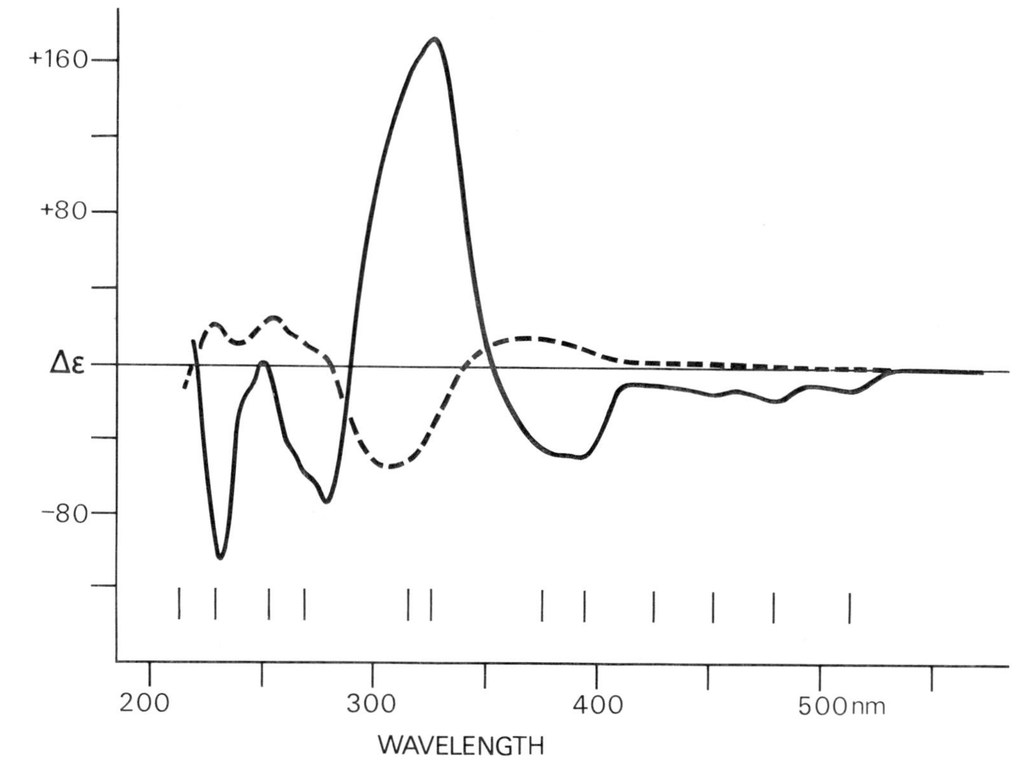

Fig. 10. C.D. spectra of (3S,3'S)-13,13'-di-*cis* astaxanthin diacetate at RT -----, at -180°C ———, bars indicate positions of absorption maxima or shoulders at -180°C.

C.D. OF CAROTENOIDS WITH NON-CONJUGATED RINGS

The "substituted β-end-ring" compounds discussed so far are, of course, only a small, although important, part of the total number of known optically active carotenoids and we will now proceed to discuss some other types.

It has been observed that the c.d. of all-*trans* and 9-*cis* violaxanthin also show a mirror-image relationship with the exception of the lowest energy band (Ref. 16) and that the spectra are very similar to those of all-*trans* and 9-mono-*cis* zeaxanthin (Fig. 12).

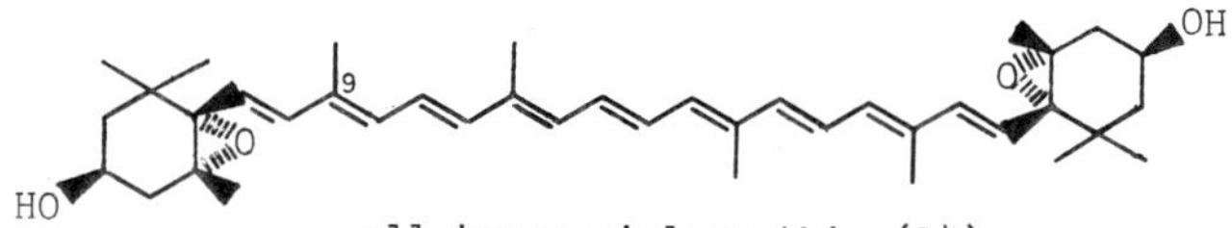

all-*trans* violaxanthin (14)
9-*cis* violaxanthin (violeoxanthin) (15)

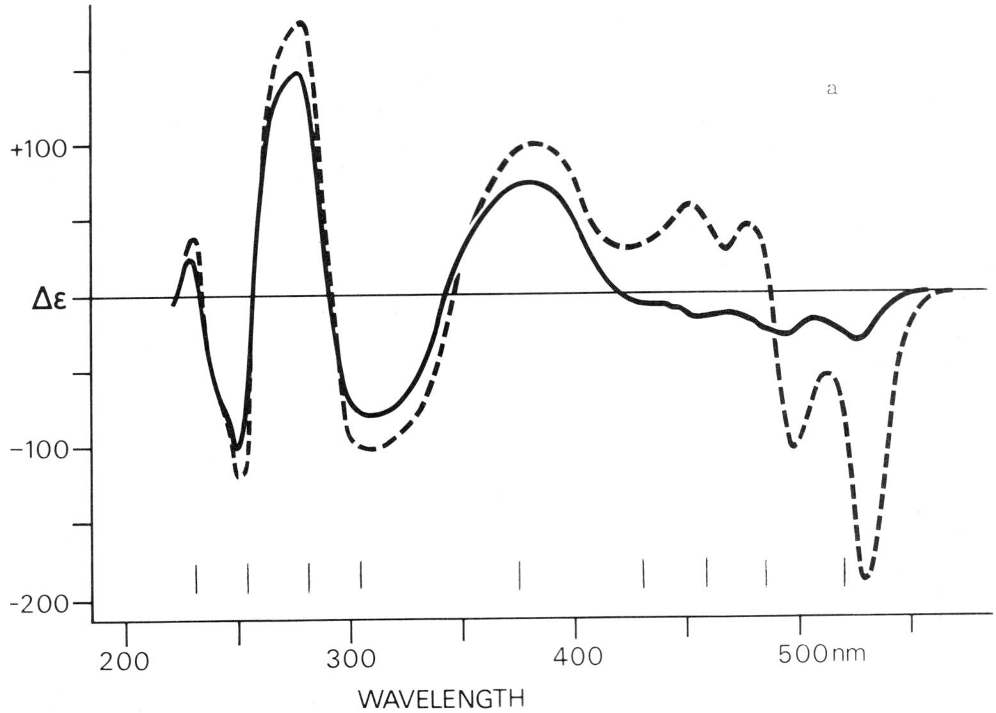

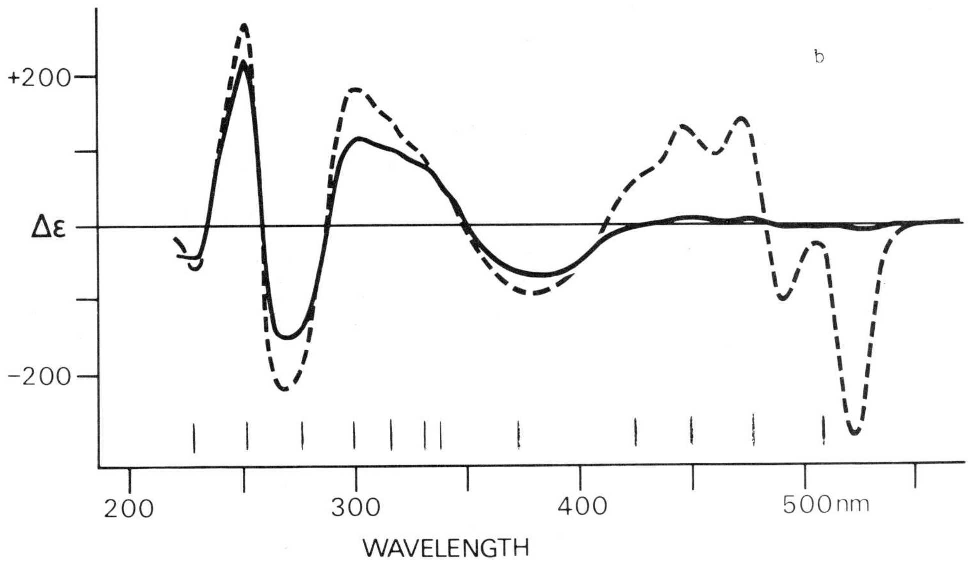

Fig. 11. C.D. spectra at -180°C.
a. (3S,3'S)-9-*cis* astaxanthin diacetate, ——— 7.2 μM, ----- 140 μM
b. (3S,3'S)-9,9'-di-*cis* astaxanthin diacetate, ——— 2.8 μM, ----- 87 μM
Bars indicate positions of absorption maxima or shoulders at -180°C.

In violaxanthin the end-rings are certainly twisted out of the plane of the conjugated chain. But how does this influence the conjugated system? It is known from c.d. spectra in the steroid field that an epoxy group does interact strongly with the π-electrons of conjugated ketones, almost as a further conjugated C=C-bond. The same is also true for a cyclopropyl group. Table 1 gives the two longest wavelength c.d. peaks of some relevant structural types.

The epoxy group produces a red-shift of the maxima almost as great as an additional double bond. It is therefore not surprising that the epoxy groups in 14 and 15 extend the conjugated system and that it becomes inherently chiral, very similar to zeaxanthin, and that the *cis*-inversion rule is obeyed.

I do not know a corresponding carotenoid with a cyclopropyl group but I would expect that its c.d. properties would be very similar to the epoxy compound.

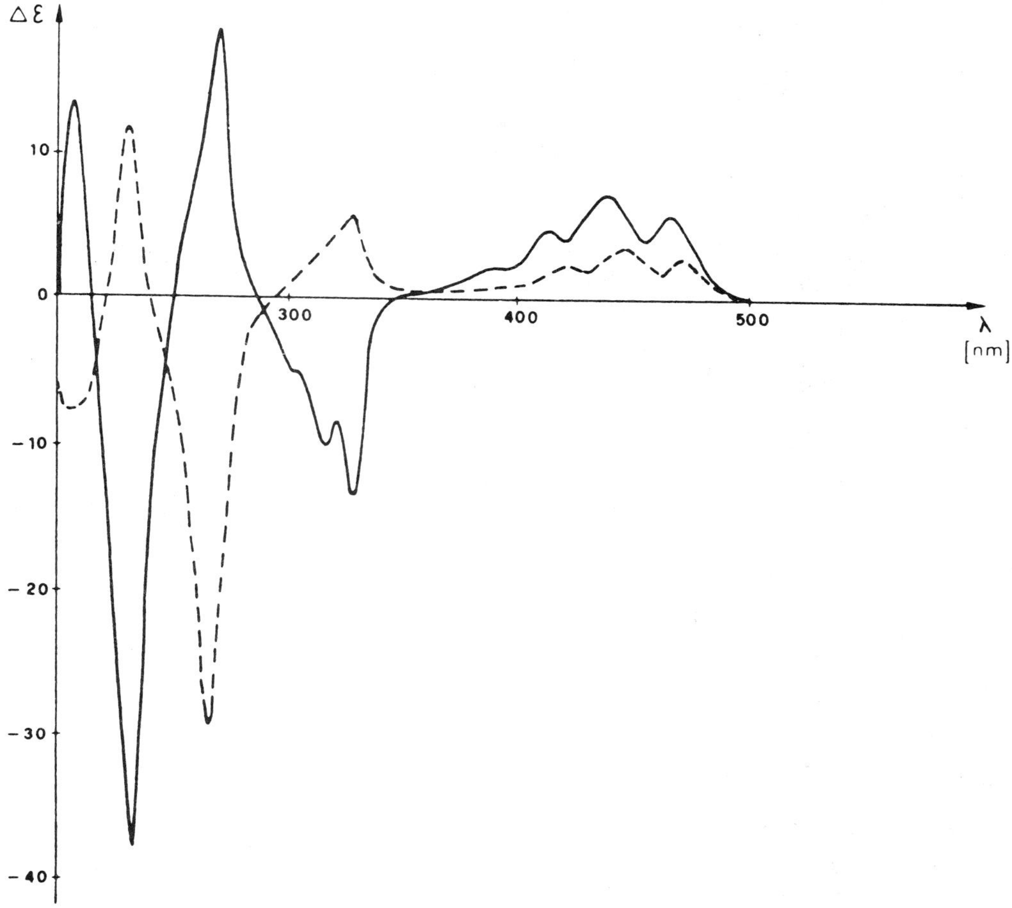

Fig. 12. C.D. spectrum of violaxanthin at room temperature in ethanol,
----- all-trans, ——— 9-cis (Ref. 6 & 16).

Antheraxanthins (Ref. 17) provide another illustration.

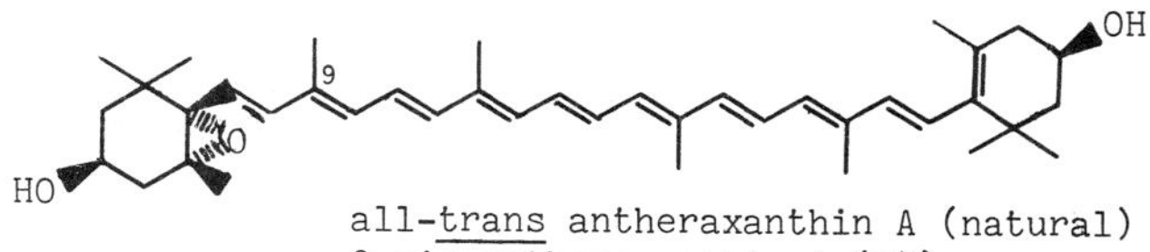

all-trans antheraxanthin A (natural) (16)
9-cis antheraxanthin A (17)

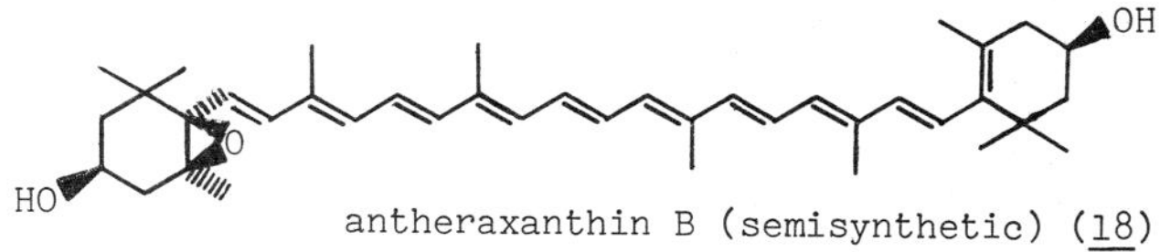

antheraxanthin B (semisynthetic) (18)

TABLE 1. C.D. of (conjugated) ketones and related epoxy or cyclopropyl ketones*

(conj.) ketones	λ_{max} (nm), $\Delta\varepsilon$	epoxy or cyclopropyl ketones	λ_{max} (nm), $\Delta\varepsilon$
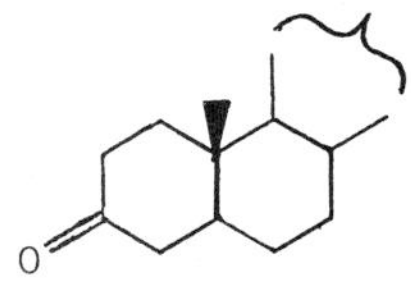	~290 +1.2		
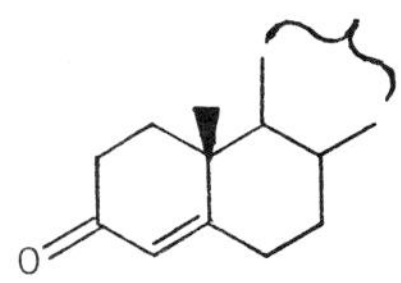	317 -1.5 ~230 +9		
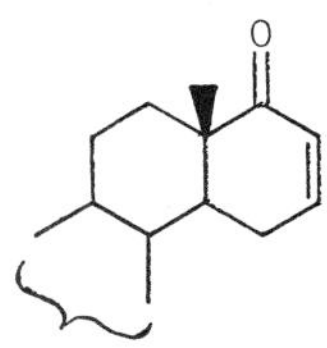	323 +1.5 ~230 -4	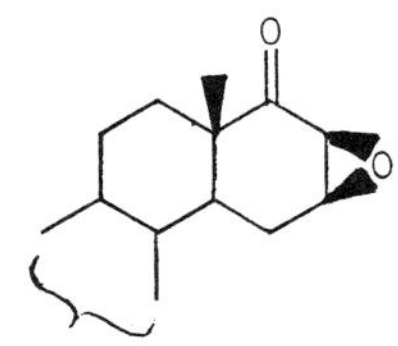	307 -1
		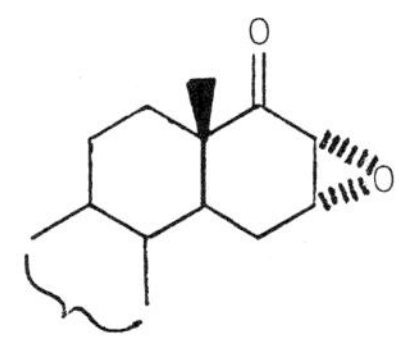	320 +2
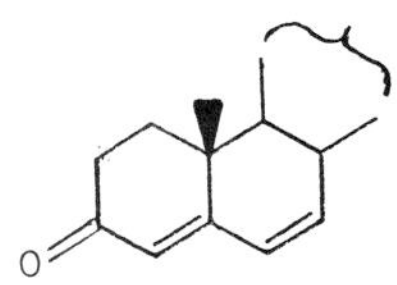	~360 +3.5 280 -4	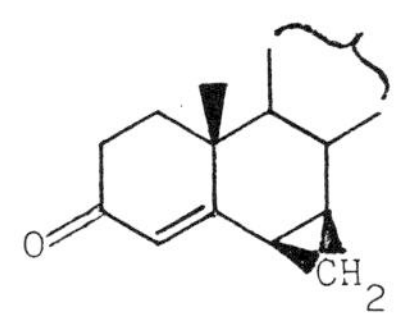	350 +1.5 260 -14
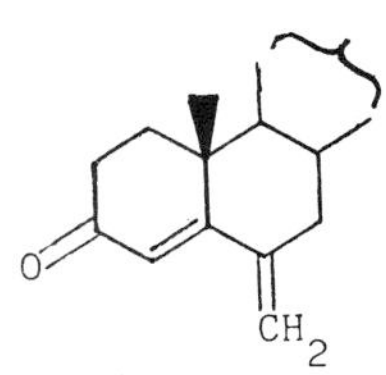	352 +1 258 +17	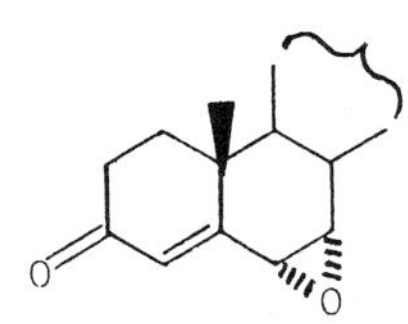	348 +2.5 224 -3.7

* The λ_{max} and $\Delta\varepsilon$ values are typical mean values of the given general structural type, drawn partly from the literature, partly from our own work. They indicate the general trend between the different structural types.

The c.d. of antheraxanthin A, except for a hypsochromic shift of ca. 10 nm, is very similar to that of zeaxanthin and the 9-*cis* antheraxanthin shows an inverted c.d., again very similar to 9-*cis* zeaxanthin, both with respect to temperature dependence, general shape and intensity of the maxima (Fig. 13).

Antheraxanthin B (18) which has an inverted epoxy group exhibits a much weaker c.d. than antheraxanthin A (16). In 16 both end groups are twisted in the same direction thus conferring true chirality to the conjugated system; in 18 due to the inverted epoxy group the epoxy-bearing end-ring adopts the opposite twist with respect to the chain which then becomes more or less non-chiral. If both end groups were identical, one would, of course, have the optically inactive meso compound. The observed weak c.d., therefore, suggests that the steric relationship of the ring with respect to the chain and not the absolute configuration at C(3) is the determining factor. The epoxy group and the double bond in the ring have a similar but not identical influence.

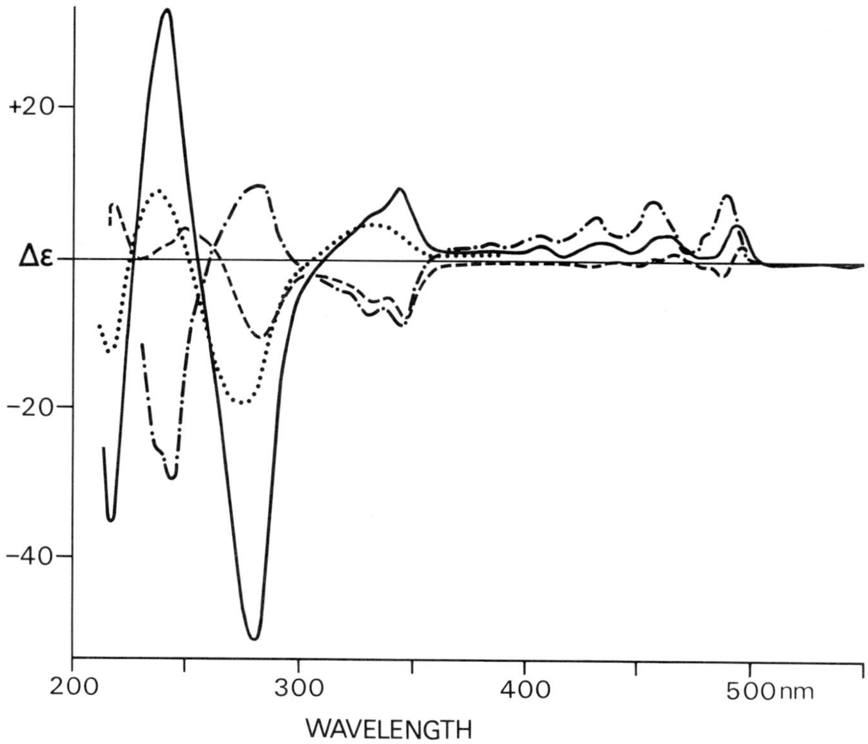

Fig. 13. C.D. spectra of antheraxanthin A (16) at RT ·····, at -180° ———. Antheraxanthin B (18) at -180°C -----. 9-*cis* antheraxanthin A (17) at -180°C -·-·-.

Another interesting series of compounds which became available recently is that of lutein and its epimers and Z-isomers (Ref. 18).

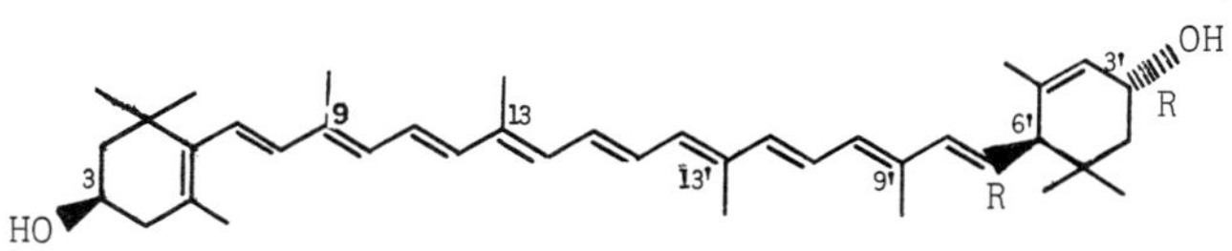

19

(3R,3'R,6'R)-lutein (19)
(3R,3'S,6'R)-lutein (3'-epi-lutein) (20)
(3R,3'S,6'S)-lutein (3',6'-epi-lutein) (21)
(3R,3'R,6'R)-9-*cis* lutein (22)
(3R,3'R,6'R)-9'-*cis* lutein (23)
(3R,3'R,6'R)-13'-*cis* lutein (24)
(3R,3'R,6'R)-13,13'-di-*cis* lutein (25)
(3R,3'R,6'R)-9,13'-di-*cis* lutein (26)
(3R,3'R,6'R)-9,13-di-*cis* lutein (27)
(3R,3'S,6'R)-13-*cis* lutein (3'-epi-13-*cis* lutein) (28)
(3R,3'S,6'R)-13'-*cis* lutein (3'-epi-13'-*cis* lutein) (29)
(3R,3'R,6'R)-13-*cis* lutein (30)

Here we have one end with a substituted β-ring as in zeaxanthin and the other end is a substituted ε-ring with two asymmetric carbons. We have measured the c.d. spectra at ambient and low temperature (-180°C) of lutein (19), its epimers 20 and 21 as well as the mono- and di-*cis* isomers 22 through 30.

Let us first examine which end, the β-ring or the ε-ring, influences the optical activity more strongly. Fig. 14 shows that the c.d. of lutein, in common with all the carotenoids measured so far, is strongly temperature-dependent. It is, however, immediately apparent that there are distinct differences in the temperature dependence of the different maxima. In this non-symmetrical molecule we appear to have several different equilibria, each with a different temperature dependence. This may arise from different temperature dependences of the conformational equilibria at each end of the molecule. One additional benefit of the low temperature spectra is that they are sharper and more distinct than those measured at ambient temperature. Therefore, we shall discuss in the next examples only the low temperature spectra. Fig. 15 shows that the c.d. of the three epimers with the same configuration at C(3) are qualitatively similar and resemble the c.d. of zeaxanthin. Even complete inversion at both centers of the ε-ring (19 vs. 21) does not change the c.d. fundamentally. Only the region around 330 nm seems to be very sensitive to the details of the structure. However, this only shows up well at low temperature since this band is weak and indistinct at room temperature. The non-conjugated ε-ring has apparently less influence than the conjugated β-ring.

Does this type of compound also obey the cis inversion rule? Figs. 16 and 17 show the c.d. spectra of some mono- and di-cis luteins. These spectra demonstrate that the situation is more complicated than with the compounds with two β-end-rings. Some of the bands invert upon introduction of one cis-bond, some do not. Regular behaviour, i.e. inversion on cis-isomerization, is exhibited by the bands at ~280 and 250 nm. The bands under the lowest energy absorption are positive for the all-trans and all the mono-cis isomers as well as the 13,13'-di-cis compound, negative only for the 9,13-di-cis and 9,13'-di-cis isomers. It does not seem possible to formulate a simple rule which could describe this behaviour.

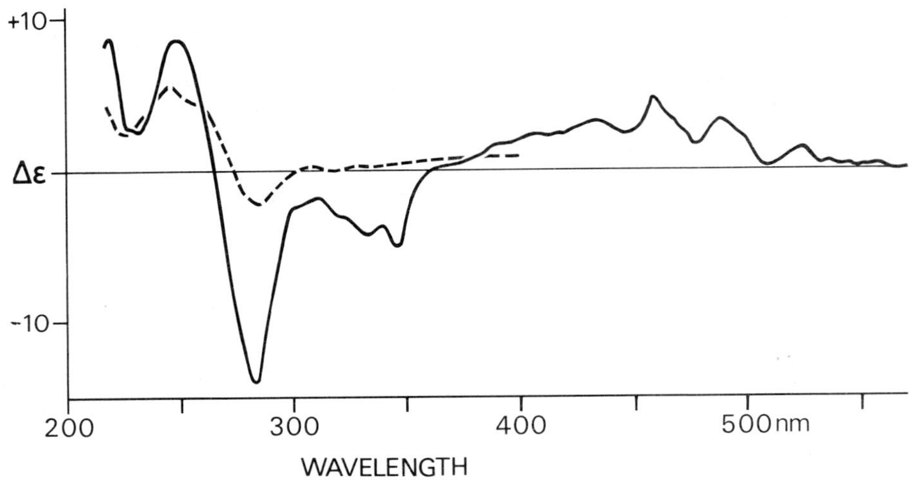

Fig. 14. C.D. spectrum of trans lutein (19) at RT -----, at -180°C ———.

In the 3'-epi lutein series the c.d. of the 13-cis and 13'-cis (28 and 29) are almost identical to the 13-cis and 13'-cis luteins (Figs. 18 and 16). (The c.d. spectrum of 13-cis lutein which is almost identical with the one of 13'-cis lutein is not shown.)

Table 2 summarizes the signs of the different c.d. bands in all these isomers. It is obvious that the ε-ring has a very distinct influence on the optical activity even if the general pattern, at least in the all-trans isomers, seems to be governed by the configuration and conformation at the β-end.

More suitable for the study of the influence of the ε-ring on the optical activity would obviously be compounds with two ε-rings. Some diastereomers of chiriquixanthin have recently been prepared in enantiomerically pure and well-defined form (Ref. 19). Unfortunately there were no Z-isomers available so far.

We show the c.d. spectra of the following three compounds (Fig. 19) all having the same absolute configuration at the centers 6 and 6'.
The spectra are again temperature-dependent but much less than the compounds with β-rings. The Δε-values are also lower. There is no alternation of sign of the c.d. bands ("non-conservative c.d.", Ref. 6). The c.d. under the longest wavelength absorption is comparatively strong. The intensities of the c.d. bands follow those of the absorption, the major c.d. peaks are under the long axis polarized bands. All these observations distinguish these compounds from those with β-end-rings and point to a different source of optical activity compared with the intrinsically chiral chromophores. The spectra are all very similar, suggesting again that it is the center at 6 which determines the optical activity.

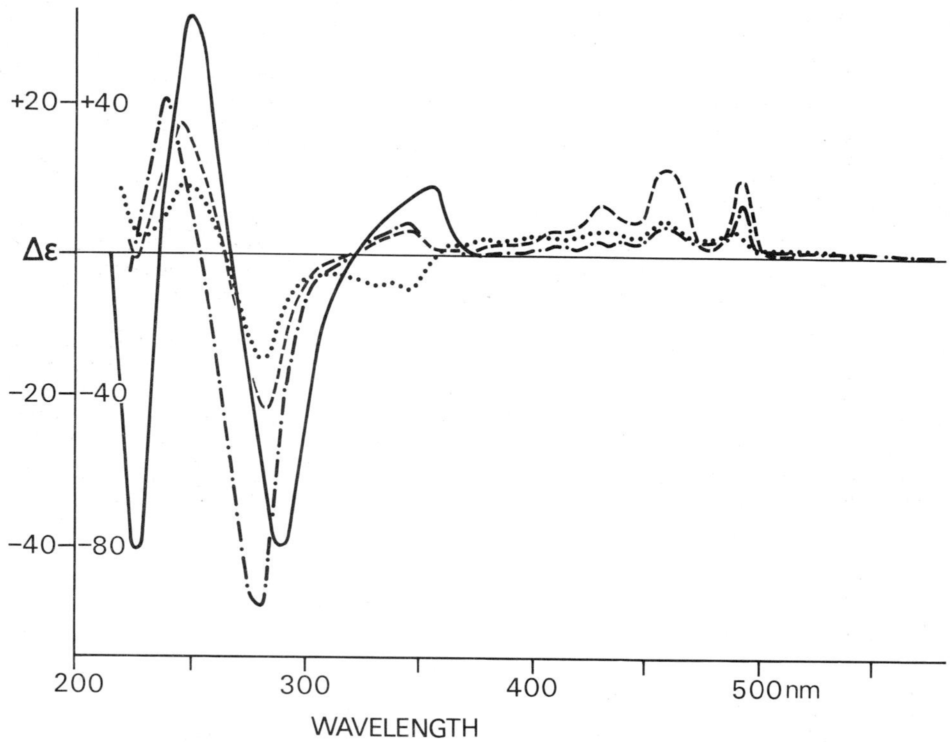

Fig. 15. C.D. spectra at -180°C of zeaxanthin (4) ——— (right hand scale), lutein (19) ·····, 3'-epi lutein (20) -----, 3',6'-epi lutein (21) -·-·-.

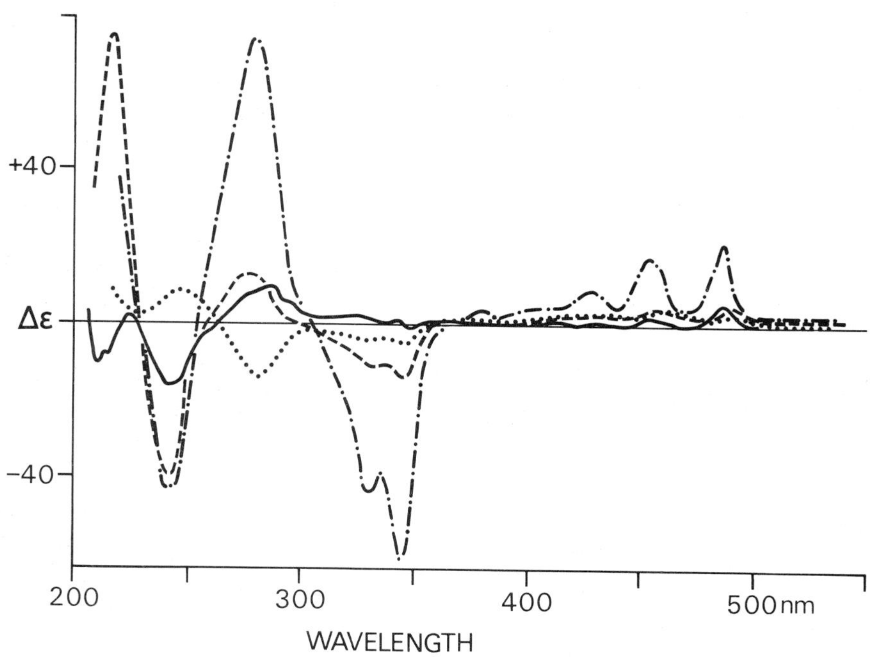

Fig. 16. C.D. spectra at -180°C of lutein (19) ·····, 9-cis lutein (22) ———, 9'-cis lutein (23) -----, 13'-cis lutein (24) -·-·-.

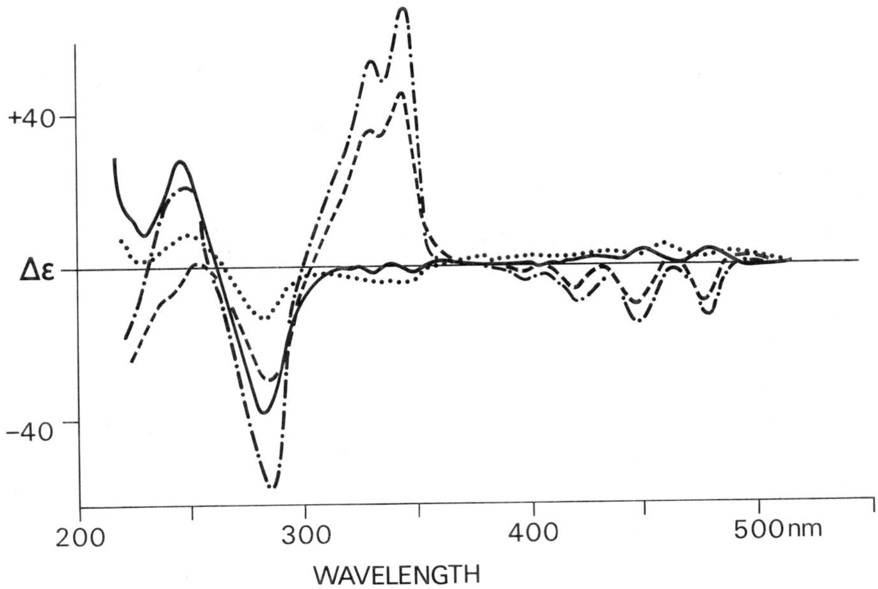

Fig. 17. C.D. spectra at -180°C of lutein (19) ·····, 13,13'-di-cis lutein (25) ———, 9,13-di-cis lutein (27) -----, 9,13'-di-cis lutein (26) -·-·-.

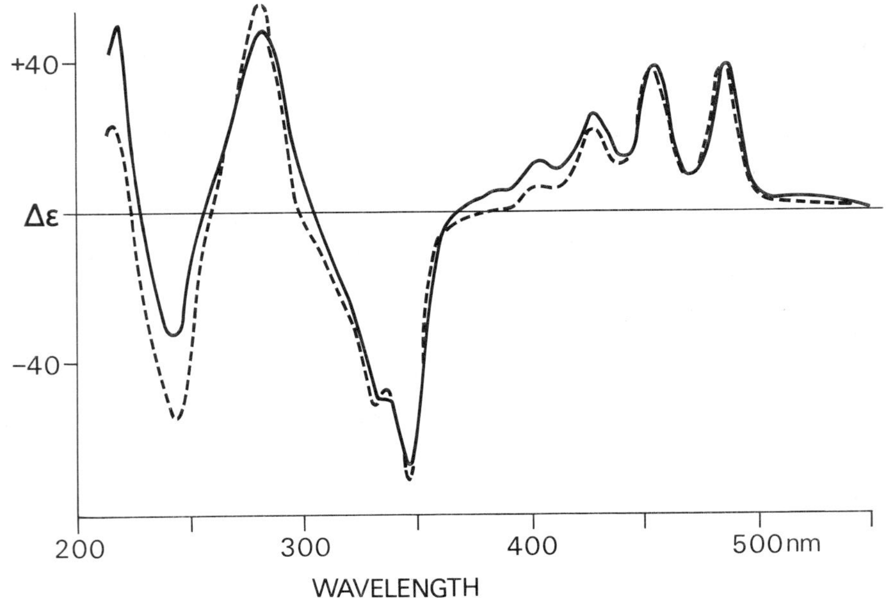

Fig. 18. C.D. spectra at -180°C of 13-cis epi-lutein (28) ———, 13'-cis epi-lutein (29) -----.

In this context the question of the conformation of the ε-ring has to be considered. Models would suggest that when the substituents are trans to each other (as in 19 and 21) both substituents would rather adopt the pseudo-equatorial position. When the substituents are cis steric 1 - 3 interaction of the OH and one of the methyls at C(1) would force the OH into the pseudo-equatorial and the side chain into the pseudo-axial position. Proton magnetic resonance measurements do, more or less, support this picture (Ref. 20) but show some additional complications.

TABLE 2. Signs of the c.d. bands (at -180°C) of lutein, its epimers and Z-isomers, as compared to zeaxanthin.

	~460 nm	~340 nm	~280 nm	~240 nm
(3R,3'R) zeaxanthin (4)	-	+	-	+
(3R,6'R,3'R) trans lutein (19)	+	-	-	+
3'-epi-lutein (3R,6'R,3'S) (20)	+	+	-	+
6',3'-epi-lutein (3R,6'S,3'S) (21)	+	+	-	+
3'-epi- 13 and 13'-mono-cis (28,29)	+	-	+	-
13-cis lutein (3R,3'R,6'R) (30)	+	-	+	-
13'-cis lutein (3R,3'R,6'R) (24)	+	-	+	-
9'-cis lutein (3R,3'R,6'R) (23)	+	-	+	-
9-cis lutein (3R,3'R,6'R) (22)	+	±	+	-
13,13'-di-cis lutein (3R,3'R,6'R) (25)	+	-	-	+
9,13'-di-cis lutein (3R,3'R,6'R) (26)	-	+	-	+
9,13-di-cis lutein (3R,3'R,6'R) (27)	-	+	-	(+)

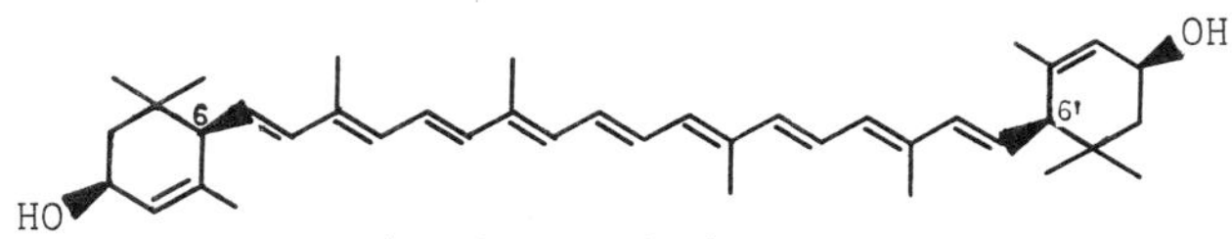

(3S,6R,3'S,6'R)-chiriquixanthin B, "cis-cis" (31)

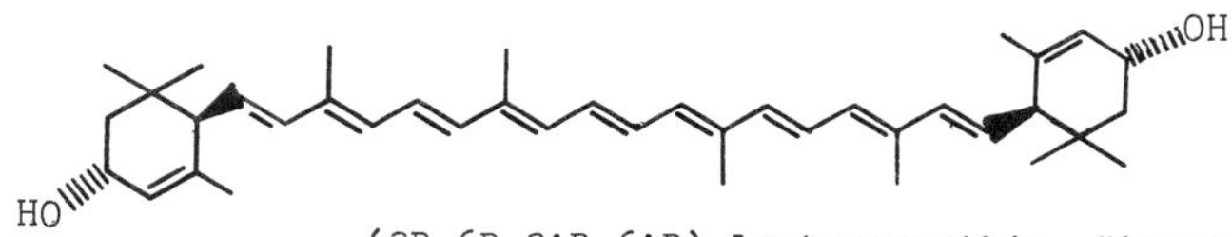

(3R,6R,3'R,6'R)-lactucaxanthin, "trans-trans" (32)

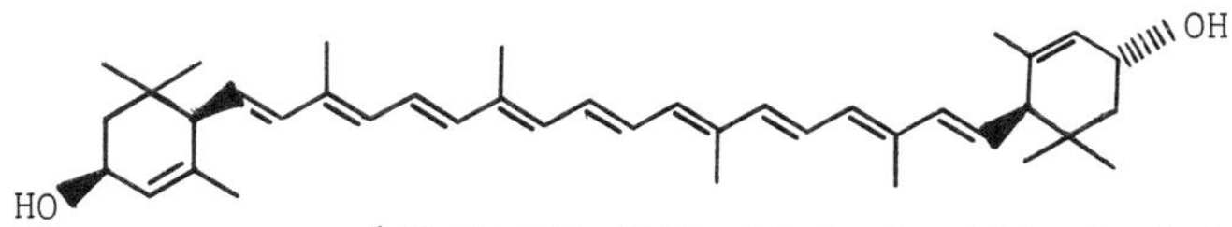

(3S,6R,3'R,6'R)-chiriquixanthin A, "cis-trans" (33)

It follows from the coupling constants of the proton on C(3) with the two protons on C(2) that in the cis-compound two of these protons are more diaxial ($J_{2,3}$ = 10 and 6 Hz) than in the trans-compound ($J_{2,3}$ = 6 and 6.8 Hz). The coupling constants of the trans-compound are, on the other hand, too large for a pure diequatorial coupling. This means that in the cis-compound the hydroxyl on C(3) is more equatorial than in the trans-compound where the ring is somewhat distorted. The chain could then be axial in the cis-compound but would not be purely equatorial in the trans-compound.

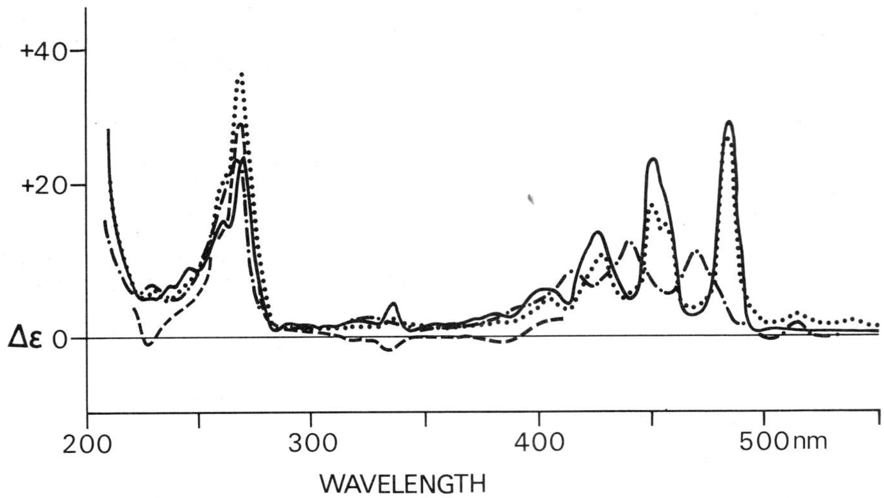

Fig. 19. C.D. spectra of chiriquixanthin A (33) at RT -·-·-, at -180°C ·····, of lactucaxanthin (32) at -180°C ----- and of chiriquixanthin B (31) at -180°C ———.

It can be seen on models that even the most extreme movement of the chain from pseudo equatorial to pseudo axial position does not change much the geometrical relationship between the chain and the homo-conjugated double bond in the ring (Fig. 20) and a major influence on the c.d. spectrum should not be expected.

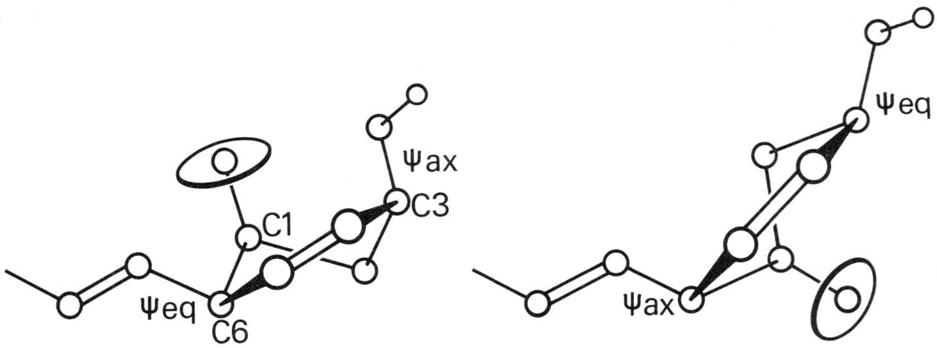

Fig. 20. Relationship of ε-ring with the chain; left side: chain Ψ_{eq}, right side: chain Ψ_{ax} (the methyl at C(5) and one of the methyls at C(1) are omitted).

CONCLUSIONS

In this work we have been able to show, by studying sets of closely related optically active carotenoids, the subtle interactions which control the form of their c.d. spectra. In all the examples studied the asymmetric centers are in the end-rings. However, the c.d. is observed in the electronic transitions of the main polyene chain. The relationship of the asymmetric center to the chain is controlled both by the conformation of the end-ring and by the steric hindrance between the end-ring and the main chain. In all cases studied there appears to be conformational mobility at both these points of the molecule. The c.d. depends critically on these conformations, since twists about the bonds joining the end-ring to the chain create the intrinsic dissymmetry of the chromophore. Without prior knowledge of the conformation it is therefore, in general, not possible to deduce the absolute configuration from the observed c.d.

A striking example is the pair zeaxanthin - astaxanthin. The room temperature c.d. spectra are deceptively similar and one could therefore be tempted to deduce just from the c.d. that both compounds have the same absolute configuration. However, if one had measured the c.d. at low temperature, the opposite conclusion would have been drawn, since astaxanthin inverts its c.d. upon cooling. Of course, it is known from chemical evidence that both compounds have the same absolute configuration.

Since the introduction of a cis double bond in the chain changes the sign of the c.d. in some classes of carotenoids, either one must know the stereo-isomeric form of the chain in order to deduce absolute configuration, or, if the latter is known, the c.d. spectrum can be used to identify the cis-trans-isomers present. There is additional warning from this work that the temperature-dependent behaviour should also be known. C.D. spectra are very sensitive to the coupling of the electrons of the end-ring with the chain and can therefore give information on the conjugation across the ring-chain junction in addition to the absorption spectrum.

The temperature dependence of the c.d. can be used to study the conformational equilibria and the concentration dependence can reveal interactions between molecules.

There are, however, still many problems and many more compounds to be studied and much interesting work to be done in the future.

Acknowledgement - I thank Dr. Thomson for fruitful discussions and for reading this manuscript and Mr. Kachler for technical assistance.

REFERENCES

1. O. Straub, Key to Carotenoids, Birkhäuser Verlag, Basel (1976).
2. G. Englert, M. Vecchi, Helv. Chim. Acta 63, 1171-1718 (1980).
3. M. Vecchi, R.K. Müller, J. High Resol. Chromatogr. & Chromatogr. Commun. 2, 195-196 (1979)
H. Rønneberg, B. Renstrøm, K. Aareskjold, S. Liaaen-Jensen, M. Vecchi, F. Leuenberger, R.K. Müller, H. Mayer, Helv. Chim. Acta 63, 711-715 (1980)
R.K. Müller, K. Bernhard, H. Mayer, A. Rüttimann, M. Vecchi, Helv. Chim. Acta 63, 1654-1664 (1980).
4. K. Noack, A.J. Thomson, Helv. Chim. Acta 62, 1902-1921 (1979).
5. S. Liaaen-Jensen, Progress in the Chemistry of Organic Natural Products, Ed. W. Herz, H. Grisebach, G.W. Kirby, Vol. 39, 123-172 (1980) Springer-Verlag, Wien, New York.
6. V. Sturzenegger, R. Buchecker, G. Wagnière, Helv. Chim. Acta 63, 1074-1092 (1980).
7. S. Hertzberg, G. Borch, S. Liaaen-Jensen, Acta Chem. Scand. B 33, 42-46 (1979).
8. G. Englert, F. Kienzle, K. Noack, Helv. Chim. Acta 60, 1209-1219 (1977).
9. K. Bernhard, G.P. Moss, G. Tóth, B.C.L. Weedon, Tetrahedron Letters, 3899-3902 (1974).
10. E. Charney, Tetrahedron 21, 3127-3139 (1965).
11. G. Wagnière, W. Hug, Tetrahedron Letters, 4765-4768 (1970).
12. A. Moscowitz, K. Wellman, C. Djerassi, J. Amer. Chem. Soc. 85, 3515-3516 (1963).
13. D.A. Lightner, E.L. Docks, Tetrahedron 35, 713-720 (1979) and literature cited therein.
14. K. Noack, A.J. Thomson, Helv. Chim. Acta (submitted for publication).
15. I. Tinoco, Adv. Chem. Phys. 4, 113-160 (1962)
I. Tinoco, Radiation Res. 20, 133-139 (1963).
16. G.P. Moss, J. Szabolcs, G. Tóth, B.C.L. Weedon, Acta Chim. Acad. Sci. Hung. 87, 301-309 (1975).
17. I thank Prof. Eugster, Zürich, for the gift of the compounds.
18. I thank Dr. Mayer for the preparation and Dr. Vecchi for the separation of the compounds.
19. I thank Dr. Mayer for the compounds; see also lecture by Dr. Mayer at this symposium.
20. Dr. Englert, personal communication.
21. B. Honig, A. Warshel, M. Karplus, Accounts Chem. Res. 8, 92-100 (1975).
22. J.C.J. Bart, C.H. MacGillavry, Acta Crystallogr. B 24, 1569-1587, 1587-1606 (1968).
23. R. Buchecker, U. Marti, C.H. Eugster, 6th International Symposium on Carotenoids, Abstracts of Papers (1981).

MASS SPECTRA OF CAROTENOIDS - LABELLING STUDIES

Herbert Budzikiewicz

Institut für Organische Chemie der Universität zu Köln, Greinstraße 4, 5000 Köln 41, Bundesrepublik Deutschland

Abstract - Mass spectroscopic data obtained from isotopically labelled carotenoids are reviewed.

Mass spectrometry has become an indispensable tool for structural studies in the carotenoid field. There are two main goals of research on the fragmentation behavior of this class of compounds, *viz.*, (a) to establish processes characteristic of the various terminal groups which is of importance for the structure elucidation of new representatives, and (b) to understand the mechanisms governing the elimination of parts of the polyene chain, an area more of academic interest. Obviously, after more than 15 years of research progress is manifested not so much any more by leading discoveries but rather by filling in gaps here and there and by tidying up loose ends. This is reflected, e.g., by only three entries for mass spectrometry of carotenoids in the latest Specialist Periodical Report on Terpenoids and Steroids (1). In view of a series of summarizing articles (2-7) which have appeared recently I decided rather to review a special aspect of carotenoid mass spectrometry, *viz.* labelling studies, since the data available are scattered widely and have not always been taken into account for the formulation of fragmentation mechanisms.

D-LABELLED CAROTENOIDS.

Fragmentation processes comprising the end groups.

Though ions formed by the loss of a (substituted) cyclohexene end group are usually of very low abundance $[M - 137]^+$ (for 1, R = H) and $[M - 153]^+$ (for 1, R = OH) are of some diagnostic value (8). To account for this loss rupture of the 7,8-bond and elimination of an additional H (originally assumed (8) to stem from C-14) has to be invoked. Variously D-labelled β-carotene derivatives (4, 9, 10) (4,4'-d_2,10,10',11,11'-d_4; 11,11'-d_2; 11,11',15,15'-d_4; 14-d_1; 15,15'-d_2) show, however, that there is no specific transfer from C-14: ~40% of the hydrogen lost stems from C-11 and the rest from various positions of the polyene chain (9) as indicated in *Scheme 1*.

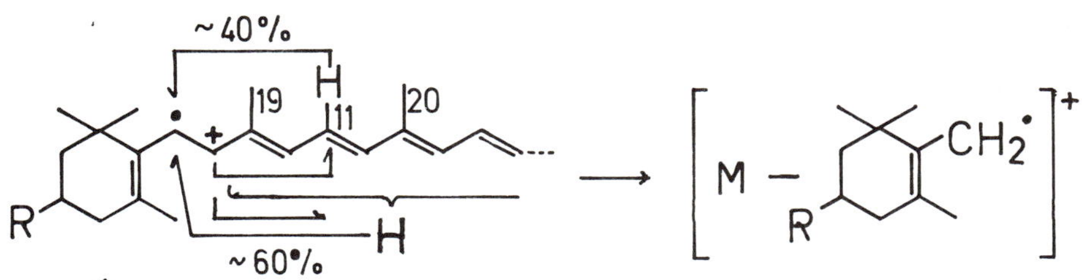

1

Scheme 1: Formation of $[M - 137]^+$

Appropriate shift of the ion formed by allylic cleavage (*Scheme 2*) upon introduction of trideuteroacetyl groups allowed localization of the hydroxyl functions in a C_{50}-carotenoid isolated from *Sarcina lutea* (11).

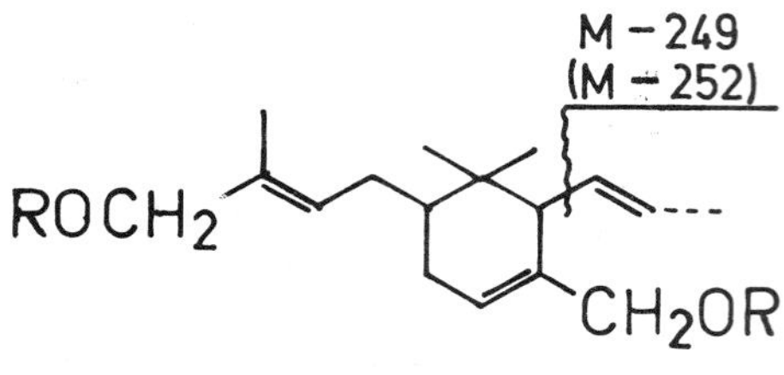

R = $COCH_3$ ($COCD_3$) + H

Scheme 2: Fragmentation of a C_{50}-carotenoid

Both, 5,6- (2) and 5,8-epoxides (3) form characteristic fragments of the mass *m/z* [164 + R]+ (a) and [204 + R]+ (b) (see *Fig. 1*) for which the following geneses and structures have been suggested (*Scheme 3*) (12):

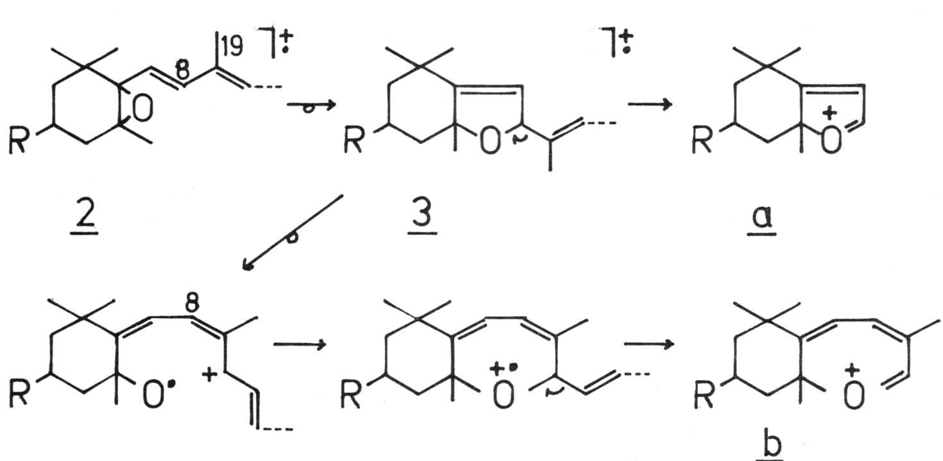

Scheme 3: Fragmentation of epoxides

The results obtained from labelled analogs (4,4,4',4'-d_4; 7,7'-d_2; 8-d_1; 8,8'-d_2; 7,7',8,8'-d_4; 8,8',15,15'-d_4; 4,4,4',4',8,8',15,15',19,19,19,19',19',19'-d_{14}; 10,10'-d_2; 10,10', 11,11'-d_4; 10,10',11,11',15,15'-d_6; 11,11'-d_2; 11,15-d_2; 11,11',12,12'-d_4; 11,11',15,15'-d_4; 12,20,20,20-d_4; 14-d_1; 15,15'-d_2) are in accordance with the formulation for a. However, the loss of about two thirds of the D from C-8 during the formation of b indicates a hydrogen exchange with other loci of the polyene chain prior to fragment formation, esp. C-15/C-15' and to some extent also C-11 and C-12 (or C-20). C-7, C-10 and C-14 are apparently not involved in the hydrogen exchange (9, 10, 13).

The species a and b are the first members of a series of ions comprising the epoxide moiety which are formed by formal cleavage of the 8,9-, 9,10-, 10,11-, etc. bond (for R = H *m/z* 165, 192, 205, etc., series c in *Fig. 1*). The formation of the higher members (cleavage of a bond beyond C-15) is accompanied by the loss of one H. One of them, *viz.* [(336 + R) - H]+ has been examined in detail: It is generated by rupture of the bond between C-13' and C-12' with H-abstraction exclusively from C-15 (see *Scheme 4*) (9):

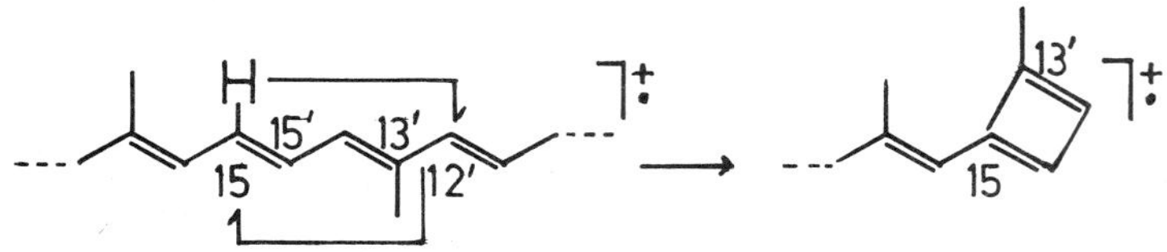

Scheme 4: Formation of the ion [(336 + R) - H]+

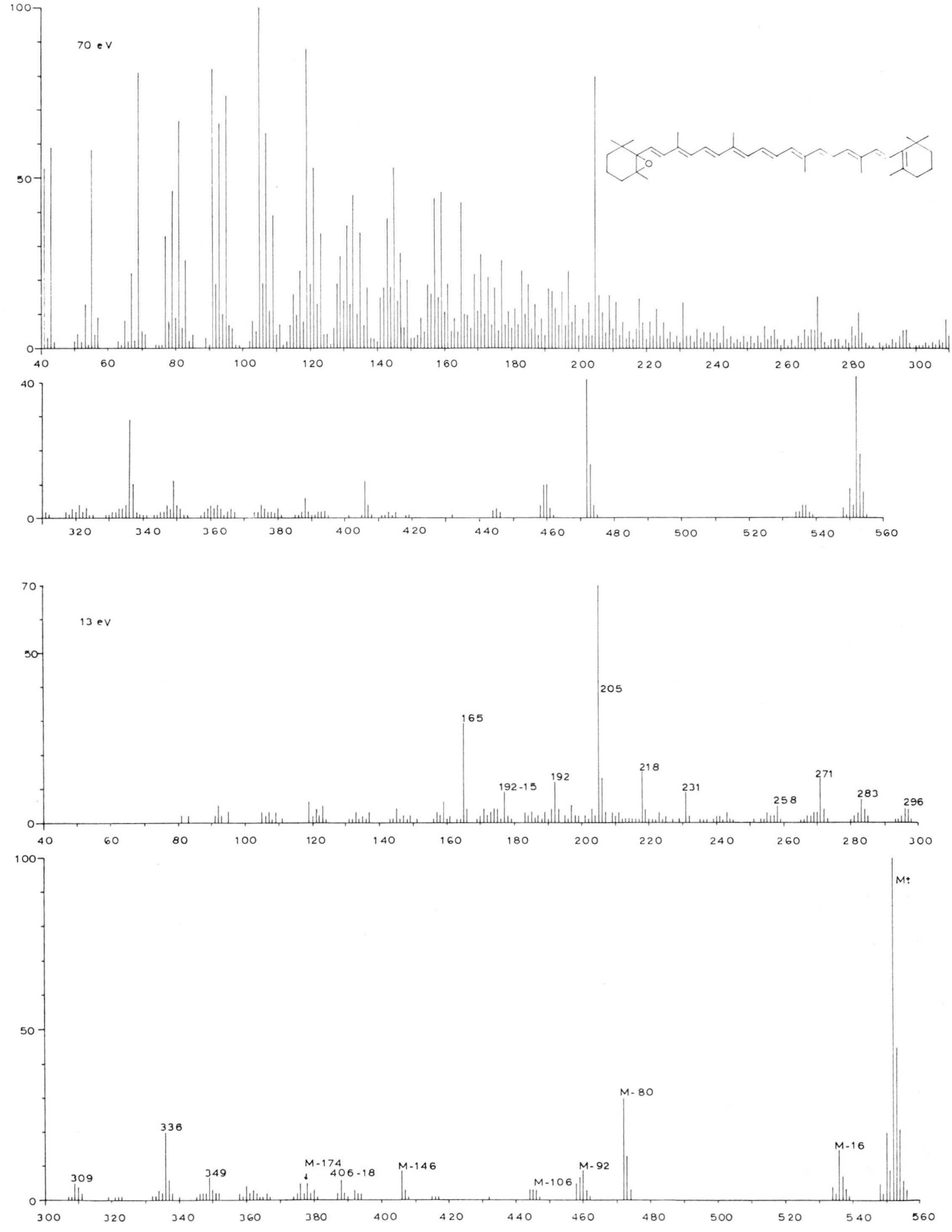

Fig. 1: Mass spectra (70 and 13 eV) of β-carotene-5,6-monoepoxide. *m/z* 165: a; *m/z* 205: b; *m/z* 165, 192, 205, 218, 231, 258, 271, 283, 296, 309, 336, 349: c-series; *m/z* 272: d; *m/z* 460: $[M - 92]^{+\cdot}$; *m/z* 446: $[M - 106]^{+\cdot}$; *m/z* 394: $[M - 158]^{+\cdot}$; *m/z* 446, 406, 380: e, f, g; *m/z* 554 $[M + 2H]^{+\cdot}$ (partially).

Substituents in the polyene chain frequently alter the fragmentation pattern observed for the parent compound. Thus, the presence of a hydroxyl group at C-8 as in fucoxanthol (4) gives rise to an abundant fragment $[M - 170]^+$ for the formation of which a hydrogen rearrangement as depicted in *Scheme 5* has been suggested (14) which is in accord with the complete retention of D at C-8 in the ionized fragment (13).

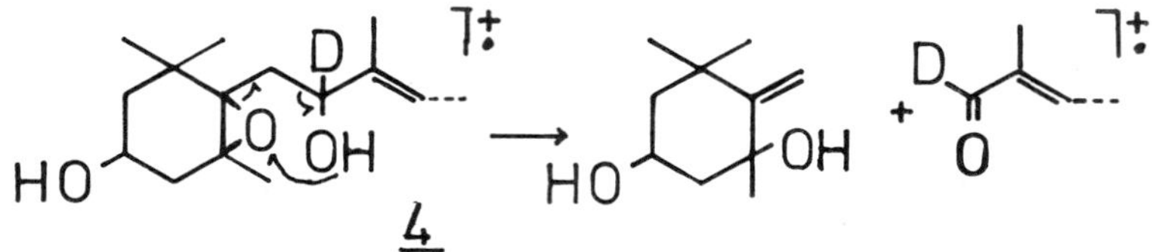

4

Scheme 5: Fragmentation of fucoxanthol

Elimination of hydrocarbon moieties from the polyene chain

Hardly any fragmentation process in mass spectrometry has attracted so much attention as the loss of toluene and of xylene from carotenoids (for a summary of the results see Ref. 7). The intensity ratio of the ions $[M - 92]^{+\cdot}/[M - 106]^{+\cdot}$ (usually referred to as R-value) is inversely proportional to the number of conjugated double bonds and is further influenced by steric and electronic factors exerted by the end groups. The mechanism generally agreed upon today (15) consists of 3 steps, *viz.* an 8 electron conrotatory, a 6 electron disrotatory electrocyclic reaction and opening of the fourmembered ring (*Scheme 6*).

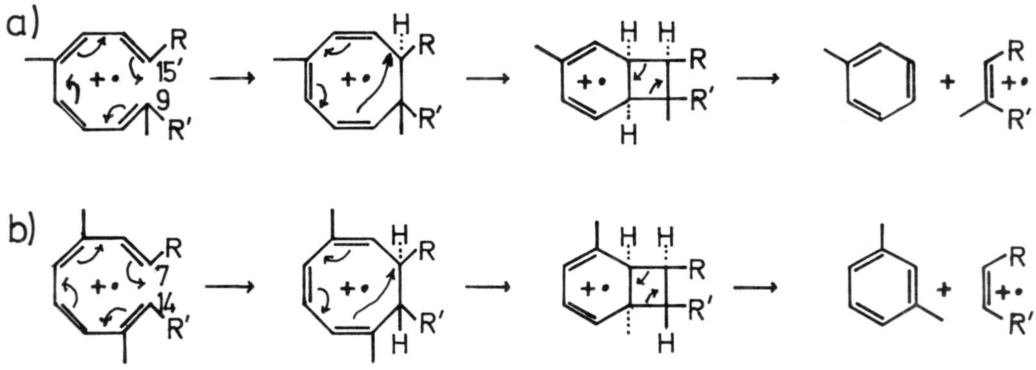

Scheme 6: Elimination of (a) toluene and (b) xylene

The first information as to from which portion of the polyene chain toluene and xylene were derived came from a comparison of the spectra of β-carotene (5) and its 15,15'-d_2 analog (2). The fact that only xylene-d_0, but toluene-d_1 and -d_2 (60:40) were lost pointed towards a formal cleavage of double bonds rather than single bonds as had been suggested originally (16) (see *Scheme 7*). It could also be shown that pyrolytic and electron impact degradation gave the same distribution of label (2).

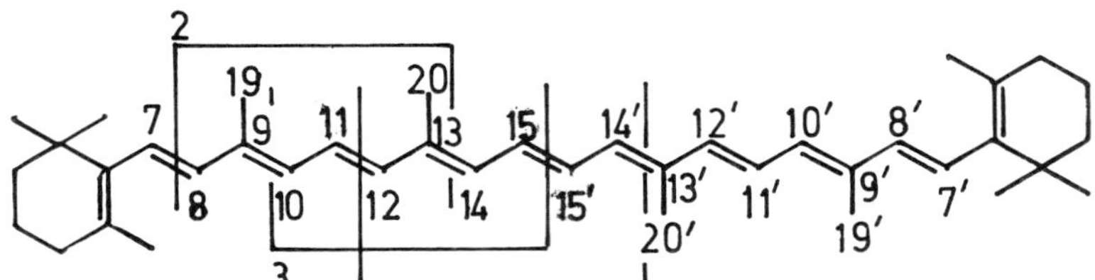

5

Scheme 7: Elimination of toluene (3, 4) and of xylene (2) from β-carotene (note: here and in the following Schemes the analogous elimination reactions from the right-hand part of the molecule have been omitted.

From 15,15'-d_2-lycopene (6) where the conjugated chain is extended by one ethylene unit on each side loss of unlabelled toluene is observed in addition

(*Scheme 8*) (2).

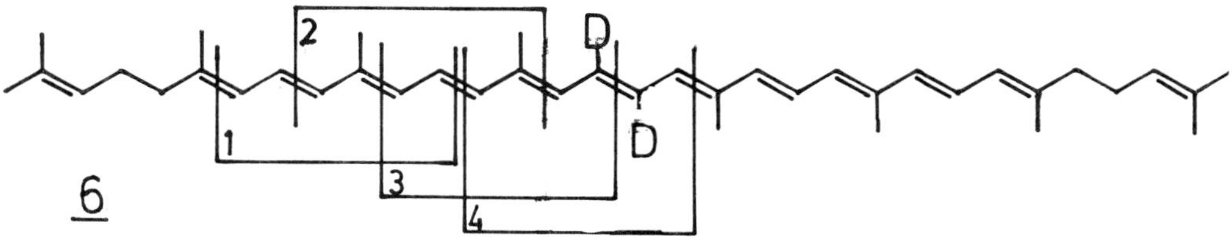

6

Scheme 8: Elimination of toluene (1, 3, 4) and of xylene (2) from lycopene.

These results were confirmed by the observation that 7,7'-d_2 aromatic carotenoids (5, trimethylbenzene instead of trimethylhexene rings) lost both unlabelled toluene and xylene only (cf. *Scheme 7*), and that 7,7'-d_2 lycopene derivatives eliminated unlabelled xylene, but toluene-d_o and -d_1 in the ratio 2:1 (cf. *Scheme 8*) (17, 18). Subsequent labelling in all positions of the polyene chain for the bicyclic (β-carotene) type (9, 18) and at the 11,11'-position for the acyclic (lycopene) type (18) are in complete agreement with the mechanism *Scheme 7* and *8* (formal cleavage of the double bonds), and they also show that there are no hydrogen migrations prior to or concomitant with the toluene and xylene elimination. The same mechanism also applies to *retro*carotenoids in which the shift of the double bonds alters the loci of rupture correspondingly. As can be seen (9, 10) from the spectrum of [11,11',12,12'-D_4]-6,7-*retro*-β,ε-carotene (7), again formally the double bonds are cleaved which results in the elimination of toluene-d_2, but xylene-d_2 and -d_o (*Scheme 9*).

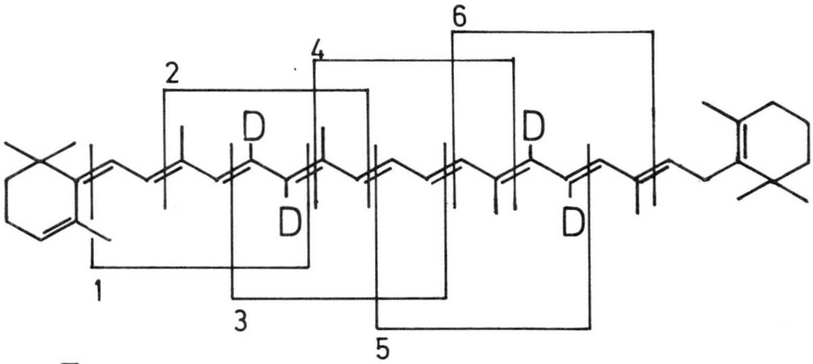

7

Scheme 9: Toluene (1, 3, 5) and xylene (2, 4, 6) elimination from a *retro*-carotene

15,15'-Didehydrocarotenoids show loss of xylene, but that of toluene is replaced by [M - 90]$^{+\cdot}$. Labelling (9, 10, 18, 19) (7,7'-d_2, 8,8'-d_2, 8,8',19,19,19,19',19',19'-d_8, 11,11'-d_2) shows that xylene lost comprises the parts C-8 to C-13 and C-8' to C-13' only, while [M - 90]$^{+\cdot}$ stems from C-12 to C-14' and C-14 to C-12'. Again, formal cleavage of double bonds (but not of the triple bond) is responsible for the loss of the hydrocarbon moieties (*Scheme 10*).

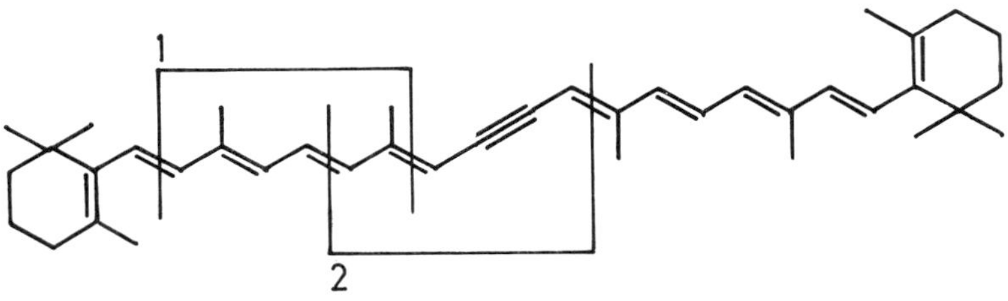

Scheme 10: Xylene (1) and C_7H_6 (2) elimination from 15,15'-didehydrocarotenoids

The labelling studies revealed also that loss of toluene does not occur at the same rate from the different parts of the polyene chain according to *Schemes 7* and *8*. If the rate constant for the loss of xylene is arbitrarily given the value $k_2 = 1$, for the toluene elimination $k_3 = 8$ and $k_4 = 4$ can be calculated. Though less complete labelling data are available for lycopene type carotenoids for the additional toluene loss $k_1 = 6$ is rather likely (7).

In order to obtain further information on the factors governing the relative rates of the competing elimination reactions a series of labelled model compounds (varying length of the polyene chain, alteration in the methyl substitution pattern, etc.) have been investigated (20). The results may be summarized as follows: (a) Loss of xylene is preferred over that of toluene; benzene (from appropriate *nor*-compounds) is not lost at all. (b) As suggested by *Francis* (15) a methyl group at the terminal carbon of the octatetraene portion undergoing the first (rate determining) cyclisation step (see *Scheme 6*, elimination of toluene) reduces the elimination rate. (c) Losses from the end of the polyene chain are sterically hindered by the end groups and hence less favourable. (d) A phenyl group conjugated with the polyene chain fosters cyclisation involving the first double bond. That even the replacement of hydrogen by deuterium shows some effect is demonstrated by the change of the R-values if normal and perdeuterated α- and β-carotene are compared (21) or if an $OCOCH_3$-substituent in an end group is replaced by $OCOCD_3$ (22, 23).

The third "classical" elimination reaction is the loss of $C_{12}H_{14}$ usually referred to as dimethyl dihydronaphthalene ($[M - 158]^{+\cdot}$), again by formal cleavage of the double bonds (*Scheme 11*). From the labelled compounds discussed in connection with the toluene/xylene loss it became evident that the $C_{12}H_{14}$ moiety lost comprises only C-10 to C-12' (C-12 to C-10') (9). From this region (C-10 to C-10') stem also the ions $[M - 78]^{+\cdot}$, $[M - 79]^{+}$ and $[M - 80]^{+\cdot}$ (loss of C_6H_{6-8}). Their low abundance and the dependence of their relative ratio upon experimental conditions do, however, not allow anything to be said about the mechanism of their formation (9).

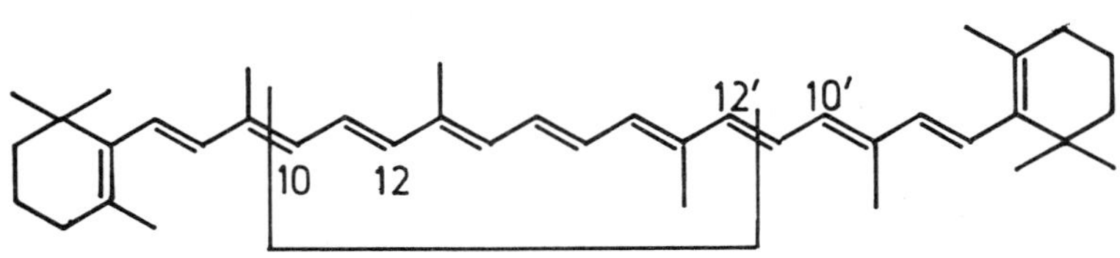

Scheme 11: Elimination of $C_{12}H_{14}$ from β-carotene

The $[M - 80]^{+}$ mentioned above which stems from various parts of the polyene chain must not be confused with the characteristic $[M - 80]^{+\cdot}$-ion (d) observed for epoxides. For this process mechanisms have been formulated (13, 14) which had to be abandoned when extensive labelling data (positions 4, 7, 8, 10, 11, 12, 14, 15, 19, 20) became available (9). The hydrogen atoms bound to the end groups and to C-7, C-10 and C-19 are retained during the elimination of C_6H_8, those from C-8, C-11, C-12, C-14, C-15 and C-20 are lost. The mechanism formulated in *Scheme 12* accounts for these observations.

In the spectra of epoxides in addition to the pronounced $[M - 80]^{+\cdot}$ ion a series of less abundant fragments $[M - 106]^{+\cdot}$; $[M - 146]^{+\cdot}$; $[M - 172]^{+\cdot}$ (e - g) is observed the geneses of which are related to that of $[M - 80]^{+\cdot}$ (*Scheme 13*). $[M - 106]^{+\cdot}$ is apparently not only formed by the typical $[M - \text{xylene}]^{+\cdot}$ mechanism (*v. supra*). Thus, $[14\text{-}D_1]$-β-carotene-5,6-monoepoxides shows (in addition to the expected $[M - 106]^{+\cdot}$) also $[M - 107]^{+\cdot}$, and $[10,10'\text{-}D_2]$-β-carotene-5,6-monoepoxide (in addition to the expected $[M - 107]^{+\cdot}$) also $[M - 106]^{+\cdot}$ neither of which can be explained by *Scheme 7*. The labelling data (9) demonstrate for $[M - 106]^{+\cdot}$ and $[M - 146]^{+\cdot}$ again H-transfer from C-8 and localize the position of the polyene chain wherefrom the elimination occurs as depicted in *Scheme 13*. For $[M - 172]^{+\cdot}$ a different mechanism has to be envisaged since H-migration occurs here from C-10.

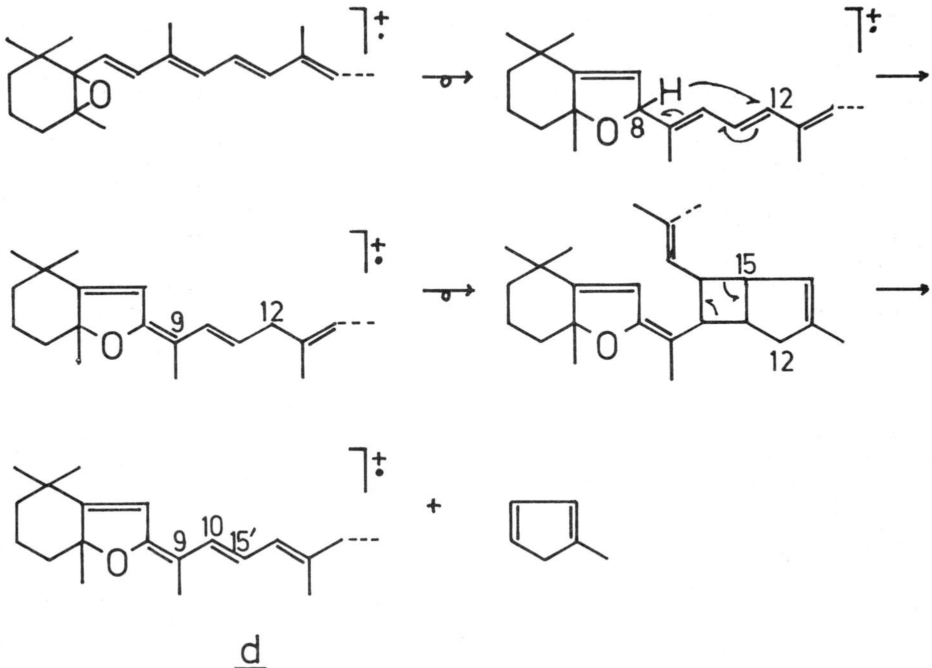

Scheme 12: Formation of [M - 80]$^{+\cdot}$ from carotene epoxides.

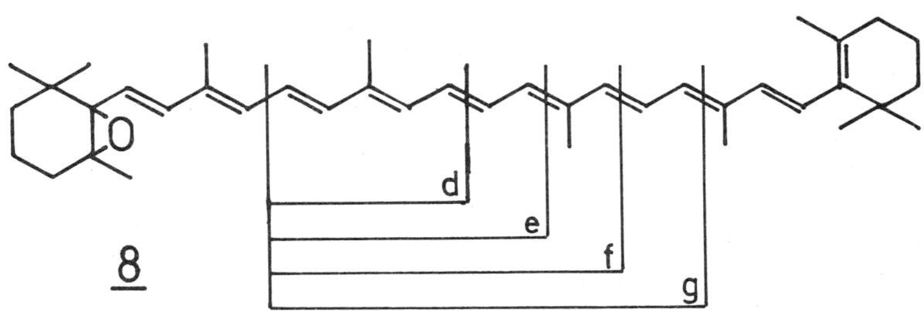

8

Scheme 13. Fragmentation of the polyene chain of carotene epoxides.

^{18}O-LABELLED CAROTENOIDS

^{18}O-labelled carotenoids are of minor importance for the elucidation of fragmentation mechanisms. In most cases the same information may be obtained by exact mass measurements and/or comparison of the mass spectra of related compounds ("substituent labelling"). They play, however, an important role in the investigation of metabolic pathways of oxygen in plant photosynthesis (24) and other processes where carotenoids are involved. As oxygen does not possess any sufficiently long-lived radioactive isotopes mainly ^{18}O is resorted to for labelling studies. Its analysis may, however, cause difficulties: Methods which measure the ^{18}O content after transformation to H_2O, O_2, CO or CO_2 as well as proton activation analysis ([^{18}O(p,n)^{18}F]) only allow one to determine mean enrichment and do not differentiate between hydroxyl, epoxide, etc. functions in the molecule. Further complications are introduced by the sensitivity of carotenoids to oxygen since oxidation products formed during the work-up and sample preparation may falsify the results (25, 28).

The obvious advantage of a mass spectroscopic analysis of the intact molecule as compared with methods yielding only the total ^{18}O content is the differentiation between ^{18}O-free, $^{18}O_1$, $^{18}O_2$, etc. species, and the possibility - within limits - to analyse only the compound one is interested in without interference from (more highly oxygenated) transformation products. In addition, characteristic fragments allow one to distinguish between the different oxygen functions in a molecule.

The indispensable prerequisite for the mass spectroscopic analysis is, however, that there is no exchange of oxygen with that of water adsorbed in the ion source. This has been checked (25) for β-carotene-5,6-mono- and 5,6,5',6'-diepoxide by adding $H_2{}^{18}O$ and subsequently $H_2{}^{16}O$ to the sample in the ion source. While the ratio *m/z* 207 : *m/z* 205 is hardly influenced and corresponds to the calculated value for the natural content of ^{18}O (~0,1), that of $[M + 2]^{+\cdot}$: $[M]^{+\cdot}$ is much too high (0,2 - 0,3) and varies considerably during the measurements. These variations are due to the fact that the ion $C_{40}H_{56}{}^{18}O$ is superimposed by $C_{40}H_{58}{}^{16}O$ (see *Fig. 1*) formed by hydrogenation in the ion source. Since this process occurs on active spots in the source the hydrogen stemming from adsorbed water (26, 27) the abundance of $[M + 2H]^+$ is a function of the partial pressure both of the sample and of water. This can be learned from *Fig. 2*: With increasing sample pressure the active spots are occupied to an increasingly higher percentage, hence the ratio $[M + 2]^+/[M]^+$ drops to a minimum at maximal sample pressure and rises again as the sample disappears slowly from the ion source. If one introduces $H_2{}^{16}O$ as soon as the minimum of the curve is reached, the ratio $[M + 2]^{+\cdot}$: $[M]^{+\cdot}$ increases in the same way for natural and ^{18}O-enriched 8. This observation and the invariance of the *m/z* 207 : *m/z* 205 ratio upon addition of $H_2{}^{18}O$ + $H_2{}^{16}O$ (*v. supra*) indicates that there is no exchange of epoxide oxygen with the water adsorbed in the ion source. The results have been corroborated by experiments with cyclohexene and isobutene epoxide where no hydrogenation is possible, and where the ratio of $[M + 2]^{+\cdot}$: $[M]^{+\cdot}$ remains unchanged even if large amounts of $H_2{}^{18}O$ are introduced into the source (25).

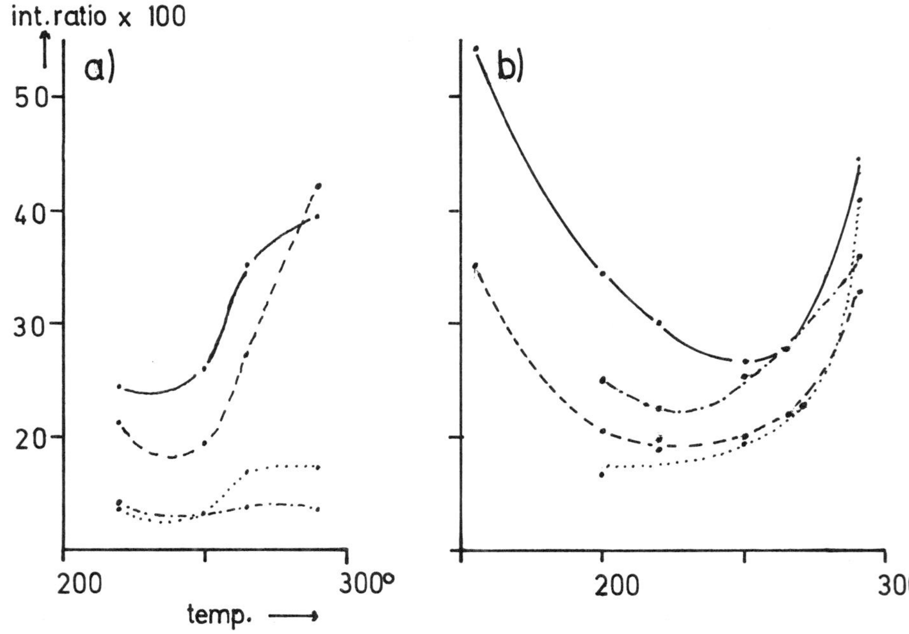

Fig. 2: Temperature dependence (a: 13 eV, b: 70 eV) of the $[X + 2]^{+\cdot}$: $[X]^{+\cdot}$-ratio for various ions from ^{18}O-enriched (11%) β-carotene-5,6-monoepoxide (8): ____ $M^{+\cdot}$, ---- d, ···· b, -·-· a.

Low Resolution Measurements.

In principle, measurements of the abundance ratios of $M^+(^{16}O_n)$: $M^+(^{16}O_{n-1}{}^{18}O)$: $M^+(^{16}O_{n-2}{}^{18}O_2)$ etc. as well as the ratio of the intensities of fragment ions which comprise definite parts of the molecule (allowing for ^{13}C correction) will allowcalculation of the ^{18}O content. Suitable fragments, e.g., both for 5,6- and for 5,8-epoxides are a (*m/z* 164 + R), b (*m/z* 204 + R) and d ($[M - 80]^{+\cdot}$). The main obstacle for the analysis of the M^+-region is the formation of hydrogenation products (*v. supra*) the amount of which depends upon so many parameters (sample preparation, source condition, sample pressure, temperature) that the contribution of $[M + 2H]^{+\cdot}$ cannot be standardized. For the same reason fragments directly connected with $M^{+\cdot}$ (as $[M - H_2O]^{+\cdot}$) cannot be used, either. Complications may arise for fragment ions if there exist isobaric species stemming from other parts of the molecule. The relative amount of these may vary with the source temperature (cf. *Fig. 1*

Table 1.

^{18}O-Content of β-carotene-5,8-monoepoxide samples

sample	ionisation energy	low resolution						high resolution		^{18}O content (%)
		P_{167}/P_{165} a)	$\%^{18}O$	P_{207}/P_{205} a)	$\%^{18}O$	P_{474}/P_{472} a)	$\%^{18}O$	P_{207}/P_{205} a)	$\%^{18}O$	
natural	13	1,7		2,4		9,2				0,20 b)
	70	2,3		6,6		10,0		1,41		
^{18}O enriched	13	13,3	10,6	13,3	10,0	19,5	9,5			
	70	22,5	12,6	14,5	10,0	20,1	9,3	12,94	10,54	11,00 c)

a) intensity ratio x 100; means from 4 measurements b) natural abundance

c) calculated from the ^{18}O content of BaO_2 used for the synthesis and 2). For a, b and d they are less pronounced at low ionisation energies (cf. *Fig. 1*). Nevertheless, correction factors from unlabelled material have to be determined considering that the minimum of the temperature-dependence curves can be reproduced best (24, 28). Typical values are given in *Table 1*.

Since M^+ cannot be used for the ^{18}O determination, evaluation of low resolution spectra is restricted to compounds giving abundant fragment ions which are not directly connected with M^+. The ubiquitous ions $[M - 92]^{+\cdot}$ and $[M - 106]^+$ are less suitable due to their complex genesis.
Chemical ionisation (H_2 and i-C_4H_{10}) (29) has also been applied to carotenoids, but due to the formation $[M + H]^+$ and $[M - H]^+$ from all molecular ions including the hydrogenation and dehydrogenation products renders the M^+-region even more complex. First results (30) with FD-spectra indicate that even with this method hydrogenation/dehydrogenation reactions do occur which in connection with the generally less reproducible ion abundances should not make this method more suitable than EI for ^{18}O analyses.

High Resolution Measurements.
The contribution of isobaric ions of different elemental composition can be excluded, hence the determination of correction factors derived from unlabelled material is not necessary. For epoxides the ion b (*m/z* 205) may be used: At a resolution of 20 000 only $^{12}C_{12}{}^{13}C_2{}^1H_{21}{}^{16}O$ and $^{12}C_{13}{}^{13}C{}^1H_{20}{}^2H{}^{16}O$ coincide with $^{12}C_{14}{}^1H_{21}{}^{18}O$ the contribution of which can be calculated. In this way the most reliable results have been obtained (see *Table 1*). Instrumental limits may, however, be reached for higher masses (resolving power, sufficient ion currents) (28).

REFERENCES

1. G. Britton, Specialist Periodical Report: Terpenoids and Steroids, Vol. 10, p. 184 ff, The Royal Society of Chemistry, London (1981).
2. U. Schwieter, G. Englert, N. Rigassi and W. Vetter, *Pure Appl. Chem.* 20, 365 (1969)
3. C.R. Enzell, *Pure Appl. Chem.* 20, 497 (1969)
4. W. Vetter, G. Englert, N. Rigassi and U. Schwieter in Carotenoids (O. Isler, ed.), p. 243 ff., Birkhäuser, Basel (1971)
5. S. Liaaen-Jensen, *Pure Appl. Chem.* 35, 81 (1973)
6. C.R. Enzell, R.A. Appleton and I. Wahlberg in Biochemical Applications of Mass Spectrometry (G.R. Waller, ed.), p. 375 ff., Wiley, New York (1972)
7. C.R. Enzell and I. Wahlberg in Biochemical Applications of Mass Spectrometry, First Supplementary Volume, (G.R. Waller and O.C. Dermer, eds.), p. 407 ff., Wiley, New York (1980)
8. C. Enzell, G. Francis and S. Liaaen-Jensen, *Acta Chem. Scand.* 23, 727 (1969)
9. B. Johannes, H. Brzezinka and H. Budzikiewicz, *Org. Mass Spectrom.* 9, 1095 (1974); see also H. Budzikiewicz, *Adv. Mass Spectrom.* 6, 163 (1974).
10. H. Brzezinka, Dissertation, TU Braunschweig, 1971
11. S. Norgård, G.W. Francis, A. Jensen and S. Liaaen-Jensen, *Acta Chem. Scand.* 24, 1460 (1970)
12. J. Baldas, Q.N. Porter, L. Cholnoky, J. Szabolcs and B.C.L. Weedon, *Chem. Commun.* 852 (1966)
13. H. Budzikiewicz, H. Brzezinka and B. Johannes, *Monatsh. Chem.* 101, 579 (1970)
14. R. Bonnett, A.K. Mallams, A.A. Spark, J.L. Tee, B.C.L. Weedon and A. McCormick, *J. Chem. Soc. C* 429 (1969)
15. G.W. Francis, *Acta Chem. Scand.* 26, 1443 (1972)
16. U. Schwieter, H.R. Bolliger, L.H. Chopard-dit-Jean, G. Englert, M. Kofler, A. König, C.v.Planta, R. Rüegg, W. Vetter and O. Isler, *Chimia* 19, 294 (1965)
17. H. Kjøsen, S. Liaaen-Jensen and C.R. Enzell, *Acta Chem. Scand.* 25, 85 (1971)
18. J.E. Johansen, R. Eidem and S. Liaaen-Jensen, *Acta Chem. Scand.* B 28, 385 (1974)
19. unpublished results
20. B. Johannes, H.Brzezinka and H. Budzikiewicz, *Z. Naturf.* 34b, 300 (1979)
21. W.A. Svec, A.L. Harkness, H.H. Strain and J.J. Katz, *Org. Mass Spectrom.* 6, 843 (1972)
22. G.W. Francis, *Acta Chem. Scand.* 23, 2916 (1969)
23. G.W. Francis, S. Norgård and S. Liaaen-Jensen, *Acta Chem. Scand.* B 28 244 (1974)

24. B. Johannes and H. Budzikiewicz, *Z. Naturf.* 33c, 116 (1978)
25. B. Johannes, Dissertation, TU Braunschweig 1971
26. H. Budzikiewicz, *Croat. Chem. Acta* 42, 567 (1970)
27. A. Weymann, *Anal. Chem.* 50, 830 (1978)
28. H. Budzikiewicz and B. Johannes, H. Weigel and M. Heimann, *Fresenius Z. Anal. Chem.* 290, 382 (1978)
29. J. Carnevale, E.R. Cole, D. Nelson and J.S. Shannon, *Biomed. Mass Spectrom.* 5, 641 (1978)
30. C.D. Watts, J.R. Maxwell, D.E. Games and M. Rossiter, *Org. Mass Spectrom.* 10, 1102 (1975)

METASTABLE ION TECHNIQUES FOR THE ANALYSIS OF CAROTENOID ISOMERS

M. E. Rose

Department of Biochemistry, University of Liverpool, P.O. Box 147, Liverpool, L69 3BX, U.K.

Abstract - Carotenoid compounds are not easily analysed by conventional mass spectrometry. The major obstacles to obtaining useful mass spectra are shown to be removed by use of a technique for observing metastable ions without interference from normal ions. The method involves linked scanning of the magnetic field and electric sector voltage of a conventional double-focussing mass spectrometer and provides a new and powerful means of identifying carotenoid compounds, even in the presence of gross contamination. This paper describes one application of linked scan mass spectra: the ready differentiation of natural isomeric carotenoid compounds which are difficult or impossible to distinguish by normal mass spectra. The reasons why metastable ion techniques provide more diagnostic information on structure than does routine mass spectrometry are also discussed.

INTRODUCTION

The use of electron impact mass spectrometry (Ref. 1) for structural elucidation of carotenoid compounds has been thoroughly reviewed (Ref. 2-6). These publications clearly identify three factors which cause difficulties in obtaining diagnostic mass spectra of carotenoid compounds. Firstly, complex thermal degradations take place prior to ionisation and as a result slightly different experimental conditions (particularly variations in the temperature and pressure of the ion source) markedly affect the mass spectra obtained. Secondly, isomeric carotenoid compounds afford similar mass spectra in which ions characteristic of the different end groups are generally of low abundance. Lastly, contaminants in natural samples obscure the differences that do exist between the mass spectra. Taken together, these factors often cause mass spectra of different carotenoid compounds to show fewer differences than the day-to-day variation in recording of the mass spectra. However, these difficulties are redressed by examining metastable ions rather than normal ions, as explained below.

Normal fragment ions result when ionisation imparts sufficiently large amounts of internal energy to the molecular ions that they decompose whilst still in the ion source. On the other hand, ions formed with low internal energy have slower rates of decomposition and therefore reach the detector before they have time to fragment. Ions having intermediate internal energy may fragment after leaving the ion source and before reaching the detector. The term applied to the ionic products of these reactions occurring during flight through the mass spectrometer is 'metastable'. Several different means of recording metastable ion spectra are known (Ref. 1,7 & 8) and their many applications have been discussed (Ref. 1,7,9 & 10). When the magnetic field ($\underline{B}$) and the voltage ($\underline{E}$) of the electric sector of a double-focussing mass spectrometer are varied such that the ratio between them is always constant, the ionic products of fragmentation of a selected precursor ion in the region between the ion source and the electric sector (the first field-free region) are detected. All other ions are 'defocussed' and are not observed. This so-called $\underline{B}/\underline{E}$ linked scanning has been described elsewhere (Ref. 1,8 & 11). Here, carotenoid compounds are identified by the $\underline{B}/\underline{E}$ linked scan spectra of their molecular ions.

Normal, electron impact mass spectra are frequently found to be less sensitive to fine differences in structure than metastable ion mass spectra (Ref.1). Hence, the latter have been used for distinguishing isomeric compounds

(Ref.12-16). The reasons why methods based on metastable ions are more diagnostic of structure are not obvious; they are discussed later. Metastable ion techniques have been used previously in the carotenoid field. The so-called 'defocussing' method (Ref. 1 & 7) was used to show that losses of 92, 106 and 158 mass units (m.u.) from polyene chains were, at least in part, true mass spectrometric processes and not solely due to thermal reactions of the neutral molecules (Ref. 17). Metastable ions have also been employed to elucidate secondary decompositions of the polyene chain of lycopene (Ref. 18). Of course, when metastable ions appear in routine mass spectra, they are frequently helpful for structural interpretation. The only disadvantages of methods for selective recording of metastable ions are that sophisticated instrumentation is needed and that ambiguities sometimes arise when interpreting the resulting data (Ref. 19 & 20). The ensuing data appear to be free of such artifacts. This publication describes the first application of a metastable ion technique for observing selectively products of molecular ions of carotenoid compounds, thereby characterising fragmentation of the end groups and differentiating the individual members of series of carotenoid isomers.

RESULTS AND DISCUSSION

A $\underline{B}/\underline{E}$ linked scan spectrum is shown in Fig. 1 for the molecular ion of zeaxanthin. It is readily apparent that linked scan spectra are very different in appearance from normal mass spectra. The selected precursor ion ($\underline{m}/\underline{z}$ 568 for zeaxanthin) and losses of hydrogen therefrom are highly abundant. These and the other product ions observed give rise to peaks which are broader than those in normal mass spectra; the reasons for this decrease in resolution have been clearly delineated (Ref. 21). Also, because $\underline{B}/\underline{E}$ linked scanning of molecular ions is selective to primary fragmentations occurring in the first field-free region, there are relatively few peaks in the mass spectra obtained (Fig. 1). The pyrolysis of carotenoid compounds which complicates their normal mass spectra makes no direct contribution to metastable ion mass spectra. Hence the spectra reported here, such as that in Fig. 1, confirm an earlier report (Ref. 17) that $[M-92]^{+\cdot}$, $[M-106]^{+\cdot}$ and $[M-158]^{+\cdot}$ ions from carotenoid compounds with conjugated polyene chains are true fragment ions and not solely due to molecular ions of thermal reaction products. The fragmentations observed for zeaxanthin (Fig. 1) are discussed below.

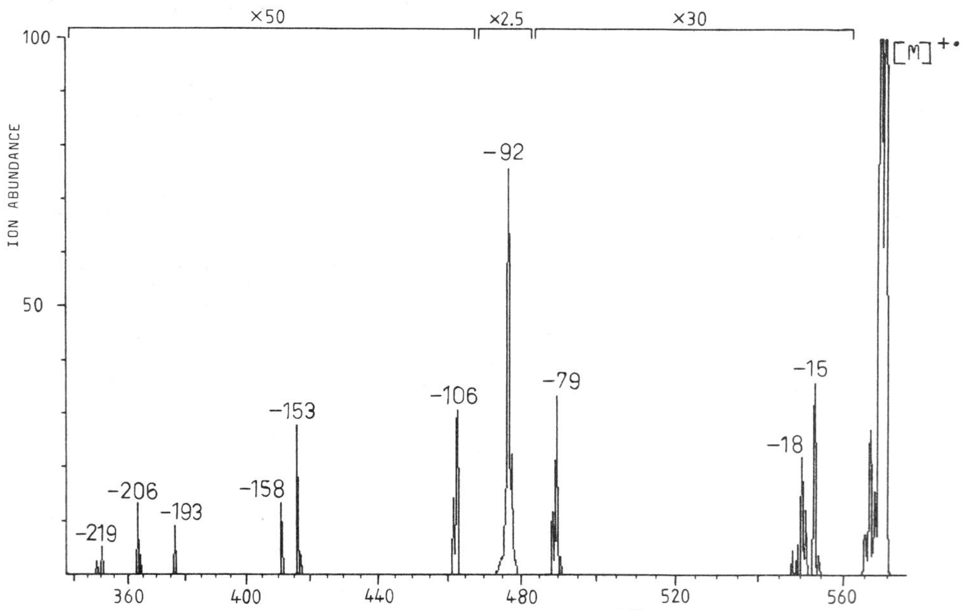

Fig. 1. $\underline{B}/\underline{E}$ linked scan spectrum of the molecular ion of zeaxanthin. Peaks are identified by the number of mass units ejected from $[M]^{+\cdot}$ at $\underline{m}/\underline{z}$ 568.

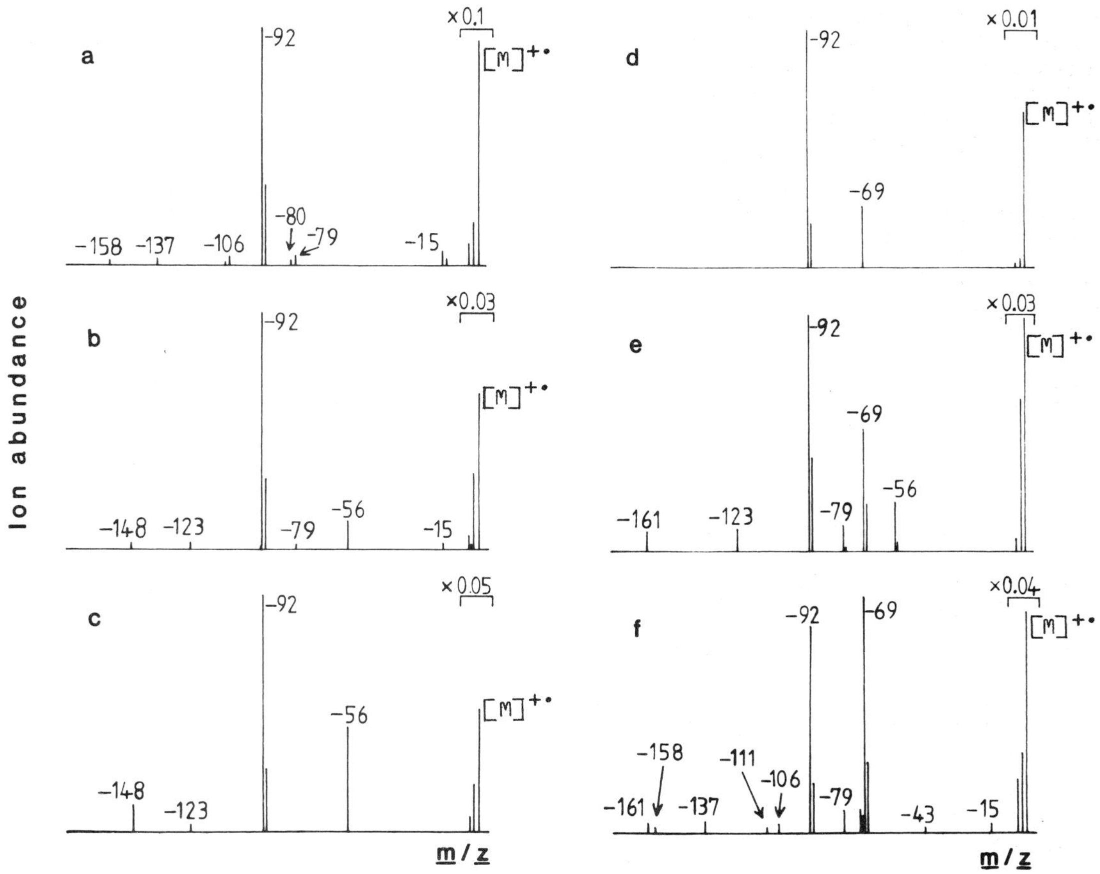

Fig. 2. B/E linked scan spectra of the molecular ions of β-carotene (a), α-carotene (b), ε-carotene (c), γ-carotene (d), δ-carotene (e) and lycopene (f).

Individual carotenes and lycopene (molecular ions at m/z 536) are readily differentiated by their linked scan spectra (Fig. 2). The spectra are normalised to the most abundant metastable ion (corresponding to loss of toluene, 92m.u., for all but lycopene) and peaks of over 1% relative abundance are included in the figure. Nearly all of the fragment ions observed have been reported previously and their origins discussed (Ref. 2-6). For the purposes of differentiating these compounds with the same polyene chain, the losses of 79, 92, 106 and 158m.u. from that common part of the structure are not useful and will not be discussed further. Decompositions characteristic of the end groups are of prime importance and are amply represented in the mass spectra. The end groups of β-carotene, (1), are known to be almost stable to mass spectrometric conditions (Ref. 3). Accordingly, only loss of the complete end group with concomitant

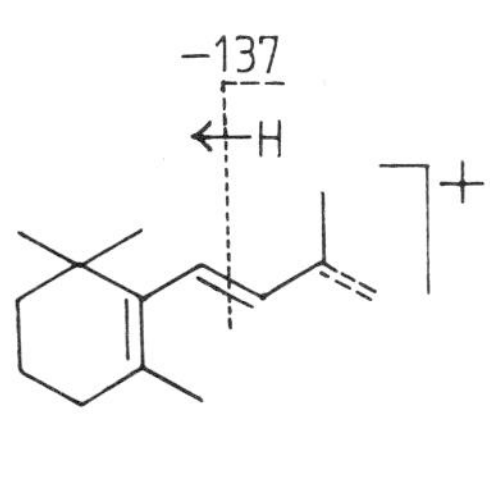

(1)

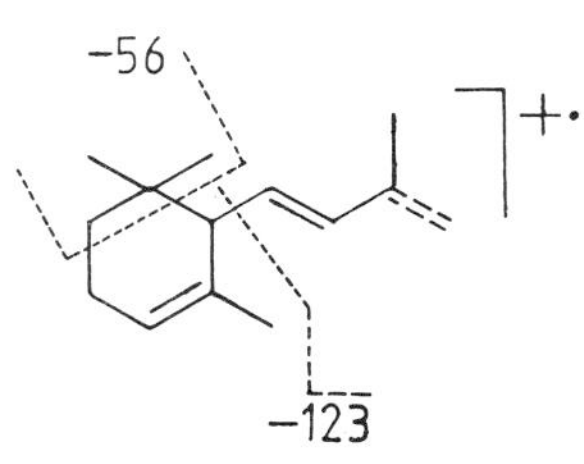

(2)

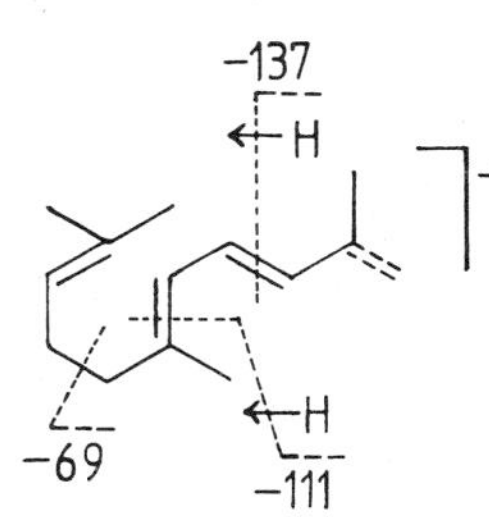

(3)

hydrogen migration as shown, (1), was observed, affording a metastable [M-137]+ ion [Fig. 2(a)]. In contrast, the unconjugated 4,5-double bond of α-carotene makes favourable the characteristic losses of 56 and 123m.u. from $[M]^{+\cdot}$ as seen in Fig. 2(b). The former process is conveniently regarded as a mass spectrometric equivalent of the *retro*-Diels-Alder reaction and the latter is an energetically favourable cleavage at the doubly allylic position (2). The loss of C_4H_8 (56m.u.) is highly diagnostic of the end group, (2), but the reaction frequently gives rise to very small or insignificant peaks in normal mass spectra (Ref. 3). As evidenced in Fig. 2(b), this is certainly not the case for linked scan mass spectra, making the metastable ion technique the preferred method of analysis. Also observed in Fig. 2(b) is a peak due to ejection of 148m.u. from $[M]^{+\cdot}$. Consecutive losses of toluene (92m.u.) and C_4H_8 (56m.u.) in the same field-free region probably account for the $[M-148]^{+\cdot}$ ion. For the sake of clarity, α-carotene is here designated as having end groups (1)/(2). Likewise, ϵ-carotene is denoted by (2)/(2). The distinction between α- and ϵ-carotene is made readily on the basis of the abundances of their $[M-56]^{+\cdot}$ and $[M-148]^{+\cdot}$ ions, as seen in Fig. 2(b) and (c). The fact that ϵ-carotene has two end groups, (2), is correlated with more prominent losses of 56 and 148m.u. In particular, the very different ratios of peak sizes, $[M-56]^{+\cdot}$/ $[M-92]^{+\cdot}$, for α-carotene (0.11) and for ϵ-carotene (0.44) are sufficient criteria for their differentiation.

Figure 2 also shows the results for three isomers containing the acyclic end group (3). All three *B/E* linked scan spectra of $[M]^{+\cdot}$ ions, Fig. 2(d), (e) and (f), are distinct from each other and from the spectra of the other isomers discussed in the previous paragraph. The very favourable direct cleavage of the acyclic end group, (3), affords abundant $[M-69]^{+}$ ions in all compounds containing this functionality. Other than losses of hydrogen, γ-carotene, (1)/(3), afforded only $[M-92]^{+\cdot}$ and $[M-69]^{+}$ ions as shown in Fig. 2(d). This is entirely expected, given the stability of the end group, (1), as noted above. The metastable ion mass spectrum of δ-carotene correlates particularly well with its structure, (2)/(3). Losses of 56 and 123m.u. from $[M]^{+\cdot}$ characterise the end group, (2), whilst $[M-69]^{+}$ and $[M-161]^{+}$ ions demonstrate the presence of the acyclic group, (3). The loss of 161m.u. can be rationalised by consecutive losses of $C_5H_9^{\cdot}$ (69m.u.) and toluene (92m.u.). In the case of lycopene, (3)/(3), ejection of $C_5H_9^{\cdot}$ can presumably occur from either end of the molecular ion and, as a result, the $[M-69]^{+}$ ion dominates the spectrum, being even more abundant than the $[M-92]^{+\cdot}$ ion. The ratio of peak sizes, $[M-92]^{+\cdot}/[M-69]^{+}$, clearly distinguishes lycopene and γ-carotene. Other peaks in the linked scan spectrum of lycopene include those corresponding to $[M-111]^{+}$, $[M-137]^{+}$ and $[M-161]^{+}$ ions. The first two of these may be generated as shown in (3), and, as already noted, consecutive losses of toluene and $C_5H_9^{\cdot}$ probably account for the $[M-161]^{+}$ ion.

All of the spectra in Fig. 2 show apparent losses of 91m.u. from $[M]^{+\cdot}$ ions, but they are more likely to be ^{13}C satellite peaks. With the instrument used, the resolution in the region of the precursor ion was not sufficient to focus only $[M]^{+\cdot}$ ions and some $[M+1]^{+\cdot}$ ions due to the natural ^{13}C isotope content were also sampled. Loss of toluene from these $[M+1]^{+\cdot}$ ions would account for the anomolous peaks in the linked scan spectra.

The utility of *B/E* linked scanning is not restricted to the hydrocarbons. In Fig. 3, the main features of the linked scan spectra of $[M]^{+\cdot}$ ions of zeaxanthin (a) and lutein (b) are illustrated. As with the examples in Fig. 2, differences between the spectra are clear and are readily rationalised in terms of the structures of the two compounds. As expected, the molecular ions of both substances eject water and undergo cleavages shown in (4) and (5) to yield $[M-153]^{+}$ and $[M-206]^{+\cdot}$ ions. However, only lutein afforded $[M-56]^{+\cdot}$, $[M-138]^{+\cdot}$ and $[M-230]^{+\cdot}$ ions. The formation of the first two of these abundant ions is thought to be as shown in (5) whilst the last is probably a result of sequential losses of toluene and 138m.u. in the first field-free region. Routine mass spectrometry can differentiate these two alcohols as long as the samples are pure. The *B/E* linked scan method not only provides a surer analysis because of its emphasis on primary fragmentations of $[M]^{+\cdot}$ ions but also tolerates large amounts of contamination.

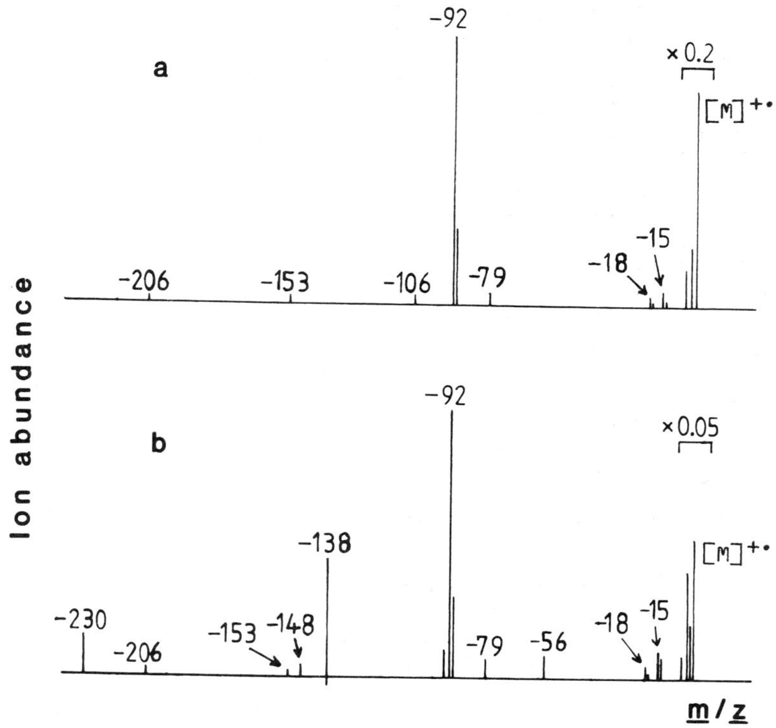

Fig. 3. B/E linked scan spectra of the molecular ions of zeaxanthin (a) and lutein (b).

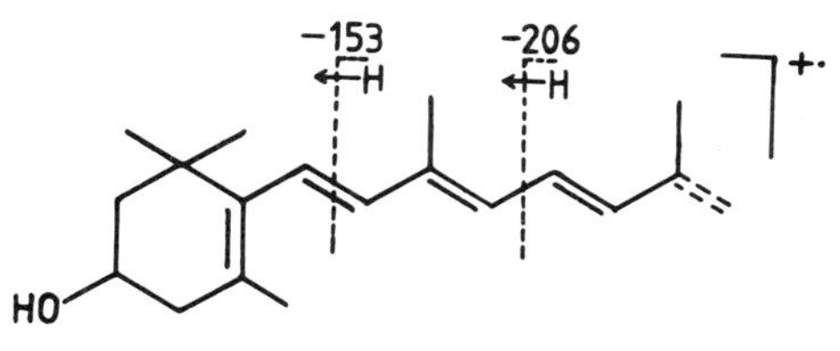

(4)

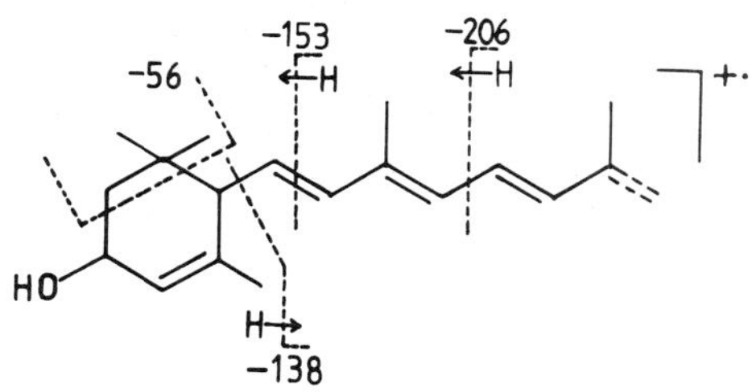

(5)

Application to contaminated samples

The data shown in Fig. 2 & 3 were obtained with synthetic or well-characterised natural samples, or both. Figure 4 depicts the normal mass spectrum of a carotenoid hydrocarbon isolated from *Mycobacterium aurum*. The sample is seen to be grossly contaminated, with all major ions being consistent with a cholestadiene impurity. The molecular ion of the carotenoid compound (m/z 536) carried only 0.3% of the total ion current with 1.2% abundance relative to the base peak at m/z 368 due to the steroid. In a pure sample of a carotenoid hydrocarbon, the molecular ion would be expected to give the largest peak in this mass range. It was not possible to identify the compound from the spectrum in Fig. 4 but further purification of the substance was considered unwise because of the small quantity obtained. Instead the B/E linked scan spectrum of the molecular ion at m/z 536 was recorded. It is shown in Fig. 5. The contamination made no contribution to the spectrum so that, despite the small quantity, the compound was readily identified as lycopene on the basis of the characteristic ratio of abundances of $[M-92]^{+\bullet}$ and $[M-69]^{+}$ ions (compare Fig. 2(f) and 5).

Ionisation and attendant fragmentation create in the ion source a mixture of ions of different masses. This occurs whether the sample is a pure compound

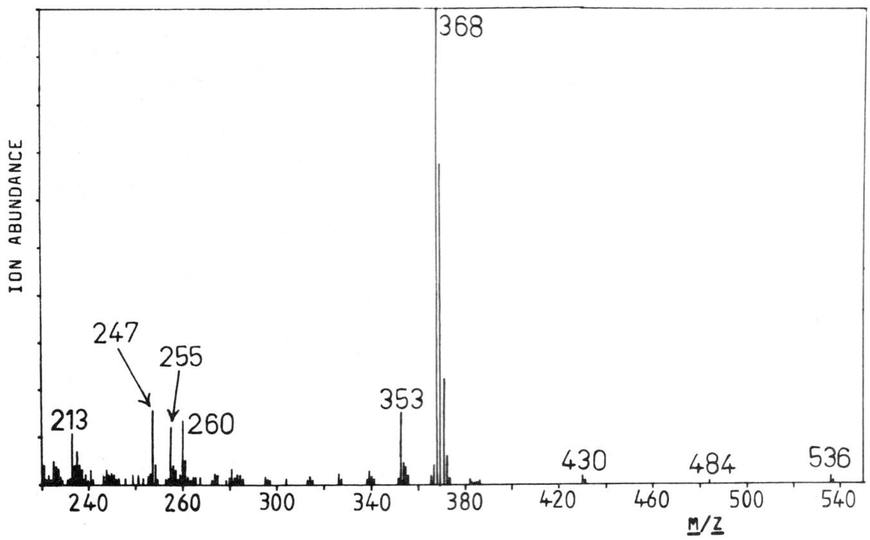

Fig. 4. Normal mass spectrum of a carotenoid hydrocarbon from *Mycobacterium aurum*.

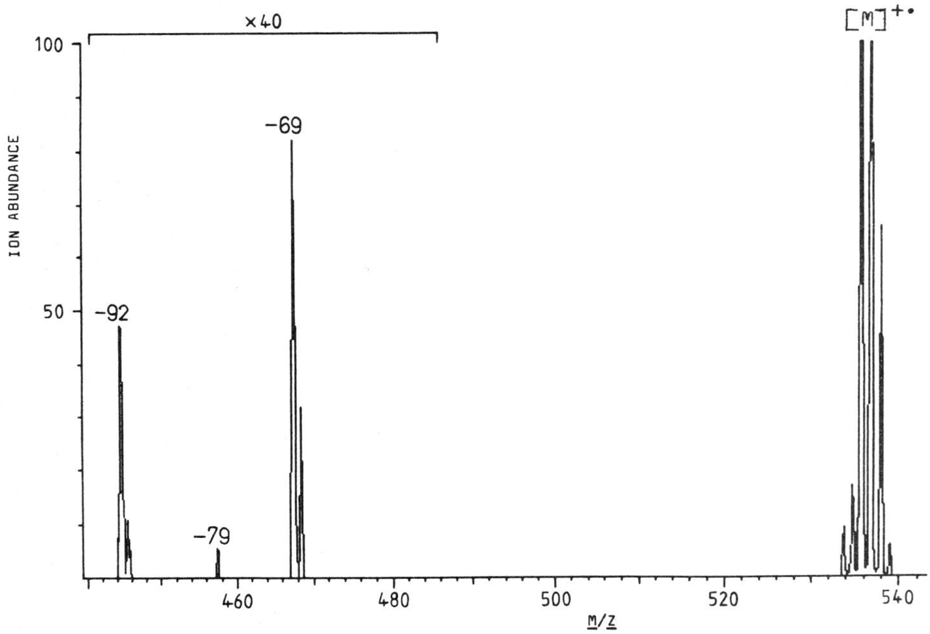

Fig. 5. *B/E* linked scan spectrum of the molecular ion of the hydrocarbon from *Mycobacterium aurum*.

or a mixture of compounds. To obtain a linked scan spectrum, ions of just one mass are selected for examination and all others are excluded. For a single compound, it is possible to study a specific portion of the molecule by appropriate choice of ion (Ref. 13). Also, the selection step allows one compound to be separated, on the basis of the *m/z* value of one of its characteristic ions, from other compounds present in the sample. In this respect, metastable ion techniques have been compared with combined chromatography and mass spectrometry and used recently for direct analysis of mixtures (Ref. 22-27). The example of structural elucidation given above illustrates that the selectivity of linked scanning permits impure carotenoid samples to be analysed as readily as pure ones. An exception occurs if the contaminants afford ions of the same mass as the ion chosen for study. At present, this effect precludes successful analysis of mixtures of isomeric carotenoid compounds.

Structural discrimination by metastable ions

It is sometimes argued that, for closely related compounds ionised by electron impact, the high-energy molecular ions fragmenting in the ion source may do so too indiscriminately to be sensitive to structural subtleties. By the same token, it is said that molecular ions with lower internal energies would be expected to undergo fragmentation more characteristic of structure. Whilst metastable ion mass spectra do distinguish successfully compounds which afford very similar routine mass spectra, as reported here and elsewhere (Ref. 12-16), the simple thermodynamic argument is not necessarily validated thereby. In fact, there are two main reasons for doubting the explanation. Ions of low internal energy content are more discriminating in that fewer reaction channels are available to them but there is no inherent reason why these reaction channels should be more diagnostic of structure than those available to high-energy ions. Secondly, because there is a long time lapse between ionisation and fragmentation in the first field-free region, many different states of an ion are accessible with the possibility of rearrangements occurring. If such rearrangements do take place, evidently they do not destroy all useful information about the structure before ionisation because the method is successful. An alternative mode of analysis has been suggested (Ref. 22) in which ions having very low internal energies are induced to fragment. (These are the ions which otherwise would have been stable and reached the detector intact). Not only do these ions experience the same time delay before fragmentation but also the method of excitation is usually "collisional activation" (CA) and this imparts to ions a very large amount of internal energy, similar to that imparted by electron impact (Ref. 1). Therefore the excited ions are expected to undergo decompositions rather like those in the ion source. Indeed, CA mass spectra are frequently similar to normal electron impact spectra so, on energetic and kinetic grounds, the use of collisional activation for differentiation of isomers is questionable. However, the CA method does provide data which are highly characteristic of structure (Ref. 22).

It is proposed here that a much simpler effect is operating and that this relies on the selectivity of metastable ion techniques such as linked scanning. Closely related compounds might be differentiated by such methods because it is possible to observe in isolation those processes which are most likely to be sensitive to fine differences in structure. For carotenoid compounds, B/E linked scanning allows the most diagnostic events - the primary fragmentations of molecular ions - to be examined selectively. The linked scan mass spectra of molecular ions thus obtained are not cluttered by the highly abundant products of subsequent reactions which have undergone extensive structural modification and are common to most carotenoid compounds. Generally, as energetic considerations suggest, the high-energy ions decomposing in the ion source may have open to them just as many, if not more, reaction channels capable of discriminating between isomeric compounds than have low-energy ions (this will be highly dependent on structure). The advantage offered by metastable ion techniques is that the mass spectrometrist, by judicious choice of precursor ion, can concentrate on those reactions which will be most characteristic of structure and ignore those which will not. This aspect is clear when a precursor ion is chosen to correspond to a specific portion of a molecule, such as the side-chain of a steroid (Ref.13). In this way, the information that is partly or totally obscured in routine mass spectra is brought to light in metastable ion spectra.

CONCLUDING REMARKS

Linked scan spectra of carotenoid compounds are simple and correlate well with structure. It is this feature that makes them particularly well suited to identification of unknown carotenoid structures isolated from their natural sources. Such work is currently under investigation in this laboratory. The method should be less sensitive than routine mass spectrometry to slight variations in experimental conditions since pyrolysis, whilst it still takes place, makes no direct contribution to the data obtained. The selectivity of linked scanning also provides the key to the problem of contamination. The method is a viable and preferable alternative to further purification, particularly when small amounts of material only are available, because loss of sample is inevitable in any extra purification stages. Whilst sensitivity tests have not yet been made, the amount of sample required for analysis is no more than that needed for routine mass spectrometry. The application of metastable ion techniques to other classes of carotenoid compounds, including aromatic ones, and to steroidal isomers is under active research in these laboratories.

EXPERIMENTAL SECTION

Materials

The following compounds were isolated from the stated sources by established methods: lutein and α- and β-carotene from *Scenedesmus obliquus*; δ-carotene from tomato; γ-carotene from *Chlorobium limicola*; lycopene from *Mycobacterium aurum*. Synthetic samples of β-carotene, lycopene and zeaxanthin were supplied by Hoffmann-La Roche & Co.

Methods

Mass spectra were obtained by electron impact with a VG Micromass 70-70F mass spectrometer coupled to a Finnigan Incos Data System. The computer controlled repetitive *B/E* linked scanning, based on readings from a Hall effect probe, as the samples evaporated from the direct insertion probe. Ion beam energy, 70*eV*; ion source temperature, 200-250°C.

Acknowledgements - The author thanks Dr. S. Pollard for her considerable help in isolating and supplying the carotenoid samples. Useful discussions with Drs. G. Britton and R.A.W. Johnstone are acknowledged. The work was supported by a grant from the Science Research Council.

REFERENCES

1. M.E.Rose and R.A.W.Johnstone, *Mass Spectrometry for Chemists and Biochemists*, Cambridge University Press, London. In press.
2. C.R.Enzell, G.W.Francis and S.Liaaen-Jensen, *Acta Chem. Scand.* 23, 727-750 (1969).
3. W.Vetter, G.Englert, N.Rigassi and U.Schwieter, in *Carotenoids*, p.189, O.Isler (ed.), Birkhäuser Verlag, Basel (1971).
4. C.R.Enzell, R.A.Appleton and I.Wahlberg, in *Biochemical Applications of Mass Spectrometry*, p.375, G.R.Waller (ed.), Wiley, New York (1972).
5. G.P.Moss and B.C.L.Weedon, in *Chemistry and Biochemistry of Plant Pigments*, p.149, T.W.Goodwin (ed.), Academic Press, London (1976).
6. C.R.Enzell and I.Wahlberg, in *Biochemical Applications of Mass Spectrometry, First Supplementary Volume*, p.407, G.R.Waller and O.C.Dermer (eds.), Wiley, New York (1980).
7. R.G.Cooks, J.H.Beynon, R.M.Caprioli and G.R.Lester, *Metastable Ions*, Elsevier, Amsterdam (1973).
8. R.K.Boyd and J.H.Beynon, *Org. Mass Spectrom.* 12, 163-165 (1977).
9. J.H.Beynon and R.M.Caprioli, in *Biochemical Applications of Mass Spectrometry, First Supplementary Volume*, p.89, G.R.Waller and O.C.Dermer (eds.), Wiley, New York (1980).
10. J.L.Holmes and J.K.Terlouw, *Org. Mass Spectrom.* 15, 383-396 (1980).
11. A.P.Bruins, K.R.Jennings and S.Evans, *Int. J. Mass Spectrom. Ion Phys.* 26, 395-404 (1978).
12. S.J.Gaskell, A.W.Pike and D.S.Millington, *Biomed. Mass Spectrom.* 6, 78-81 (1979).
13. M.H.Bozorgzadeh, A.G.Brenton, J.L.Weibers and J.H.Beynon, *Biomed. Mass Spectrom.* 6, 340-344 (1979).
14. T.L.Kruger, R.W.Kondrat, K.T.Joseph and R.G.Cooks, *Analyt. Biochem.* 96, 104-112 (1979).
15. B.Shushan, S.H.Safe and R.K.Boyd, *Analyt. Chem.* 51, 156-158 (1979).
16. B.Shushan and R.K.Boyd, *Org. Mass Spectrom.* 15, 445-453 (1980).
17. U.Schwieter, G.Englert, N.Rigassi and W.Vetter, *Pure Appl. Chem.* 20, 365-420 (1969).
18. C.R.Enzell, G.W.Francis and S.Liaaen-Jensen, *Acta Chem. Scand.* 23, 727-750 (1969).
19. M.Lacey and C.Macdonald, *Org. Mass Spectrom.* 15, 484-485 (1980).
20. M.E.Rose, *Org. Mass Spectrom.* 16, 323-324 (1981).
21. C.J.Porter, A.G.Brenton and J.H.Beynon, *Int. J. Mass Spectrom. Ion Phys.* 36, 69-83 (1980).
22. P.F.Bente, III and F.W.McLafferty, in *Mass Spectrometry, Part B*, p.253, C.Merritt, Jr. and C.N.McEwen (eds.), Marcel Dekker, New York (1980).
23. A.G.Brenton and J.H.Beynon, *Eur. Spectrosc. News* 29, 39-42 (1980).
24. F.W.McLafferty, *Acc. Chem. Res.* 13, 33-39 (1980).
25. D.H.Russell, E.H.McBay and T.R.Mueller, *Intern. Lab.* 49-61 (1980).
26. G.L.Glish and R.G.Cooks, *Anal. Chim. Acta* 119, 145-149 (1980).
27. F.W.McLafferty and E.R.Lory, *J. Chromatog.* 203, 109-116 (1981).

A CHEMIST'S VIEW OF ANIMAL CAROTENOIDS

Richard Buchecker

Institute of Organic Chemistry, University of Zurich, Winterthurerstrasse 190, CH-8057 Zurich, Switzerland

Abstract - Carotenoids occurring predominantly or exclusively in animals are presented by means of the following representative endgroups:

- 3-Hydroxy-4-keto-β-endgroup (including 3,4-dihydroxy-, 4-hydroxy- and 4-keto-endgroups).
- 3-Hydroxy-2-nor-4-keto-β-endgroup.
- 3-Hydroxy-6,8-diketo-κ-endgroup.
- 3-Hydroxy-ε-endgroup.
- Sporadic endgroups.

Where possible, their stereochemistry and metabolic formation is discussed.

1. INTRODUCTION

Carotenoids belong to the most widely distributed pigments in the animal kingdom. Reviews are to be found in the books by Fox (1), Goodwin (2)(3) and Karrer (4). However, many earlier investigations using the analytical methods then available are incomplete or not beyond all doubt. In more recent investigations with modern methods, new interesting structures have come to light. A few of these have so far only been found in the animal kingdom. Although it is generally assumed that animals are not able to synthesise carotenoids de novo, they are apparently able to modify plant carotenoids taken up in their food. These are frequently highly oxidised metabolites. In this lecture it is not possible to classify the animal carotenoids according to taxonomic aspects. However, in this context I can refer you to the excellent review by Prof. Liaaen-Jensen (5) which comprises the most important newer works on marine animals. Non-marine animals have been far less investigated with modern methods. Exceptions though are insects, a few amphibia and freshwater fish. Investigations on birds and mammals are mostly of early origin.

Being a chemist, I would like to place the emphasis on a few carotenoid structures which play an important part in animals or are exclusively found in animals. I will take the liberty of effecting a classification according to endgroups. The stereochemistry will be considered and conclusions drawn on the possible consequences for the animal metabolism. I will not, however, deal with the caroteno proteins, which are frequently found in animals. For this topic I will refer you to the lecture given by Dr. Britton.

2. THE 3-HYDROXY-4-KETO-β-ENDGROUP

These represent the most widely distributed carotenoids with animal-metabolised endgroups (Schemes 1 and 2). However, the oxidised diosphenols such as astacenes were not taken into consideration. Of the carotenoids with this endgroup, whose absolute configuration has so far been determined, most exhibit the (3S)-configuration. Since the total syntheses of both enantiomeric astaxanthins and the meso-form it is possible to separate these chromatographically as the camphanate esters (6). Corresponding investigations on astaxanthin from lobster eggs revealed the natural co-occurrence of both enantiomers and of meso-astaxanthin (7). This is the first occurrence on record of enantiomeric carotenoids in the

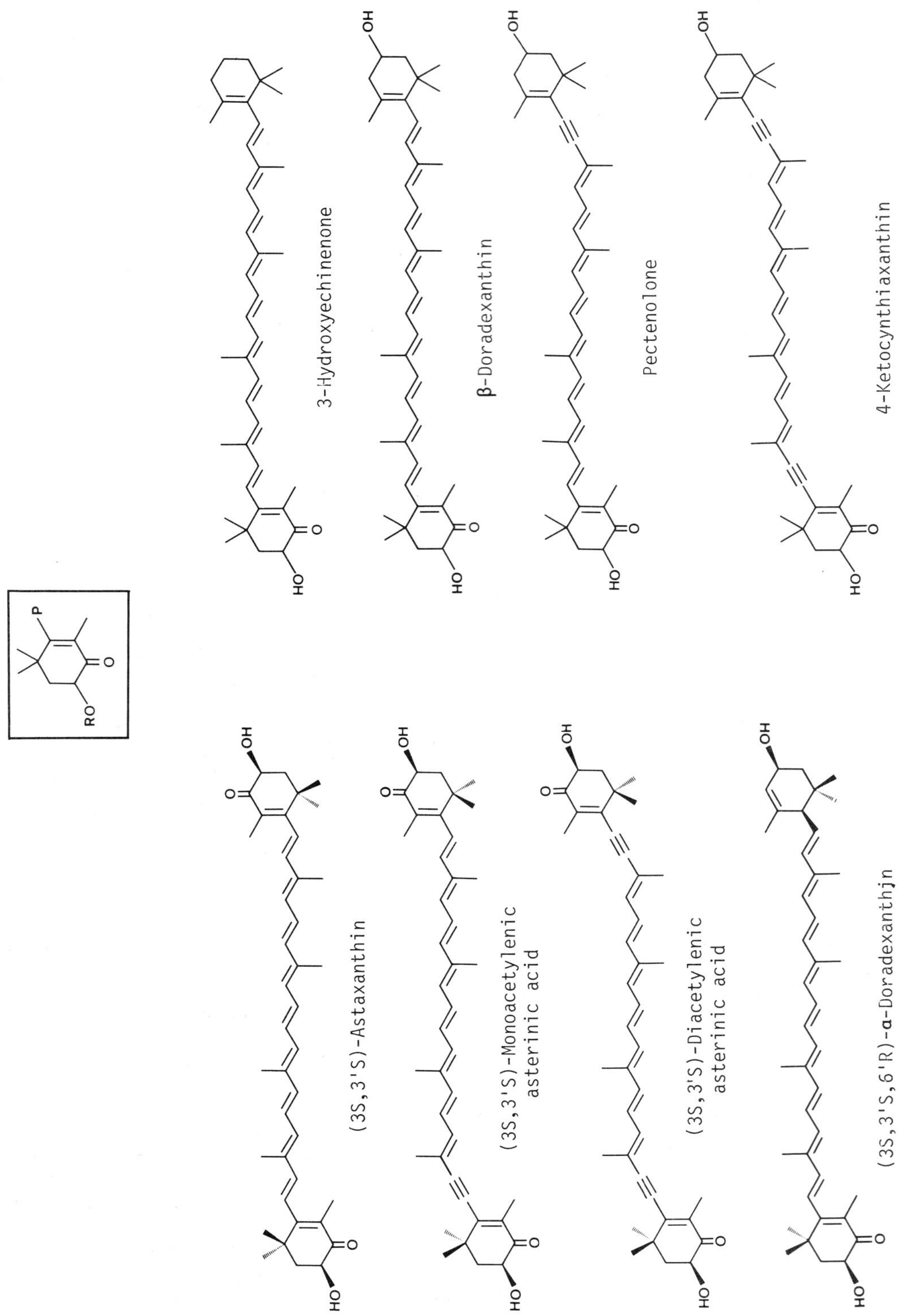
RO
P
O
3-Hydroxyechinenone
β-Doradexanthin
Pectenolone
4-Ketocynthiaxanthin
(3S,3'S)-Astaxanthin
(3S,3'S)-Monoacetylenic asterinic acid
(3S,3'S)-Diacetylenic asterinic acid
(3S,3'S,6'R)-α-Doradexanthin

Scheme 1

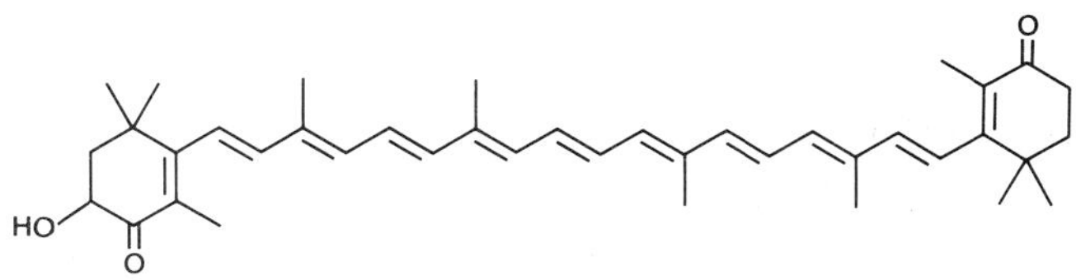

Adonirubin, Phoenicoxanthin, Metridene

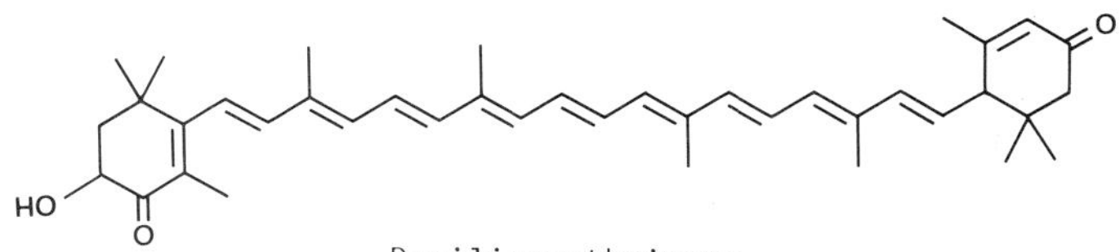

Papilioerythrinone

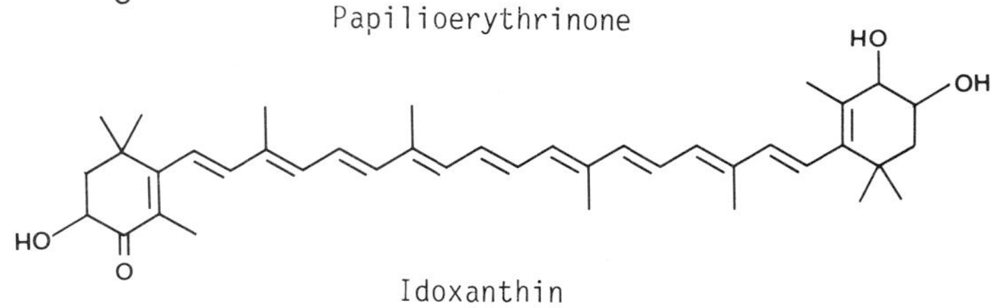

Idoxanthin

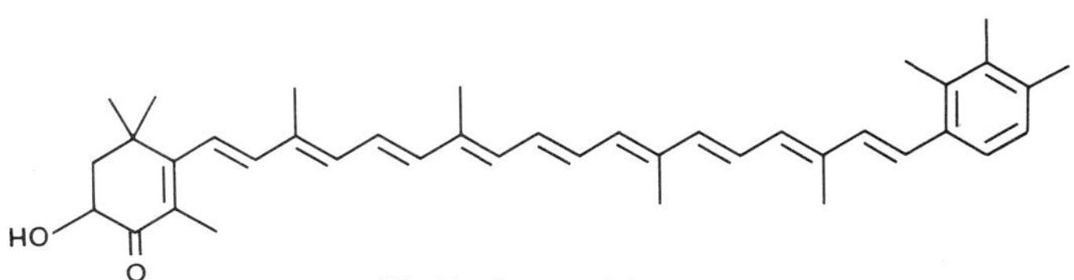

Clathriaxanthin

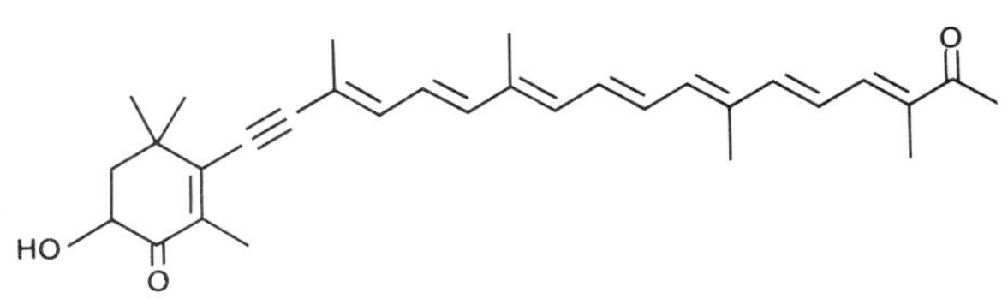

Hopkinsiaxanthin

Scheme 2

same organism and of meso-carotenoids at all. Since by its total synthesis (8) the chiroptical data of optically pure astaxanthin are now known beyond doubt, it is easy to estimate the optical purity of natural astaxanthin in each case. This is, however, not yet possible for the other carotenoids with only one astaxanthin endgroup. The enantiomeric purity is also open to doubt here. The question is, how does the formation of the enantiomeric endgroups arise at all?

A partial racemisation through the enol of the α-OH-ketone in the cell environment is possible (Scheme 3). However, it could be shown that the 3,3'-hydroxyl groups of astaxanthin are configuratively remarkably stable (7). During the synthetic sequence, the chiral endgroup survived strongly acidic and basic conditions with essentially no racemisation. For complete racemisation, treatment with sodium ethoxide at room temperature for at least twenty four hours is required. A parallel synthesis with an enantiomeric enzyme can be excluded. Further possibilities though include formation via the diosphenol astacene with subsequent enzymatic reduction. Furthermore, the enantiomeric astaxanthin could be formed by two different metabolic pathways as postulated by Andrewes et al. (9) in Phaffia rhodozyma (Scheme 4).

This raises the general question of the biogenesis of the astaxanthin endgroup. A great deal of work has been done on the biogenesis of astaxanthin itself,

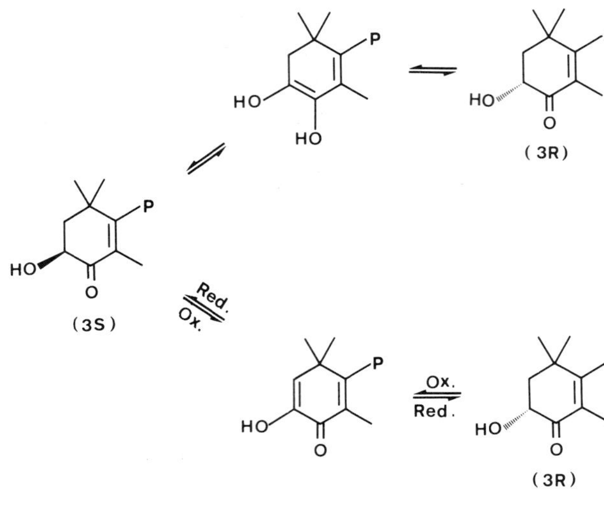

Scheme 3

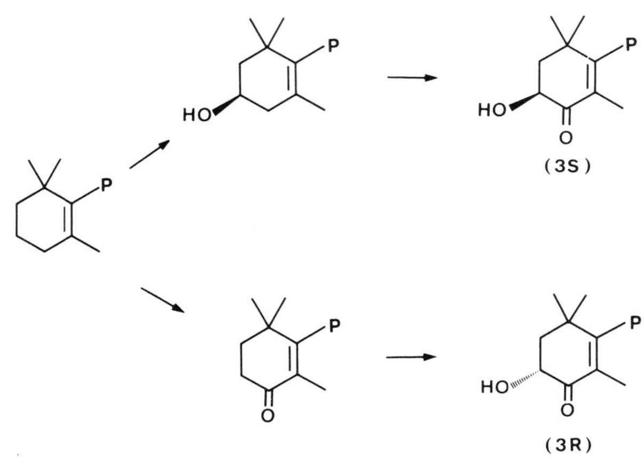

Scheme 4

particularly on animal organisms (10). It seems undisputed that animals are able to form these endgroups from other cyclic endgroups. In general, the β-endgroup (e.g. β-carotene) is accepted as being the first precursor. Thus for astaxanthin the sequence depicted in Scheme 5 was found, based on feeding experiments on the prawn Penaeus japonicus (11) and the lobster Panulirus japonicus (12). In goldfish, besides astaxanthin, isozeaxanthin is also formed from β-carotene (13). However, it appears that no astaxanthin arises from isozeaxanthin (14). Another route starting from zeaxanthin was found in Fancy Red Carp (15). The authors also regard this as the major pathway in goldfish, whereas the formation of astaxanthin via echinenone and canthaxanthin represents at most a minor route (16). Correspondingly, the formation of the monoacetylenic and diacetylenic asterinic acids could also result from plant diatoxanthin and alloxanthin, respectively or from zeaxanthin with subsequent dehydrogenation. The stereochemistry at C(3) and C(3') is known to be identical in all these compounds (17). Possible intermediates could be 4-keto-cynthiaxanthin (4-keto-alloxanthin?) and pectenolone.

It is still unclear whether astaxanthin can be formed from lutein. Corresponding labelling experiments gave contradictory results. Hsu et al. (18) found incorporation of ^{14}C-labelled lutein into α-doradexanthin, β-doradexanthin and astaxanthin in goldfish. Hata and Hata (15)(16) confirm this incorporation only

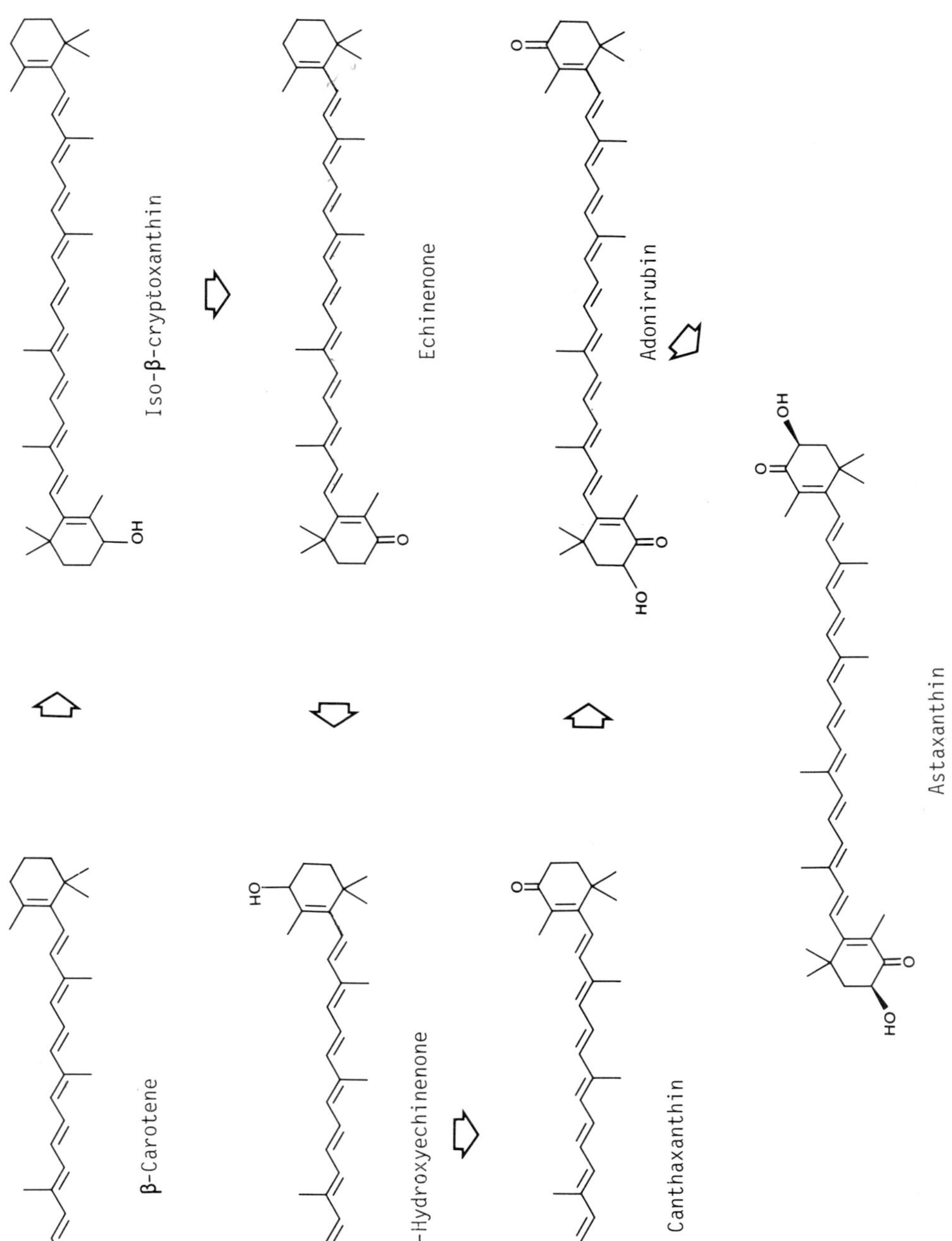

Iso-β-cryptoxanthin
Echinenone
Adonirubin
β-Carotene
4'-Hydroxyechinenone
Canthaxanthin
Astaxanthin

Scheme 5

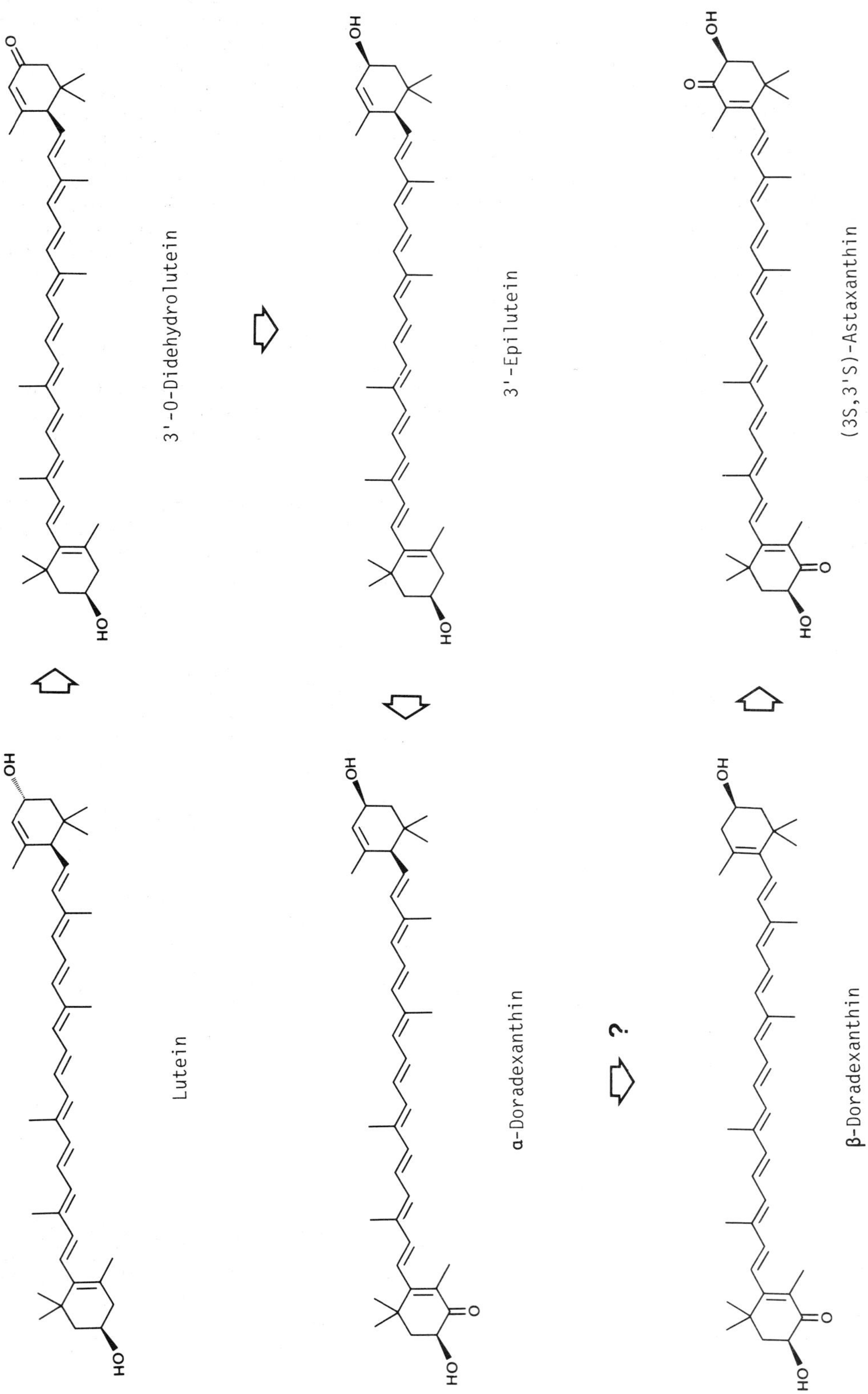
3'-O-Didehydrolutein
Lutein
3'-Epilutein
α-Doradexanthin
(3S,3'S)-Astaxanthin
β-Doradexanthin
?

Scheme 6

into α-doradexanthin and not into astaxanthin. Their experiments were performed on goldfish and on Fancy Red Carp. Previously also the opposite chirality at C(3') in lutein (19)(20) and at C(3) in astaxanthin (21) seemed to speak against this biogenetic pathway. However, we were recently able to show that α-doradexanthin from goldfish has the same chirality at both C(3) atoms as astaxanthin, and also the "lutein" isolated from goldfish is in reality 3'-epilutein (22). Since the incorporation of labelled lutein into α-doradexanthin has been proved (15)(16)(18) we regard the sequence lutein, 3'-O-didehydrolutein, 3'-epilutein, α-doradexanthin (Scheme 6) as probable. The formation of astaxanthin from β-doradexanthin is also undisputed (15)(16). The critical step is consequently only the formation of β-doradexanthin from α-doradexanthin, in other words the isomerisation of an ε-ring into a β-ring. As we shall also see later, this question turns out to be more and more of central importance in animal carotenoid metabolism. On the basis of the co-occurrence of lutein, α-doradexanthin and astaxanthin, the biogenetic pathway lutein ⟶ astaxanthin was also recently postulated for crustaceae(23)(24). Unfortunately, the stereochemistry of the compounds involved was not discussed.

Thus, generally, it can be said that the transformation of the 3-hydroxy-ε-endgroup into the 3-hydroxy-4-keto-β-endgroup is not assured, since contradictory results exist. Furthermore, both endgroups are also known in the enantiomeric forms. Consequently, when identifying molecules with these endgroups and deriving conclusions on their biogenesis, far more consideration must be paid to the stereochemical assignments.

Besides the 4-keto-β- and 4-hydroxy-β-endgroups already referred to, I would like to mention crustaxanthin in this context, which can be formally interpreted as reduction product from astaxanthin (Scheme 7). To my knowledge it has

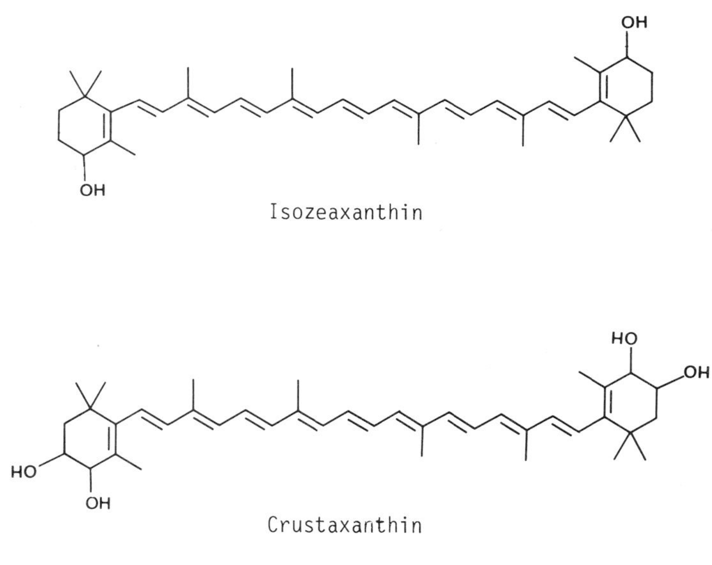

Scheme 7

only been found with certainty in the crustacean copepod Arctodioptomus salinus (25). Although semi-synthetically prepared from astaxanthin (21), only the 3,4-trans substitution of the natural product has so far been stereochemically assured. The absolute stereochemistry of isozeaxanthin is also outstanding. Andreas Haag from our group has recently finished his synthesis of optically pure (4R,4'R)-isozeaxanthin (25a). The chiroptical data of the natural product however, are not yet known.

2. THE 3-HYDROXY-2-NOR-4-KETO-β-ENDGROUP

Carotenoids with this typical animal endgroup (Scheme 8) have so far only been met with in sea anemones (5). The most important representative is actinioerythrin (R_1,R_2=acyl). Its constitution was elucidated by the Liaaen-Jensen

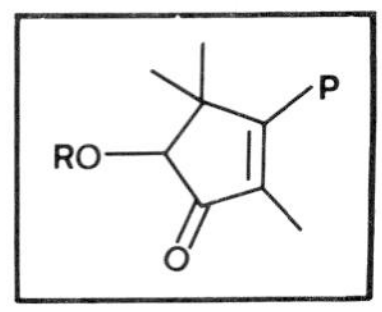

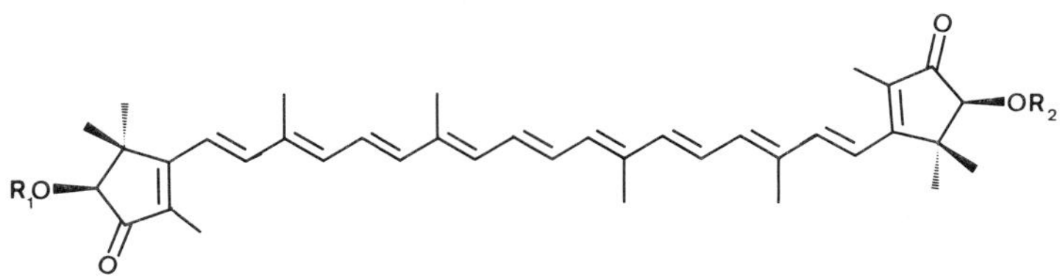

R_1=R_2=acyl: (3S,3'S)-Actinioerythrin

R_1=acyl, R_2=H: Actinioerythrolmonoester

R_1=R_2=H: Actinioerythrol

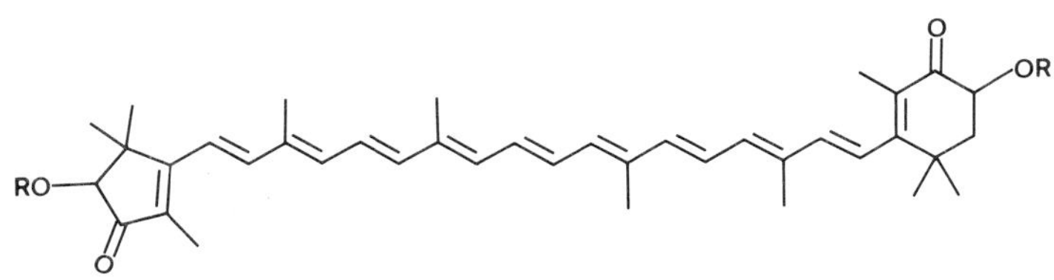

R=acyl: 2-Nor-astaxanthin

Scheme 8

research group in Trondheim (26)(27). Recently, actinioerythrol (R_1=R_2=H) and its C(3)-monoester were found for the first time (28). The absolute configuration of actinioerythrin was determined to be 3S,3'S, on the one hand by total synthesis of both enantiomers (29), and on the other by chemical and chiroptical correlation with 2-hydroxy-3,3-dimethylsuccinate (30).

Biogenetically, the formation from astaxanthin has been suggested by a type of benzylic acid rearrangement of a hypothetical achiral triketone (26) (Scheme 9).

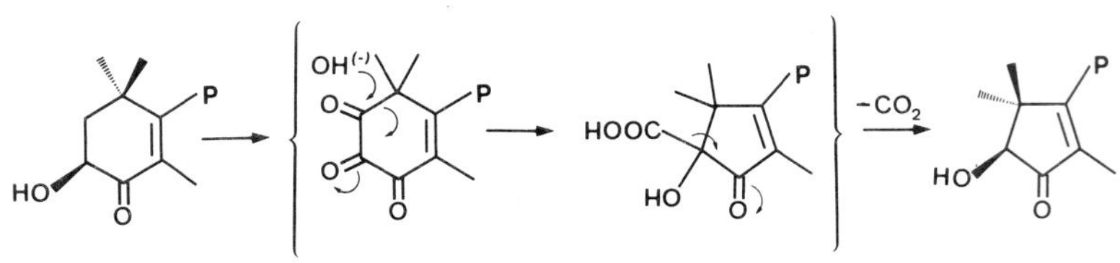

Scheme 9

This would mean that the chirality of astaxanthin is not directly transferred. Since the triketone was not found, it is nevertheless possible that the astaxanthin remains bound at the same enzyme complex during the entire process until actinioerythrol. In the newly found astaxanthins with diverse configurations (R,R, S,S and R,S), presumably only the one enantiomer and perhaps one ring of the meso-compound would then be metabolised. 2 -Norastaxanthin can be regarded as an intermediate in the formation of actinioerythrin from astaxanthin. It was found in small amounts in *Actinia equina* (31) and *Actinia tenebrosa* (28), but its absolute configuration has not yet been determined. It would be interesting to clarify whether the endgroup of actinioerythrin also occurs in both enantiomeric forms, analogous to the astaxanthin endgroup.

4. THE 3-HYDROXY-6,8-DIKETO-κ-ENDGROUP

The combination of a κ-endgroup with a 6,8-diketone was found for the first time in mytiloxanthin from *Mytilus californianus* (32) and *M. edulis* (elucidation of constitution) (33) (Scheme 10). Agelaxanthin C from the sponge *Agelas schmidtii* (34) is structurally related and has as special feature a hydroxylated 19-methyl group and a methoxy group in the β-ring. Finally, the endgroup is also found in sponges in combination with aromatic endgroups as trikentriorhodin (34)(35) and trikentriophidin (36). The absolute configuration of tri-

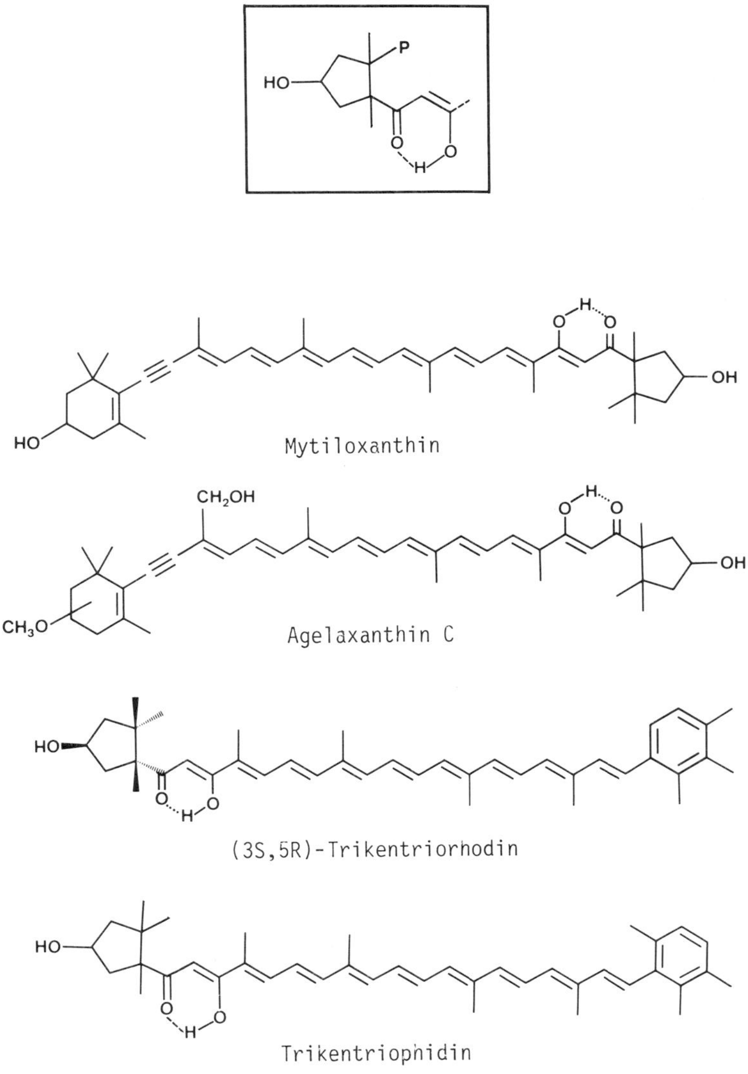

Scheme 10

kentriorhodin from the sponge Agelas schmidtii (34) could be determined by chiroptical comparison with partly optically active synthetic trikentriorhodin (37). Assuming the same absolute configuration in the other compounds, the formation of this endgroup can be visualised by pinacol rearrangement from a carotenoid with a fucoxanthin endgroup (33) (Scheme 11). Such a mechanism was al-

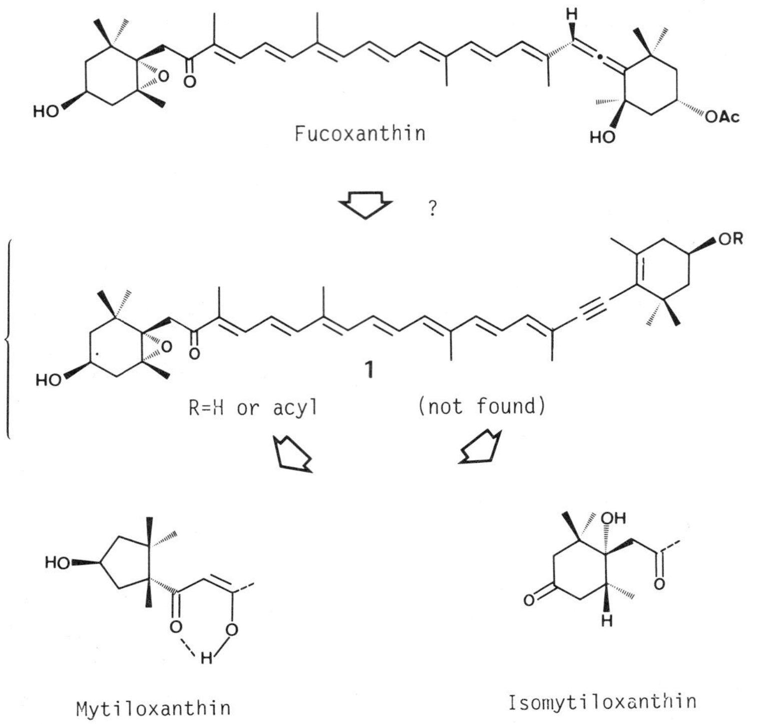

Scheme 11

ready previously suggested for the formation of capsorubin from zeaxanthin (38). The formation of isomytiloxanthin, also isolated from M. edulis with hitherto unknown stereochemistry, can be formulated from the same 5,6-epoxy-8-keto endgroup by hydride reduction at C(5) and oxidation at C(3) (33). Whether the formation of the κ-endgroup in trikentriorhodin or trikentriophidin occurs before or after formation of the aromatic endgroup is still open to speculation due to lack of suitable precursors.

5. THE 3-HYDROXY-ε-ENDGROUP

During the last few years, the stereochemically most interesting modifications were observed in carotenoids with this endgroup (Scheme 12). For some years only the 3'R,6'R (trans) stereochemistry (19)(20) was known, as found in lutein. Also in plants, a deviation from this stereochemistry has so far been observed only once. Calthaxanthin from Caltha palustris is 3'-epilutein (39)(40). In animals, the circumstances are different. Recently, carotenoids with 3-OH-ε-endgroups have repeatedly been found whose stereochemistry deviates from that of lutein. For example in 3'-epilutein and α-doradexanthin from goldfish (22), 3'-epilutein from various types of trout (41), chiriquixanthins A and B from the skin of the frog Atelopus chiriquiensis (42) and from the fish Sebastes flavidus (only B) (43). Furthermore in the three isomeric tunaxanthins from the fish Oxyjulis californica (43), Amanses modestus, Thunnus thynnus and Seriola quinqueradiata (44). These three 3,3'-dihydroxy-ε,ε-carotenes all have 6S,6'S chirality with cis-cis, cis-trans and trans-trans ring substitution. Together with 6S,6'S-ε,ε-carotene, found in the retina of turkey (45), the tunaxanthins are

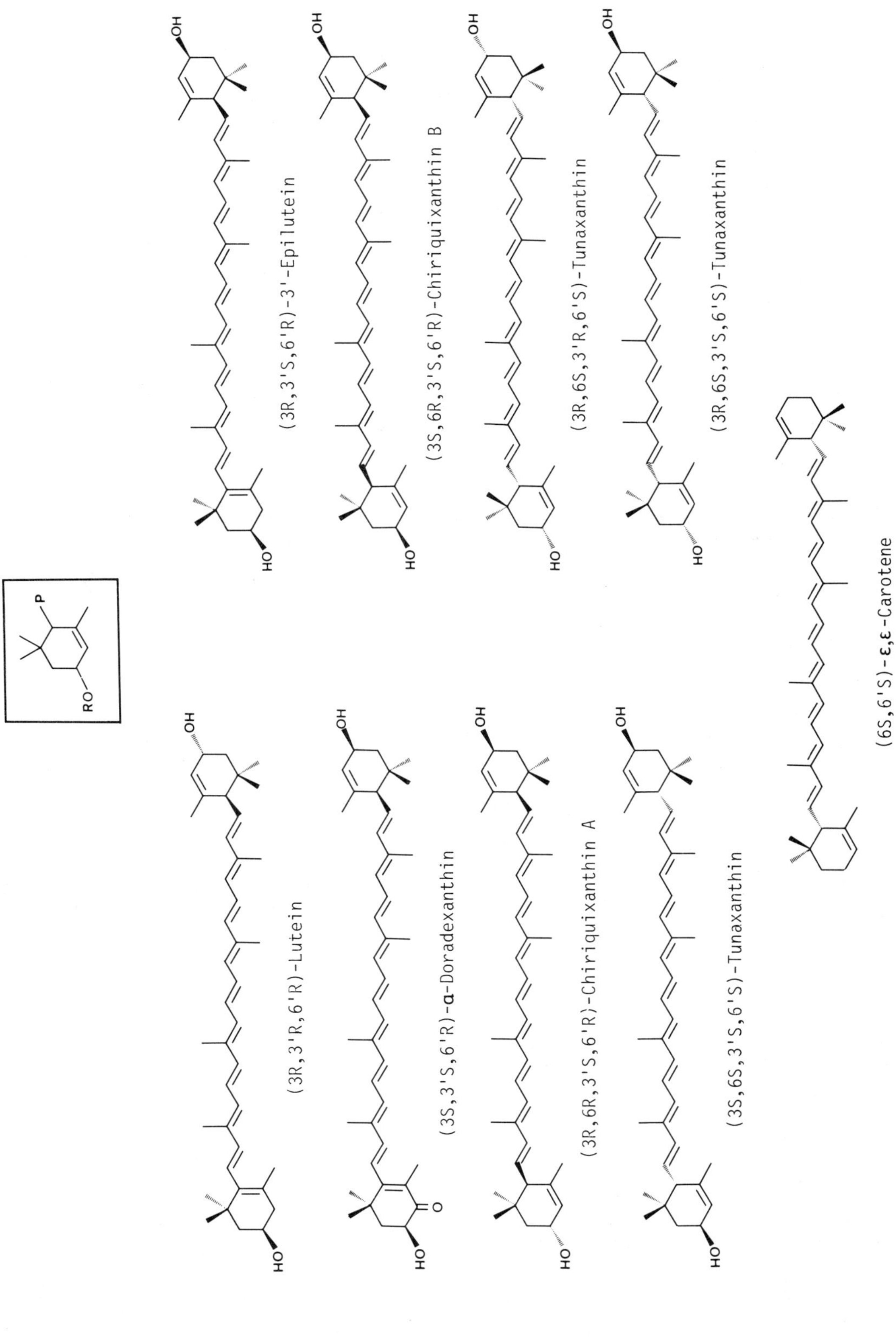
(3R,3'R,6'R)-Lutein
(3S,3'S,6'R)-α-Doradexanthin
(3R,6R,3'S,6'R)-Chiriquixanthin A
(3S,6S,3'S,6'S)-Tunaxanthin
(3R,3'S,6'R)-3'-Epilutein
(3S,6R,3'S,6'R)-Chiriquixanthin B
(3R,6S,3'R,6'S)-Tunaxanthin
(3R,6S,3'S,6'S)-Tunaxanthin
(6S,6'S)-ε,ε-Carotene
RO
P

Scheme 12

so far the only C_{40}-carotenoids with a 6S-chirality of the ε-ring. In particular, all C_{40}-carotenoids of plant origin with ε-ring show the 6R-chirality, so far as they have been investigated (46)(47) (see Note a). Two important biogenetical questions result from these stereochemical facts:

1. How is the 6S ε-ring formed in animals?
2. By which pathway does the formation of the unusual 3,6-cis-substitution in the 3-hydroxy-ε-ring ensue?

As I mentioned before, there is no reason to assume that animals have the ability to biosynthesize carotenoids. In particular, it is probable that animals are also unable to cyclise acyclic precursors. The increased emergence of ε-endgroups with S-chirality suggests that animals are able to rearrange β-endgroups into ε-endgroups. This hypothesis is still considered improbable for plants (49)(50). Circumstantial evidence for such a rearrangement is above all provided by the discovery of 6S,6'S-ε,ε-carotene in turkey embryo, although no trace of ε,ε-carotene was found in the egg yolk (45). If one assumes that the chiriquixanthins A and B with 6R,6'R-chirality also arise by such Δ5,4 rearrangements from lutein and zeaxanthin, respectively (44), then both the 6S and some of the 6R configurated ε-rings could be formed in this way (Scheme 13). The

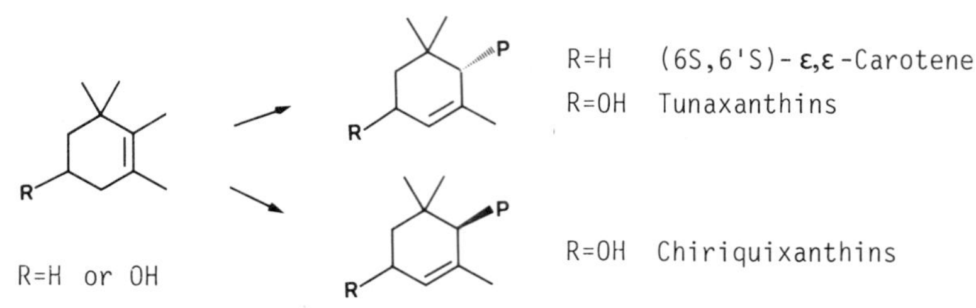

Scheme 13

various published diverse Δε-values from CD-measurements (42)(43)(44), lend weight to the supposition that some of the 3,3'-dihydroxy-ε,ε-carotenes mentioned occur together with their enantiomers or meso-compounds. A similar pathway for the formation of the tunaxanthins was proposed by Bingham et al. (43) (Scheme 14). Accordingly the unsubstituted β-endgroup is initially isomerised to the 6S-ε-endgroup and subsequently cis-hydroxylated at C(3). The 3-hydroxy-β-endgroup, however, gives the 3,6-trans 3-hydroxy-ε-endgroup directly by allylic rearrangement. If this is applied to β-carotene, β-crypto-

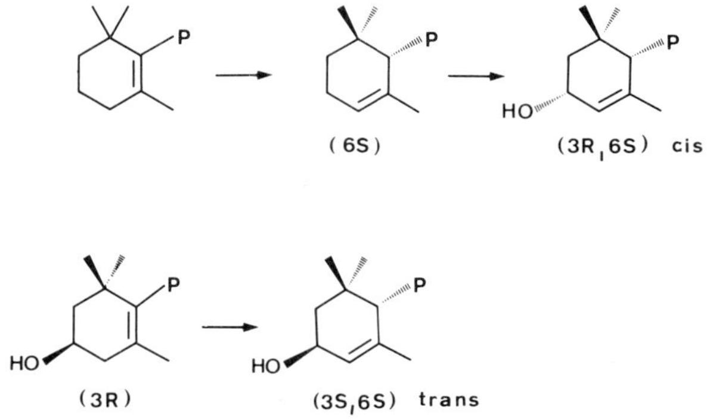

Scheme 14

Note a. According to new CD-measurements (48) the ε,ε-carotene from *Ulva lactuca* has 6R,6'R-chirality and not 6S,6'S as previously suggested (45).

xanthin and zeaxanthin, three tunaxanthins would arise. Thereby, the question of the 3,6-cis-substitution is also partly answered. However, there must still be another route to the cis-hydroxylated ε-endgroup (Scheme 15). In the gold-

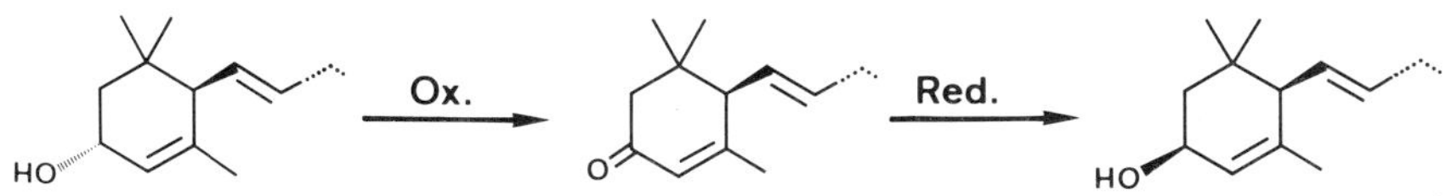

Scheme 15

fish, labelled lutein (3',6'-trans) was unequivocally converted into α-doradexanthin (3',6'-cis) (16)(18). More exact investigation though showed that also the "lutein" stored in goldfish is in fact 3'-epilutein (22). Accordingly, lutein from the food is initially epimerised at C(3) and then either stored or further metabolised to α-doradexanthin. We have found 3'-O-didehydrolutein, which is a possible intermediate product of the epimerisation (22). It is interesting to note that we were also able to identify this compound in Caltha palustris and in egg yolk, from the latter, however, without 3'-epilutein. It is to be suspected that many further carotenoids hitherto identified as lutein from the animal kingdom are, in fact, identical with 3'-epilutein. Equally, the presumed intermediate 3'-O-didehydrolutein has probably remained undetected in most instances due to its instability to bases. Apart from the occurrences mentioned, its discovery has so far only been reported in Philosamia cynthia (silkworm) as philosamiaxanthin (51) and in a few species of moth (52). No details on the absolute configuration are given in these publications. We have investigated the reaction properties of 3'-O-didehydrolutein (40). An ethereal solution of 3'-O-didehydrolutein when left to stand with an equal amount of 10% methanolic KOH (as normally used for the saponification of carotenoid esters) shows the complete disappearance of the 3'-O-didehydrolutein within three hours. In its place are a whole number of more polar substances, including one main product of somewhat higher polarity than the educt. With the help of UV/VIS, MS, ^{1}H-NMR and ^{13}C-NMR we were able to elucidate the structure of this product (2) (Scheme 16). The facile oxidisability of 3'-O-didehydrolutein suggests that

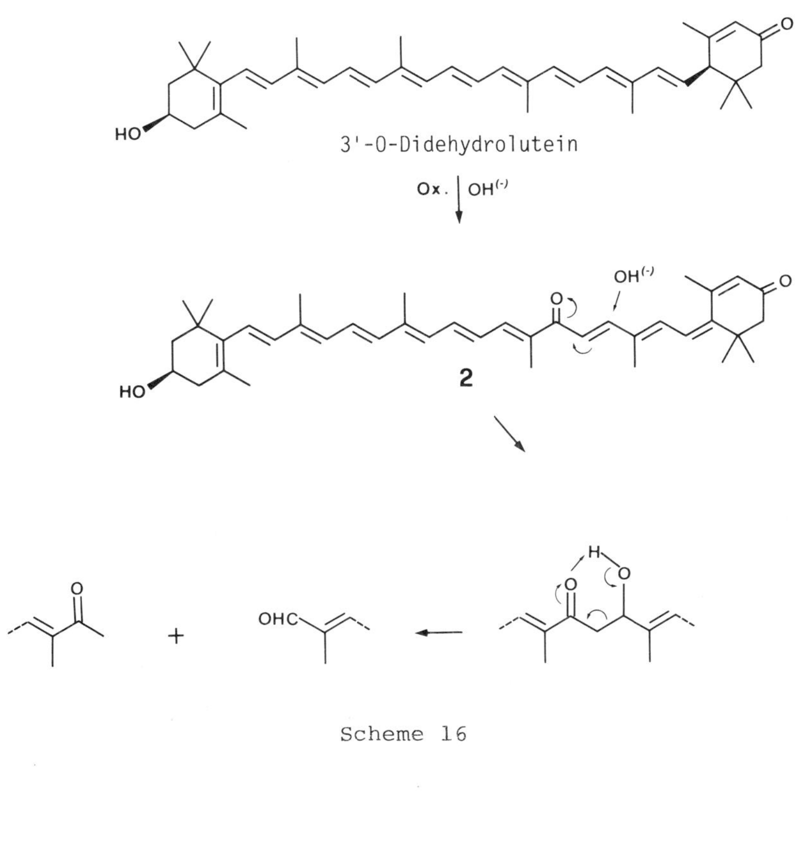

Scheme 16

lutein undergoes a similar degradation also in vivo. The carbonyl group is conceivable at various positions. Apocarotenones and apocarotenals would be the products of a metabolic reaction according to this mechanism.

In concluding the 3-hydroxy-ε-endgroup carotenoids, it must be noted that with the configurational variations encountered to date, it is insufficient to carry out identifications only by comparison of Rf-values and visible spectra. In future, it will be essential to also include NMR and chiroptical methods. Recently, a 3-hydroxy-ε,ε-carotene constitution was proposed for a new carotenoid from Neothunnus albacora (53). If its absolute configuration were known, it might be possible to deduce an intermediate in the tunaxanthin synthesis according to Bingham et al. (43).

6. AROMATIC ENDGROUPS

Carotenoids with aromatic endgroups have been most frequently found in sponges. I will, therefore, refer you to the lecture by Prof. Yamaguchi: "Carotenoids in sponges".

7. SPORADIC ENDGROUPS

At this point, I would like to deal with a few carotenoids which have hitherto only sporadically appeared in animals. I will mention the C_{40}-carotenoids with the γ-endgroup only briefly (Scheme 17). β,γ- and γ,γ-carotene were earlier found in the aphids Macrosiphum liriodendri (54). Both have been synthesised in optically active form (55)(56), but the absolute configuration of nat. γ,γ-carotene is not yet known due to the lack of chiroptical data. Of interest are also

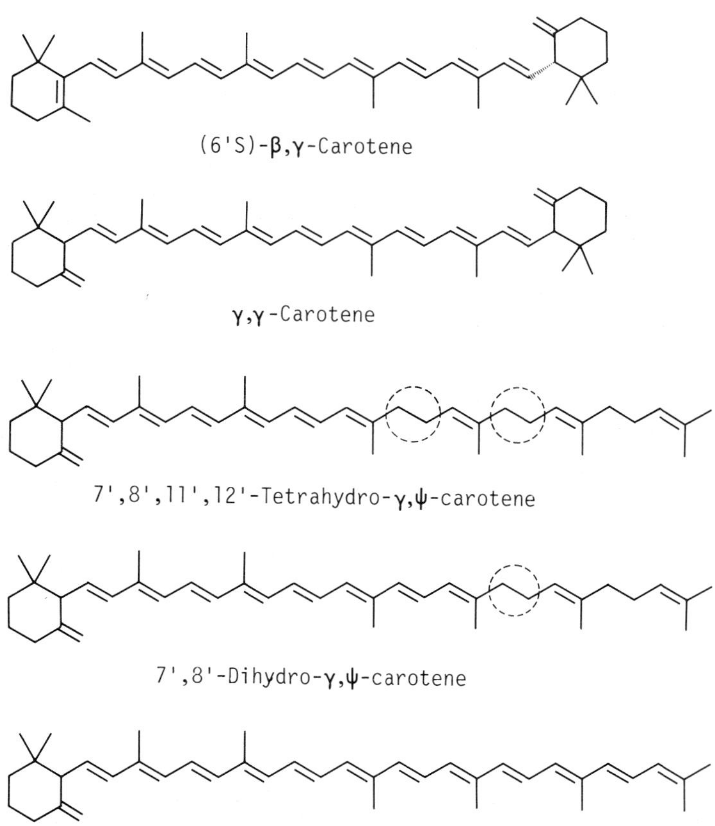

(6'S)-β,γ-Carotene

γ,γ-Carotene

7',8',11',12'-Tetrahydro-γ,ψ-carotene

7',8'-Dihydro-γ,ψ-carotene

3',4'-Didehydro-γ,ψ-carotene

Scheme 17

the carotenes with the γ-endgroup which were discovered a few years ago in the lady-bird beetle Coccinella septempunctata: besides β,γ- and γ,γ-carotene also 7',8',11',12'-tetrahydro-γ,ψ-carotene, 7',8'dihydro-γ,ψ-carotene and 3',4'-didehydro-γ,ψ-carotene (57). It is hinted that these carotenoids are either formed by microorganisms in the beetle or originate from the nutriment (aphids, rusts and other fungi). The γ-endgroup is also typical for fungi (58).

Recently an aromatic carotene with a dehydrogenated γ-endgroup was found in the sponge Microciona prolifera: 3,4(2,3)-didehydro-γ,χ-carotene (59) (Scheme 18).

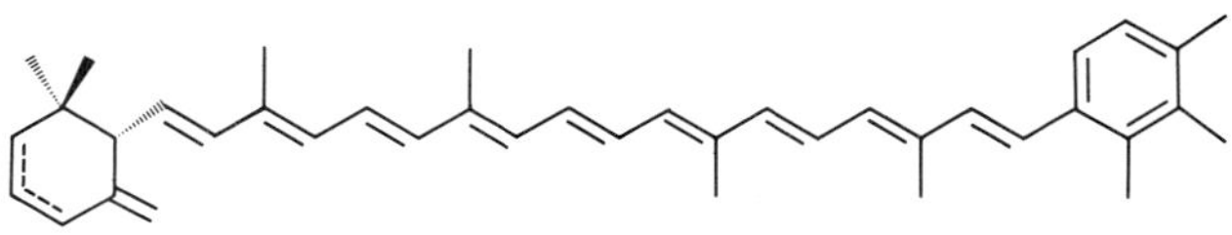

(6S)-3,4(2,3)-Didehydro-γ,χ-carotene

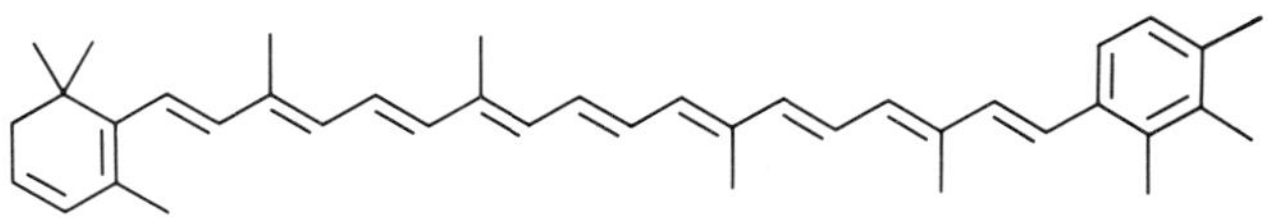

Tethyatene

Scheme 18

The position of the endocyclic double bond has not yet been localised exactly. Since the CD is in good agreement with that of natural (6'S)-β,γ-carotene (55), the same absolute configuration is probable. The authors emphasize that this endgroup could possibly ensue by dehydration of a carotenoid with a (6S)-3-OH-ε-ring. In a similar way, the related structure tethyatene with a 3,4-didehydro-β-endgroup could also have arisen. Tethyatene was previously found by Tanaka et al. (60) in the sponge Tethya amamensis and has recently been synthesised (61). It could be that both compounds represent intermediate or side-products of the aromatisation reaction (59).

Carotenoids hydroxylated at C(2) are known mainly from algae (62)(63) and yeast (64) (Scheme 19). It is surprising, therefore, that the 2-hydroxy-β-endgroup is also found in a crustacean (Idotea) as β,β-caroten-2-ol (65) and, above all, in insects (66)(67). It could be shown that the two moth species Cerura vinula L. and Phalera bucephala L. as well as the stick insect Carausius morosus metabolise β,β-carotene in this way (67)(68). Further oxidised endgroups were also found here, e.g. in 3,4,3',4'-didehydro-β,β-carotene-2,2'-dione. The metabolic pathway proposed is briefly illustrated on an endgroup (Scheme 20). The β-endgroup is oxidised at C(2) directly to the ketone. Hydride reduction then leads to the 2-hydroxy endgroup, while 3,4-dehydrogenation gives the conjugated ketone. Subject to only the dehydrogenation of the diketo compound, all combinations are imaginable starting from β,β-carotene and these have apparently also been found (68). Suggested biogenetic mechanisms for the 2-hydroxy-β-ring to date comprise:

a) Cyclisation of an open-chain 1,2-epoxide (62);
b) Cyclisation with the electrophile OH^+ (69);
c) Direct hydroxylation of the β-ring (63)(45).

Thus we have as a further possibility the reduction of a carbonyl group at C(2). Unfortunately, to date nothing is known about the stereochemistry of the 2-hydroxy-carotenoids formed by insects. The absolute configurations at C(2) in carotenoids from Trentepohlia iolithus (70) and Anacystis nidulans (63) are known to be opposite.

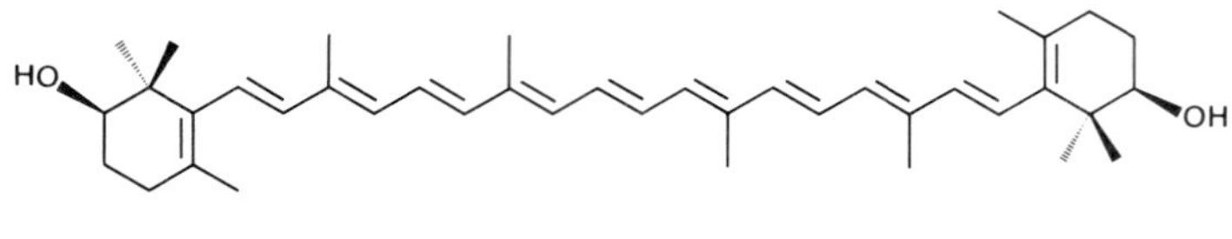

(2R,2'R)-β,β-carotene-2,2'-diol

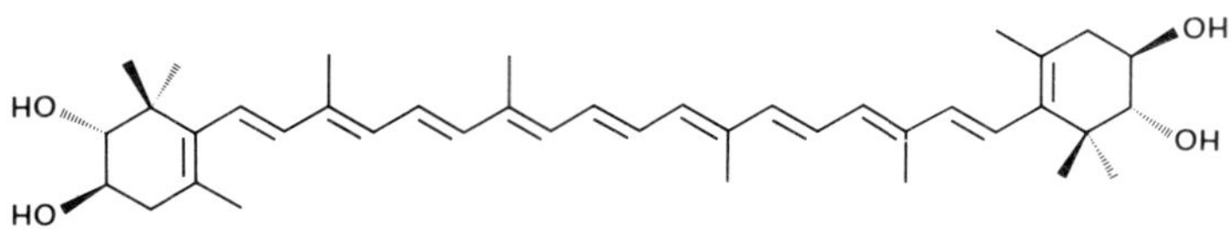

Nostoxanthin

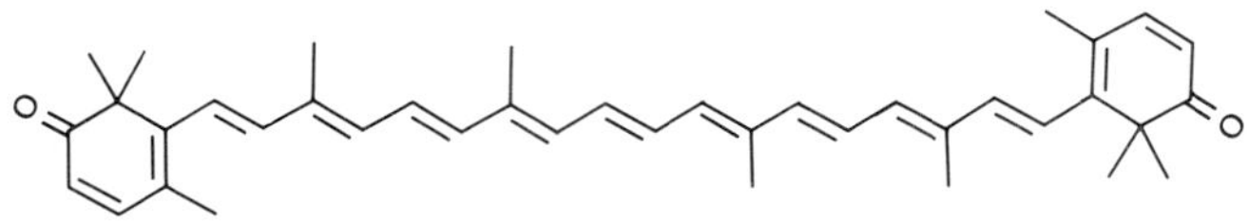

3,4,3',4'-tetradehydro-β,β-carotene-2,2'-dione

Scheme 19

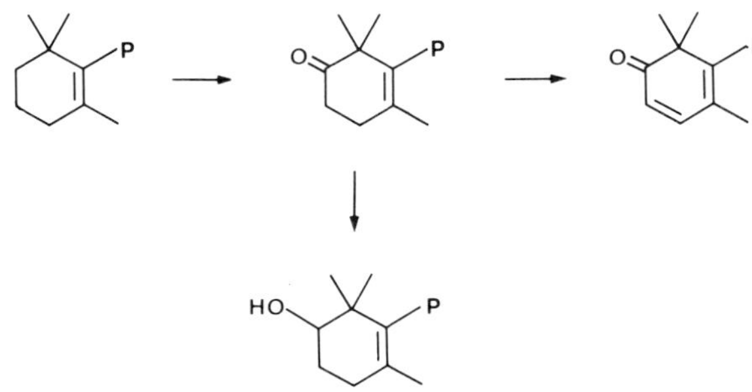

Scheme 20

Recently, Japanese authors (71) reported four new carotenoids from the red tilefish Branchiostegus japonicus japonicus. In addition to tunaxanthin, the carotenoids were isolated and designated as tilefishxanthin I-IV (Scheme 21). Their constitutions were proposed only on the basis of chromatographic properties, visible spectra and behaviour on saponification, reduction and S_N1-methylation. They should not, therefore, be considered as certain. The new endgroups are worthy of note, e.g. the 2-hydroxy-ε-endgroup in tilefishxanthin I and II, the 2-hydroxy-4-keto-β-endgroup in tilefishxanthin III and the 2-keto-3-hydroxy-ε-endgroup in tilefishxanthin IV. However, verification by MS and NMR is necessary and a chiroptical characterisation desirable.

Two other animal carotenoids are worthy of further mention here: parasiloxanthin and 7,8-dihydroparasiloxanthin (Scheme 22). They were isolated a few years ago from the Japanese common catfish Parasilus asotus (72). 7,8-dihydro-cyclic endgroups are unusual in carotenoids. In contrast to squalene, the lycopene skeleton is generally only cyclised at the half where the ψ-endgroup is through-conjugated. It is therefore to be assumed that the original 7,8-double bond (or acetylenic bond) of the cyclic carotenoid, e.g. zeaxanthin (alloxanthin, diato-

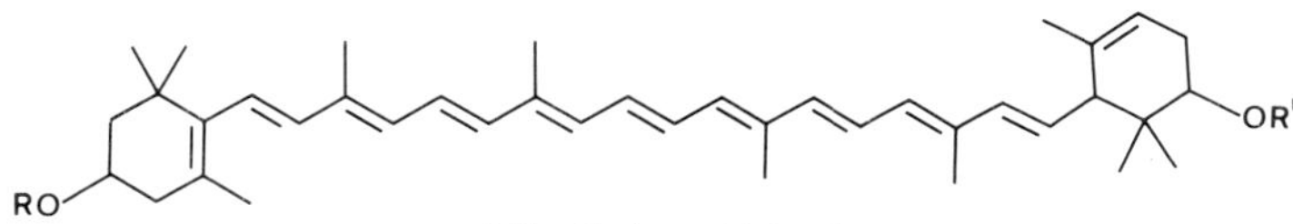

Tilefishxanthin I

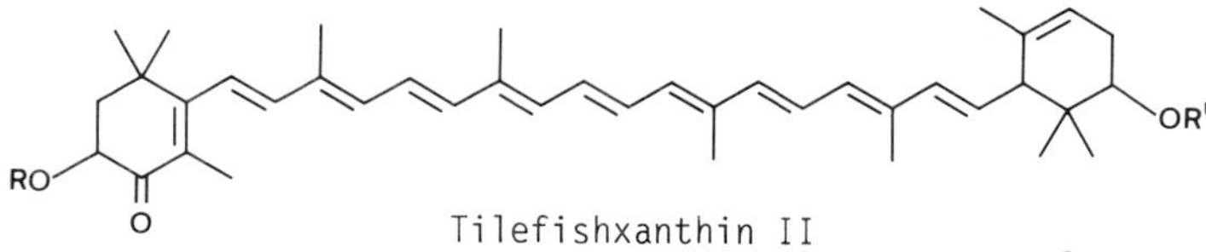

Tilefishxanthin II

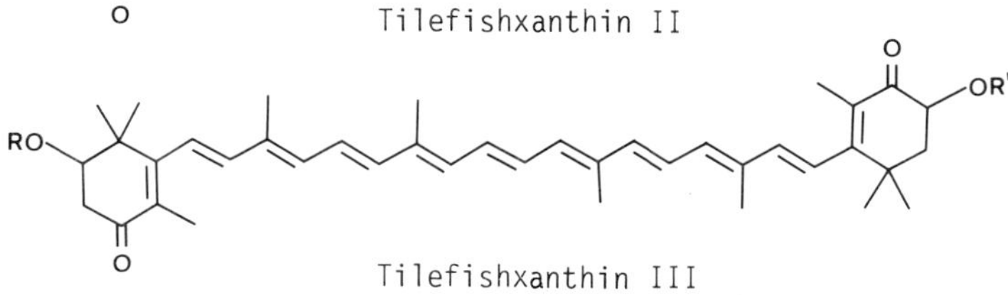

Tilefishxanthin III

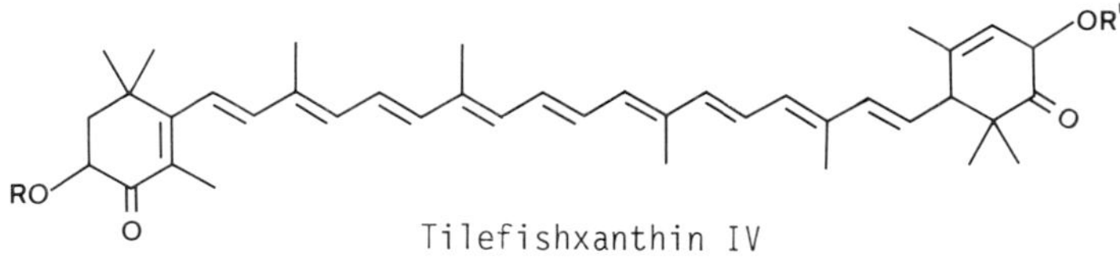

Tilefishxanthin IV

Scheme 21

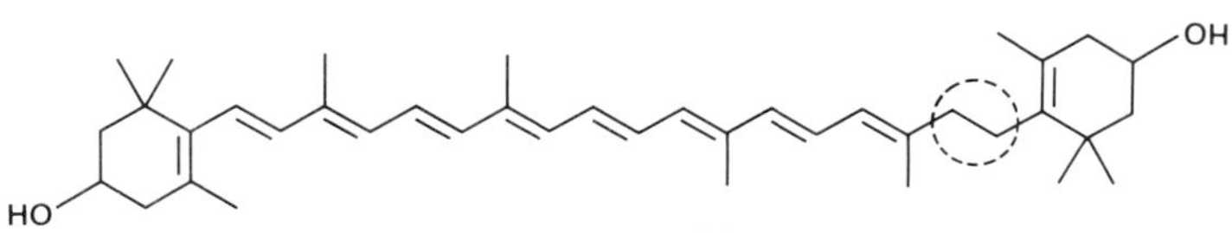

Parasiloxanthin

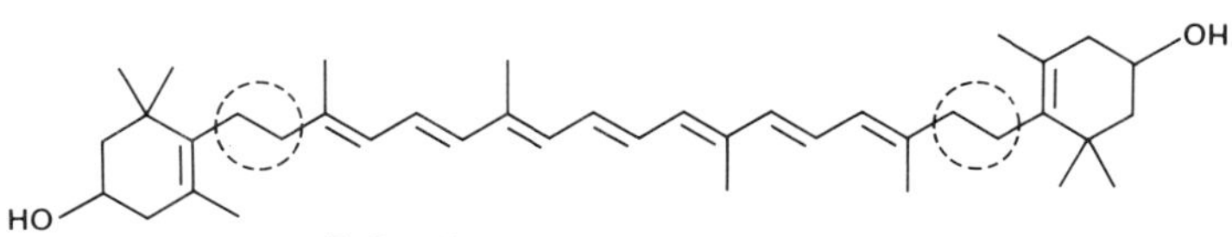

7,8-Dihydro-parasiloxanthin

Scheme 22

xanthin) was subsequently hydrogenated in the fish. For several cyclic carotenoids mentioned in the literature with a 7,8-dihydro structure, unequivocal proof is lacking (73).

In conclusion I would like to mention that a growing number of publications on carotenoids in various animals has appeared in the last few years. These deal mostly with the identification of already known carotenoids by Rf-values and UV/VIS-spectra. However, because of the ever-increasing number of new carotenoids with very similar chromatographical behaviour and sometimes the same photospectroscopical properties, the possibility of incorrect identification is becoming more and more likely. The potential presence of cis/trans isomers complicates matters even further. In addition, we have the recent appearance of enantiomers and diastereomers. Chiroptical methods and NMR should therefore be used to a greater extent for identification purposes. Also, the application of HPLC-techniques opens up new possibilities here. Combined with the diastereomeric derivatisation of chiral carotenoids excellent results were achieved, for example with astaxanthin (7). As far as the metabolism of carotenoids in animals is concerned, only a limited amount of reliable information is available to date. It would be desirable if the hypothetical mechanisms could be investigated by means of labelling experiments.

REFERENCES

1. D.L. Fox, "Animal Biochromes and Structural Colours", University of California Press, Berkeley (1976).
2. T.W. Goodwin, "The Comparative Biochemistry of the Carotenoids", Chapman and Hall, London (1952).
3. T.W. Goodwin in "Chemical Zoology" (M. Florkin and B.T. Scheer eds.), Vol. 2, Academic Press, New York (1971).
4. P. Karrer and E. Jucker, "Carotenoids", Elsevier, London (1950).
5. S. Liaaen-Jensen in "Marine Natural Products" (P. Scheuer ed.), Vol. 2, Academic Press, London (1978).
6. R.K. Müller, K. Bernhard, H. Mayer, A. Rüttimann and M. Vecchi, Helv. Chim. Acta 63, 1654 (1980).
7. H. Rønneberg, B. Renstrøm, K. Aareskjold, S. Liaaen-Jensen, M. Vecchi, F. Leuenberger, R.K. Müller and H. Mayer, Helv. Chim. Acta 63, 711 (1980).
8. F. Kienzle and H. Mayer, Helv. Chim. Acta 61, 2609 (1978).
9. A.G. Andrewes and M.P. Starr, Phytochem. 15, 1009 (1976).
10. H. Thommen in "Carotenoids" (O. Isler ed.), p. 637, Birkhäuser, Basel (1971).
11. T. Katayama, M. Shimaya, M. Sameshima and C.O. Chichester, Int. J. Biochem. 4, 223 (1973).
12. T. Katayama, T. Kamata, M. Shimaya, O. Deshimaru and C.O. Chichester, Bull. Jap. Soc. Sci. Fish. 38, 1171 (1972).
13. D.B. Rodriguez, K.L. Simpson and C.O. Chichester, Int. J. Biochem. 4, 213 (1973).
14. D.B. Rodriguez, K.L. Simpson and C.O. Chichester, Int. J. Biochem. 5, 157 (1974).
15. M. Hata and M. Hata, Bull. Jap. Soc. Sci. Fish. 41, 653 (1975), 42, 203 (1976
16. M. Hata and M. Hata, Bull. Jap. Soc. Sci. Fish. 38, 331 (1972).
17. R. Berger, G. Borch and S. Liaaen-Jensen, Acta Chem. Scand. B 31, 243 (1977).
18. W.-J. Hsu, D.B. Rodriguez and C.O. Chichester, Int. J. Biochem. 3, 333 (1972).
19. R. Buchecker, P. Hamm and C.H. Eugster, Chimia 25, 192 (1971), 26, 134 (1972); Helv. Chim. Acta 57, 631 (1974).
20. A.G. Andrewes, G. Borch and S. Liaaen-Jensen, Acta Chem. Scand. B 28, 139 (1974).
21. A.G. Andrewes, G. Borch, S. Liaaen-Jensen and G. Snatzke, Acta Chem. Scand. B 28, 730 (1974).
22. R. Buchecker, C.H. Eugster and A. Weber, Helv. Chim. Acta 61, 1962 (1978).
23. R. Castillo and R. Lenel, Comp. Biochem. Physiol. 59 B, 67 (1978).
24. R. Lenel, R. Castillo and G. Negre-Sadargues, Biochem. Syst. and Ecology 6, 251 (1978).
25. E. Nicoara, G. Illyes, M. Şuteu and C. Bodea, Rev. Roum. Chim. 12, 547 (1967).

25a. A. Haag, Ph. D. Thesis in preparation.

26. S. Hertzberg and S. Liaaen-Jensen, Acta Chem. Scand. 22, 1714 (1968).
27. S. Hertzberg, S. Liaaen-Jensen, C.R. Enzell and G.W. Francis, Acta Chem. Scand. 23, 3290 (1969).
28. J.D. Tauber, A. Fiksdahl and S. Liaaen-Jensen, Biochem. Syst. and Ecology 8 437 (1980).
29. R.K. Müller, H. Mayer, K. Noack, J.J. Dali, J.D. Tauber and S. Liaaen-Jense Helv. Chim. Acta 61, 2881 (1978).
30. P.S. Foss, P.J. Green and R.W. Rickards, Aust. J. Chem. 31, 1981 (1978).
31. G.W. Francis, S. Hertzberg, R.R. Upadhyay and S. Liaaen-Jensen, Acta Chem. Scand. 26, 1097 (1972).
32. B.T. Sheer, J. Biol. Chem. 136, 275 (1940).
33. A. Khare, G.P. Moss and B.C.L. Weedon, Tetrahedron Letters 40, 3921 (1973).

34. R. Buchecker, C.H. Eugster and C. Litchfield, Helv. Chim. Acta 60, 2780 (1977).
35. M. Aguilar-Martinez and S. Liaaen-Jensen, Acta Chem. Scand. B 28, 1247 (1974).
36. C. Litchfield and S. Liaaen-Jensen, Comp. Biochem. Physiol. 66 B, 359 (1980).
37. A.K. Chopra, G.P. Moss and B.C.L. Weedon, Chem. Commun. 1977, 467.
38. M.E. Barber, L.M. Jackman, C.K. Warren and B.C.L. Weedon, Proc. Chem. Soc. 1960, 19.
39. A.G. Dabbagh and K. Egger, Z. Pflanzenphysiol. 72, 177 (1974).
40. R. Buchecker and C.H. Eugster, Helv. Chim. Acta 62, 2817 (1979).
41. M. Takao, N. Seiichi, K. Masaaki, M. Hisako, M. Takashi and A. Toshiko, Nippon Suis. Gakk. 46, 473 (1980); C.A. 93, 22941 (1980).
42. A. Bingham, H.S. Mosher and A.G. Andrewes, Chem. Commun. 1977, 96.
43. A. Bingham, D.W. Wilkie and H.S. Mosher, Comp. Biochem. Physiol. 62 B, 489 (1979).
44. H. Rønneberg, G. Borch, S. Liaaen-Jensen, H. Matsutaka and T. Matsuno, Acta Chem. Scand. B 32, 621 (1978).
45. B.H. Davies, Pure Appl. Chem. 51, 623 (1979).
46. C.H. Eugster, R. Buchecker, Ch. Tscharner, G. Uhde and G. Ohloff, Helv. Chim. Acta 52, 1729 (1969), 56, 2548 (1973).
47. R. Buchecker and C.H. Eugster, Helv. Chim. Acta 56, 1124 (1973).
48. B.H. Davies, S. Pollard, A.J. Summerfield, R.J. de B. Apps, P.M. Scopes, R. Buchecker and C.H. Eugster, to be published.
49. T.J. Walton, G. Britton and T.W. Goodwin, Biochem. J. 112, 383 (1969).
50. T.W. Goodwin, Biochem. J. 123, 293 (1971).
51. K. Harashima, Int. J. Biochem. 1, 523 (1970).
52. H. Kayser, J. Comp. Physiol. 104, 27 (1975).
53. Y. Tanaka, F. Shimamura and T. Katayama, Kogoshima Daigaku Suisangakubu Kiyo 26, 33 (1977).
54. A.G. Andrewes, H. Kjøsen, S. Liaaen-Jensen, K.H. Weisgraber, R.J.J.C. Lousberg and U. Weiss, Acta Chem. Scand. 25, 3878 (1971).
55. M. Hallenstvet,R. Buchecker, G. Borch and S. Liaaen-Jensen, Phytochem. 16, 583 (1977).
56. H.P. Märki and C.H. Eugster, Helv. Chim. Acta 64, in press.
57. G. Britton, T.W. Goodwin, G.E. Harriman and W.J.S. Lockley, Insect Biochem. 7, 337 (1977).
58. N. Arpin, J.L. Fiasson, M.P. Bouchez-Dangye-Caye, G.W. Francis and S. Liaaen-Jensen, Phytochem. 10, 1595 (1971)
59. C. Litchfield and S. Liaaen-Jensen, Comp. Biochem. Physiol. 66 B, 359 (1980).
60. Y. Tanaka and T. Katayama, Bull. Jap. Soc. Sci. Fish. 43, 1229 (1977).
61. A. Shimada, Y. Ezaki, J. Inanaga, T. Katsuki and M. Yamaguchi, Tetrahedron Letters 22, 773 (1981).
62. H. Kjøsen, N. Arpin and S. Liaaen-Jensen, Acta Chem. Scand. 26, 3053 (1972).
63. R. Buchecker, S. Liaaen-Jensen, G. Borch and H.W. Siegelman, Phytochem. 15, 1015 (1976).
64. I.-S. Liu, T.H. Lee, H. Yokoyama, K.L. Simpson and C.O. Chichester, Phytochem. 12, 2953 (1973)
65. W.L. Lee and B.M. Gilchrist, Comp. Biochem. Physiol. B 51, 247 (1975).
66. H. Kayser, Z. Naturforsch. 31 c, 121, 646 (1976).
67. H. Kayser, Comp. Biochem. Physiol. 58 B, 177 (1977).
68. H. Kayser, Z. Naturforsch. 32 c, 327 (1977).
69. G. Britton, Pure Appl. Chem. 47, 223 (1976).
70. R. Buchecker, C.H. Eugster, H. Kjøsen and S. Liaaen-Jensen, Helv. Chim. Acta 56, 2899 (1973); Acta Chem. Scand. B 28, 449 (1974).
71. M. Asahara, S. Matsuno and S. Matsumori, Bull. Jap. Soc. Sci. Fish. 45, 485 (1979).
72. T. Matsuno, S. Nagata and K. Kitamura, Tetrahedron Letters 1976, 4601.
73. O. Straub, "Key to Carotenoids", Birkhäuser, Basel (1976).

CAROTENOIDS IN INSECTS

Hartmut Kayser

Abteilung für Allgemeine Zoologie (Biologie I),
Universität Ulm, Postfach 4066, D-7900 Ulm/Donau, F.R.G.

Abstract - The distribution and origin of carotenoids in insects is critically reviewed. In insects the presence of carotenoids and their structural types primarily depends on specific feeding habits. The carotenoid pattern reflects group- or even species-specific capacities in selective absorption and/or metabolic transformations of dietary carotenoids rather than phylogenetic relations. Though some structural types are frequently found within certain taxonomic groups carotenoids do not appear to be useful chemosystematic markers for insects. This review focuses on the structures of those carotenoids which are obviously produced in the insects themselves. Direct evidence for such capacities which are not widespread among insects has been obtained in only few cases. Insects are able to introduce oxygen functions at carbon(s)-2,-3, and/or -4 of a β-end ring. The 3'-hydroxyl in lutein may be dehydrogenated. The occurrence of fungal carotenoids in some insects reflects the presence of microbial symbionts or complex food chains. The proposed metabolic pathways for carotenoid transformations in insects are discussed with special emphasis on the biogenesis of 2-hydroxy carotenoids. The stereochemistry of 2-hydroxy β,β-type carotenols has been studied by CD and NMR. All of them proved to be partly racemic. Two different metabolic pathways are offered to interpret these results.

INTRODUCTION

Two facts may have stimulated very early the study of insect carotenoids: the most widespread occurrence of this class of pigments in nature and the predominance of insects among known animal species. A large number of carotenoids in insects has been reported since then; however, many early "identifications" of these pigments suffer from insufficient analytical tools. This situation changed when about twenty years ago modern methods for structural research such as nuclear magnetic resonance spectroscopy and mass spectrometry were introduced into the carotenoid field and allowed precise assignments (cf. Refs. 1,2). Especially mass spectrometry has become a routine method. Much of the recent progress in insect carotenoids is due to this analytical tool. Many interesting earlier reports on insects carotenoids should be regarded as a stimulus for thorough reinvestigations rather than as established facts. Such weakly based and therefore tentative identifications will be referred to only when considered stimulating or when more reliable information is not available. A good compilation of papers related to insect carotenoids has been given by Feltwell (Ref. 3) some years ago.

The aim of this review is to concentrate on the more recent work on insect carotenoids, roughly published since 1950. Modern work in this field began in Liverpool in the late fifties when Goodwin started a research program on the biochemistry of locust pigmentation. In 1952 (Ref. 4), he expressed the generally accepted view that insect carotenoids are of dietary origin, are accumulated in the body, and in some cases the carbon skeleton of a preformed carotenoid can be modified. These aspects of insect carotenoids are used as a guideline in this lecture. First, the distribution of carotenoids in the various insect orders will be reviewed under the aspect of the origin of these pigments. Then, I want to concentrate on the structures of those carotenoids which are considered as genuine insect products, and finally the proposed metabolic schemes for transformations of carotenoids in insects will be discussed together with recent results on the stereochemistry of one type of insect carotenoids, which is the focus of my own work.

DISTRIBUTION AND ORIGIN OF CAROTENOIDS IN INSECTS

General aspects

Up to date, there is no convincing report on any *de novo* formation of carotenoids in an animal. Insects therefore depend on exogenous supply of the carotenoid skeleton which is derived from *de novo* carotenoid producers such as green plants, fungi, bacteria and others. These producers need not necessarily be outside the insects' body as in the case of endosymbiotic microorganisms being well known in some insect groups. The carotenoids, once being within the alimentary channel of an insect, can be treated in four different ways: 1. carotenoids are totally rejected, 2. carotenoids are absorbed indiscriminately, 3. only a few carotenoids are selectively absorbed, 4. the sequestered carotenoid(s) are structurally modified e.g. by introduction of oxo-groups by which the colour of the precursor carotenoid may change.

According to this outline, profound knowledge on the biology and principally on the feeding habits of an insect is a prerequisite in considering the origin of an insect carotenoid. Examples will be presented to illustrate this important point.

Carotenoid distribution

Orthoptera (*Saltatoria*). The best studied species are the locusts, *Locusta migratoria migratoriaides* and *Schistocerca gregaria* which according to Goodwin and Srisukh (Refs. 5,6,7) have only ß,ß-carotene (A-A) and astaxanthin (N-N). ß,ß-Carotene was found in all body parts, astaxanthin in the integument, wings, and eyes. Astaxanthin was not present in the food but shown to be formed at the expense of β,β-carotene during egg development (Ref. 8). Both pigments were largely complexed with proteins (Ref. 9). Other workers (Ref. 10) did not find astaxanthin but lutein in *Schistocerca*. No explanation can be presented for this difference.

The presence of astaxanthin-proteins in the red, blue, and yellow hind wings of *Oedipoda* spp. and other locusts have been reported (Refs. 7,11). In the pink form of *Amblycorypha* sp. the presence of α-cryptoxanthin (?)(Ref. 12) and in *Tettigonia viridissima* that of cryptoxanthin (A-L)(Ref. 13) was claimed. Both reports need to be reinvestigated.

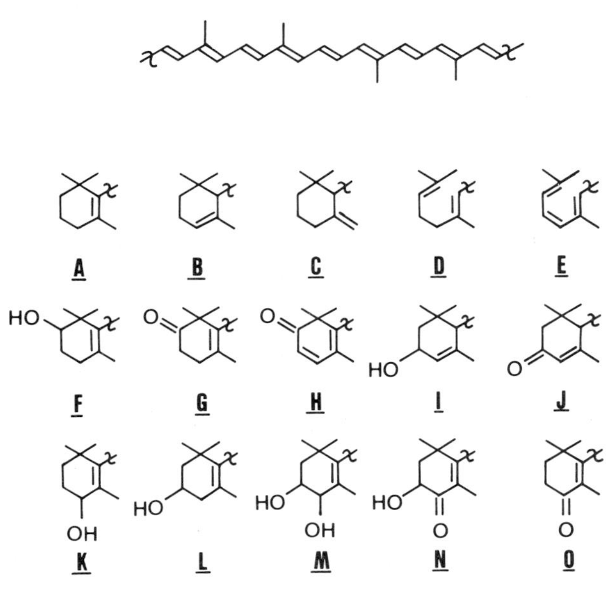

Fig. 1 Structural features of carotenoids from insects.

Phasmida. The study on stick insects revealed a series of novel carotenoids. In *Carausius morosus* the presence of isocryptoxanthin (A-K) and isozeaxanthin (K-K) together with an unidentified red keto-carotenoid had been claimed by Willig (Ref. 13). A reinvestigation by Kayser (Ref. 14), however, revealed β,β-caroten-2-ol (A-F) and β,β-carotene-2,2'-diol (F-F) which had been isolated before from a green alga (Ref. 15). The red keto-carotenoid of Willig was assigned to 3,4,3',4'-tetradehydro-β,β-carotene-2,2'-dione (H-H) (Ref. 16) which had not yet been found in nature. The structure of this pigment with a chromophore extending over fifteen conjugated double bonds has been confirmed by total synthesis carried out by Liaaen-Jensen's group (Ref. 17). In addition, some other hitherto unknown β,β-type carotenoids were isolated (Ref. 16): 2-one (A-G), 2,2'-dione (G-G), 2'-hydroxy-2-one (F-G), 3,4-didehydro-2,2'-dione (G-H), and 2'-hydroxy-3,4-didehydro-2-one (F-H).
In a comparative study on other Phasmids the same β,β-type carotenoids have been established in *Ectatosoma tiaratum*, *Ctenomorphodes brieveus*, and *Acrophylla wulfingi* (Refs. 18,19). In all stick insects, except for *Carausius*, β,ε-carotene (A-B) was also present together with its 2-oxo (B-G) and 2-hydroxy (B-F) derivatives (Refs. 18,19). β,ε-Caroten-2-ol (B-F) had only once been found in nature before (Ref. 15). Another stick insect, *Sipyloidea sipylus*, contained no trace of a carotenoid at all (Ref. 19) though feeding on the same leaves. So, this species seems to totally reject carotenoids in the gut while the other stick insects absorb almost selectively the common leaf carotenes which obviously are metabolized to the series of hydroxy- and oxo-carotenoids as presented above.

Hemiptera. Let us consider now bugs (Heteroptera) and plant lice (Homoptera). Concerning bugs there is an early report by Lederer (Ref. 20) on lycopene (ψ,ψ-carotene)(D-D) in the red bug, *Pyrrhocoris apterus*, which is interesting and needs confirmation by modern methods. *Nezara viridula* contains β,β-carotene (A-A) as a protein complex in the haemolymph (Ref. 21), and *Eurydema ornata* is reported to accumulate preferably β,β-carotene from its food plant (Ref. 22). In *Dysdercus* sp. the presence of "oxo-carotenoids" has been claimed (Ref. 23).

Among the Homoptera the occurrence of carotenoids appears to be restricted to aphids and some coccids (Refs. 24,25). The most thoroughly studied species is the aphid *Macrosiphum liriodendri* (Refs. 12,26) which is known to display a colour dimorphism with a green and a pink variant. In the pink form the principal carotenoids were the two mono-cyclic pigments, torulene (A-E) and γ-carotene (A-D); their acyclic isomers, 3,4-didehydro lycopene (D-E) and lycopene (D-D), were the minor carotenoids. The green variety contains β,γ-carotene (A-C) and small amounts of γ,γ-carotene (C-C). β,β-Carotene (A-A) was found in both colour forms.
Aphids are well known to be obligatorily associated with endosymbiotic microorganisms (Ref. 27). Since torulene and γ-ring carotenoids are typical fungal products (Ref. 28) the authors reached the conclusion (Refs. 12,26) that these aphid carotenoids are actually synthesized by the microbial symbionts. Whether aphids are at all able to modify preformed carotenoids remains to be established.
Czeczuga (Refs. 29,30) screened twenty species of aphids for their carotenoid composition. Apart from those pigments found also in the host plants the following carotenoids should be mentioned: isocryptoxanthin (A-K), isozeaxanthin (K-K), echinenone (A-O), canthaxanthin (O-O), astaxanthin (N-N) resp. astacene, eschscholtzxanthin, torulene (A-E), and rhodopin (1-hydroxy-1,2-dihydrolycopene). The latter two carotenes again point to a biogenetic contribution to the aphid carotenoids by microbial symbionts. Astaxanthin and its presumed precursors may be formed by the aphids themselves since these pigments are typical animal products. Valadon and Mummery (Ref. 31) failed in their study of *Aphis fabae* to detect any of those carotenoids (astaxanthin, torulene, isozeaxanthin) identified by Czeczuga (Ref. 30) in this aphid.

Coleoptera. We now proceed to the beetles and start with the Coccinellid family, since, typically, their members are predators feeding on aphids.
A detailed study by the Liverpool group (Refs. 32,33) on the carotenoids of the ladybird beetle, *C.septempunctata*, recently confirmed the presence of lycopene (D-D) which had been identified by Lederer (Ref. 34) more than forty years ago. In addition, seventeen other carotenoids were reported: these were intermediates of the desaturation series from phytoene to lycopene, furthermore 3,4-dehydrolycopene (D-E), mono-cyclic carotenoids such as γ-carotene (A-D) and torulene (A-E), and β,γ-carotene (A-C) and γ,γ-carotene

(C-C). In contrast, Valadon and Mummery (Ref. 35) were unable to find lycopene in this beetle, however, they state the presence of "red bands". Because most of the pigments, found by Britton and co-workers (Refs. 32,33), are known intermediates in the de novo biosynthesis of carotenoids, and since other compounds are typical fungal carotenes, the authors conclude that these carotenoids are produced neither by the beetles nor by the aphids per se they prey upon but most likely by the microbial symbionts associated with the aphids. It appears also possible that the beetles sometimes feed on fungi directly (cf. Ref. 33).

This example nicely demonstrates that the biology of an insect must be well known if anything on the biogenesis of its carotenoids can be concluded.

In some cases complex food chains may be responsible for the presence of unusual carotenoids.

In contrast to Coccinella and most other Coccinellid beetles the members of the genus Subcoccinella are not predators but plant feeders. It is interesting to see from the study of Tamas and co-workers (Ref. 36) on S.vigintiquatuorpunctata that this species contained only the carotenoids of its food plant (alfalfa). A predominance of epoxy-carotenoids demonstrated some selectivety in accumulation.

The Chrysomelid family comprises beetles that typically feed on leaves of green plants. The Colorado beetle, Leptinotarsa decemlineata, has been reported by four agreeing papers (Refs. 37,38,39,40) to contain echinenone (A-O) and canthaxanthin (O-O) in addition to β,β-carotene and lutein (I-L). Isocryptoxanthin (A-K) has been tentatively identified in the beetles by one of these authors (Ref. 39). The oxo-carotenoids are already present in the eggs and larvae of this species (Ref. 38). Poff (Ref. 41) working also on other Leptinotarsa species identified astaxanthin (N-N) in addition to echinenone and canthaxanthin. All the oxo-carotenoids are supposed to be formed by the beetles since their food plant lacks them.

Another Chrysomelid, Phytodecta fornicata, feeding exclusively on alfalfa is reported (Ref. 42) to contain echinenone (A-O), 3,4-diketo-ß-carotene(resp. A-N), 3,4,4'-triketo-ß-carotene (resp. N-O), and astacene (resp. N-N), but no canthaxanthin (O-O). The ketones amounted to about 70% of total carotenoids in the beetles. In eggs and larvae, however, only plant carotenoids could be identified.

In the lily beetle, Lilioceris (Crioceris) lilii, studied by Mummery and Valadon (Ref. 43), β,β-carotene (A-A), isocryptoxanthin (A-K), echinenone (A-O), isozeaxanthin (K-K), and canthaxanthin (O-O) were identified. The predominance of echinenone in larvae and of canthaxanthin in adults is suggested to reflect the biogenetic pathway of these pigments.

In preliminary work on lily beetles collected in Southern Germany (Ref. 44) a large percentage of astaxanthin (N-N) as a diester was found in addition to canthaxanthin (O-O). It may well be that different populations or subspecies of insects have different capacities to metabolize carotenoids.

In contrast to the lily beetle the carotenoids of the related species, Crioceris duodecimpunctata, paralleled those of the food plant, asparagus (Ref. 45). No oxo-carotenoids were found. The elytra were only rich in β,β-carotene (A-A). Similarily, in Cassida murraea only β,β-carotene (A-A) and lutein (I-L) have been identified (Refs. 46,47).

As to other beetle families, the presence of unidentified oxo-carotenoids in Tenebrio molitor (Tenebrionidae)(Ref. 23), and of isocryptoxanthin (A-K) and isozeaxanthin (K-K) in a number of water beetles (Dytiscidae)(Ref. 48) has been claimed. The latter report, however, is based only on chromatographic comparison with the carotenoids from the stick insect, Carausius, as falsely identified by Willig (Ref. 13), so they may be the 2-hydroxy isomers (Ref. 14) in truth.

Diptera. Carotenoids of Dipteran insects have been studied in only few cases. The eggs of Chironomus annularius contain β,ε-carotene (A-B), lutein (I-L), cryptoxanthin (A-L), and echinenone (A-O)(Ref. 49), in the larvae β,β-carotene (A-A), canthaxanthin (O-O), and astaxanthin (N-N) resp. astacene were found in addition,but no echinenone (A-O)(Ref. 50).

β,β-Carotene and cryptoxanthin have also been identified in Chironomus larvae by others (Ref. 51). In Pollenia sp. cryptoxanthin was found together with β,β-carotene, lutein, and zeaxanthin (L-L)(Ref. 52). In the house fly, Musca domestica, there is only a very tentative description of "xanthophylls" in the heads (Ref. 53).

The most reliable results concerning Dipteran carotenoids have been recently obtained by Terra and co-workers (Refs. 54,55,56) in their studies on three Rhynchosciara species and mutations affecting carotenoid metabolism.

The major pigments were echinenone (A-O), canthaxanthin (O-O), cryptoxanthin (A-L), and ß,ß-carotene (A-A); isocryptoxanthin (A-K) and 4'-hydroxy-ß,ß-caroten-4-one (K-O) were present in minor amounts. The carotene predominated in the midgut, the other carotenoids were bound to haemolymph proteins. There is a yellow lipoprotein associated with β,β-carotene, cryptoxanthin, and echinenone, and a violet true carotenoprotein (without lipid) that stoichiometrically binds echinenone and canthaxanthin at a 3:1 ratio. The authors propose that β,β-carotene is absorbed from the diet, oxidized in the midgut, and the products are loaded directly onto haemolymph proteins to form the chromoproteins that principally determine the colour of the larvae.

Lepidoptera. The Lepidopteran order is the last large group of insects being reviewed here. As to carotenoid pigments 64 species from 15 families have been looked at up to date. These families were:

Papilionidae: 8 spp. (Refs. 57,58,59,60,61)
Pieridae: 10 spp. (Refs. 21,62,63,64,65,66,67)
Nymphalidae: 5 spp. (Refs. 64,67,68,69)
Lycaenidae: 1 sp. (Ref. 70)
Sphingidae: 7 spp. (Refs. 64,67,71)
Notodontidae: 2 spp. (Refs. 64,67,72,73,74)
Saturniidae: 9 spp. (Refs. 64,67,71,75,76,77,78,79)
Lasiocampidae: 1 sp. (Ref. 67)
Lymantriidae: 4 spp. (Refs. 64,67)
Noctuidae: 6 spp. (Refs. 21,64,80)
Geometridae: 2 spp. (Ref. 64)
Arctiidae: 5 spp. (Ref. 64)
Zygaenidae: 3 spp. (Refs. 64,81)
Tortricidae: 1 sp. (Ref. 21)

Despite the large number of species being studied the results can be easily summarized by saying that in most Lepidoptera the carotenoid composition simply reflects the food usually taken up by the larvae. As most of them feed on green leaves of higher plants β,β-carotene (A-A) and lutein (I-L) are typically encountered as the predominant carotenoids. Epoxy-carotenoids and other leaf carotenoids are frequently established in minor amounts depending probably on type and quality of the food (cf. Ref. 82).
Two types of Lepidoptera may be discerned: one type absorbs β,β-carotene and lutein in roughly equal amounts (e.g. *Pieris brassicae*; Ref. 65), the other type absorbs lutein with a high preference (e.g. *Aglais urticae*; Ref. 68).

Some Papilionid species are the only butterflies (as opposed to moths) containing carotenoids that are not present in the food. Most of this work has been done on *Papilio xuthus* from East Asia initiated by Ohnishi (Ref. 57) and performed in detail by Harashima and co-workers (Refs. 59,60). Apart from β,β-carotene (A-A), β,ε-carotene (A-B), and lutein (I-L) they isolated canthaxanthin (O-O), astaxanthin (N-N), and papilioerythrin (4-ketolutein; I-N) from the orange-type (diapausing) pupae. Similar pigments are reported from *P.protenor demetrius* (Ref. 57). In *P.alcinous* echinenone (A-O) and crustaxanthin (M-M) were identified in addition to canthaxanthin (O-O) and leaf carotenoids (Ref. 61). In a comparative study only *Papilio* species from East Asia were found to contain oxo-carotenoids at all (Ref. 61).
In *P.xuthus* 3'-dehydrolutein (philosamiaxanthin; J-L), too, has been identified (cf. Ref. 60) which had been first reported from a moth, *Philosamia cynthia* (Refs. 75,76) and later from two other species, *Actias selene* and *Cerura vinula* (Ref. 79). This pigment occurs probably in other moths, too (cf. Refs. 76, 67). From *P.xuthus* also papilioerythrinone (J-N) has been isolated (Ref. 60).
Cerura was the first insect from which a carotenoid with an oxygen function at C-2 could be isolated and characterized by all relevant methods: this was ß,ß-carotene-2-ol (A-F)(Ref. 72) later followed by the corresponding 2-one (A-G)(Ref. 74) which is now also confirmed by FD mass spectrometry (Ref. 44). As already shown this type of carotenoid is typical of stick insects. In an other moth, *Phalera bucephala*, as *Cerura* belonging to the Notodontid family, the isomeric cryptoxanthin (A-L) was identified (Refs. 64, 73). This case exemplifies that the same type of carotenoids (not present in the food) may be found in widely different orders and different types of carotenoids within even the same family. Therefore, carotenoids are not considered as useful taxonomic markers in insects.

Hymenoptera. The Hymenoptera have been poorly investigated for carotenoids. In the honey bee, Apis mellifica, these pigments are derived from the collected pollen and hence their composition is very variable. For example, β,β-carotene, lutein (I-L), zeaxanthin (L-L), and mutatochrome have been tentatively identified in heads of bees (Ref. 83). Apanteles glomeratus, which is an endoparasite of the large white butterfly, was found to mirror the host's carotenoids, predominantly β,β-carotene and lutein (Ref. 66).

FATES OF CAROTENOIDS IN INSECTS

Carotenoids, once absorbed in the gut, can be handled along various lines by the insects. These pigments may be conjugated in a reversible way not affecting the carbon skeleton, or new functional groups may be introduced into the preformed C_{40}-compound, or the tetraterpene may be decomposed into smaller units.

Reversible modifications

The type of reversible modifications of carotenoids includes the formation of carotenoproteins and of carotenoid esters. Complexing of a carotenoid to a protein or lipoprotein to render these pigments watersoluble is frequently observed in integument and haemolymph (Refs. 7,11,51,55,56,75,80,84). So far the best studied insect carotenoproteins are those from the moth, Philosamia (Ref. 75), and the fly, Rhynchosciara (Ref. 55,56). Hydroxy carotenoids may be easily esterified with long-chain fatty acids as preferably observed in the fat body (Refs. 14,16,59,65,68,85). Detailed work has been performed on the diesters and isomeric mono-esters of lutein from Aglais and Pieris (Refs. 68,85). In both species polyunsaturated fatty acids predominated in the esters as revealed by mass spectrometry. The same holds for the ester of a 2-hydroxy carotenoid from Carausius (Ref. 16).

Modifications of the carbon skeleton

A carotenoid which is found in an insect but not in its food is generally presumed to be produced in the insect by a transformation of a diet-derived C_{40}-precursor. The situation of microbial symbionts has already been considered and cannot be treated more in this chapter. Most modifications by insects, as obvious so far, refer to introductions of hydroxyl- and/or oxo-groups at various positions of a β-end ring.

Oxygen function at C-4 or C-(3+4). β,β-Type carotenoids with 4-hydroxy-, 4-oxo-, and/or 3-hydroxy-4-oxo-end rings (isocryptoxanthin→astaxanthin series) are typical animal pigments which in insects are preferentially found in locusts, Chrysomelid beetles, many aphids, in some midges and Papilionid butterflies. This type has not been encountered in Phasmids (stick insects) and Hymenoptera so far. As to β,ε-type carotenoids papilioerythrin (I-N) and its 3'-dehydro derivative, papilioerythrinone (J-N), have been isolated from a Papilionid.

Oxygen function at C-3. This refers to cryptoxanthin (A-L), possibly also to zeaxanthin (L-L). Cryptoxanthin has been found in some Lepidoptera, aphids, Diptera, and in a locust but not yet in Coleoptera and Phasmida. The occurrence of philosamiaxanthin (3'-dehydrolutein; J-L) appears to be restricted to a number of moth species.

Oxygen function at C-2. This group of carotenoids is typical for stick insects (Phasmida) where β,β-type and β,ε-type carotenoids with 2-hydroxy-, 2-oxo-, and 3,4-didehydro-2-oxo-β-end rings are present in various combinations. Outside the Phasmid order β,β-caroten-2-ol (A-F) and β,β-caroten-2-one (A-G) are known from a single moth species, Cerura.

Other type C_{40}-carotenoids. The series of acyclic, mono-cyclic, and γ-ring (C) carotenoids, identified in Hemiptera (bugs and aphids) and in Coccinellid beetles feeding on aphids, are most probably synthesized de novo by microbial symbionts associated with many Hemipteran insects as discussed above. These pigments will therefore not be considered further. The contribution to carotenoid biogenesis, if any, by these insects remains to be clarified.

Degradation to smaller compounds

The most important degradation product of β,β-carotene (and possibly also of other carotenoids) is the C_{20}-compound retinal$_1$ (I in Fig. 2) which serves as the light absorbing prosthetic group in all insect visual pigments being studied (Ref. 86).

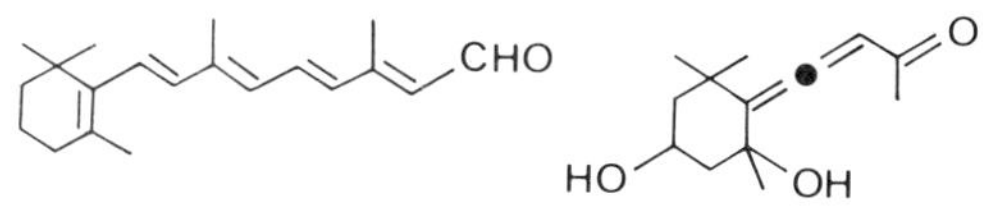

I II

Fig. 2 Compounds derived from carotenoids in insects.

A sesquiterpenoid ($C_{13}H_{20}O_3$) has been isolated from the defence secretion of the grasshopper, *Romalea microptera* (Ref. 87). The compound (II in Fig. 2) proved to be a conjugated allenic ketone and therefore is suggested to derive from dietary neoxanthin (or fucoxanthin).

TRANSFORMATIONS OF CAROTENOIDS IN INSECTS

Evidence for transformations

The carotenoids considered before are obviously produced from dietary precursors by the insects themselves. However, direct evidence for the presumed transformations has been achieved in only few cases studied in our laboratory. So, it has been unequivocally demonstrated that $[^{14}C]$β,β-carotene is incorporated into β,β-caroten-2-ol (A-F) by *Cerura* (Ref. 73), into β,β-caroten-3-ol (A-L) by the related moth, *Phalera* (Ref. 73), and into a series of β,β-type carotenoids with 2-hydroxy- (F), 2-oxo- (G), and 3,4-didehydro-2-oxo-rings (H) by the stick insects, *Carausius* (Ref. 88) and *Ectatosoma* (Ref. 18).
A more indirect demonstration is the formation of astaxanthin (N-N) at the expense of β,β-carotene (A-A) during egg development in locusts as shown by Goodwin (Ref. 8). That was the first study related to this problem.
A similar approach has recently been used to analyze carotenoid interconversions in eggs of a stick insect (Ref. 89) to be discussed later in this chapter.

Presumed metabolic pathways

Transformation of β,β-carotene to 4-oxo carotenoids. As to the presumed oxidation of β,β-carotene to canthaxanthin (O-O) and astaxanthin (N-N) in insects possible pathways have been suggested by a number of authors (Refs. 38,42,43,59). All follow the same obvious pattern which has also been proposed for similar transformations in crustacea, vertebrates, and others (cf. Ref. 90). According to this scheme (Fig. 3) hydroxyls are introduced at C-4 of one or both β-end rings and then oxidized to oxo-groups to form echinenone (A-O) and canthaxanthin (O-O). In the biogenesis of astaxanthin (N-N) hydroxylation at C-3 may proceed either before or after the oxidation of the 4-hydroxyls to the 4-ones. Obviously, hydroxylation at C-4 requires an unmodified end ring since zeaxanthin (L-L) is seemingly not involved in the biogenesis of astaxanthin in insects. As deduced from the presence or absence of possible intermediates the sequence of steps (cf. Fig. 3) may vary among the species and proceed symmetrically or not. In those cases where only oxo-carotenoids have been reported (Refs. 38,40,59) the hydroxylated pigments may have escaped detection or occur short-lived within the enzyme complex (cf. Ref. 91). Up to date, there is no experimental support for this pathway in insects by feeding them a radiolabelled precursor or a pure cold compound on a synthetic diet. This contrasts to the situation in fish (e.g. Refs. 92,93) and crustacea (e.g. Refs. 94,95).

Transformation of lutein to astaxanthin and papilioerythrinone. Dietary lutein has been proposed as a precursor for 3'-dehydrolutein (philosamiaxanthin; J-L)(Refs. 76,79) and papilioerythrin (4-ketolutein; I-N)(Ref. 59) as outlined in Fig. 4. Papilioerythrinone (J-N) could be formed by introduction of a 4-oxo group into philosamiaxanthin or by allylic oxidation of papilioerythrin (Ref. 60). Astaxanthin (N-N) in *Papilio* may be derived (Ref. 59) either from canthaxanthin (O-O) and hence from β,β-carotene, or from papilioerythrin *via* an isomerization of the ε-end ring to a β-ring (β-doradexanthin), or from both possible precursors (Fig. 4).

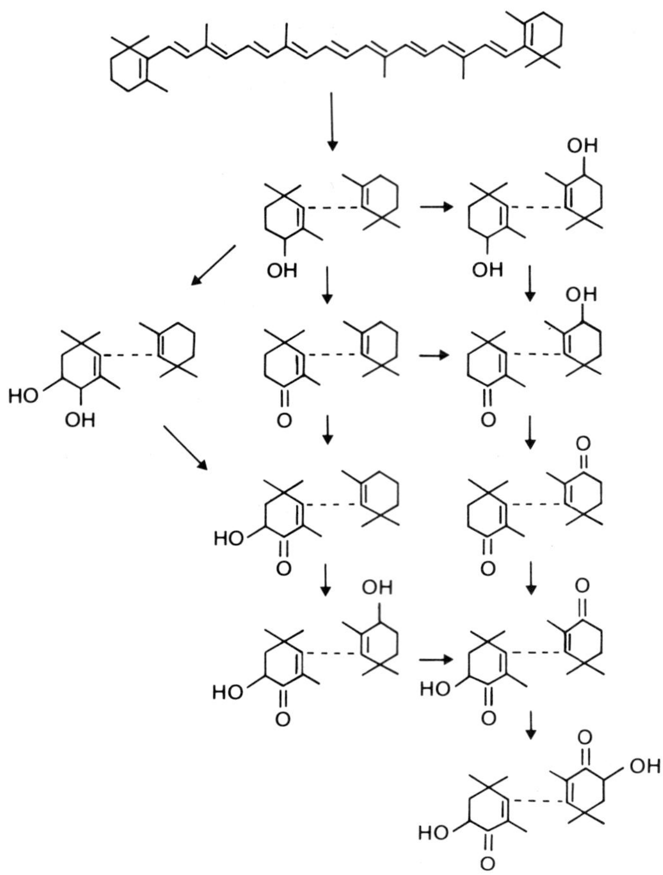

Fig. 3 Proposed metabolic pathways from ß-carotene to astaxanthin in insects.

The presumed pathways starting from dietary lutein are highly interesting in the light of recent information on the absolute configuration of the carotenoids involved.
The proposed conversion of lutein(I-L) into astaxanthin (N-N) by goldfishes (Ref. 96) had been rejected on stereochemical grounds (Ref. 97) until recently goldfish "lutein" was shown to be pure 3'-epilutein (3R,3'S,6'R) by Eugster's group (Ref. 98). Furthermore, α-doradexanthin (I-N) from goldfishes (Ref. 96) proved to be a derivative of 3'-epilutein (Ref. 98) making acceptable its transformation into (3S,3'S)-astaxanthin (Ref. 98). The transformation of radiolabelled lutein to astaxanthin *via* α-doradexanthin (I-N) and β-doradexanthin (L-N) by goldfishes has already been demonstrated (Ref. 92).
Whether this pathway operates in *Papilio*, too, is completely open since the chirality of the carotenoids involved has not been studied up to date. Therefore, the claimed identity of papilioerythrin with α-doradexanthin (Ref. 59) has yet to be demonstrated.

Considering astaxanthin formation generally the recent finding (Refs. 99, 100,101) that astaxanthin from various animal sources occurs as a mixture of both enantiomers and the *meso*-compound is of prominent importance for biogenetic considerations and should stimulate similar work in the insect field.

The structure of 3-hydroxy-β,ε-caroten-3'-one (J-L) has been assigned to a carotenoid from various moths and termed "3'-dehydrolutein". However, its chiral identity with 3',O-didehydrolutein which displays (3R,6'R)-configu-

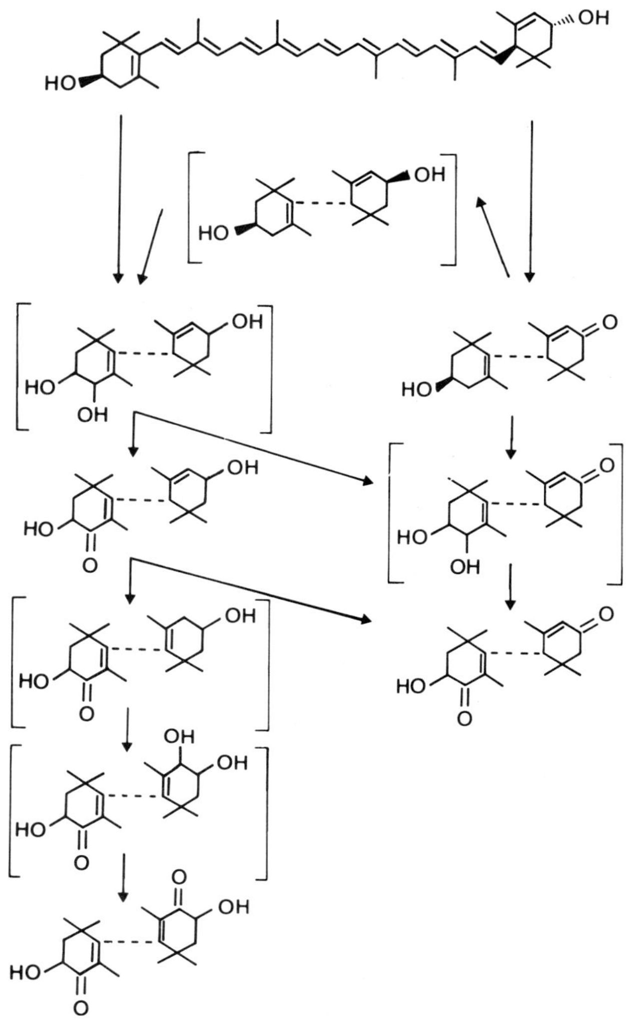

Fig. 4 Possible transformation of plant lutein into 3'-epilutein, papilioerythrinone, and astaxanthin in insects. Compounds in brackets have not yet been reported from insects.

ration (Refs. 98,102) remains to be established. In these insects it would be highly interesting to study the chirality of the "lutein". It may well be to find 3'-epilutein or a mixture of this epilutein and lutein since epimerization could be achieved via the 3'-one (3'-dehydrolutein) in these species (Fig. 4). Such a reversible process may provide a redox system which could be of physiological interest.

Transformation of β,β-carotene to 2-oxo carotenoids. Let us turn back to β,β-carotene the incorporation of which into carotenoids with 2-hydroxy and/or 2-oxo groups has been shown in stick insects (Refs. 18,88) and in a moth (Ref. 73). As to the metabolic pathway underlying these transformations the hypothesis has been offered (Refs. 16,18, 74) that the hydroxy carotenoids are derived from the corresponding ketones rather than synthesized directly. According to this proposed scheme (Fig. 5) β,β-carotene-2,2'-dione (G-G) should be at a central position since it can both be reduced to the 2,2'-diol (F-F) and also be oxidized to 3,4,3',4'-tetradehydro-2,2'-dione (H-H). These two products are in fact the predominant carotenoids in stick insects (Ref. 19).
In order to confirm this hypothetical pathway a kinetic study was performed on the incorporation of radiolabel from β,β-carotene into the various

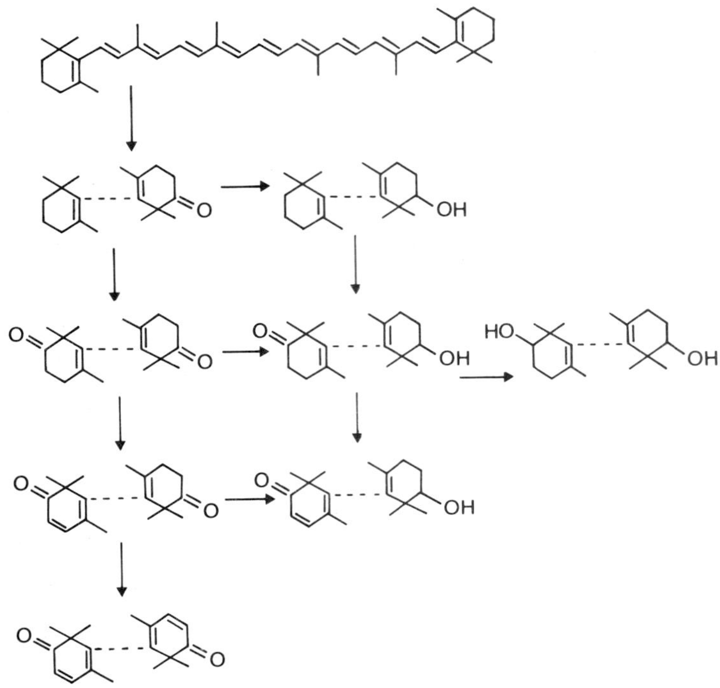

Fig. 5 Hypothetical scheme for the transformation of ß-carotene into 2-oxo and 2-hydroxy carotenoids in stick insects. (From Ref. 16)

β,β-type carotenoids in Carausius (Ref. 88). However, this experiment provided no direct support either for the hypothetical "reversed" pathway or for the commonly accepted hydroxy→oxo-scheme. Not even a monohydroxy→dihydroxy-sequence could be derived from this study.
Comparative studies (Refs. 18,19) had revealed that Ectatosoma would be more favourable for those aims. So, we decided to follow carotenoid changes during embryonic development in this stick insect because the egg provided a closed system (except for gas exchange) not dependent on exogenous carotenoid supply. The results of one study consistent with further five series (Ref. 89) are presented in Fig. 6. The most striking features of carotenoid metabolism during egg development in Ectatosoma were the following:

- there was no oxidation of β,β-carotene as observed in locust eggs but rather interconversions of the various carotene metabolites.
- carotenoid transformations started with embryonic development; in non-developing eggs the carotenoid pattern remained unchanged.
- in the beginning the major carotenoids were β,β-caroten-2-ol (A-F) and β,β-carotene-2,2'-dione (G-G) which decreased during development as did 2'-hydroxy-β,β-caroten-2-one (F-G).
- increasing carotenoids were β,β-carotene-2,2'-diol (F-F), 3,4,3',4'-tetradehydro-β,β-carotene-2,2'-dione (H-H), and 2'-hydroxy-3,4-didehydro-β,β-caroten-2-one (F-H).

It is evident from these results that the 2-ol is converted into the 2,2'-diol and that the 2,2'-dione is a precursor of the tetradehydro-dione. However, this does not discriminate between the two metabolic pathways under consideration. The obvious result that the diol is not converted to the diones might be even in favour of the "reversed" pathway (Fig. 5).

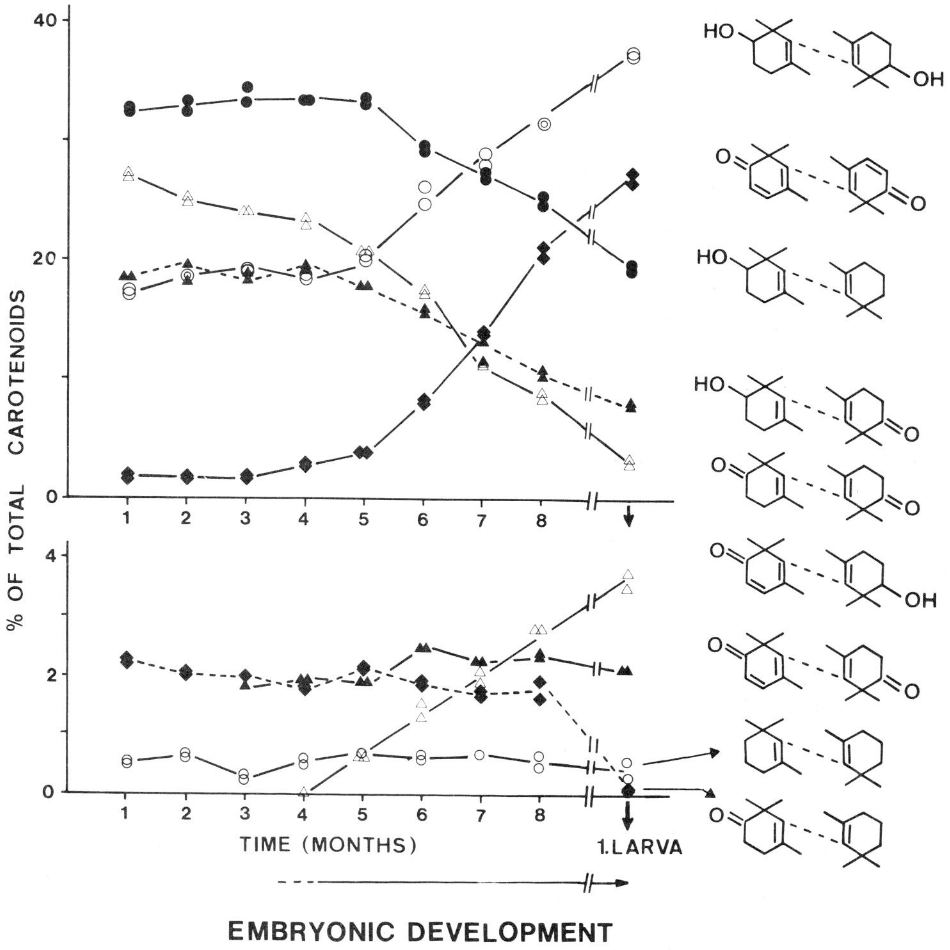

Fig. 6 Changes in the carotenoid composition during embryonic development in Ectatosoma tiaratum (stick insect). 1.Larva: newly hatched first instar larva. Duplicate measurements from one series (out of five; Ref. 89).

Stereochemistry of 2-hydroxy carotenoids from insects

Stereochemical aspects are of decisive importance in considering biogenetic pathways. The work on the absolute configuration of β,β-type 2-hydroxy carotenoids from the stick insect, Ectatosoma, and the moth, Cerura, was performed as a joint project with Liaaen-Jensen's group and G. Borch. This is the first study dealing with the chirality of insect carotenoids. The results (Ref. 103) are compiled in Table 1.

TABLE 1. Enantiomeric composition of 2-hydroxy carotenoids.

Source	Carotenoid (β,β-type)	S/R ratio†	Number of different lots examined	Methods
Cerura sp.	2-ol	77-68% S	3	CD, ^{1}H-NMR
Ectatosoma sp.	2-ol	61-34% S	3	CD
"	2'-hydroxy-2-one	37-36% S	2	CD
"	2,2'-diol	77-33% S	3	CD, ^{1}H-NMR

† accuracy ± 10 rel. %

All 2-hydroxy carotenoids examined from the two insect sources proved to be partly racemic according to their CD spectra. In the Ectatosoma pigments there was no preferred configuration in contrast to the Cerura 2-ol which displayed 2S dominance with a rather constant proportion in all lots studied. In the latter carotenoid and in the 2,2'-diol from Ectatosoma the CD results were confirmed by a ^{1}H-NMR method developed by K. Aareskjold and S. Liaaen--Jensen (Ref. 104).

The demonstration of having partly racemic 2-hydroxy carotenoids fits the proposed pathway in stick insects and Cerura: the most obvious explanation is that these caroten-2-ols are derived from the corresponding 2-ones by a reduction process lacking stereospecificity. The variable degree of racemization may depend on the enzyme's microenvironment that may change with the physiological status.This type of reduction is shown in Fig. 7A.

However, there is still another interpretation for the occurrence of partly racemic carotenoids which circumvents the problems inherent in a direct introduction of oxo-groups. According to this hypothesis (Fig. 7B) the carotene is oxidized by a direct hydroxylation mechanism providing an optically pure 2-hydroxy carotenoid but this may be now epimerized via the 2-one. (Figure 7B shows the sequence of reactions for the two enantiomers of the 2-ol only one of which should be formed by the hydroxylation mechanism.)

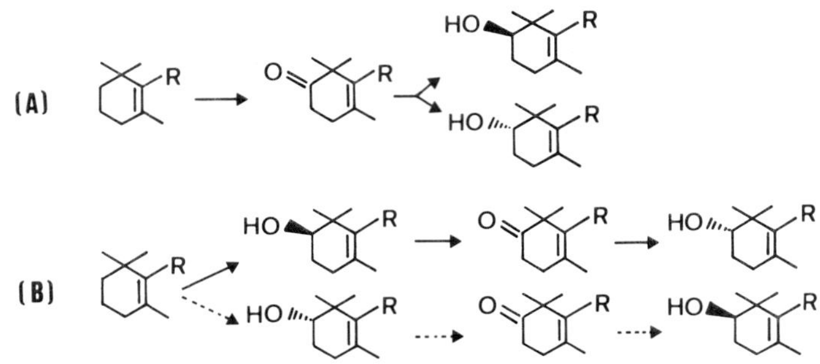

Fig. 7 Two explanations for the occurrence of partly racemic caroten-2-ols.
(A) non-stereoselective reduction of 2-one(cf. Fig. 5)
(B) epimerization of a 2-ol via 2-one (cf. Fig. 8)

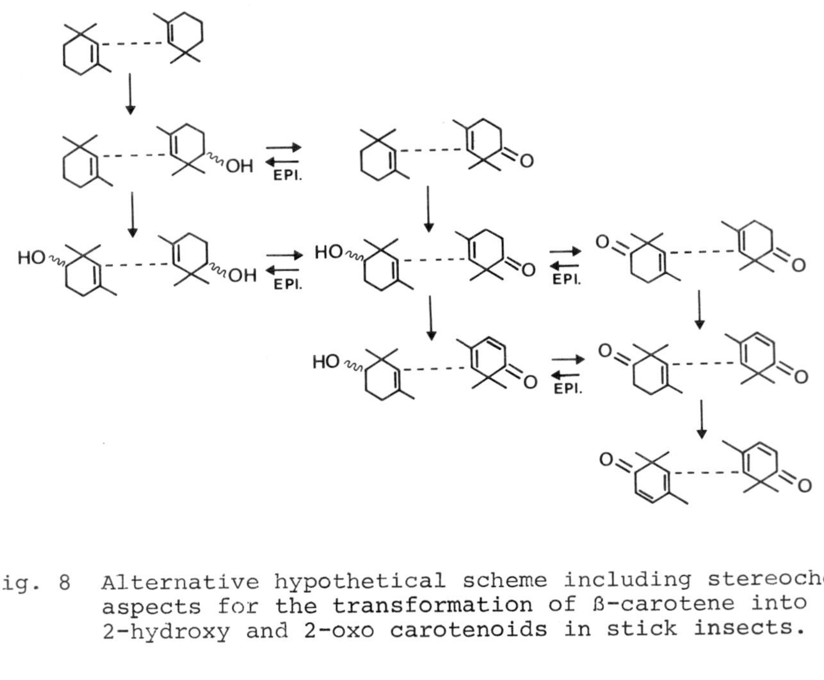

Fig. 8 Alternative hypothetical scheme including stereochemical aspects for the transformation of ß-carotene into 2-hydroxy and 2-oxo carotenoids in stick insects.

Based on this principle another carotenoid pathway is now offered (Fig. 8) for the biogenesis of 2-hydroxy carotenoids in stick insects and in the moth, Cerura (which forms only the 2-ol and 2-one). This scheme is a combination of the commonly accepted hydroxy→oxo-sequence and the "reversed" pathway (cf. Fig. 5): the important point is that the 2*S* and 2*R* enantiomers result from two different enzymatic mechanisms.
The formation of β,ε-caroten-2-ol and β,ε-caroten-2-one from dietary β,ε-carotene is thought to follow this novel scheme, too.
Further studies on the chirality of the 2-hydroxy carotenoids from insects are expected to lend support to this stereochemical aspect of insect carotenoid metabolism.
An analogous reaction sequence has already been proposed for the presumed 3'-epimerization of lutein *via* 3'-dehydrolutein (cf. Fig. 4).

Enzymic aspects

Carotenoid transformation in stick insects appears to be a complex network involving ten different metabolites but only three different modified β-end rings (2-hydroxy; 2-oxo; 3,4-didehydro-2-oxo). If one includes stereochemical differences a maximum of even sixteen different carotenoids is expected. In considering this situation it seems convenient to apply the "half-molecule substrate" hypothesis for carotenoid biosynthesis in plants (Refs. 105,106) to carotenoid metabolism in animals. Then the picture at least in stick insects becomes simpler and more rational: not more than four different enzymes are required to produce the many combinations of end rings as observed. The two end rings of a carotenoid would be metabolized independently because each enzyme would accept only one end ring as a substrate at a time. In insects (except Papilio) the enzymes involved in carotenoid transformations should be specific for β-end rings since ε-rings are not modified as we know so far.

The half molecule model could also hold for the transformation of β,β-carotene to astaxanthin and of lutein to the set of related carotenoids. One might speculate that this type of enzymic recognition is unique both to later reactions of carotenoid biosynthesis and transformations of preformed carotenoids.

FINAL CONSIDERATIONS AND SUGGESTIONS

As compared to crustacea being another arthropod class, in insects the capacity to transform dietary carotenoids is far less common. On the other hand the diversity of metabolic reactions of carotenoids is seemingly greater. Both may be due to the fact that the insects represent the most evolved group of arthropods.

There are great differences in distribution and structural types of carotenoids in insects not only between different orders but also within much lower taxons. The consequence is that carotenoids cannot successfully be used as chemosystematic markers in insects.

Further studies on insect carotenoids should concentrate on the following aspects:

- the carotenoids from selected insects known for special feeding habits or for symbiosis
- the contribution of microbial symbionts to carotenoid biogenesis and transformation in insects associated with them
- the biochemistry of carotenoid transformations using enzyme extracts
- the stereochemistry of insect carotenoids since considering the chirality of a compound is essential in determining the enzymic mechanism of its biogenesis.

Especially in this last point the study of insect carotenoids seems to contribute interesting aspects of carotenoid transformations in animals.

Acknowledgements - The work in the author's laboratory has received financial support from the Deutsche Forschungsgemeinschaft.
I acknowledge the collaboration in the stereochemical field of Prof. Liaaen-Jensen, K. Aareskjold and G. Borch. Furthermore, I am grateful to F. Hoffmann-La Roche, Basel, for generous gifts of carotenoids both labelled and unlabelled.

REFERENCES

1. S. Liaaen-Jensen, Pure Appl. Chem. 47, 129-145 (1976).
2. B.C.L. Weedon, Pure Appl. Chem. 51, 435-445 (1979).
3. J. Feltwell, in J.B. Harborne: Biochemical Aspects of Plant and Animal Coevolution, Academic Press, London (1978), pp. 277-307.
4. T.W. Goodwin, The Comparative Biochemistry of the Carotenoids, Chapman and Hall, London (1952).
5. T.W. Goodwin and S. Srisukh, Nature 161, 525-526 (1948).
6. T.W. Goodwin and S, Srisukh, Proc. Int. Congr. Biochem. 1, Cambridge (1949), p. 65.
7. T.W. Goodwin and S. Srisukh, Biochem. J. 45, 263-267 (1949).
8. T.W. Goodwin, Biochem. J. 45, 472-479 (1949).
9. T.W. Goodwin and S. Srisukh, Biochem. J. 48, 199-203 (1951).
10. M. Rothschild, B. Gardiner, R. Mummery and G. Valadon, J. Zool., Lond. 181, 475-494 (1977).
11. S. Okay, Bull. Soc. Zool. France 74, 11-15 (1949).
12. K.H. Weisgraber, R.J.J.C. Lousberg and U. Weiss, Experientia 27, 1017-1018 (1971).
13. A. Willig, J. Insect Physiol. 15, 1907-1927 (1969).
14. H. Kayser, Z. Naturforsch. 31c, 646-651 (1976).
15. H. Kjøsen, N. Arpin and S. Liaaen-Jensen, Acta Chem Scand. 26, 3053-3067 (1972).
16. H. Kayser, Z. Naturforsch. 32c, 327-336 (1977).
17. K. Aareskjold and S. Liaaen-Jensen, Proc. 5th Int. Symposium on Carotenoids, Madison (1978), p. 1.
18. H. Kayser, Z. Naturforsch., in press.
19. H. Kayser, Comp. Biochem. Physiol., to be published.
20. E. Lederer, C. R. Séanc. Soc. Biol. Filiales Ass. 117, 413-416 (1934).
21. R.H. Hackman, Arch. Biochem. Biophys. 41, 166-174 (1952).
22. V. Tamas, V. Ciurdaru, K.L. Simpson and T. Perju, Stud. Cercet. Biochim. 20, 197-201 (1977).
23. K.H. Trautmann and H. Thommen, quoted by H. Thommen, in O. Isler: Carotenoids, Birkhäuser, Basel (1971), p. 658.
24. H.J. Banks and D.W. Cameron, Insect Biochem. 3, 139-162 (1973).
25. J. Seuge and M. Vuillaume, C. R. Soc. Biol. France 164, 525-527 (1970).
26. A.G. Andrewes, H. Kjøsen, S. Liaaen-Jensen, K.H. Weisgraber, R.J.J.C. Lousberg and U. Weiss, Acta Chem. Scand, 25, 3878-3880 (1971).
27. A. Koch, in S.M. Henry: Symbiosis, Vol. 2, Academic Press, New York (1967).
28. T.W. Goodwin, The Biochemistry of the Carotenoids, 2nd edition, Vol. 1, Chapman and Hall, London (1980).
29. B. Czeczuga, Zool. Pol. 24, 5-10 (1974).
30. B. Czeczuga, Zool. Pol. 25, 27-46 (1976).
31. L.R.G. Valadon and R. Mummery, Comp. Biochem. Physiol. 46B, 427-434 (1973).
32. G. Britton, W.J.S. Lockley, G.A. Harriman and T.W. Goodwin, Nature 266, 49-50 (1977).
33. G. Britton, T.W. Goodwin, G.E. Harriman and W.J.S. Lockley, Insect Biochem. 7, 337-345 (1977).
34. E. Lederer, Bull. Soc. Chim. Biol. 20, 567-610 (1938).
35. L.R.G. Valadon and R. Mummery, Comp. Biochem. Physiol. 46B, 427-434 (1973).
36. V. Tamas, V. Ciurdaru, K.L. Simpson and T. Perju, Stud. Cercet. Biochim. 21, 95-97 (1978).
37. L. Merlini and G. Cardillo, Gazz. Chim. Ital. 93, 949-952 (1963).
38. F. Leuenberger and H. Thommen, J. Insect Physiol. 16, 1855-1858 (1970).
39. B. Czeczuga, J. Insect Physiol. 17, 2017-2025 (1971).
40. F.-C. Czygan, Z. Pflanzenphysiol. 67, 33-42 (1972).
41. J.M. Poff, Thesis, Utah State Univ. (1977).
42. V. Tamas, V. Ciurdaru and T. Perju, Stud. Cercet. Biochim. 19, 209-214 (1976).
43. R. Mummery and L.R.G. Valadon, J. Insect Physiol. 20, 429-433 (1974).
44. H. Kayser, unpublished results.
45. V. Tamas and T. Perju, Stud. Cercet. Biochim. 19, 121-123 (1976).
46. G. Turian, Mitt. Schweiz. Ent. Ges. 25, 47-48 (1952).
47. G. Turian, Mitt. Schweiz. Ent. Ges. 33, 83-87 (1960).
48. K. Dettner and B. Hopstätter, Ent. Zeitschrift 90, 225-232 (1980).
49. B. Czeczuga and R. Czerpak, Experientia 25, 1037-1038 (1969).
50. B. Czeczuga, Hydrobiol. 36, 353-360 (1970).
51. J. Gross and P. Budowski, Biochem. J. 101, 747-754 (1966).
52. J. Feltwell et al., quoted in Ref. 3.

53. J.J. Wolken, J.M. Bowness and I.J. Scheer, Biochim. Biophys. Acta 43, 531-537 (1960).
54. W.R. Terra, A.G. de Bianchi, M. Paes de Mello and R. Basile, Experientia 32, 432-434 (1976).
55. W.R. Terra, C. Ferreira and A.G. de Bianchi, Comp. Biochem. Physiol. 66B, 491-497 (1980).
56. W.R. Terra, C. Ferreira, A.G. de Bianchi and K. Zinner, Comp. Biochem. Physiol. 68B, 89-93 (1981).
57. E. Ohnishi, J. Insect Physiol. 3, 132-145 (1959).
58. S.M. Oldroyd, Entomologist 104, 111-123 (1971).
59. K. Harashima, T. Ohno, T. Sawachika, T. Hidaka and E. Ohnishi, Insect Biochem. 2, 29-48 (1972).
60. K. Harashima, J. Nakahara and G. Kato, Agr. Biol. Chem. 40, 711-717 (1976).
61. L.R.G. Valadon and R.S. Mummery, Comp. Biochem. Physiol. 61B, 371-374 (1978).
62. T. Ohtaki and E. Ohnishi, J. Insect Physiol. 13, 1569-1574 (1967).
63. J.S.E. Feltwell and L.R.G. Valadon, J. Insect Physiol. 18, 2203-2215 (1972).
64. J. Feltwell and M. Rothschild, J. Zool., Lond. 174, 441-465 (1974).
65. H. Kayser, J. Insect Physiol. 20, 89-103 (1974).
66. M. Rothschild, G. Valadon and R. Mummery, J. Zool., Lond. 181, 323-339 (1977).
67. H. Nagel, Thesis, Univ. Giessen (1970).
68. H. Kayser, Z. Naturforsch. 30c, 369-378 (1975).
69. M. Rothschild, B. Gardiner and R. Mummery, J. Zool., Lond. 186, 351-358 (1978).
70. J. Feltwell and L.R.G. Valadon, Nature 225, 969 (1970).
71. R. Mummery, L.R.G. Valadon and M. Rothschild, Physiol. Entomol. 1, 51-54 (1976).
72. H. Kayser, Z. Naturforsch. 31c, 121-128 (1976).
73. H. Kayser, Comp. Biochem. Physiol. 58B, 177-181 (1977).
74. H. Kayser, Z. Naturforsch. 34c, 483-484 (1979).
75. H. Chino, S. Murakami and K. Harashima, Biochim. Biophys. Acta 176, 1-26 (1969).
76. K. Harashima, Int. J. Biochem. 1, 523-531 (1970).
77. R.S. Mummery, M. Rothschild and L.R.G. Valadon, Comp. Biochem. Physiol. 50B, 23-28 (1975).
78. G. Valadon, R. Mummery and M. Rothschild, J. Ent. (A) 50, 169-173 (1975).
79. H. Kayser, J. Comp. Physiol. 104, 27-31 (1975).
80. T.W. Goodwin, Biochem. J. 55, 834-838 (1953).
81. T. Bornefeld and F.-C. Czygan, Z. Naturforsch. 30c, 298-299 (1975).
82. J.S.E. Feltwell and L.R.G. Valadon, J. agric. Sci., Camb. 83, 19-26 (1974).
83. T.H. Goldsmith and L.T. Warner, J. Gen. Physiol. 47, 433-441 (1964).
84. L.P.S. van der Geest, J. Insect Physiol. 14, 537-542 (1968).
85. H. Kayser, Insect Biochem. 5, 861-875 (1975).
86. R.H. White, Adv. Insect Physiol. 13, 35-67 (1978).
87. J. Meinwald, K. Erickson, M. Hartshorn, Y.C. Meinwald and T. Eisner, Tetrahedron Letters 1968, 2959-2962.
88. H. Kayser, Z. Naturforsch., to be published.
89. H. Kayser and B. Dursch, in preparation.
90. H. Thommen, in O. Isler: Carotenoids, Birkhäuser, Basel (1971), pp. 637-668.
91. B.H. Davies, W.-J. Hsu and C.O. Chichester, Comp. Biochem. Physiol. 33, 601-615 (1970).
92. W.-J. Hsu, D.B. Rodriguez and C.O. Chichester, Int. J. Biochem. 3, 333-338 (1972).
93. T. Katayama, T. Miyahara, M. Shimaya and C.O. Chichester, Int. J. Biochem. 3, 569-572 (1972).
94. T. Katayama, Y. Kunisaki, M. Shimaya, K.L. Simpson and C.O. Chichester, Comp. Biochem. Physiol. 46B, 269-272 (1973).
95. T. Katayama, M. Shimaya, M. Sameshima and C.O. Chichester, Int. J. Biochem. 4, 223-226 (1973).
96. T. Katayama, H. Yokoyama and C.O. Chichester, Int. J. Biochem. 1, 438-444 (1970).
97. A.G. Andrewes, G. Borch, S. Liaaen-Jensen and G. Snatzke, Acta Chem. Scand. B28, 730-736 (1974).
98. R. Buchecker, C.H. Eugster and A. Weber, Helv. Chim. Acta 61, 1962-1968 (1978).

99. H. Rønneberg, B. Renstrøm, K. Aareskjold, S. Liaaen-Jensen, M. Vecchi, F.J. Leuenberger, R.K. Müller and H. Mayer, Helv. Chim. Acta 63, 711-715 (1980).
100. K. Schiedt, F.J. Leuenberger and M. Vecchi, Helv. Chim. Acta 64, 449-457 (1981).
101. K. Aareskjold, B. Renstrøm, G. Borch and S. Liaaen-Jensen, Proc. 6th Int. Symposium on Carotenoids, Liverpool (1981).
102. R. Buchecker and C.H. Eugster, Helv. Chim. Acta 62, 2817-2824 (1979).
103. H. Kayser, K. Aareskjold, G. Borch and S. Liaaen-Jensen, Insect Biochem., to be published.
104. K. Aareskjold and S. Liaaen-Jensen, Acta Chem. Scand., to be published.
105. J.C.B. McDermott, D.J. Brown, G. Britton and T.W. Goodwin, Biochem. J. 144, 231-243 (1974).
106. G. Britton, Pure Appl. Chem. 47, 223-236 (1976).

GENERAL SURVEY OF THE CAROTENOIDS IN CRUSTACEA

René Castillo, Geneviève Nègre-Sadargues and Roland Lenel

Centre de Physiologie des Invertébrés, Université des Sciences et Techniques du Languedoc, Place E. Bataillon, 34060 Montpellier Cedex (France)

Abstract - Carotenoids are widely represented in crustaceans ; the list of these pigments is enhanced by the detection of new structures. Crustaceans cannot synthesize carotenoids "*de novo*" but they are able to transform these substances into endogenous forms. β-Carotene appears as the most common precursor in the different metabolic pathways; however other carotenoids are supposed to play such a role. The metabolism of carotenoids in Crustacea is closely related to environmental factors, food in particular. Controlled feeding experiments using labelled pigments have permitted the metabolic schemes as well as the different intermediates involved to be determined. Physiological cycles like molting and vitellogenesis and the metabolic alterations induced by parasitic infections are found to affect the metabolism of carotenoids in these animals. Several possible functions of carotenoids in Crustacea are discussed.

INTRODUCTION

Our purpose is not to provide a broad review of carotenoids in Crustacea but to draw a clear and coherent survey of almost all that is already established in this field. As far as we know the first data on the occurrence of carotenoids in Crustacea are those reported by Pouchet (1) in 1872 concerning some changes on the color of lobsters. Since then, a large number of investigations on various other species have been carried out. For this reason it is not possible to mention all the studies concerning this subject.
The class of crustaceans includes a wide variety of forms like crabs, lobsters, shrimps, prawns, barnacles, woodlice, etc... Some groups are strictly marine like stomatopods, cirripeds, euphausiids, etc... Others, although predominantly marine, have a more diversified range of occurrence; amphipods, copepods, decapods and ostracods have brackish and fresh water species as well as terrestrial and semiterrestrial ones.

BIOLOGICAL CONSIDERATIONS

One of the most common features of crustaceans is the presence of an all enveloping exoskeleton that varies from a thin flexible membrane in copepods and cirripeds to a thick hard shell in most decapods. This circumstance implies that crustaceans must leave their exoskeleton periodically, that is what permits the growth. Hence the process of molting is the most common and important metabolic event in these animals. The term "molting" means all the process of preparation of the animal when leaving its old cuticle at ecdysis.
The ecdysis may be taken as the starting point of the intermolt cycle, the stages being the number of days from this event. The following scheme (fig*) based on the classification outlined for brachyurans (2) and adapted for other crustaceans (3) allows us to visualize this phenomenon.

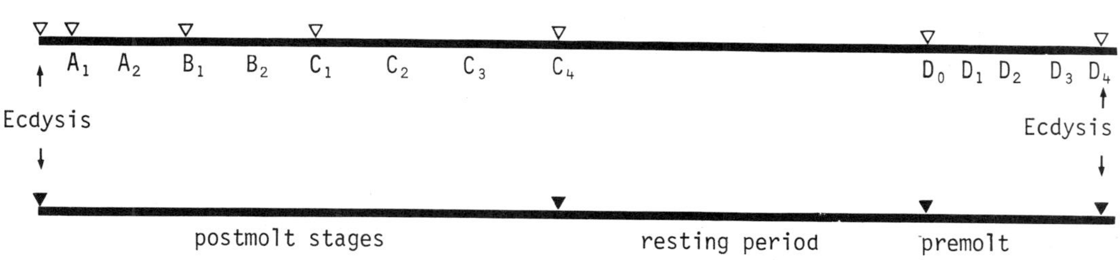

* Figure

Basically crustaceans are never free from molting. Vitellogenesis, carrying of developing eggs and hibernation are the only interruptions in the periodicity of molts. However, in certain species molting stops when the animal reaches a limit of size, whereas in others this process continues but its frequency diminishes in senescent individuals.

NATURE AND CLASSIFICATION

The choice of analytical methods permitting the determination of the nature of the carotenoids in crustaceans often depends on the quantities of pigment available and on its chemical stability. Often only a few traces of pigment can be isolated. In general, esterified forms are more readily extracted than unesterified ones, however the use of more accurate spectroscopic methods permitting the identification is often hindered by the esterified condition, since oxidative alterations and isomerizations may result during saponification and purification attempts.
The carotenoids of Crustacea are basically C_{40} structures with β- and ε- cyclic end groups. The location of hydroxyls, ketones and/or hydroxy-keto substituents in one or both of the terminal rings determines the main different forms which have been observed in these animals. Many other carotenoids represented by new structural types have been proposed and isolated in several cases.

Classification

The carotenoids of crustaceans may be sorted into three main groups : esterified carotenoids, unesterified forms and protein complexes.
The esterified forms generally considered as the more active structures in carotenoid metabolism are present in almost all organs and tissues.
The protein complexes contribute to a wide variety of colorations. The carotenoid represents the prosthetic group ; the link between carotenoid and protein gives to the compound a water-soluble character. The non enolized ketonic substituents of astaxanthin and canthaxanthin allow the formation of conjugated bonds with terminal protein amino groups ; echinenone was found to form a chitin-bound complex (4).
The red carotenovitellin of the crab *Cancer pagurus* is a mixture of all the carotenoids occurring in the eggs (5).
The unesterified forms have also been found to occur in the organs and tissues of most crustaceans.
Crustaceans generally contain the same major carotenoids, these are :

- β-carotene (β,β-carotene)
- astaxanthin (3,3'-dihydroxy-β,β-carotene-4,4'-dione)
- echinenone (β,β-caroten —4-one)
- canthaxanthin (β,β-carotene-4,4'-dione)
- phoenicoxanthin (3-hydroxy-β,β-carotene-4,4'-dione)
- cryptoxanthin (β,β-caroten —3-ol)
- isocryptoxanthin (β,β-caroten —4-ol)
- zeaxanthin (β,β-carotene-3,3'-diol)
- isozeaxanthin (β,β-carotene-4,4'-diol)
- lutein (β,ε-carotene-3,3'-diol) ;

astacene (β,β-carotene-3,3',4,4'-tetrone) and phoeniconone (β,β-carotene-3,4,4'-trione), oxidized forms of astaxanthin and phoenicoxanthin respectively, seem not to occur in the animal.
Small quantities of minor carotenoids have also been detected ; often they are important intermediates in metabolism, furthermore one may also admit that their low concentrations could be due to a rapid transformation (6). Minor hydroxyl forms having β-configuration are represented by :

- crustaxanthin (β,β-carotene-3,3',4,4'-tetrol)
- 2-hydroxy-β-carotene (β,β-caroten —2-ol)
- violaxanthin (5,6,5',6'-diepoxy-5,6,5',6'-tetrahydro-β,β-carotene-3,3'-diol)

while hydroxy-ketonic forms are :

- 4'-hydroxy-echinenone (4'-hydroxy-β,β-caroten —4 -one)
- 3'-hydroxy-echinenone (3'-hydroxy-β,β-caroten —4 -one)
- β-doradexanthin (3,3'-dihydroxy-β,β-caroten —4-one)
- idoxanthin (3,3',4'-trihydroxy-β,β-caroten —4-one) ;

as far as we know β-doradecin (3'-hydroxy-β,β-carotene-3,4-dione), the oxidized form of β-doradexanthin is not reported in Crustacea.
Other carotenoids like α-carotene (β,ε-carotene) and related compounds often occur in amounts too small to be identified with certainty ; however five structures have been reported :

- phoenicopterone (β,ε-caroten —4-one)
- 3,4-diketo-α-carotene (β,ε-carotene-3,4-dione)
- α-doradexanthin (3,3'-dihydroxy-β,ε-caroten —4-one)
- lutein epoxide (5,6-epoxy-5,6-dihydro-β,ε-carotene-3,3'-diol)
- flavoxanthin (5,8-epoxy-5,8-dihydro-β,ε-carotene-3,3'-diol)

α-doradecin (3'-hydroxy-β,ε-carotene-3,4-dione) oxidized form of α-doradexanthin is not reported.

More particular structures like :
γ-carotene (β,ψ-carotene)
rubixanthin (β,ψ-caroten -3-ol)
gazaniaxanthin (5'-cis-β,ψ-caroten -3-ol)
δ-carotene (ε,ψ-carotene)
ε-carotene (ε,ε-carotene)
the allenic fucoxanthin (5,6-epoxy-3,3',5'-trihydroxy-6',7'-didehydro-5,6,7,8,5',6'-hexahydro-β,β-caroten -8-one-3'-acetate) and the acetylenic zeaxanthin analogues, diatoxanthin (7,8-didehydro-β,β-carotene-3,3'-diol) and alloxanthin (7,8,7',8'-tetradehydro-β,β-carotene-3,3'-diol) have also been observed in crustaceans, nevertheless their participation in metabolic schemes has not yet been considered.
The elucidation of the nature of "unknown" carotenoids, often observed during analytical procedures, could enhance the list of these substances in Crustacea.
There is little information concerning the distribution and amounts of vitamin A in crustaceans, however its occurrence in these animals has been confirmed by several authors.

Chemical reactions

Besides esterification and deesterification processes, the main chemical reactions observed in Crustacea are oxidative changes by which carotenes are transformed into hydroxy —keto and epoxy-derivatives. The reduction of keto and/or hydroxyketo carotenoids has also been suggested in crustaceans (7).
Although there is no experimental evidence supporting the conversion of epsilon cyclic end groups into beta ones, that such a reaction could occur in these animals is not excluded.
As far as we know, other reactions like cyclization and addition of conjugated double bonds have not been reported.
Our poor knowledge of carotenoprotein formation and enzymatic activities does not allow us to discuss this field.

Concentration

There is no doubt that the relative proportions of carotenoids occurring in different organs and tissues fluctuate according to the species, moreover the variations in the content of pigment are dependent on numerous physiological and ecological parameters.
Basically, carotenoid levels reflect the availability of pigment in food and the appetite of the animal for it. Besides this, it appears that females are often found to contain more pigment than males (8) and the nature and concentration of pigments may vary according to the particular geographic distribution of the animals.

LOCALIZATION AND MOVEMENTS OF CAROTENOIDS IN CRUSTACEA

Teguments

Carapace

The exoskeleton secreted by the subepithelial layer or epidermis shows two main strata as follows :

(A) Epicuticle		Pre-ecdysial layers
(B) Endocuticle	pigmented layer	Pre-ecdysial layers
	main calcified layer membranous layer	Post-ecdysial layers

Generally the carapace as well as the ecdysial exoskeleton contain mainly unesterified astaxanthin and lutein ; astaxanthin represents 90 % of the total pigment in the carapaces of the shrimps *Pandalus borealis* (9) and *Penaeus japonicus* (10), whereas lutein and β-carotene are the major pigments in the shell of the prawn *Metapenaeus affinis* (11). The investigations about the carotenoids of the carapace of the crab *Portunus trituberculatus* (12), have confirmed the presence of canthaxanthin, 4'-hydroxyechinenone, 3-ketocanthaxanthin and astaxanthin. The same pigments have also been found to occur in the carapace of the lobster *Panulirus japonicus* (13) ; canthaxanthin is also reported in the cuticle of certain Idothea (14). The fractions recovered from the carapace of the crab *Emerita analoga* show a predominance of ketonic forms (15). More recently the occurrence of a particular structure , papilioerythrinone, has been reported in the carapace of the crab *Paralithodes brevipes* (16). Only traces of esterified forms occur in the carapace of the hermit crab *Pagurus prideauxi* (17).

Besides this, the coloration of the exoskeleton is often due to the presence of protein complexes. This has been observed in most malacostracans as well as in branchiopods and maxillopods. The carotenoids are probably conveyed to the exoskeleton in the form of carotenoprotein or lipoprotein carried by the blood that, besides astacene, contains all the carotenoids of the animal (18). A yellowish carotenoprotein containing astaxanthin and canthaxanthin is observed in the carapace of the crayfish *Orconectes limosus* (19) ; lutein is found to form lipoprotein complexes in the carapace of some idotheids (20).

Therefore the change of colour which most crustacean carapaces undergo on boiling is generally due to the denaturation of the carctenoprotein complexes (21)(22)(23).

Epidermis

Contrary to the situation in the carapace, esterified forms seem to predominate in the epidermis and subepithelial connective tissue (24). Most of the carotenoids of the epidermis occur in the chromatophores. The analyses made on the nature of epidermal carotenoids in the shrimp *Plesiopenaeus edwardsianus* (25), the lobster *Homarus vulgaris* and the Norwegian lobster *Nephrops norvegicus* (26) have revealed the presence of astaxanthin esters as the only carotenoid observed in this tissue. However, unesterified astaxanthin occurs in the epidermis of the shrimps *Aristeomorpha foliacea* and *Aristeus antennatus* (27). Although the epidermis secretes the carotenoids of the carapace, the pigments in these layers are different. Therefore the main problem met with, is to know how and when carotenoid is transferred from epidermis to the new teguments . The study of carotenoid variations in the crab *Carcinus maenas* throughout the intermolt cycle, has demonstrated a transfer of pigments from internal organs to the epidermis through haemolymph during the D_2 stage. The analysis of carotenoids in the different layers indicates that modifications do not occur immediately. In D_2 the pigmentation of the epidermis and that of new teguments are identical. During the period between D_3 and D_4 the teguments contain epidermal carotenoids and some pigments typical of the carapace. Finally the transformation of carotenoids of new teguments into typical pigments, occurs after the ecdysis, more exactly during the period between A_1 and B intermolt stages (24). The transfer of esterified carotenoids from the epidermis to the teguments in the crab *Pachygrapsus marmoratus*, is likewise found to occur between D_1 and D_2 ; further transformations into carapace carotenoids take place after ecdysis (28). A discoloration of the carapace at different stages of intermolt cycle and a not well-defined "stades couleur" have been reported for the crab *Carcinus maenas* ; the green colour observed during early premolt (A_2) is replaced in C_1 by a yellow tone which becomes reddish in D_1 during premolt. In regard to the quantitative variations observed in both sexes, it appears that the carotenoid content of cephalothorax remains constant, whereas that of the abdominal region seems to increase. Thereupon, the variability of coloration could be due to changes undergone by carotenoproteins (29). This type of compound has also been reported in the epidermis of the isopod *Idothea granulosa* in which canthaxanthin represents the prosthetic carotenoid (30).

Internal organs

Hepatopancreas

This gland of various shapes and sizes, plays a major role in the absorption of carotenoids from food. During later premolt and early postmolt stages, the organ exhibits a reduced size, it becomes less coloured owing to the depletion of lipid and other reserves required for the elaboration of the new teguments. Moreover, the carotenoid content of the hepatopancreas fluctuates during vitellogenesis.
For most brachyurans and almost all decapods, stage C_4 is the part of the intermolt cycle in which tissue growth and mineralization of the cuticle are achieved. During the period between C_1 and D_1, the level of lipid in the gland increases and the organ becomes highly coloured. In general the accumulation of organic reserves is achieved at D_2 stage, at which the animal ceases feeding (31). The hepatopancreas of the crab *Pachygrapsus marmoratus* in D_0 is found to contain unesterified lutein, astaxanthin and "carcinoxanthin" as well as canthaxanthin. The presence of the latter is not reported throughout the postmolt stages, therefore, one may suppose that this pigment could be either absorbed directly from diet or partially synthetized in the digestive gland during early premolt (28). β-Carotene is the main carotenoid in the hepatopancreas of the crabs *Carcinus maenas* (24)(32), *Carcinus mediterraneus* (33) and *Xantho poressa* (8). On the other hand only traces of this pigment are reported in the digestive gland of the lobster *Homarus vulgaris* (26). The hepatopancreas of the hermit crab *Pagurus prideauxi* appears invariably poor in carotenoids (17) whereas that of the shrimp *Penaeus japonicus* contains all the carotenoids of the animal (34). The gut diverticula of three varieties of the isopod *Idothea granulosa* present an analogous condition (30).
Vitellogenesis also affects the hepatopancreas whose carotenoid content decreases during ovarian activity.

Gut and stomach epithelium

The carotenoids from food pass across gut walls into body fluids to be distributed to other tissues and organs. Therefore in certain species, the gut wall may likewise act as a carotenoid storage organ. In fact, carotenoids are found to occur in fat globules in the cells of the gut walls in *Daphnia* (35) and in the pigmented fat body of *Simocephalus vetulus* ; the green colour of fat cells is replaced by an orange one, owing to the disruption of carotenoprotein (36). The presence of carotenoproteins is also reported in the stomach walls of the shrimp *Aristeus antennatus* (37). The transfer of carotenoids from gut to the hepatopancreas is accomplished through "slow glycoprotein intermediates" and varies according to molting stage and vitellogenesis (38). This kind of protein presents a striking resemblance to α-crustacyanin, the pigment of the lobster shell (22). The mid gut may also be considered as a site of carotenoid storage and the way of transfer of pigment into the blood (39). The stomach connective tissue of the shrimp *Plesiopenaeus edwardsianus* is found to contain free and esterified astaxanthin as well as a protein complex (25). β-Carotene is the major carotenoid in the intestine of the crayfish *Astacus leptodactylus* (40).

Haemolymph

The main function of haemolymph is to transport materials between hepatopancreas and integument ; it may also act as a storage organ. The changes in hepatopancreas and integument carotenoid content cause the modifications observed in the blood. The carotenoid levels of the haemolymph rise during the premolt stages, however the main fluctuations are observed during vitellogenesis owing to the transfer of pigment to the ovaries.

Eggs and evolution of carotenoids during vitellogenesis and embryonic development

Generally, crustacean ovaries become colored during vitellogenesis, due to the development of oocytes. During this period, most of the carotenoids of ovigerous individuals are found to occur in the eggs ; protein complexes, in particular (41), having a lipoglycocarotenoprotein composition, constitute the crustacean lipovitellins. The vitellogenin, often called female protein since its presence is not reported in the male, occurs in the ovaries during vitellogenesis.

The various colorations given by these complexes result from different particular compositions depending on the species and probably on the stages of development of the eggs.

Often, a single carotenoid is bound to the lipoprotein ; the green or blue complexes are often found to contain astaxanthin as prosthetic group, for example, the ovoverdin in the eggs of the lobster *Homarus gammarus* (21). However, there are other complexes in which canthaxanthin is the prosthetic carotenoid. In such cases the resulting coloration may be green in certain anostracans (42) and in some isopods (14)(30), orange-red in the eggs of the brine shrimp *Artemia salina* (43) or blue in the egg yolk of *Branchipus stagnalis* (44). The only carotenoid observed in the yellow complex of the eggs of the crab *Callinectes sapidus* is β-carotene (45). However a mixture of all the carotenoids of the eggs is observed in the red lipovitellin in the eggs of the crab *Cancer pagurus* (5).

The studies concerning the evolution of the different pigments throughout vitellogenesis and embryonic development are too fragmentary and the results are far too variable. The first observations, made on the eggs of the lobster, have shown the presence of astaxanthin which was not utilized during vitellogenesis (46) ; other investigations indicate that much of the carotenoid of the cladoceran *Simocephalus vetulus* is transferred to the eggs just before molt, moreover the females of cladocerans put 40 to 50 % of their carotenoids into the developing embryos (36) ; analogous observations have been made in *Daphnia magna* (47). Esterified astaxanthin, the major carotenoid in the eggs of *Artemia salina*, is also found to occur in the developing nauplii (6), since the carotenoids of the animal are transferred to the eggs at one precise stage of their development (48) ; furthermore, synthesis of canthaxanthin (49) and the occurrence of echinenone (50) have been reported for the developing embryos. Large quantities of β-carotene, lutein and astaxanthin occur in the eggs of the crayfish *Orconectes rusticus* suggesting that pigments might be required for teguments and/or vitamin A formation (51). Simultaneous increase of weight and carotenoid content is observed during vitellogenesis in the shrimp *Plesiopenaeus edwardsianus* (25). Lutein is supposed to act as a stabilizing factor of protein in the eggs of certain crustaceans (52). A decrease of lutein and esterified astaxanthin is observed during egg development of the barnacle *Pollicipes polymerus* (53). Carotenoids are accumulated by female copepods *Diaptomus sicilis* and *Diaptomus nevadensis* and concentrated in their eggs and nauplii (54). Finally, it is noteworthy that a protein complex dissociation occurs at the end of the embryonic development of various crustaceans (49).

ORIGIN AND PIGMENTARY PHYSIOLOGY

Crustaceans cannot synthesize their carotenoids "*de novo*" but they can transform the pigments of their diet into endogenous forms (55). It is indeed clear that certain animals can obtain all their carotenoids directly from their diet without any further transformation (56), however crustaceans can elaborate their own pigments from ingested precursors. Consequently in regard to their origin, two types of carotenoids may occur in Crustacea :

Those obtained directly from food.
Those resulting after transformation of exogenous pigments.

It seems very hard to establish which of these two processes is predominant. In fact, if one of them prevails, this does not discard a simultaneous action, therefore alternative processes are possible according to certain ecological conditions, food in particular, and to the physiological state of the animal. Moreover, alternative changes may arise throughout the life cycle of the individuals. In the copepod *Meganyctiphanes couchii* for example, these two processes exist according to either the herbivorous habit of young individuals or to the adult carnivorous state (57). Metabolic changes are mainly due to oxidative reactions whose sequence is not yet well-defined, however, three types of transformations are possible :

Direct introduction of hydroxyl or ketonic groups into β-rings
Introduction of hydroxyl groups only, with further oxidation to ketonic forms in one or both terminal rings
Reduction of ketonic groups to hydroxyl groups.

Metabolic pathways

The most common metabolic pathway starts from β-carotene, ending either at astaxanthin, or at the canthaxanthin level. Indeed certain crustaceans do not contain astaxanthin which is the major carotenoid in this class ; this is what happens in *Artemia* (58)(50)(59)(48)(60), in *Chirocephalus diaphanus* (61) in *Daphnia* (62)(63)(59)(64) and in certain malacostracan isopods (14)(30)(20)(65). On the other hand, astaxanthin has however been further reported in *Artemia* (6)(66) in *Daphnia* (35)(39) and in other anostracans (42). Besides this, astaxanthin is invariably detected in Decapoda.
Ketonic forms like echinenone and canthaxanthin are also widely distributed in crustaceans, being considered as intermediate forms involved in oxidative transformations of β-carotene into astaxanthin (6)(67)(63)(68).
It must be emphasized that large amounts of other pigments detected in almost all crustaceans are not included in this pathway (lutein, α and β-doradexanthin), but they might participate in other accessory metabolic routes which will be discussed later.
The following scheme proposes some hypothetical steps in the formation of astaxanthin from β-carotene :

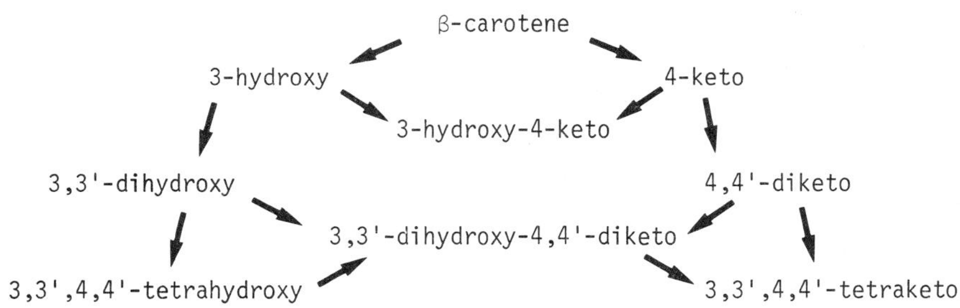

It is outlined that "this does not exhaust the list of possible intermediates but indicates those which are most likely to be involved" (49). The 4-hydroxy and 4,4'-dihydroxy isomers (isocryptoxanthin and isozeaxanthin) as well as 4-hydroxy-4'-keto and phoenicoxanthin are also considered as important intermediates. Several pathways, based upon the nature and localization of carotenoids in Crustacea have been suggested, however, the experiments using depigmented animals followed by a repigmentation with a diet containing well-defined carotenoids, have permitted only certain intermediates to be identified. The results of investigations made on *Artemia salina* are not clear enough, since astaxanthin is not found to occur systematically in this crustacean.
The utilization of precise diets containing β-carotene or echinenone (58)(60), canthaxanthin or zeaxanthin (60) as well as the use of labelled pigments ($[^{14}C]$-β-carotene)(69) have permitted the demonstration that *Artemia* is able to synthesize canthaxanthin from β-carotene *via* echinenone. These steps have been confirmed up to the canthaxanthin level (48) ; other authors outlined the fact that the Californian strain of *Artemia* was unable to synthesize astaxanthin (60), moreover it has been shown that the Californian strain cannot metabolize carotenoids beyond the canthaxanthin level, whereas they are transformed into astacene by the Canadian strain in which ketonic derivatives are considered as final products but not as intermediates (66). In the same way *Daphnia* can transform β-carotene into astaxanthin through echinenone and canthaxanthin ; nevertheless astaxanthin formation appears unnecessary since further transformation of β-carotene beyond the canthaxanthin level might not occur (39).
The researches on the pigmentary metabolism of idotheids indicate the transformation of β-carotene into canthaxanthin according to the following sequence :

β-carotene → isocryptoxanthin → echinenone → 4-hydroxy-4'-keto-β-carotene → canthaxanthin

The monohydroxy-monoketo form is indeed present in *Idotea granulosa* as well as in *Idotea montereyensis* (14)(30), while isocryptoxanthin (monohydroxy-β-carotene) is found to occur in *Idotea granulosa* only.
Furthermore, the isopod *Idotea resecata* fed with ^{14}C labelled β-carotene is also able to transform this pigment into canthaxanthin through ketonic and hydroxyketonic intermediates (65). This confirms unequivocally the role of hydroxyl forms as steps in the formation of canthaxanthin.

β-carotene → 4-hydroxy → echinenone → 4-hydroxy-4'-keto → canthaxanthin

The use of either labelled algal carotenoids (15) or pure labelled β-carotene in the diet of the decapod crustaceans has also permitted to demonstrate the participation of monohydroxy (isocryptoxanthin) and monohydroxy-monoketo carotenoids in the lobster *Panulirus japonicus* (70) and in the crab *Portunus trituberculatus* (71) and that of phoenicoxanthin in the prawn *Penaeus japonicus* (72), in the lobster *Panulirus japonicus* (70), in the crab *Portunus trituberculatus* (71) and the hermit crab *Clibanarius erythropus* (73).
The following scheme represents the most complete metabolic pathway from β-carotene to astaxanthin. It has been established for *Panulirus japonicus* and *Portunus trituberculatus*.

β-carotene → isocryptoxanthin
↓
echinenone → 4-hydroxy-echinenone
↓
canthaxanthin → 3-hydroxy-canthaxanthin
↓
astaxanthin

Nevertheless only ketonic intermediates have been isolated and identified in the sand crab *Emerita analoga* (15)

β-carotene → echinenone → canthaxanthin → astaxanthin

Closely related organisms may exhibit different metabolic features ; in fact, idoteid isopods having been fed with an algal diet can transform β-carotene into canthaxanthin (14)(30)(20)(65) whilst the omnivorous species *Idothea metallica* fed with an astaxanthin-containing diet, reduces this pigment to crustaxanthin *via* idoxanthin (7).

astaxanthin → idoxanthin → crustaxanthin

On the other hand, the results obtained with the lobster *Panulirus japonicus* differ. According to certain authors the metabolic pathway involves all the hydroxy, keto and hydroxyketo intermediates (70). However two other pathways have been proposed (74).

1. β-carotene → echinenone → canthaxanthin → phoenicoxanthin → astaxanthin.
2. zeaxanthin → 4-ketozeaxanthin → astaxanthin.

All these results seem contradictory, however they reflect the great diversity of physiological responses in Crustacea. Furthermore, these differences are probably due to the particular enzymatic systems involved in this metabolism, or merely to the availability of carotenoids in the natural environment.
In certain cases, one or more intermediates may be absent, this could be due to the fact that the pigment occurs at a too low concentration to be detected (14)(75). Finally, isolation and elucidation attempts are often hindered by a mixture of the intermediate with a closely related pigment (7)(14).

Other carotenoids are involved into this scheme ; isozeaxanthin and canthaxanthin for example, are found to be simultaneously formed from 4-hydroxyechinenone (30) ; isozeaxanthin is a normal intermediate in the metabolic scheme concerning *Daphnia* (39) ; in fact, isozeaxanthin is probably oxidized into canthaxanthin. On the other hand, the use of labelled pigments indicates that *Artemia salina* is able to absorb isozeaxanthin but cannot transform it (69). Finally, since this dihydroxy intermediate has not been detected, it is merely proposed as a step between whether β-carotene and canthaxanthin or between isocryptoxanthin and canthaxanthin in the commensal crab *Pinnotheres pisum* (75), as well as in certain anostracans (42).

isozeaxanthin
β-carotene ⇢ isozeaxanthin ⇢ canthaxanthin
β-carotene → isocryptoxanthin → canthaxanthin
isocryptoxanthin ⇢ isozeaxanthin

Isozeaxanthin could be an intermediate between monohydroxy and trihydroxy-β-carotene in other species like *Artemia salina*.

4-hydroxy → 4,4'-dihydroxy → 3,4,4'-trihydroxy → 3,3',4,4'-tetrahydroxy (66).

β-Carotene appears as the common precursor in the different metabolic pathways, but it seems likely that other carotenoids may represent the start point of transformations. The simultaneous occurrence of zeaxanthin, β-doradexanthin and astaxanthin has been observed in various crustaceans like *Panulirus japonicus* (74) *Scyllarides squamosus* (76) *Geryon quinquedens* (77) *Pagurus prideauxi* (17) and the amphipod *Arctodiaptomus bacillifer* (78).Therefore, the following metabolic scheme has been proposed (74)(77)(72)(17)(78)

Zeaxanthin → 4-ketozeaxanthin → astaxanthin

This scheme has recently been confirmed by the use of labelled pigments in the fishes *Carassius auratus* (79) and *Cyprinus carpio* (80) ; free zeaxanthin seems to arise at the integument level, to be further metabolized after esterification (81)(80). Thereupon, β-doradexanthin (adonixanthin)(78) might have been formed either from zeaxanthin or from hydroxyechinenone according to the following scheme

Zeaxanthin → adonixanthin → astaxanthin
hydroxyechinenone → adonixanthin

However, food zeaxanthin seems not to be metabolized to either canthaxanthin or astaxanthin (60). Two different origins have been proposed for these pigments:

- ingestion and absorption after an eventual esterification
- absorption and oxidative transformations into astaxanthin through β-doradexanthin (77).

The introduction of lutein in the scheme of metabolic transformations needs, in addition to oxidative alterations, the modification of the ε-cyclic end group into a β-type. The metabolism of lutein into astaxanthin through α and β-doradexanthins has been confirmed in the fish *Carassius auratus* (82)(83)

lutein → α-doradexanthin → β-doradexanthin → astaxanthin

These results do not agree with those of other authors which have shown that lutein was not converted into astaxanthin but into 4-ketolutein (79)(84)(85).
The simultaneous determination of astaxanthin, lutein and α-doradexanthin in various crustaceans (86)(87)(88) as well as the occurrence of α-doradexanthin in nineteen freshwater species (89) support the metabolic scheme proposed above. However, no experimental evidence about the presence of both α and β- doradexanthin in one given species has been reported up till now. The radioactive lutein observed in *Idotea resecata* (65) and in *Clibanarius erythropus* (73) after feeding experiments using labelled precursors, is more probably due to a contamination of this pigment during the analytical procedure. Lutein might participate in the formation of caroteno–lipoprotein complexes in the teguments of certain idoteids (14)(32) ; besides this, *Daphnia* cannot metabolize the lutein of its algal food into derivatives having two β-ionone terminal rings (39).
It appears from all these studies that astaxanthin is not formed *via* a unique and immutable transformation pathway ; sometimes, this pigment may be absorbed directly with the diet; this is also indeed plausible for all the carotenoids of the animal, for example 7, 8 - didehydroastaxanthin, 7, 8, 7', 8' - tetradehydroastaxanthin (90), alloxanthin (91), fucoxanthin (92), and peridinin. Concerning the 2 - hydroxy compound the opinion of the authors is that there is no reason to believe that it is involved in carotenoid metabolism nor to think that it is taken in the diet (65). Nevertheless, the experimental observations have shown that the crustaceans can metabolize at least some part of their food pigments.
Finally, although the knowledge of carotenoid metabolism in crustaceans is considerable, it is however not possible to draw a general pattern valid for all the species so far studied. According to the site of metabolic transformations, crustaceans may be divided into two different groups (70). Within the first, one can find individuals converting β-carotene into astaxanthin through all the possible intermediates in the internal organs like hepatopancreas and gut. This kind of animal generally has a digestive gland containing all the carotenoids of the organism ; this is the case of the prawn *Penaeus japonicus* (34). The second group embraces animals converting β-carotene into echinenone in the hepatopancreas, however the formation of astaxanthin as well as that of the intermediates seems likely to occur in the cells of other organs or tissues like the epidermis ; this is what has been observed in the lobster *Panulirus japonicus* (70), in the crab *Portunus trituberculatus* (71) and in the hermit-crab *Pagurus prideauxi* (17). The transformation of β-carotene into echinenone *via* isocryptoxanthin in the shrimp *Panulirus japonicus* and in the crab *Portunus trituberculatus* occurs in the internal organs while further oxidations occur in the carapace.

Several authors suggest that esterified hydroxylated pigments are the most active forms in the metabolism of carotenoids in fishes. One may suppose that it is so in crustaceans. Nevertheless, in certain cases, it has been observed that carotenoids of artificial diet are not transformed ; the excretion products contain large amounts of non-transformed pigment, thus the animals remain unpigmented. These results support the view that the transformations are possible only if the ingested carotenoids induce appropriate biochemical reactions within the animal. Thereupon, two questions rise from this topic :
first, are crustaceans able to transform the ε-cyclic end groups into the β type ?
second, are they able to metabolize "trans" structures into the "cis" isomers ?
These observations suggest the existence of a specific enzymatic activity according to the taxonomic position of the animals, however, as far as we know, knowledge on the series of enzymatic reactions of carotenoid metabolism in Crustacea is still fragmentary and uncertain.

Excretion

Two main processes may be considered : the elimination of carotenoids in the excretion products (94) and the loss of pigment through molting and vitellogenesis. In the first case, it is logical to suppose that the rejected pigments have not been assimilated owing either to a high concentration of carotenoids in the food or to the absence of appropriate enzymatic responses in the animal. The presence of lutein, β-carotene and astaxanthin has been reported in the excretion products of the crab *Carcinus maenas* (24).
Molting and oviposition may also be considered as periodic rejection of carotenoids by the animal ; in addition to the loss of inorganic materials when molting, the integument may also act as a carotenoid excretory organ. Hence, the question is why important amounts of pigment are periodically neglected by crustaceans ? More interesting is the fact that carotenoids seem not to have a particular function in the evolution of the eggs, since the amounts remain constant all along larval development (46)(15). So these two phenomena may appear as a "cheaper" way to clear the surplus of carotenoids from the organism. It seems probable that the canthaxanthin content in the eggs of certain anostracans comes from the ovary, so the laying produces a considerable diminution of body canthaxanthin (42).

Endocrine control

Carotenoid metabolism in Crustacea has been found to be under endocrine control, the neurosecretory complex of eyestalks as well as the activity of the androgenic gland appear to have a marked influence on various physiological cycles related to carotenoid metabolism like vitellogenesis and molting.

Eyestalks

The removal of eyestalks leads to the disruption of the carotenoprotein complex in the pigmented layer (95) due to the action of molting hormone on the epidermis. During the premolt stages, carotenoids are transferred from the cuticle to the hepatopancreas, where they are often stored. This transfer is made through haemolymph. The results of a number of workers have allowed the demonstration of carotenoid deposition in internal organs as well as the breakdown of astaxanthin protein complex in the pigmented layer are due to the influence of molting hormone (31). The bilateral ablation of sinus glands induces flagrant modifications in the carotenoid composition of haemolymph, hepatopancreas and epidermis (24). The same surgical action in the crab *Uca pugilator* is responsible for a decrease of the total carotenoid content ; besides this, an increase of pigment in hepatopancreas and epidermis is observed just before molting (96). The experiments made on the shrimp *Palaemon serratus* have shown a decrease of astaxanthin as well as of other xanthophylls after the ablation (97)(98)(99), whereas β-carotene appears to increase. These results have permitted the precise differences between the pigmentary reactions of Brachyura and those of Macrura-natantia to be defined (100). The bilateral eyestalk ablation in the hermit crab *Dardanus arrosor* has shown a decrease in the content of esterified forms while unesterified appear predominant (101).
On the other hand, a large increase of astaxanthin and its esters is observed in the eyestalkless prawn *Macrobrachium rosembergii* fed with a diet containing carotenoids ; however, a small decrease in the total carotenoid content is observed after eyestalk ablation in individuals having a diet free of these pigments. Therefore it would appear that the lack of pigment in the diet does not allow the maintenance of carotenoid levels necessary for such an increase after ablation (102).
The experiments thus described suggest a direct action of the endocrine system on the metabolism of carotenoids. Besides this the endocrine activity because of its influence on the different physiological processes like molt and vitellogenesis, exerts an indirect action on pigmentation.
Eyestalk ablation modifies the molting cycle by diminishing the intermolt period ; thus if one considers ecdysis as an important loss of carotenoids, the fact that eyestalk ablation increases the carotenoid content suggests an action of molting effectors on the reconstitution of the stock of carotenoids in the animal when hormonal activity is stopped.
Eyestalk ablation in the female crab *Rhithropanopeus harisii* during slow vitellogenesis shows an increase in the ovarian weight as well as a change of colour which becomes darker. Nevertheless if the ablation is made during the resting phase of the ovary, the increase of

weight occurs but no colour changes are observed (103).
The reduction of the number of pigmented granules and their localization at the edge of chromatophores in the eyestalk-ablated prawn *Palaemon serratus* (104) seem to be induced by the metabolic alterations produced by the suppression of the neurosecretory complex of the eyestalks.

Androgenic gland

The grafting of an androgenic gland in the females of the amphipods *Talitrus saltator* and *Orchestia gammarella* has shown the appearance of a bright red colour in the antennae of these animals. On the other hand, the antennae of the males lose their coloration after ablation of the androgenic gland. It seems thus possible that the male hormone controls the astaxanthin content in the antennae (105). The injections of androgenic gland extracts are also found to induce an increase of colour in malacostracans (106).

Seasonal and diurnal variations

Crustacean carotenoid internal rhythms may be modified by environmental factors like light, temperature, food, etc... It has been shown that the carotenoid content of two species of calanidae *Diaptomus claripes* and *Diaptomus pallidus* increases during the winter when the transparency of water reaches a maximum and decreases in the summer when the water becomes turbid (107). Analogous correlations have been made for cladocerans (36)(47) in which light induces the accumulation of carotenoids by the animals. The red colour of the copepod *Acanthodiaptomus denticornis* exhibits marked variations according to the seasons : the carotenoid content decreases in the winter, probably owing to transfer of pigments to the eggs and to the utilization of lipids during this period (108). The copepods *Diaptomus sicilis* and *Diaptomus nevadensis* are more pigmented in the surface waters than the individuals living in the deep zone (109) ; during the winter and the early spring, the adults tend to be much more coloured than in the summer (110). Quantitative and qualitative circadian changes of carotenoids have been observed in the shrimp *Penaeus japonicus* suggesting possible interconversions of pigments in organs and tissues at different times of the day (111). In the same way, the carotenoid content of the copepods *Acanthodiaptomus denticornis* (112) and *Daphnia longispina* shows significant diurnal variations following a night/day rhythm (113). The diminution of carotenoid content during the day reflects the utilization of the lipid reserves required for migrating activities (113).

Carotenoids in cavernicolous animals

The loss of pigmentation of hypogean species could be ascribed to particular conditions of caves like absence of light, low temperature and lack of food, as well as low oxygen content in subterranean waters. Nevertheless, the influence of all these parameters is still controversial and available data appear contradictory. It seems indeed clear that, in the absence of light, colour has no apparent significance and may be regarded as of neutral survival value (114)(115). However it has been assumed that darkness could be responsible for a low pigmentation, since carotenoids occur in sedimentary food in caves (116). The hypogean crayfish *Cambarus bartonii tenebrosus* is found to contain astaxanthin whereas *Orconectes pellucidus pellucidus* contains only β-carotene and lutein (68). Furthermore the colourless amphipod *Gammarus duebeni* becomes coloured when exposed to light (117).
On the other hand, the observations made on the amphipod *Gammarus pulex subterraneus* (118) and on the crayfish *Procambarus simulans* (119) indicate that the less pigmented appearance is a result of a lack of pigmented food, and that the absence of light has no effect on the carotenoid pigmentation of the isopod *Asellus aquaticus cavernicolus* in which the predominant carotenoid pigments are β-carotene and cryptoxanthin (120). The authors conclude that the reduced pigmentation is more probably due to the genetic constitution of the animal than to other environmental factors. The amphipod *Niphargus virei* fed with a diet containing pure carotenoids is unable to accumulate the absorbed pigments (121).

Parasitic relationships

It seems indeed clear that parasitic infections are closely related to the endocrine relationships between the parasite and its host (122).
The parasite living at the expense of its host may obtain carotenoids directly from it ; thus it appears interesting to consider these relationships. The different parasitic constitutions may influence the fat metabolism of the hosts, however this varies according to the species of both host and parasite. The deterioration of the ovaries and the alteration of intermolt cycles of the crab *Inachus mauritanicus*, due to a parasitic infection by the rhizocephalan crustacean *Sacculina neglecta* (123), are concomitant with the increase of carotenoids in the haemolymph of the crab. More interesting appears the selective absorption of pigments by the parasite. *Sacculina carcini* seems not to absorb carotenoids other than β-carotene (124) while its host *Carcinus maenas* contains several carotenoids in the haemolymph and in the other tissues (24). The same phenomenon is observed in the acanthocephalan worm *Polymorphus minutus* which is coloured by the astaxanthin absorbed from its host the amphipod

Gammarus pulex (125).
In the case of crustacean parasites of other species, the parasitic relationships concerning the metabolism of carotenoids are not yet well-defined. *Argulus foliaceus* the external parasite of the fish *Gasterosteus aculeatus*, contains some pigments taken from its host ; however, specific parasite carotenoids can be found (126).

GENETIC VARIATIONS

There are few papers concerning the inheritance of carotenoid pigmentation in Crustacea, and available data are too fragmentary. Although it has been demonstrated that the carotenoid pigmentation depends upon external sources, it is also logical to think that pigmentation may be under genetic control. However this kind of segregation is very complex for Mendelian analysis.
The observations made on the colour of the eggs of the amphipod *Gammarus crinicornis* have shown a genetic determinism on the polychromatism of this species (127) the pigmentation of which seems not to be essentially dependent upon food.
Populations of the hypogean isopod *Asellus aquaticus cavernicolus* exhibit different appearances varying from a dark color to an almost lack of coloration. This range of pigmentation, being due to the segregation of characters determining the different colours, is not affected by light. The pigmented features are not only due to a phenotypic effect of ecological factors but also to the presence of a permanent element in the genetic configuration of the species (114). The absence of astaxanthin in the branchiopod *Chirocephalus diaphanus* and the blocking of the transformation of β-carotene at the canthaxanthin level (128) suggest a particular genetic constitution that hinders the formation of astaxanthin within the animal.
So far one may thus conceive that the differences of pigmentation in individuals of the same species, having different geographic distribution like the crabs *Eriphia spinifrons*, *Pachygrapsus marmoratus*, *Carcinus maenas* (129)(130)(88) and the hermit crab *Clibanarius erythropus* (*misanthropus*)(131)(87) could be ascribed to the peculiar genetic configuration of individuals rather than to the phenotypic effect of environment.

FUNCTIONS

It is still not clear, however, whether carotenoids have or have not precise biological function in crustaceans. Very little is known on the participation of carotenoids in reproduction; could carotenoids act as fertilizing hormones ? (132). Moreover, there is no evidence that carotenoids are necessary in developing eggs ; *Daphnia magna* is able to grow and reproduce without carotenoids (47) ; little or no change in the total carotenoid content of the lobster eggs takes place during the development of the embryos (46) and carotenoids appear unutilized during the development of the eggs of the sand crab *Emerita analoga* (15). Besides this, certain hypothetical functions have been ascribed to these pigments. Although carotenoids appear not to be necessary in low solar radiation, they might be utilized as a protective screen against higher illumination (47). Although the role of carotenoids in the stabilization of polypeptide configuration has been suggested in molluscs (133), it seems not illogical to suppose such a role in Crustacea. Carotenoids might act as a cross-link between lipid and protein to stabilize the lipoprotein, exerting thereby a control in the permeability of membranes (134) ; furthermore the carotenoid is supposed to protect the protein from the catalytic action of enzymes (49). The carotenoprotein complex might also act as attenuator of light ; furthermore in the case of crustacyanin and ovoverdin, the prosthetic pigment is protected against photooxidation and at the same time it stabilizes the protein structure (135)(134).
Carotenoprotein content in *Daphnia* is found to increase under intensive illumination (35). The bluish colour due to a carotenoprotein complex in pelagic invertebrates screens the organs against solar radiations (136) ; carotenoprotein acts as a possible protecting coloration in idotheid isopods (14)(30)(32) and constitutes the main protein reserve of the crustacean eggs (137)(29). Finally carotenoids are supposed to act as final electron acceptors in molluscs (138); is it so in Crustacea ?

CONCLUSIONS

Crustaceans represent one class of animals in which carotenoids are particularly abundant ; this could explain the interest of scientists and thereby the wide number of papers concerning these substances.
Satisfactory results have been obtained in the determination of the nature, the localization and the metabolic transformations in various species. However the data already established on the pigmentary physiology and ecophysiology of these animals are still too fragmentary and often incoherent. A review of several hypotheses and other theoretical demonstrations thus seems necessary. Furthermore, efforts should be made to determine the precise roles of carotenoids in this class.
Consequently, a considerable number of new studies must be carried out, in order to elucidate some of the questions inherent in the presence of carotenoids in Crustacea.

Acknowledgement - We would like to thank Ms Sonia Landrein for manuscript advising and Mrs Chistiane Sibleyras for typing the manuscript.

REFERENCES

1. G. Pouchet, C. R. Acad. Sci., Paris 74, 757-760 (1872).
2. P. Drach, Annls Inst. Océanogr., Monaco 19, 103-391 (1939).
3. P. Drach and C. Tchernigovtzeff, Vie Milieu A 18, 595-610 (1967).
4. D.L. Fox, Comp. Biochem. Physiol. 44B, 953-962 (1973).
5. P.F. Zagalsky, D.F. Cheesman and H.J. Ceccaldi, Comp. Biochem. Physiol. 22, 851-871 (1967).
6. B.M. Gilchrist and J. Green, Proc. R. Soc. B 152, 118-136 (1960).
7. P.J. Herring, J. mar. biol. Ass. U.K. 49, 767-779 (1969).
8. C. Bilaus, E. Nicoara, C. Bodea and I. Petrescu, St. Cerc. Biochim. 15, 5-8 (1972).
9. N. Tsukuda, Bull. Japan Sea Reg. Fish. Res. Lab. 11, 109-115 (1963).
10. T. Katayama, T. Kamata and C.O. Chichester, Int. J. Biochem. 3, 363-368 (1972).
11. A.V. Narsubai and Y.R. Mohanrao, Curr. Sci. 42, 107-108 (1973).
12. T. Katayama, Y. Kunisaki, M. Shimaya, M. Sameshima and C.O. Chichester, Bull. Jap. Soc. scient. Fish. 39, 283-287 (1973).
13. T. Katayama, M. Shimaya, M. Sameshima and C.O. Chichester, Bull. Jap. Soc. scient. Fish. 39, 215-220 (1973).
14. W.L. Lee, Comp. Biochem. Physiol. 18, 17-36 (1966).
15. B.M. Gilchrist and W.L. Lee, Comp. Biochem. Physiol. 42B, 263-294 (1972).
16. K. Harashima, J. Nakahara and G. Kato, Agr. Biol. Chem. 40, 711-717 (1976).
17. R. Castillo, R. Lenel and G. Nègre-Sadargues, Comp. Biochem. Physiol. 66B, 483-489 (1980).
18. H. Nakagawa, M. Kayama and S. Asakawa, J. Fac. Fish. Anim. Husb., Hiroshima, Univ. 14, 61-67 (1975).
19. B. Czeczuga and S. Krywuta, Comp. Biochem. Physiol. 68B, 339-343 (1981).
20. W.L. Lee and B.M. Gilchrist, J. exp. mar. Biol. Ecol. 10, 1-27 (1972).
21. R. Kuhn and N.A. Sorensen, Ber. dt. chem. Ges. 71, 1879-1888 (1938).
22. G. Wald, N. Nathanson, W.P. Jencks and E. Tarr, Biol. Bull. 95, 249-250 (1948).
23. P.F. Zagalsky and D.F. Cheesman, Biochem. J. 89, 21 p. (1963).
24. R. Lenel, Bull. Soc. lorr. Sci. 1, 1-134 (1961).
25. R. Establier, Investigacion Pesq. 30, 207-222 (1966).
26. T.W. Goodwin and S. Srisukh, Biochem. J. 45, 268-270 (1949).
27. R. Massonet, Thèse Doct. Sci. Nat., Lyon 1-147 (1958).
28. G. Nègre-Sadargues, Thèse 3ème cycle, Montpellier 1-247 (1974).
29. H.J. Ceccaldi, Thèse Doct. Sci. Nat., Aix-Marseille 1-479 (1968).
30. W.L. Lee, Comp. Biochem. Physiol. 19, 13-27 (1966).
31. L.M. Passano, The Physiology of Crustacea, in Waterman 1. Academic Press, 473-536 (1960).
32. B.M. Gilchrist and W.L. Lee, J. Zool. Lond. 151, 171-180 (1967).
33. E. Nicoara, C. Bilaus, C. Bodea and J. Petrescu, St. Cerc. Biochim. 13, 65-68 (1970).
34. T. Katayama, T. Kamata, M. Shimaya, O. Deshimaru and C.O. Chichester, Bull. Jap. Soc. scient. Fish. 38, 1171-1175 (1972).
35. J. Green, Proc. R. Soc. B 147, 392-401 (1957).
36. J. Green, J. Zool. Lond. 149, 174-187 (1966).
37. P.F. Zagalsky, H.J. Ceccaldi and R. Daumas, Comp. Biochem. Physiol. 34, 579-607 (1970).
38. H.J. Ceccaldi, C. R. Soc. Biol. 161, 1105-1110 (1967).
39. P.J. Herring, Comp. Biochem. Physiol. 24, 187-203 (1968).
40. B. Czeczuga, Comp. Biochem. Physiol. 39B, 945-953 (1971).
41. P.F. Zagalsky, Pure & Appl. Chem. 47, 103-120 (1976).
42. B.M. Gilchrist, Comp. Biochem. Physiol. 24, 123-147 (1968).
43. A.H. Warner, J.G. Puodziukas and F.J. Finamore, Expl. Cell. Res. 70, 365-375 (1972).
44. P.F. Zagalsky and B.M. Gilchrist, Comp. Biochem. Physiol. 55B, 195-200 (1976).
45. M.S. Kerr, Devl. Biol. 20, 1-17 (1969).
46. T.W. Goodwin, Nature 167, p. 559 (1951).
47. P.J. Herring, Comp. Biochem. Physiol. 24, 205-221 (1968).
48. M. Hata and M. Hata, Comp. Biochem. Physiol. 29, 985-994 (1969).
49. J. Green, Biol. Rev. 40, 580-600 (1965).
50. N.I. Krinsky, Comp. Biochem. Physiol. 16, 181-187 (1965).
51. D.A. Wolfe and D.G. Cornwell, Comp. Biochem. Physiol. 16, 205-213 (1965).
52. P.F. Zagalsky, Ph. D.,Thesis, University of London (1964).
53. A.R. Holter, Comp. Biochem. Physiol. 28, 675-684 (1969).
54. N.G. Hairston Jr, Limnol. Oceanogr. 24, 38-44 (1979).
55. T.W. Goodwin, The comparative biochemistry of carotenoids, p. 356, Chapman and Hall Ltd, London (1952).
56. P.J. Herring, J. mar biol. Ass. U.K. 53, 539-562 (1973).
57. L.R. Fisher, S.K. Kon and S.Y. Thompson, J. mar biol. Ass. U.K. 33, 589-612 (1954).
58. B.H. Davies, W.J. Hsu and C.O. Chichester, Biochem. J. 94, 26 (1965).
59. F.C. Czygan, Z. Naturf. 21, 801-805 (1966).

60. W.J. Hsu, C.O. Chichester and B.H. Davies, Comp. Biochem. Physiol. 32, 69-79 (1970).
61. R. Lenel and M. Nourisson, C. R. Acad. Sci., Paris 253, 2143-2145 (1961).
62. H. Euler, H. Hellstrom and E. Klussmann, Hoppe-Seyler's, Z. physiol. Chem. 228, 77-89 (1934).
63. H. Thommen and H. Wackernagel, Naturwissenschaften 51, 87-88 (1964).
64. J. Gross and P. Budowski, Biochem. J. 101, 747-754 (1966).
65. B.M. Gilchrist and W.L. Lee, Comp. Biochem. Physiol. 54B, 343-346 (1976).
66. F.C. Czygan, Z. Naturf. 23, 1367-1368 (1968).
67. R. Lenel, C. R. Acad. Sci., Paris 236, 1448-1450 (1953).
68. D.A. Wolfe and D.G. Cornwell, Science 144, 1467-1469 (1964).
69. B.H. Davies, W.J. Hsu and C.O. Chichester, Comp. Biochem. Physiol. 33, 601-615 (1970).
70. T. Katayama, M. Shimaya, M. Sameshima and C.O. Chichester, Int. J. Biochem. 4, 223-226 (1973).
71. T. Katayama, Y. Kunisaki, M. Shimaya, K.L. Simpson and C.O. Chichester, Comp. Biochem. Physiol. 46B, 269-272 (1973).
72. Y. Tanaka, H. Matsuguchi, T. Katayama, K.L. Simpson and C.O. Chichester, Bull. Jap. Soc. Soc. scient. Fish. 42, 197-202 (1976).
73. R. Castillo, Comp. Biochem. Physiol. 66A, 695-697 (1980).
74. T. Matsuno, T. Kusumoto, T. Watanabe and Y. Ishihara, Bull. Jap. Soc. scient. Fish 39, 43-50 (1973).
75. S.A. Campbell, Comp. Biochem. Physiol. 30, 803-812 (1969).
76. T. Matsuno, T. Watanabe and S. Nagata, Bull. Jap. Soc. scient. Fish. 40, 619-624 (1974).
77. H.C. Kuo, T.C. Lee, C.O. Chichester and K.L. Simpson, Comp. Biochem. Physiol. 54B, 387-390 (1976).
78. H. Seefried and F.C. Czygan, Z. Naturf. 33, 671-674 (1978).
79. M. Hata and M. Hata, Bull. Jap. Soc. scient. Fish. 38, 331-338 (1972).
80. M. Hata and M. Hata, Bull. Jap. Soc. scient. Fish. 42, 203-205 (1976).
81. M. Hata and M. Hata, Bull. Jap. Soc. scient. Fish. 38, 339-343 (1972).
82. W.J. Hsu, D.B. Rodriguez and C.O. Chichester, Int. J. Biochem. 3, 333-338 (1972).
83. T. Katayama, H. Yokoyama and C.O. Chichester, Bull. Jap. Soc. scient. Fish 36, 702-708 (1970).
84. M. Hata and M. Hata, Bull. Jap. Soc. scient. Fish. 41, 653-655 (1975).
85. M. Hata and M. Hata, Bull. Jap. Soc. scient. Fish. 44, 83-84 (1978).
86. T. Matsuno and T. Watanabe, Bull. Jap. Soc. scient. Fish. 40, 767-774 (1974).
87. R. Castillo and R. Lenel, Comp. Biochem. Physiol. 59B, 67-74 (1978).
88. R. Lenel, R. Castillo and G. Nègre-Sadargues, Biochem. Syst. Ecol. 6, 251-253 (1978).
89. B. Czeczuga, Bull. Acad. pol. Sci. C II ser. Sci. biol. 28, 59-63 (1980).
90. H. Thommen, F. Leuenberger, R. Berger and S. Liaaen-Jensen, Biochem. Syst. Ecol. 4, 131-132 (1976).
91. Y. Tanaka, H. Matsuguchi, T. Katayama, K.L. Simpson and C.O. Chichester, Comp. Biochem. Physiol. 54B, 391-393 (1976).
92. P.J. Herring, Experientia 27, 1027-1028 (1971).
93. D.L. Fox and G.F. Crozier, Experientia 23, 12-13 (1967).
94. E. Fischer, C. r. Soc. Biol. 96, 850-852 (1927).
95. R. Lenel and A. Veillet, C. R. Acad. Sci., Paris 233, 1064-1065 (1951).
96. M. Hariharan, Amer Zool. 6, 507 (1966).
97. C. Chassard-Bouchaud and P. Noël, C. R. Acad. Sci., Paris 273, 1024-1027 (1971).
98. G.C. Genofre, C. R. Acad. Sci., Paris 276, 2269-2272 (1973).
99 G.C. Genofre, Anais Acad. bras. Cienc. 48, 301-304 (1976).
100. F.A. Brown Jr, Hormones in Crustacea, edited by G. Pincus and K.V. Thimann 1 Acad. Press N.Y. 159-199 (1948).
101. R. Castillo and R. Lenel, C. R. Acad. Sci., Paris, 277, 329-332 (1973).
102. P. Maugle, T. Kamata, S. Mc Lean, K.L. Simpson and T. Katayama, Bull. Jap. Soc. scient. Fish. 46, 901-904 (1980).
103. A. Bomirski and E. Klek, Mar. Biol. 24, 329-337 (1974).
104. M. Hubert and C. Chassard-Bouchaud, Archs Zool. exp. gén. 117, 117-138 (1976).
105. M. Barbier, H. Charniaux-Cotton and M.C. Fried-Montaufier, C. R. Acad. Sci., Paris 263, 1508-1510 (1966).
106. J. Berreur-Bonnenfant, J.J. Meusy, J.P. Ferezou, M. Devys, A. Quesneau-Thierry and M. Barbier,C. R. Acad. Sci., Paris 277, 971-974 (1973).
107. M. Siefken and K.B. Armitage, Comp. Biochem. Physiol. 24, 591-596 (1968).
108. J.L. Berthon, C. R. Acad. Sci. Paris 286, 899-900 (1978).
109. N. Hairston Jr,Ph. D. Thesis, Univ. Wash. 230 p. (1977).
110. N. Hairston Jr, Limnol. Oceanogr. 24, 38-44 (1979).
111. M. Otazu-Abrill and H.J. Ceccaldi, C.r. Soc. Biol. 172, 684-690 (1978).
112. J. Ringerberg and G.M. Hallegraeff, Hydrobiologia 51, 113-118 (1976).
113. G.M. Hallegraeff, I.J. Mous, R. Veeger, B.J.G. Flick and J. Ringelberg, Comp. Biochem. Physiol. 60B, 59-62 (1978).
114. C. Kosswig, Zool. Anz. 112, 148-155 (1935).
115. C. Kosswig, Züchter, 91-101 (1937).
116. R.A. Beatty, J. exp. Biol. 18, 144-152 (1941).
117. R.A. Beatty, J. exp. Biol. 26, 125-130 (1949).

118. F. Anders, Z. indukt. Abstamm. u. VererbLehre 87, 567-579 (1956).
119. B. Maguire Jr, Tex. J. Sci. 13, 363-370 (1961).
120. E. Baldwin and R.A. Beatty, J. exp. Biol. 18, 136-143 (1941).
121. J. Gibert, Crustaceana 4, 45-57 (1977).
122. A.M. Nadakal, J. scient. ind. Res. 22, 401-408 (1963).
123. G.C. Robson, Q. Jl microsc. Sci. 57, 267-278 (1911).
124. R. Lenel, C. R. Acad. Sci., Paris 238, 948-949 (1954).
125. J. Barrett and P.E. Butterworth, Comp. Biochem. Physiol. 27, 575-581 (1968).
126. B. Czeczuga, Acta parasit. pol. 19, 185-194 (1971).
127. B. Brun, Bull. Soc. zool. Fr. 96, 49-52 (1971).
128. R. Lenel, C. R. Acad. Sci., Paris 260, 3483-3485 (1965).
129. B. Czeczuga, Int. Rev. ges. Hydrobiol. 59, 87-93 (1974).
130. B. Czeczuga, Comp. Biochem. Physiol. 51B, 309-311 (1975).
131. B. Czeczuga and R. Czerpak, Marine Biology 4, 24-27 (1969).
132. T.W. Goodwin, Biol. Rev. 25, 391-413 (1950).
133. D.F. Cheesman, Proc. R. Soc. B 149, 571-587 (1958).
134. D.F. Cheesman, W.L. Lee and P.F. Zagalsky, Biol. Rev. 42, 131-160 (1967).
135. D.F. Cheesman, P.F. Zagalsky and H.J. Ceccaldi, Proc. R. Soc. B 164, 130-151 (1966).
136. P.J. Herring, Nature 205, 103-104 (1965).
137. H.J. Ceccaldi, Recl.Trav. Stn mar. Endoume 37, 19-24 (1965).
138. E.T. Zavras and H. James, J. Invert. Pathol. 34, 276-284 (1979).

CAROTENOIDS IN SPONGES

Masaru Yamaguchi

Department of Chemistry, Kyushu University 33, Hakozaki, Higashi-ku, Fukuoka 812, Japan

Abstract - Though the beautiful yellow to red coloration of sponges has long been known to be due to the presence of carotenoids, it is quite recently that the authentic identification or characterization of these pigments has revealed their chemically and biogenetically very interesting features. In this lecture, the important carotenoids isolated from sponges are listed, their distributions are summarized, and some developments in the synthesis of aromatic carotenoids which are one of the characteristic groups of sponge pigments are described.

INTRODUCTION

In the last decade, chemistry of marine natural products has evoked an increasing interest to organic chemists and a wide variety of marine plants and animals have been examined in chemical as well as biochemical aspects. Among them, the most striking results have been obtained from the sponges. The sponges are rich in variety (about 5.000 species) though there are still some taxonomical problems in identifying individual species, and they have really strange biochemistry to produce compounds of unusual structures and functions. Thus, over two hundred novel compounds have so far been isolated (*1*), not a few of them being biologically active.
In carotenoids, the sponges also show a quite remarkable ability to modify the pigments originated from marine plants which they mainly feed on, and carotenoids specific to this class of animals have successively been isolated and characterized in recent years (*2*).

The lipochrome nature of the yellow to deep red pigments of sponges was first described by Kruckenberg (*3*) and then by MacMunn (*4*) at the end of the last century. They examined the following sponges in qualitative way as summarized in Palmer's monograph (*5*): *Aplysina aerophoba*, *Chondrosia reniformis*, *Cocospongia*, *Grantia coriacea*, *Halichondria albescens*, *H. caruncula*, *H. incrustans*, *H. panicea*, *H. rosea*, *H. sanguinea*, *H. seriata*, *Halma bucklandi*, *Hircina spinosula*, *Hymeniacidon albescens*, *Leuconia gossei*, *Pachymatisma johnstonia*, *Pipillina suberea*, *Reniera aquaeductus*, *Suberites domuncula*, *S. flavus*, *S. massa*, *Tedania muggiana*, and *Tethya lyncureum*. Lönnberg (*6*) also studied the pigments of several sponges and described their UV-absorption properties. They were *Axinella rugosa*, *Dysidea fragilis*, *Esperia foliata*, *Halichondria panicea*, *Radiera spinolaria*, *Suberites ficus*, *S. massa*, and *Thetorium semisuberites*. The hydrocarbon nature of the major carotenoids of *Microciona prolifera* was described by Bergmann et al. (*7*).
With the increase in knowledge of carotenoids, attempts were made to identify animal carotenoids by comparing their UV-spectral and adsorptive properties with those of the known carotenoids. Thus, Karrer described the presence of the crustacean pigment, astacene, in the red sponge of the Mediterranean Sea, *Axinella crystagalli* (8). Lederer (*9*) observed that the red sponge *Suberites domuncula* and *Ficulina ficus* contained the following pigments; epiphasic carotenoids with the absorption maxima similar to those of α-, β-, and γ-carotene, respectively, the corresponding oxygenated carotenoids, and a more hypophasic pigment with its absorption maxima similar to those of torulene. Drumm et al. reported that α-, β-, and γ-carotene, and echinenone were isolated in crystalline state from a red sponge, *Hymeniacidon sanguineum* (*10*). They are summarized in Karrer's monograph (*11*). However, some of these results should be accepted with some reservation because, as we know now, the reliable identification of carotenoids is often difficult without the aid of modern spectroscopic methods.
At the end of 1950's, carotenoids of a Japanese sea sponge, *Reniera japonica*, were studied in detail and the presence of new, very unsaturated carotenoids, renieratene 26, isorenieratene 25, and renierapurpurin 27, which exhibited UV-spectra very reminiscent of β-carotene, γ-carotene, and lycopene, respectively, was reported (*12*). Classical degradation studies which required several hundred miligrams of the samples revealed that they had quite novel structures with aromatic terminal groups at both ends of the polyene chain (*13*, *14*, *16*). The

structures were soon verified by total syntheses (*15*, *16*, *17*, *18*). Introduction of NMR and MS spectroscopy techniques has brought about a revolutionary development in the structural study of carotenoids as well as other natural products and coupled with the accumulation of the knowledge on isolation, reaction, and synthesis of this class of compounds as reviewed in the Isler's book (*19*), it has become quite possible to draw an accurate structural conclusion with even a minute quantity of pigment. Thus, since 1971, carotenoids of various sponges have been investigated or reinvestigated using these modern spectroscopic methods and carotenoids having cyclopentane end group, triple bond, diosphenol end group, didehydro-β-ring, didehydro-γ-ring, hydroxylated in-chain methyl group, and even sulfate structure have successively been added to the family of sponge carotenoids.

CAROTENOIDS ISOLATED FROM SPONGES

Important carotenoids isolated from sponges are listed in Table 1 (*20*). Those recorded in the older literatures in which the accurate identification of the pigments has not been done are omitted from the list.

TABLE 1. Some carotenoids isolated from sponges

Structure	Carotenoid [IUPAC Name]	(Reference)
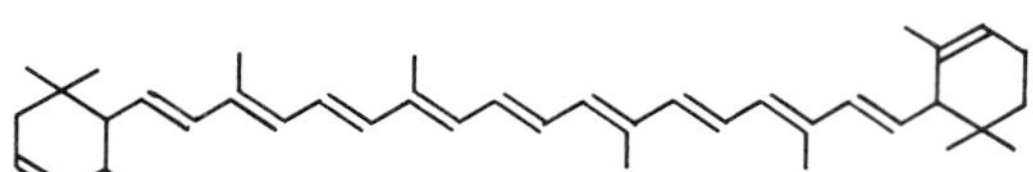 1	ε-carotene [ε,ε-carotene]	(*21*)
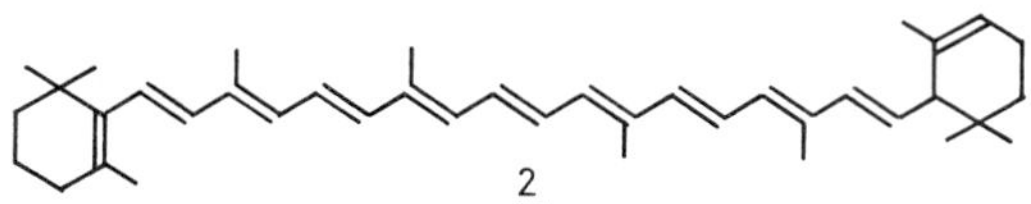 2	α-carotene [β,ε-carotene]	(*12,21,22,23*)
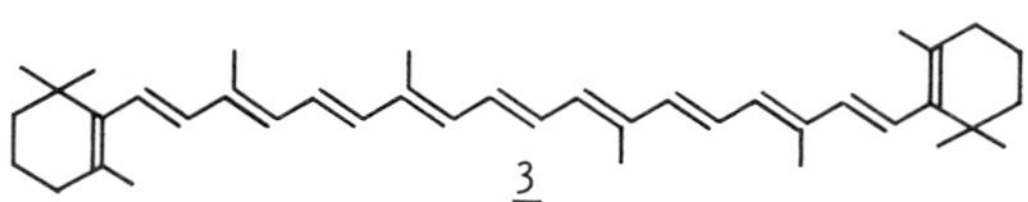 3	β-carotene [β,β-carotene]	(*12,21,23,24*)
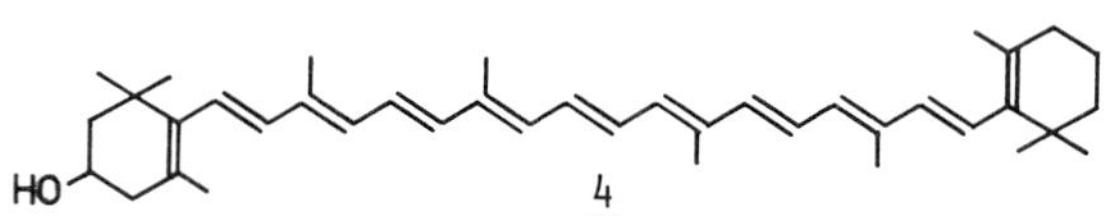 4	cryptoxanthin [β,β-caroten-3-ol]	(*21*)
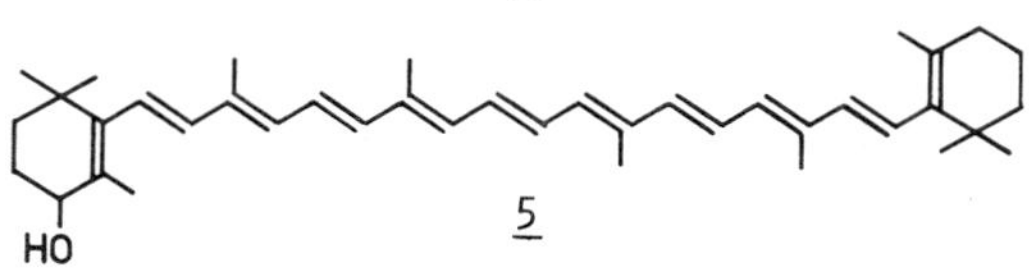 5	isocryptoxanthin [β,β-caroten-4-ol]	(*21*)
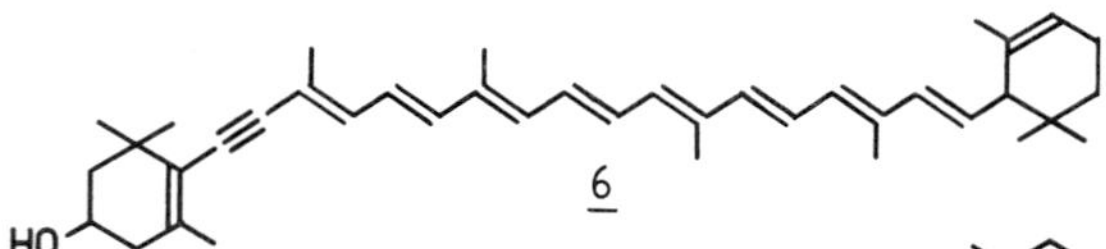 6	crocoxanthin [7,8-didehydro-β,ε-caroten-3-ol]	(*23*)
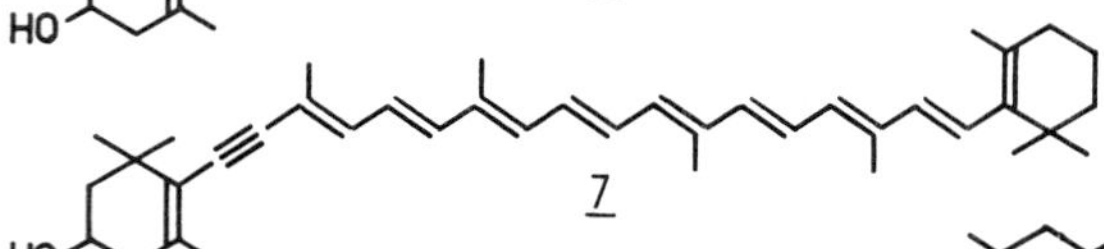 7	allobetaxanthin [7,8-didehydro-β,β-caroten-3-ol]	(*23*)
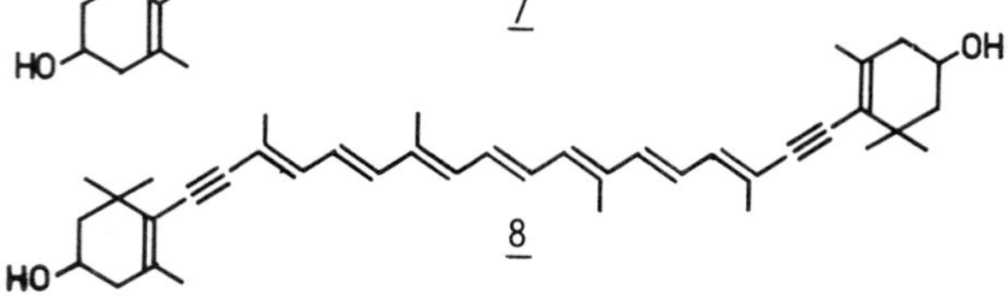 8	alloxanthin [7,8,7',8'-tetradehydro-β,β-carotene-3,3'-diol]	(*23*)
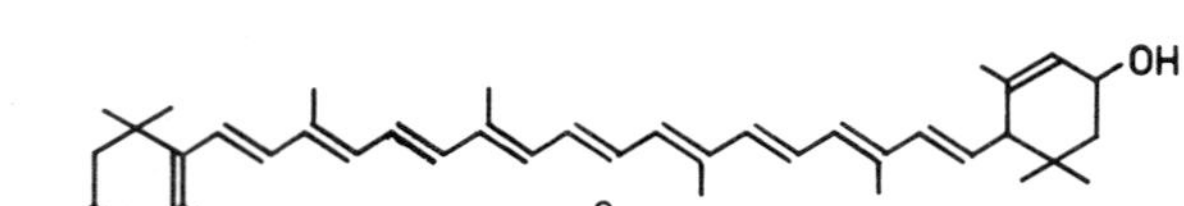 9	lutein [β,ε-carotene-3,3'-diol]	(*21*)

Table 1. Continued

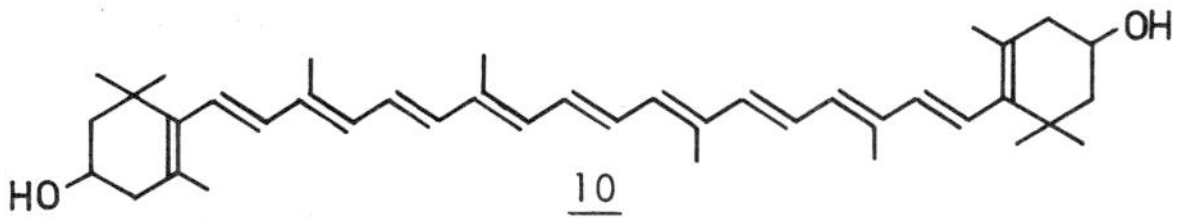

10

zeaxanthin (*21,22*)
[β,β-carotene-3,3'-diol]

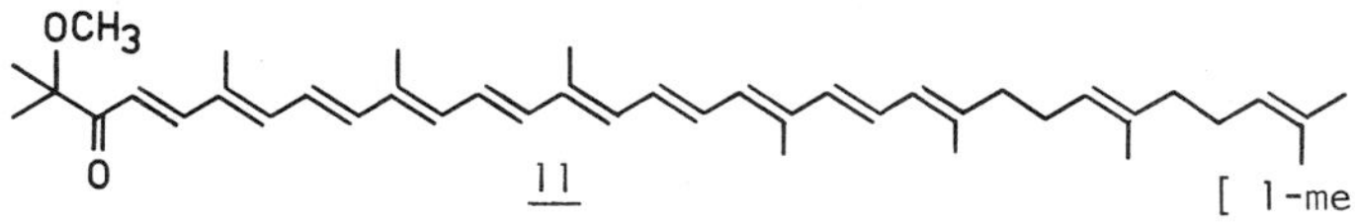

11

spheroidenone = renieraxanthin (*12,37*)
[1-methoxy-3,4-didehydro-1,2,7',8'-tetrahydro-ψ,ψ-caroten-2-one]

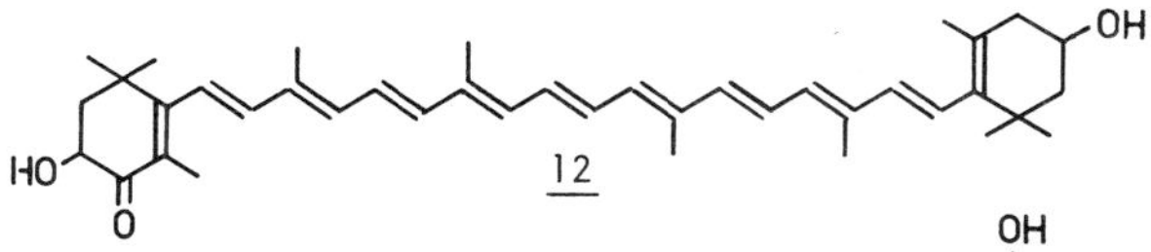

12

β-doradexanthin (*21*)
[3-hydroxy-β,β-caroten-4-one]

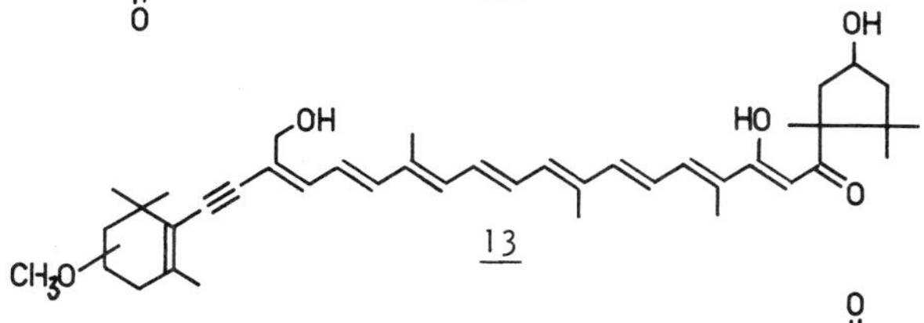

13

agelaxanthin C (*22*)
[7,8-didehydro-19,3',8'-trihydroxy-3(?)-methoxy-β,κ-caroten-6'-one]

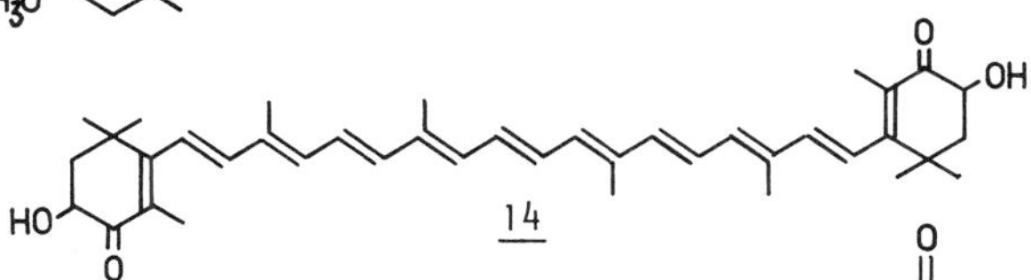

14

astaxanthin (*21*)
[3,3'-dihydroxy-β,β-carotene-4,4'-dione]

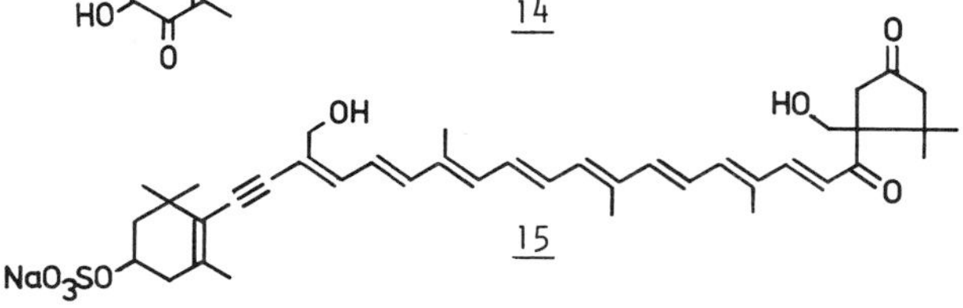

15

sodium 3-0-sulfate of 7,8-didehydro-3,19,18'-trihydroxy-β,κ-carotene-3',6'-dione (*25*)

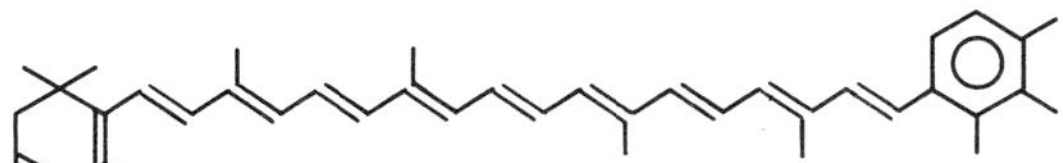

16

tethyatene (*21,26*)
[3,4-didehydro-β,χ-carotene]

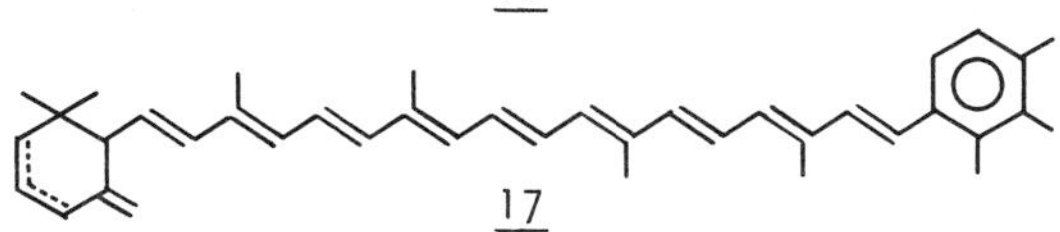

17

[didehydro-γ,χ-carotene] (*23*)

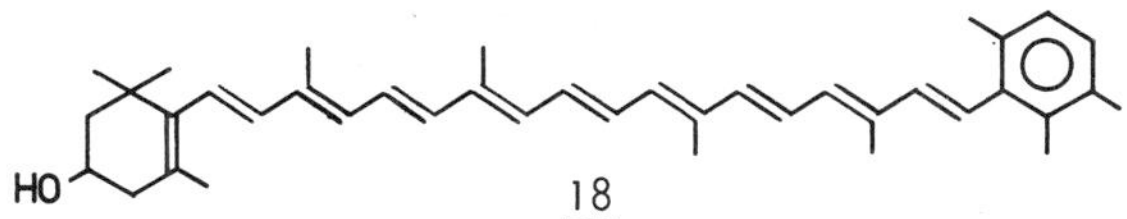

18

agelaxanthin A (*22*)
[β,φ-caroten-3-ol]

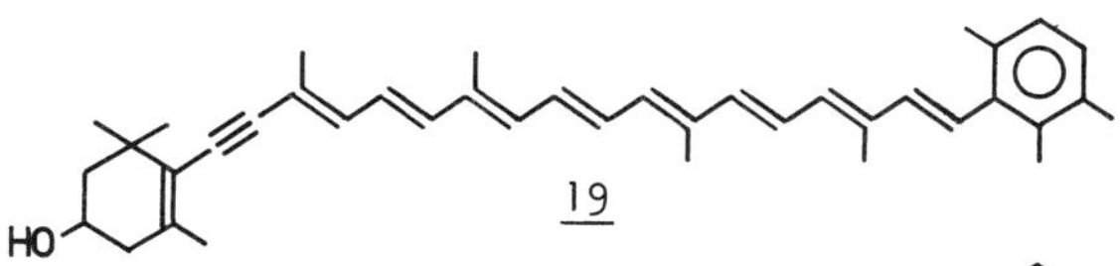

19

isotedaniaxanthin (*29*)
[7,8-didehydro-β,φ-caroten-3-ol]

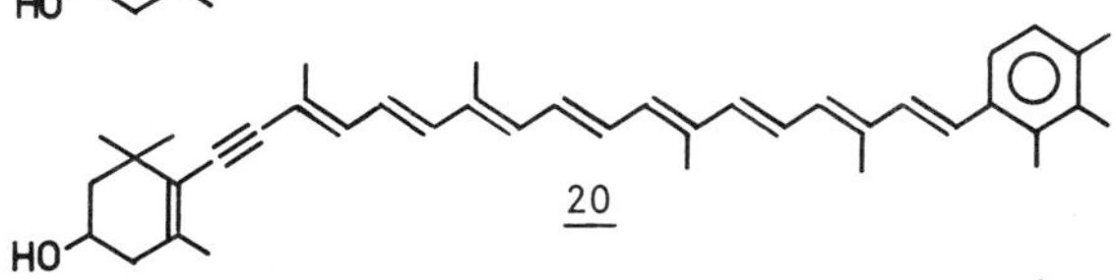

20

tedaniaxanthin = allopurpurin (*21,23,27,28*)
[7,8-didehydro-β,χ-caroten-3-ol]

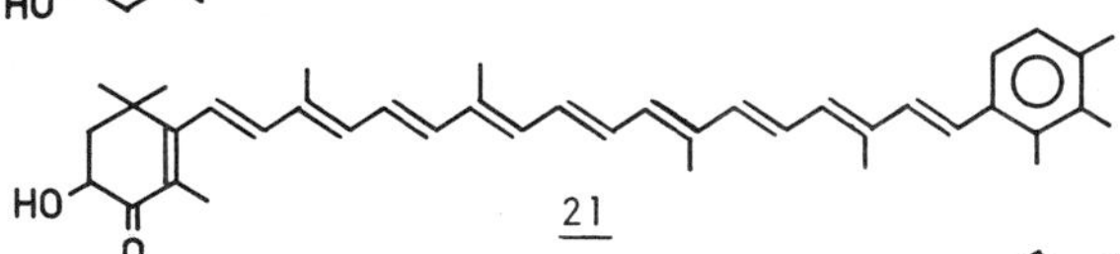

21

clathriaxanthin (*21,23,29,30*)
[3-hydroxy-β,χ-caroten-4-one]

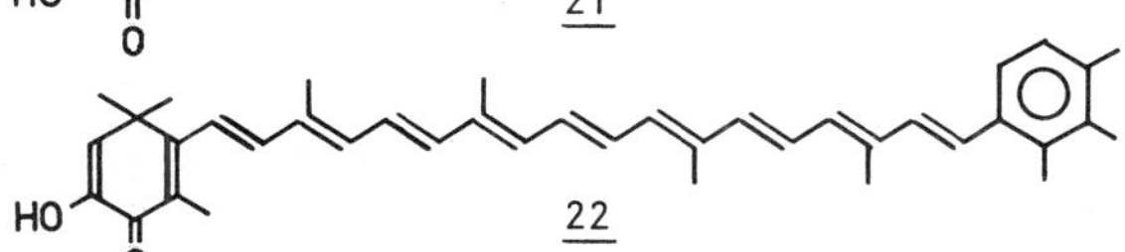

22

tedanin (*21,23,31*)
[β,χ-carotene-3,4-dione]

Table 1. Continued

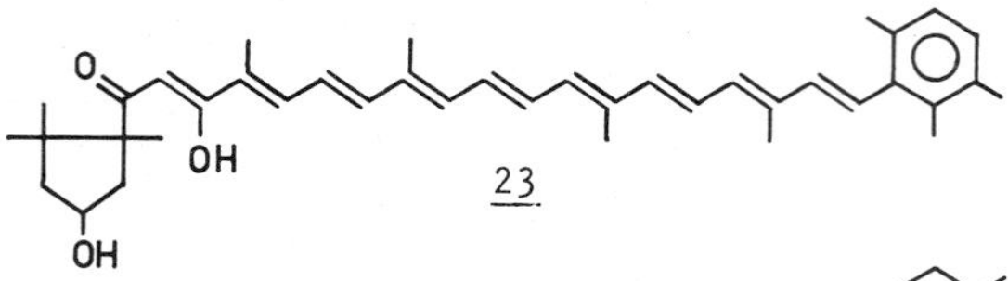

23

trikentriophidin (*23*)
[3-hydroxy-7,8-dihydro-κ,ϕ-carotene-6,8-dione]

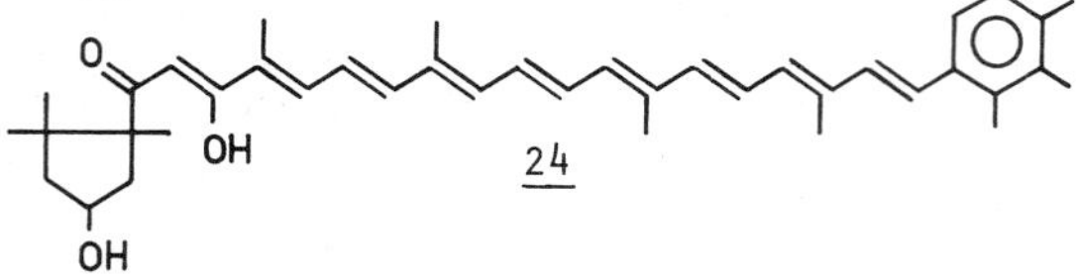

24

trikentriorhodin (*21,22,23,32,33*)
[3-hydroxy-7,8-dihydro-κ,χ-carotene-6,8-dione]

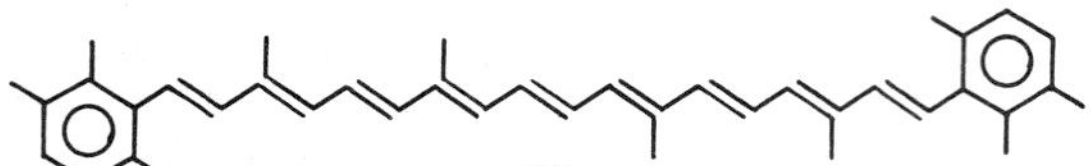

25

isorenieratene (*12,14,21,22*)
[ϕ,ϕ-carotene]

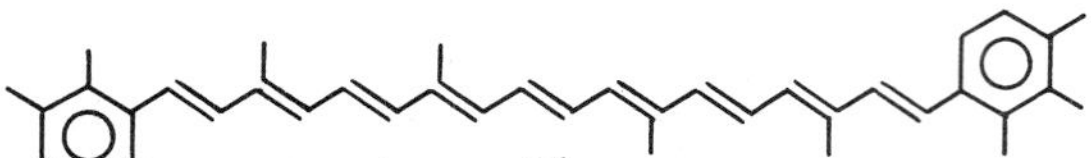

26

renieratene (*12,13,21*)
[ϕ,χ-carotene]

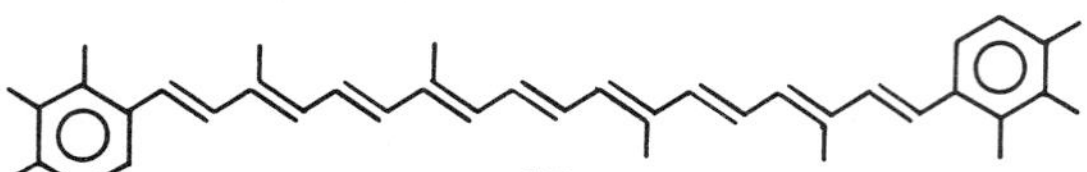

27

renierapurpurin (*12,16*)
[χ,χ-carotene]

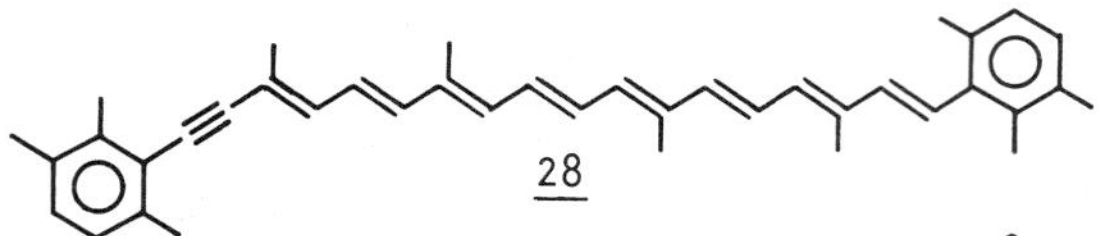

28

didehydroisorenieratene (*12,34*)
[7,8-didehydro-ϕ,ϕ-carotene]

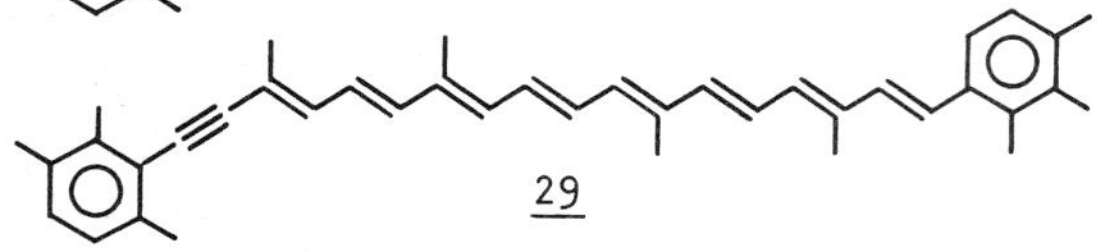

29

didehydrorenieratene (*12,34*)
[7,8-didehydro-ϕ,χ-carotene]

Some recent work on sponge carotenoids is briefly summarized below.

Verongia aerophoba.
The sponge of the Adriatic Sea was investigated by Czeczuga (*24*). By comparison of UV-spectra, Rf-values on TLC, and partition coefficients of the pigments separated by chromatography, the occurrence of β-carotene 3, γ-carotene, isozeaxanthin, lutein 9, zeaxanthin 10, violaxanthin, neoxanthin, and astaxanthin 14 was observed. β-Carotene and astaxanthin were identified by comparison with authentic samples.
Trikentrion helium.
Carotenoids of this sponge were first investigated by Smith (*32*). The main pigment, trikentriorhodin, which occurs both in esterified and unesterified forms, was structurally elucidated to be 24 by Aguilar-Martinez et al. (*33*). The unique cyclopentyl β-dicarbonyl structure had been previously encountered in a mussel carotenoid, mytiloxanthin 30 (*35*), and is considered to be related to the epoxide end group of the algal pigment, fucoxanthin 31.

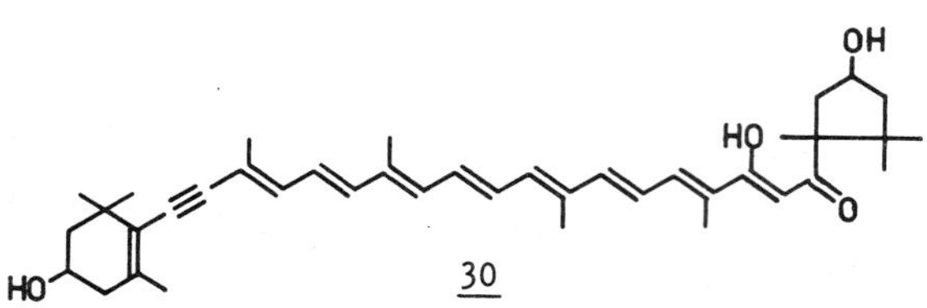

30

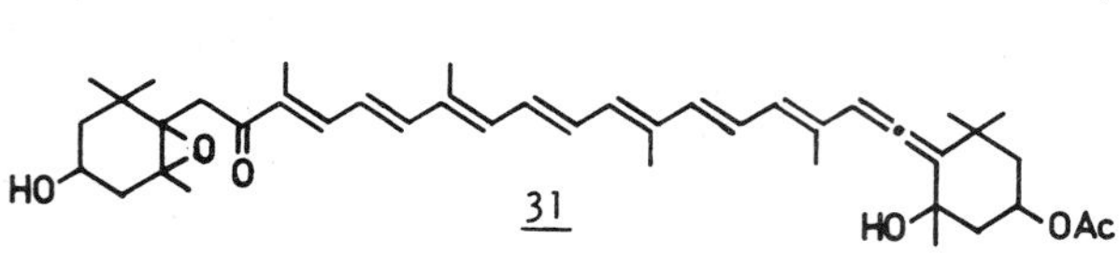

31

Reniera japonica.
In addition to α-carotene, β-carotene, and three aromatic carotenoids, 25, 26, and 27, the presence of at least ten minor pigments was recognized in the earlier report (*12*). Two of them were later shown to be acetylenic aromatic carotenoids, 28 and 29 (*34*), and strangely enough, a carotenoid named renieraxanthin (ca. 1.5% of total carotenoids) is now considered to be identical with the *Rhodopseudomonas* pigment, spheroidenone 11 (*36*) on the basis of UV, IR, CH-analysis, and LAH reduction (*37*). The presence of an acyclic carotenoid is very rare in sponges. It is obviously a product synthesized by symbiotic bacteria.
Tedania digitata.
Tedanin 22 was isolated from this deep red sponge and shown to possess an aromatic and a diosphenol end group by Okukado (*31*). Tanaka et al. also studied the sponge more precisely and in addition to tedanin and three known pigments (Table 2) they discovered two new alicyclic aromatic carotenoids, tedaniaxanthin 20 (*27, 28*) and isotedaniaxanthin 19 (*29*).
Tethya amamensis.
Tanaka and Katayama isolated a new hydrocarbon carotenoid, tethyatene, besides other carotenoids(Table 2) and proposed a structure of didehydro-β,χ-carotene 16 (*26*). The structure was later supported by partial synthesis as described in the following section.
Agelas schmidtii.
The red brown sponge of the West Indies was studied by Buchecker and Eugster (*22*). In addition to the known carotenoids, α-carotene 2, isorenieratene 25, trikentriorhodin 24, and zeaxanthin 10, three new carotenoids, agelaxanthin A, B, and C were isolated. On the basis of spectral and chemical evidence, structures 18 and 13 were assigned to agelaxanthin A and C, respectively.
Agelas mauritiana, Callyspongia confoederata, Clathria frondifera, Haliclona permollis, Hymeniacidon penicillata, and *Spirastrella insignis.*
In addition to *Tedania digitata* and *Tethya amamensis*, Tanaka et al. (*21*) examined the carotenoid composition of these six sponges from southern Japan and classified them into two groups, sponges rich in hydrocarbon carotenoids and those rich in xanthophylls (Table 2).
Microciona prolifera.
Litchfield and Liaaen-Jensen (*23*) carried out a precise study on this sponge distributed along the Atlantic coast of the United States. They isolated clathriaxanthin 21, β-carotene 3, α-carotene 2, crocoxanthin 6, alloxanthin 8, allopurpurin (tedaniaxanthin) 20, trikentriorhodin 24, and three new carotenoids, allobetaxanthin 7, didehydro-γ,χ-carotene 17, and trikentriophidin 23. The major carotenoid, clathriaxanthin, occurred in esterified form and was identified as tedanin 22 after saponification in the presence of oxygen. From biogenetic considerations, the authors classified these pigments into three categories; algal type, 2, 3, 6, 7, and 8; sponge type, 17, 21, 23, and 24; hybrid algal-sponge type, 20; and discussed the possible precursors of these carotenoids.
Ianthella basta.
Liaaen-Jensen (*25*) recently isolated a unique, water-soluble carotenoid sulfate from this sponge, besides other carotenoids of related structures, and elucidated the structure to be 15 by spectroscopic and chemical means. Sulfates of lycoxanthin and zeaxanthin were synthesized for characterization of this type of compound (*38*).

Table 2 was compiled from the data in the literature cited above. Though only a limited number of sponges are compared here, there seems to be a remarkable tendency that nine sponges which produce aromatic carotenoids can be divided into two groups, sponges which mainly produce aromatic hydrocarbon carotenoids and those which mainly produce oxygenated aromatic carotenoids, as has been suggested by Tanaka et al. (*21*), and that the two groups clearly correspond to those producing diaryl carotenoids and those producing monoaryl carotenoids, respectively. In the second group, trikentriorhodin 24 is the very common carotenoid (isomeric trikentriophidin 23 may also have a wide occurrence) and clathriaxanthin 21 (or tedanin 22) is also an important constituent. When the likeliness of the proposed precursors, the epoxide end group of fucoxanthin 31 for the 3-hydroxy-κ-ring of 24 (*35*) and the 3-hydroxy-β-ring for the diosphenol end group of 21 (*39, 40*), is considered, the formation of an aryl group at the other end of the pigment 24 or 21 is quite intriguing. If the 3-hydroxy-β-ring is also the starting terminal group for aromatization, prior introduction of carbonyl group at the other end of polyene chain may induce the fast dehydration of the 3-hydroxy-β-ring to the didehydro-β-ring. However, this mode of dehydration cannot be considered for the dual aromatization in the first diaryl carotenoid-producing group. A different mechanism may operate in the formation of diaryl carotenoids. Anyway, carotenoid biogenesis in sponges is not simple. The complex nature of sponge carotenoids as well as other metabolites seems to come from symbiosis with other living things. It is well known that aromatic carotenoids are encountered in some bacteria (*41*). In this connection, Eimhjellen's work (*42*) on the isolation of photosynthetic bacteria from a sea sponge *Halichondria panicea* is very interesting. Though the result of this investigation could not prove that the carotenoids extractable from *H. panicea* are wholly or partly derived from these bacteria, one of the isolated bacteria proved to be a good source for cross-conjugated aldehydic carotenoids (*43*). This kind of approach may give a clue for the elucidation of the unique biochemistry of sponges.

TABLE 2. Carotenoid composition in some sponges

Sponge	Relative abundance of carotenoid[#]																	
	1	2	3	16*	25*	26*	5	18*	20*	21* or 22*	23*	24*	13	9	10	12	14	Other carotenoids (Reference)
Hymeniacidon penicillata	+	+	++++		++++	++												(*21*)
Reniera japonica		+	++		+++	++++												11, 27* (*12*) 28*, 29*
Tethya amamensis	++	+	++	++		+++												(*21*)
Agelas schmidtti		++			++			++				+++	++		++			(*22*)
Agelas mauritania		+	+							++		++++						(*21*)
Clathria frondifera		+	+						+	++++		++						(*21*)
Haliclona permollis			+++									++		+	+	++	++++	(*21*)
Microciona prolifera		+	+						+	++++	++	++						6, 7, 8 (*23*)
Tedania digitata		+	+		+				++	++++		+++						19* (*21*)
Spirastrella insignis		++													++++			4 (*21*)
Callyspongia confoederata			++++				++++								++++			(*21*)

\# Relative abundance was given by: +, up to 9.9% of total carotenoids; ++, 10-19.9%; +++, 20-29.9%; ++++, over 30%.
* Aromatic carotenoid.

SYNTHESIS OF AROMATIC CAROTENOIDS

Aromatic carotenoids are one of the most interesting group of pigments produced by sponges and considerable efforts have been directed also to the synthesis of this class of compounds. Out of fourteen aromatic carotenoids listed in Table 1, nine have so far been totally or partially synthesized. The early synthesis of renieratene 26, isorenieratene 25, and renierapurpurin 27 have been summarized by Mayer and Isler (*44*). Some further developments will be described here.

7,8-Didehydrorenieratene 29 and 7,8-Didehydroisorenieratene 28.
These highly unsaturated pigments have been synthesized by Ike et al. (*45*) in 9-*cis* as well as all-*trans* form by Wittig condensation of the appropriate phosphoranes and polyene aldehydes.

Trikentriorhodin 24.
Chopra et al. (*46*) synthesized this pigment in an optically active form. The problem in the construction of the β-dicarbonyl structure attached on the end of the polyene chain was solved by Claisen type condensation of the methyl ketone 33 and the polyene ester 34. The methyl ketone was derived from (+)-camphor. Mytiloxanthin 30 was also synthesized in a similar manner.

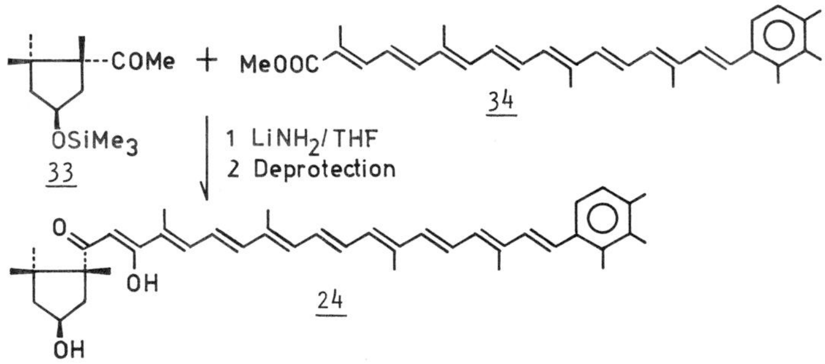

Tedanin 22.
The pigment has been synthesized by Yasuhara et al. (*47*) from β,χ-carotene via its 4-hydroxy 35 and 4-oxo derivatives 36. An isomeric carotenoid β,φ-carotene-3,4-dione has also been synthesized.

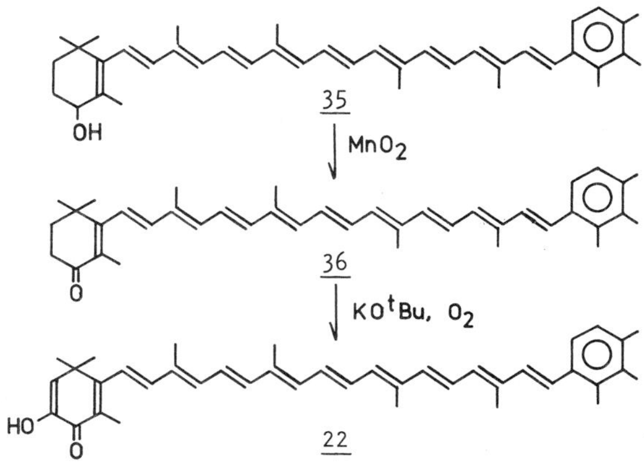

Isorenieratene 25.
Akiyama et al. (*48*) utilized 4-(*t*-butylthio)-3-buten-2-one 37 (*49*) as a synthon for the extension of the isoprenoid polyene chain and synthesized isorenieratene 25 according to the scheme below.

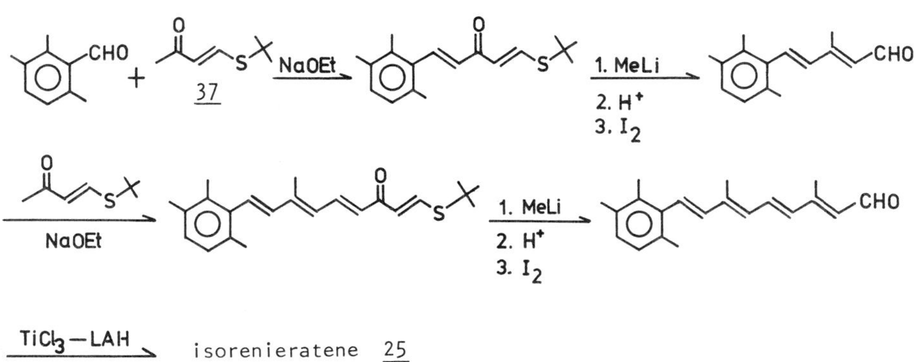

Partial Synthesis of Agelaxanthin A 18, Tedanin 22, and Tethyatene 16.
Shimada et al. (*50*) carried out the partial synthesis of these aromatic carotenoids starting with O-acetyl-β-citraurin 38 derived from natural zeaxanthin by permanganate oxidation of the diacetate (*51*). Condensation of 38 with 2,3,6-trimethylbenzyltriphenylphosphonium bromide in 1,2-epoxybutane followed by saponification gave agelaxanthin A 18. A similar condensation using the 2,3,4-trimethylbenzyl analogue and subsequent hydrolysis led to β,χ-caroten-3-ol 39, isomeric with agelaxanthin A. It is highly probable that 39 exists in sponges. Moffat oxidation of the alcohol 39 gave a ketone 40. The ketone was then smoothly converted into the corresponding enol acetate 41 but the epoxidation of the 3,4-double bond was unsuccessful. Oxidation of the acetate with *t*-butyl hydroperoxide gave tedanin 22 albiet in low yield. Alternatively, direct oxidation of the ketone 40 with oxygen in the presence of strong base such as sodium methylsulfinylmetide gave 22 in good yield. β,χ-Caroten-3-ol 39

was converted into the corresponding N-(methoxycarbonyl)sulfamate (*52*) and then treated with sodium *t*-butoxide to give 3,4-didehydro-β,χ-carotene. Examination of the spectral data showed that identity of the compound with tethyatene 16 is very probable.

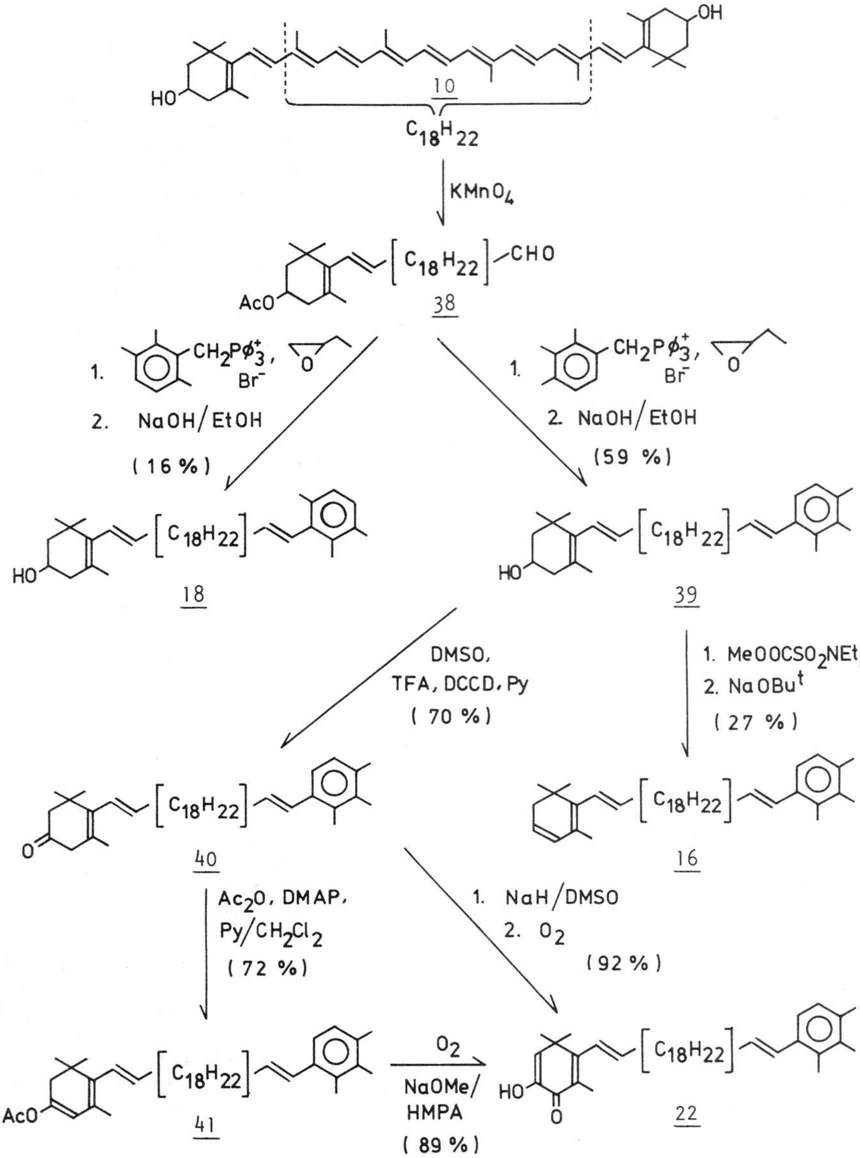

<u>Conversion of Tethyatene 16 into Renieratene 26.</u>
There is little doubt that the ϕ-ring (2,3,6-trimethylphenyl) or the χ-ring (2,3,4-trimethylphenyl) of aromatic carotenoids is formed from the appropriately oxidized or dehydrogenated β-ionone ring in sponges, though the actual biogenetic pathway is quite obscure. However, it is not difficult to find precedents for aromatization accompanied by one methyl migration leading to the formation of 2,3,6-trimethylphenyl ring *in vitro* as well as *in vivo* in non-carotenoid terpenoids as has been discussed by Karrer (*17*) or by Weedon (*18*). For example, didehydro-β-ionone was converted into 42 by tetrachloro-1,2-benzoquinone (*53*) and α-ionone into the same compound by successive treatment with NBS and silver oxide (*54*). The use of active manganese dioxide has also been reported as can be seen in the following example (*55*).

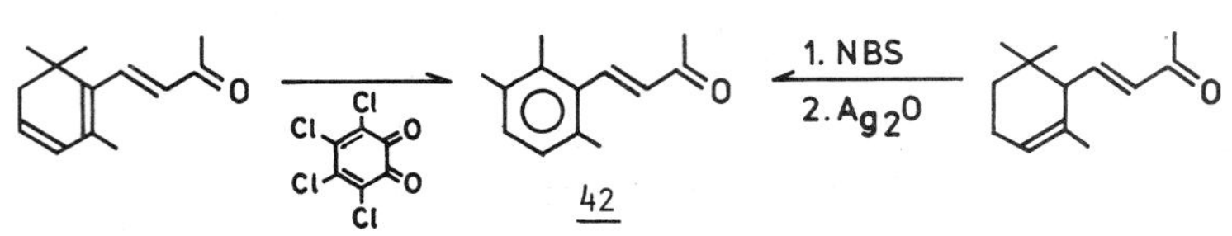

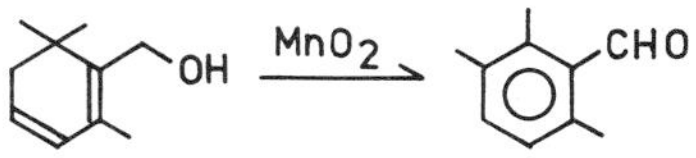

However, no such conversion has so far been realized with carotenoids as substrates except for one very suggestive example reported by Trondheim group. In their study on the structure of an algal carotenoid, myxoxanthophyll 43, Hertzberg and Liaaen-Jensen (*56*) observed that on treatment of the pigment with dry chloroform containing hydrogen chloride, it gave a hydrocarbon carotenoid very reminiscent of 3',4'-didehydrochlorobactene 45 as a major product. Its mass spectrum exhibited, besides other peaks, m/z 530 which corresponded to the molecular ion of 45, and a strong peak m/z 133 characteristic of aromatic carotenoids (*57*). UV-spectra and stereomutation behaviour also showed good agreement with a sample of didehydrochlorobactene derived from chlorobactene (ϕ,ψ-carotene) by the action of NBS. The authors suggested that the successive allylic elimination to 45 might have occurred as depicted below. Though unfortunately the complete characterization of the product could not be achieved because of difficulty in purification, the experiment is very interesting because the path seems to be biogenetically very likely. Further confirmation and, especially, experiments using authentic 44 is desirable.

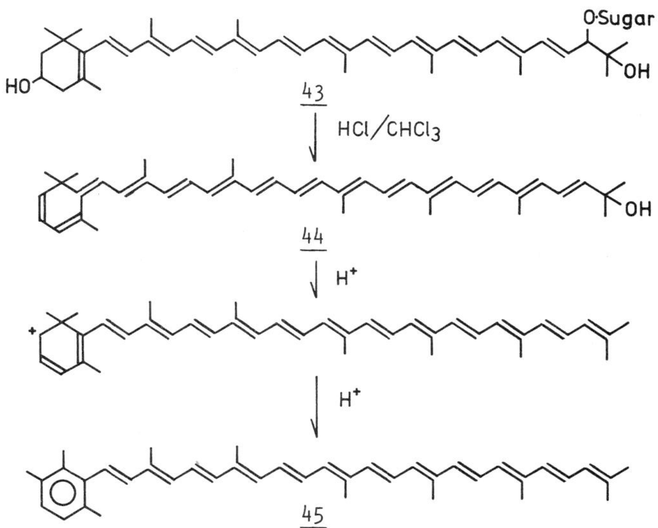

As mentioned in the previous section, a carotenoid hydrocarbon with a 3,4-didehydro-β-ring, tethyatene 16, has been isolated from a sponge (*26*) and the possibility of this end group being a precursor of aromatization to the ϕ-ring has been discussed by Tanaka et al. (*40*) and by Liaaen-Jensen et al. (*23*). Tethyatene also seemed to be a very adequate substrate for *in vitro* aromatization because an aromatic ring already present at the other terminal of the molecule prevents the disposal of the intermediary cation or radical formed at C-2 through α,ω-elimination across the conjugated double bond system. Such an elimination usually results in a mere extension of the chromophore to a retro-type structure. Thus, the oxidation of 16 on the sample obtained by the partial synthesis described above was examined under varied conditions. While NBS, DDQ, ferric chloride, mercuric acetate or mercuric trifluoroacetate gave no aromatization, oxidation with active manganese dioxide (*58*) in acetone afforded some aromatized product. The best result was obtained by γ-manganese dioxide (*59*) and renieratene was obtained in 10% yield as the sole isolable product. The identity was verified by comparison of UV, IR, NMR, and MS spectra with an authentic specimen

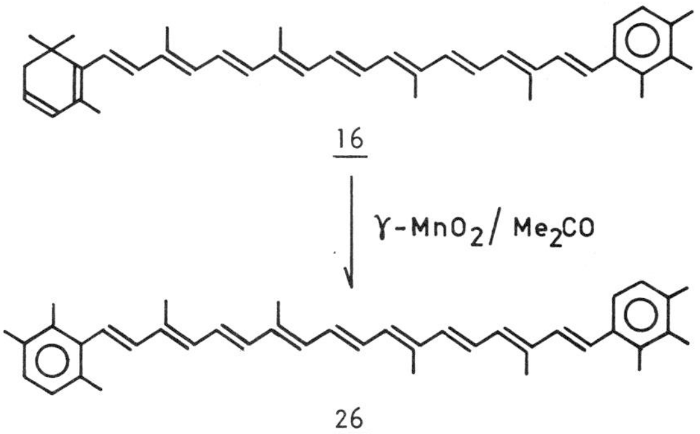

and by mixed mp. However, no trace of renierapurpurin 27 was detected in the reaction mixture, at least on TLC analysis. A similar treatment of 41 did not give an aromatized product. This aromatization is considered to proceed through radical abstraction of allylic hydrogen (*60*) and though such a mechanism might be far from the actual mode of aromatization in sponges, there is no doubt that the didehydro-β-ring is now considered one of the most probable precursors of φ-ring *in vivo*. The production of the χ-ring in sponges is very intriguing. Liaaen-Jensen (*61*) once made an attractive proposal for the formation of the χ-ring in photosynthetic bacteria, that it might be formed by photochemical valence isomerization of the φ-ring as shown below. However, no carotenoids having aromatic terminal group isomeric with the φ- or χ-ring have so far been found in nature though some such carotenoids have been synthesized for reference (*62*).

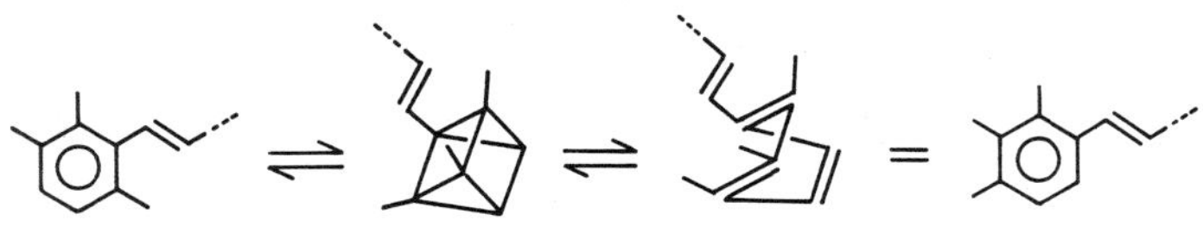

If χ-ring is formed not by phototransposition but by the usual carbonium ion mechanism common in the terpenoid field, a skeletal rearrangement of β-ring must be involved. Though it is very tempting to postulate an intermediary five membered precursor such as 47, for example, in a sense as depicted in the scheme below, no carotenoids having the terminal group, 46, 47, or 48 have been isolated. Biogenetically it is rather likely that both the φ-ring and χ-ring are formed directly from a common precursor such as 49.

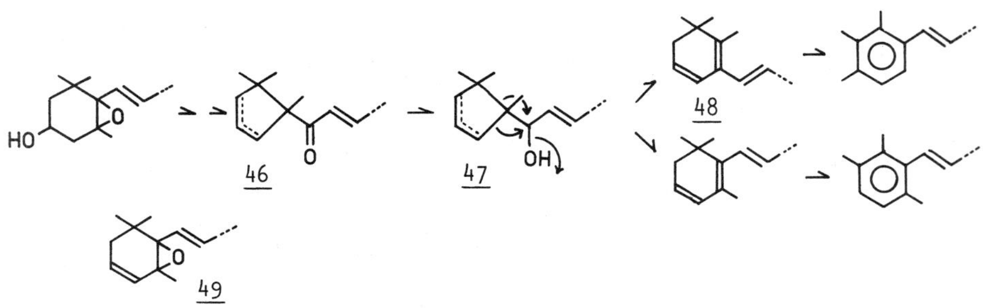

Acknowledgement - The author wishes to thank Professor S. Liaaen-Jensen of University of Trondheim for sending me information on her recent work. Thanks are also due to Professor T. Katayama and Dr. Y. Tanaka for valuable discussions.

REFERENCES

Numbers of references are common throughout the text, Table 1, and Table 2.

1. D.J. Faulkner, *Tetrahedron*, 33, 1421-1443 (1977).
2. For recent reviews: S. Liaaen-Jensen, In *NATO Conference on Marine Natural Products* (Edited by D.J. Faulkner and W.H. Fenical), p.239-260, Plenum Press, New York (1977); S. Liaaen-Jensen, In *Marine Natural Products*, Vol. 2 (Edited by P.J. Schuer), p.1-73, Academic Press, New York (1978).
3. C.Fr.W. Kruckenberg, *Vergleichend-Physiol. Studien*, Ser.1, Part 2, 65-77 (1880); Ser.2, Part 3, 108-115 (1882).
4. C.A. MacMunn, *J. Physiol.*, 9, 1-25 (1888).
5. L.S. Palmer, *Carotinoids and Related Pigments*, p.169-170, Chemical Catalog, New York (1922).
6. E. Lönnberg, *Arkiv. Zool.*, 22, A, No. 14, 1-49 (1931); E. Lönnberg and H. Hellström, *ibid.*, 23, A, No. 15, 1-74 (1931).
7. W. Bergmann and T.B. Johnson, *Z. Physiol. Chem.*, 222, 220-226 (1933).
8. P. Karrer and U. Solmssen, *Helv. Chim. Acta*, 18, 915-921 (1935).
9. E. Lederer, *Bull. Soc. Chim. Biol.*, 20, 567-610 (1938).
10. P.J. Drumm, W.F. O'Connor, and L.P. Renouf, *Biochem. J.*, 39, 208-210 (1945).
11. P. Karrer and E. Jucker, *Carotinoide*, p.95, Birkhäuser Verlag, Basel (1948).
12. T. Tsumaki, M. Yamaguchi, and T. Tsumaki, *J. Chem. Soc. Jpn. Pure Chem. Sect.*, 75, 297-300 (1954); M. Yamaguchi, *Bull. Chem. Soc. Jpn.*, 30, 111-114 (1957).
13. M. Yamaguchi, *Bull. Chem. Soc. Jpn.*, 30, 979-983 (1957); 31, 739-742 (1958).
14. M. Yamaguchi, *Bull. Chem. Soc. Jpn.*, 31, 51-55 (1958).
15. M. Yamaguchi, *Bull. Chem. Soc. Jpn.*, 32, 1171-1173 (1959).

16. M. Yamaguchi, *Bull. Chem. Soc. Jpn.*, 33, 1560-1562 (1960).
17. M.C. Khosla and P. Karrer, *Helv. Chim. Acta*, 43, 453-457 (1960).
18. R.D.G. Cooper, J.B. Davis, and B.C.L. Weedon, *J. Chem. Soc.*, 1963, 5637-5641.
19. O. Isler (Editor), *Carotenoids*, Birkhäuser Verlag, Basel (1971).
20. For convenience, trivial names of carotenoids were used in this article. IUPAC names were added in Table 1 in parentheses.
21. Y. Tanaka, T. Soejima, and T. Katayama, *Bull. Jap. Soc. Sci. Fish.*, 44, 1283-1285 (1978).
22. R. Buchecker and C.H. Eugster, *Helv. Chim. Acta*, 60, 2780-2788 (1977).
23. C. Litchfield and S. Liaaen-Jensen, *Comp. Biochem. Physiol* 66B, 359-365 (1980).
24. B. Czeczuga, *Marine Biol.*, 10, 254-257 (1971).
25. S. Liaaen-Jensen, *Proc. 12th Int. IUPAC Symp. Chem. Natur. Prod.*, L23, p.47, Tenerife (1980).
26. Y. Tanaka and T. Katayama, *Bull. Jap. Soc. Sci. Fish.*, 43, 1229-1232 (1977).
27. Y. Tanaka, Y. Fujita, and T. Katayama, *Bull. Jap. Soc. Sci. Fish.*, 43, 761-765 (1977).
28. Y. Tanaka and T. Katayama, *Bull. Jap. Soc. Sci. Fish.*, 45, 633-634 (1979).
29. Y. Tanaka and T. Katayama, *Bull. Jap. Soc. Sci. Fish.*, 46, 381-383 (1980).
30. Y. Tanaka and T. Katayama, *Bull. Jap. Soc. Sci. Fish.*, 42, 801-805 (1976).
31. N. Okukado, *Bull. Chem. Soc. Jpn.*, 48, 1061-1062 (1975).
32. V.E. Smith, *Comparative Cytology and Biochemistry of Two Marine Sponges*, Thesis, Univ. California, San Diego (1968).
33. M. Aguilar-Martinez and S. Liaaen-Jensen, *Acta Chem. Scand.*, B28, 1247-1248 (1974).
34. T. Hamasaki, N. Okukado, and M. Yamaguchi, *Bull. Chem. Soc. Jpn.*, 46, 1884-1885 (1973).
35. A. Khare, G.P. Moss, and B.C.L. Weedon, *Tetrahedron Lett.*, 1973, 3921-3924 (1973).
36. J.B. Davis, L.M. Jackman, P.T. Siddons, and B.C.L. Weedon, *Proc. Chem. Soc.*, 1961, 261; O. Straub, *Key to Carotenoids*, p.67, Birkhäuser Verlag, Basel (1976).
37. T. Inazu and M. Yamaguchi, unpublished result.
38. T. Ramdahl and S. Liaaen-Jensen, *Acta Chem. Scand.*, B34, 773-774 (1980).
39. T. Katayama, H. Yokoyama, and C.O. Chichester, *Int. J. Biochem.*, 1, 438-444 (1970); T. Katayama, M. Shimaya, M. Sameshima, and C.O. Chichester, *Int. J. Biochem.*, 4, 223-226 (1973).
40. Y. Tanaka, *Comparative Biochemical Studies on Carotenoids in Aquatic Animals*, Mem. Fac. Fish. Kagoshima Univ., 27, No.2, 355-422 (1978).
41. S. Liaaen-Jensen, In *The Photosynthetic Bacteria* (Edited by R.K. Clayton and W.R. Sistrom), p.233-245, Plenum Press, New York (1978).
42. K.E. Eimhjellen, *Acta Chem. Scand.*, 21, 2280-2281 (1967).
43. A.J. Aasen and S. Liaaen-Jensen, *Acta Chem. Scand.*, 21, 2185-2204 (1967).
44. H. Mayer and O. Isler, In *Carotenoids* (Edited by O. Isler), p.325-575, Birkhäuser Verlag, Basel (1971).
45. T. Ike, J. Inanaga, A. Nakano, N. Okukado, and M. Yamaguchi, *Bull. Chem. Soc. Jpn.*, 47, 350-354 (1974).
46. A.K. Chopra, G.P. Moss, and B.C.L. Weedon, *J. Chem. Soc. Chem. Commun.*, 1977, 467-468.
47. M. Yasuhara, K. Inanaga, T. Kumae, H.R. Brahmana, N. Okukado, and M. Yamaguchi, *Bull. Chem. Soc. Jpn.*, 53, 1629-1631 (1980).
48. S. Akiyama, S. Nakatsuji, S. Eda, M. Kataoka, and M. Nakagawa, *Tetrahedron Lett.*, 1979, 2813-2816.
49. S. Akiyama, S. Nakatsuji, T. Hamamura, M. Kataoka, and M. Nakagawa, *Tetrahedron Lett.*, 1979, 2809-2812.
50. S. Shimada, Y. Ezaki, J. Inanaga, T. Katsuki, and M. Yamaguchi, *Tetrahedron Lett.*, 22, 773-774 (1981).
51. P. Karrer, A. Rüegger, and U. Solmssen, *Helv. Chim. Acta*, 21, 448-451 (1938).
52. P. Crabbé and C. Léon, *J. Org. Chem.*, 35, 2594-2596 (1970): Application to carotenoid alcohols; S. Takimoto, K. Chin, N. Okukado, and M. Yamaguchi, *Mem. Fac. Sci. Kyushu Univ.*, Ser.C, 8, 197-202 (1973); *Chem. Abstr.*, 79, 42706 w (1973).
53. E.A. Braude, L.M. Jackman, R.P. Linstead, and G. Lowe, *J. Chem. Soc.*, 1960, 3123-3132.
54. G. Büchi, K. Seitz, and O. Jeger, *Helv. Chim. Acta*, 32, 39-46 (1949).
55. B. Bächli and P. Karrer, *Helv. Chim. Acta*, 38, 1863-1869 (1955). Some further examples of dehydrogenative aromatization of cyclohexene or cyclohexadiene derivatives bearing a side chain with an α-oxo functionality by active MnO_2: J.C. Leffingwell and H.J. Bluhm, *J. Chem. Soc. Chem. Commun.*, 1969, 1151-1152; S. Danishefsky and R. Cunningham, *J. Org. Chem.*, 30, 3676-3679 (1965).
56. S. Hertzberg and S. Liaaen-Jensen, *Phytochemistry*, 8, 1259-1280 (1969).
57. W. Vetter, G. Englert, N. Rigassi, and U. Schwieter, In reference 19, p.189-266.
58. J. Attenburrow, A.F.B. Cameron, J.H. Chapman, R.M. Evans, B.A. Hems, A.B.A. Jansen, and T. Walker, *J. Chem. Soc.*, 1952, 1094-1111.
59. L.I. Vereschchagin, S.R. Gainulina, S.A. Podskrebysheva, L.A. Gaiboronskii, L.L. Okhapkina, V.G. Voro'eva, and V.P. Latyshev, *J. Org. Chem. USSR*, 8, 1143-1147 (1972).
60. E.F. Pratt and S.P. Suskind, *J. Org. Chem.*, 28, 638-642 (1963).
61. S. Liaaen-Jensen, *Pure Appl. Chem.*, 20, 421-448 (1969).
62. T. Hamasaki, K. Chin, N. Okukado, and M. Yamaguchi, *Bull. Chem. Soc. Jpn.*, 46, 1553-1554 (1973).

CAROTENOPROTEINS

George Britton, Gillian M. Armitt, Stephen Y. M. Lau

Ashvin K. Patel and Clifford C. Shone

Department of Biochemistry, University of Liverpool, P.O. Box 147, Liverpool, L69 3BX, U.K.

Abstract - Carotenoids frequently occur *in vivo* in association with protein. Carotenoid-protein complexes have been isolated from many sources, e.g. photosynthetic membranes. The most striking and intriguing are the carotenoproteins, from marine invertebrate animals, in which binding to protein causes a large shift in the carotenoid light absorption spectrum so that the complexes are purple, blue or green in colour. This article will review work on carotenoid-protein complexes published since Zagalsky's survey at the Bern Symposium. Particular emphasis will be placed on a description of some new carotenoproteins, new information about the primary and quaternary structures of some carotenoproteins, studies of the reconstitution of complexes from apoproteins and selected carotenoids, and investigations by spectroscopic methods. Some ideas about the mechanism of binding and the spectral shift will be discussed.

INTRODUCTION

At the Bern meeting in 1975, Zagalsky (Ref. 1) presented a comprehensive survey of carotenoid-protein complexes. This review is now intended to report on progress in the field during the six years since then.

In living tissues, carotenoids frequently occur in association with protein. In the photosynthetic apparatus of plants, algae and bacteria, for example, carotenoids are associated with chlorophyll and protein in the various functional units, and some specific pigment-protein complexes have been isolated and studied, e.g. a violaxanthin-protein from *Scenedesmus obliquus* (Ref. 2) and peridinin - chlorophyll - proteins from dinoflagellates (Ref. 3). Complexes such as these, and their functioning mechanisms, are more appropriate to the 'Photosynthesis' section of the Symposium and will not be discussed further here. In many ways the most interesting of the carotenoid-protein complexes are the carotenoproteins which are found primarily in invertebrate animals and are characterised by a very large bathochromic shift in the light absorption spectrum, giving rise to purple and blue colours, in contrast to the orange of the free carotenoid. A well known example of this phenomenon is provided by the lobster, *Homarus gammarus*, which in its natural state is blue, due to the presence of the carotenoprotein pigment, α-crustacyanin. Boiling causes the lobster to change from blue to red, as the protein is denatured and the free carotenoid astaxanthin (3,3'-dihydroxy-β,β-carotene-4,4'-dione) is liberated. Crustacyanin has been investigated extensively, and many similar complexes have been found in a range of animals and tissues. Generally the carotenoid composition of these complexes is specific and the carotenoid-protein ratio is stoichiometric. The carotenoproteins are water-soluble and much more stable than the free carotenoid or protein alone.

This article, like that of Zagalsky (Ref. 1) will concentrate on these special animal carotenoproteins. No attempt will be made to attribute particular functions to carotenoproteins or to speculate about their possible evolutionary relationships or significance. The approach will be chemical and biochemical, and will deal largely with structures and the mechanism of binding. It is not intended to be an exhaustive survey. For this the reader should consult the review by Zagalsky (Ref. 1), the earlier survey by Cheesman, Lee and Zagalsky (Ref. 4), and the papers compiled in the book of Lee (Ref. 5). This progress report will concentrate on certain aspects:- a brief survey of some new carotenoproteins which have been described since 1975, new information about the protein structures, spectroscopic studies, and studies of the reconstitution of complexes from proteins and selected carotenoids. Some ideas about the mechanism of binding and of the spectral shift will be discussed.

SOME NEW CAROTENOPROTEINS

Details have been published of the characterisation of the blue astaxanthin-protein from the chondrophore *Velella velella* (Ref. 6) and the canthaxanthin-protein from the crustacean *Branchippus stagnalis* (Ref. 7), both of which were discussed in the review by Zagalsky (Ref. 1). In addition, several carotenoproteins have been described in detail for the first time.

Yellow lobster proteins.

The blue crustacyanins from lobster (*Homarus gammarus*) carapace are well characterised, and further work on their quaternary structures will be discussed below. Lobster carapace has also yielded a yellow pigment, λ_{max} 409 nm, in which some twenty astaxanthin molecules appear to be stacked like a pile of plates (Ref. 8). Photoacoustic spectroscopy of the lobster shell has provided evidence of yellow carotenoproteins both at the outer surface and in the interior of the endocuticle (Ref. 9). Zagalsky (Ref. 10) has now isolated from lobster carapace two new yellow astaxanthin-proteins absorbing in the 400 and 470 nm regions. 'Pigment Y_1' with λ_{max} at 398, 470 nm had a Stokes radius of 130Å, i.e. was rather larger than α-crustacyanin, whereas 'pigment Y_2', λ_{max} 401, 470 nm, was smaller, with Stokes radius 60Å. On SDS-PAGE (sodium dodecyl sulphate polyacrylamide gel electrophoresis), both gave predominantly two subunits, identical in size to those of α-crustacyanin.

Starfish carotenoproteins.

Asterias rubens. The occurrence of a carotenoprotein in the dorsal skin of the starfish *Asterias rubens* was first reported by von Euler and Hellström in 1934 (Ref. 11), and the carotenoids present were later characterised as astaxanthin and its acetylenic analogues 3,3'-dihydroxy-7,8-didehydro-β,β-carotene-4,4'-dione and 3,3'-dihydroxy-7,8,7',8'-tetradehydro-β,β-carotene-4,4'-dione (Ref. 12). Detailed studies of the *Asterias* carotenoprotein have now been reported by two groups (Ref. 13-15). This pigment, referred to as asteriarubin by the Trondheim group, is purple with λ_{max} between 550 and 570 nm depending on the relative proportions of the three carotenoid prosthetic groups. The protein is much smaller and simpler than most other carotenoproteins that have been described, having molecular weight 43000 and four apparently identical subunits. Extensively purified samples retain a small amount of carbohydrate and lipid. The amino acid composition has been determined (Table 1). It is an acidic protein, I.E.P. 4.5, with a high content of aspartic and glutamic acids but, interestingly, little or no tyrosine or tryptophan, so that there is little u.v. light absorption at 280 nm. Because the *Asterias* pigment is such a small protein with simple subunits it lends itself well to structural investigation, and the first stages of amino acid sequence determination will be outlined below. It is also amenable to reconstitution studies. Treatment with suitable organic solvent detaches the carotenoid, and the colourless apoprotein (40000 daltons) can be recombined with a range of carotenoids. Such reconstitution work will also be described later.

TABLE 1. Amino acid composition of the *Asterias rubens* carotenoprotein.
The figures indicate the number of times each amino acid occurs per subunit (total 129 amino acid residues)

Lysine - 8	Glutamic acid - 10	Isoleucine - 6
Histidine - 2	Proline - 5	Leucine - 14
Arginine - 5	Glycine - 5	Tyrosine - 1
Aspartic acid - 17	Alanine - 10	Phenylalanine-7
Threonine - 10	Valine - 10	Cysteine - 6
Serine - 8	Methionine - 5	Tryptophan-0

Marthasterias glacialis. The much larger spiny starfish *Marthasterias glacialis* has dorsal skin which ranges in colour from brown to grey or blue-black, due to the presence of pigments which were first referred to as carotenoproteins by Fox and Vevers (Ref. 16). Recent work in our laboratory (Ref. 17,18) has now led to the isolation of two carotenoproteins, one purple, one blue, which are quite different in their characteristics. The purple pigment, which has an absorption spectrum with λ_{max} at 555 nm and vestiges of vibrational fine structure, is very soluble in water or low ionic strength buffer between pH 3.5 and 8.5, and is very stable in the presence of 0.5*M* NaCl. The major carotenoid component (90-95%) is (3*S*,3'*S*)-astaxanthin, with some (5-10%) adonirubin (3-hydroxy-β,β-carotene-4,4'-dione) and traces of other carotenoids. Preliminary gel filtration and SDS-PAGE analysis shows a molecular weight of 43000 and four subunits, i.e. similarities with the *Asterias* protein, though other properties, such as a carotenoid: protein ratio of 4:1 as opposed to 1:1 for *Asterias*, are quite distinct. Isoelectric focusing revealed the presence of ten protein bands, all with pI between 3.58 and 4.59.

The Marthasterias blue protein has a more complex absorption spectrum with λ_{max} at 463, 489 and 600 nm, with the position of the longest wavelength band showing a dependency on NaCl concentration, i.e. being at 612 nm at 1.0M NaCl. This protein has a substantial lipid content, and is not very soluble in aqueous solution, aggregating to form a blue precipitate even at low ionic strengths. This tendency to precipitate, and the apparent hydrophobic nature of the complex, make it rather a difficult protein to purify and analyse. However, gel filtration indicates a molecular weight of 72000, with four carotenoid molecules present. The main carotenoid is again astaxanthin (60-70%) with adonirubin (3-6%) and several other carotenoids, including canthaxanthin (β,β-carotene-4,4'-dione) and zeaxanthin (β,β-carotene-3,3'-diol), contributing the remaining 25-35%. SDS-PAGE revealed the presence of two types of protein subunit, the major one (16000 daltons) with no carbohydrate, the minor one (13000 daltons) staining for carbohydrate. The amino acid composition showed unusually high threonine and arginine contents, whereas the glycine and leucine contents were low and proline appeared to be absent.

Of the two Marthasterias carotenoproteins, the purple one appears to be similar in some ways to the purple pigment of Asterias rubens. The blue protein, however, is quite different in properties. Its absorption spectrum is somewhat similar to that of ovoverdin from lobster eggs, which has two main absorption peaks at 460 and 640 nm, due to carotenoid molecules in different protein environments. It seems likely that the same is true for the Marthasterias blue pigment.

Coral carotenoproteins - alloporin.
The coral Allopora californica has attracted attention because of its deep violet colour, which Fox and coworkers (Ref. 19) tentatively attributed to a complex involving an enol-diester structure between the carotenoid astaxanthin and $CaCO_3$ of the coral's aragonite skeleton. It has now been established that the violet colour is produced by a water-soluble carotenoprotein, alloporin, with λ_{max} 545 nm (Ref. 20). The prosthetic group is astaxanthin, mainly the (3S,3'S)-isomer (at least 75%, from the CD spectrum), and no other lipid is present. Alloporin has four similar or identical subunits and a total molecular weight of 68000, with a carotenoid:protein ratio of 1:1. The high content of acidic amino acids in alloporin may account for its stable arrangement in the $CaCO_3$ skeleton.

Other corals. Carotenoproteins have also been isolated from other corals of the order Hydrocorallinae (Ref. 21). Stylaster roseus (purple-red) yielded a violet complex, λ_{max} 540 nm, with astaxanthin as the only carotenoid present. The pale red or pink S. elegans and S. sanguineus, however, gave complexes with λ_{max} (448), 470, (498) nm and (450), 474, (500) nm respectively, each containing both astaxanthin and zeaxanthin (1:1). Three Distichopora species also gave coloured aqueous extracts. A red extract (λ_{max} 488 nm) from D. coccinea contained astaxanthin and traces of a zeaxanthin-like compound. D. nitida gave a yellow complex, λ_{max} 430, 452, 482 nm, containing approximately equal amounts of astaxanthin and zeaxanthin, whereas the dark red D. violacea extract yielded astaxanthin with traces of zeaxanthin.

Orconectes limosus pigment.
A yellow-red carotenoprotein from the crayfish Orconectes limosus has a complex absorption spectrum with λ_{max} at 335, 460, 675 nm. The carotenoid prosthetic group is a mixture of astaxanthin and canthaxanthin. No molecular weight studies were reported, but the amino acid composition has been determined; no tyrosine or phenylalanine were detected (Ref. 22).

The pigment of Salpa cylindrica.
The pale blue oceanic tunicate Salpa cylindrica changes irreversibly to purple on freezing, and yields a water-soluble purple pigment, λ_{max} 560 nm (Ref. 23). Like a typical carotenoprotein this pigment is denatured by treatment with acetone and yields a yellow product with a carotenoid-like absorption spectrum, λ_{max} (ethanol) 443 nm. Reduction with $NaBH_4$ or saponification with KOH gives products with absorption maxima at lower wavelengths. The 'free carotenoid' is extremely polar and it has not yet been possible to purify and characterise it, but the reasonance Raman spectrum of the complex is typical of the carotenoid chromophore of carotenoproteins (Ref. 24). The prosthetic group is obviously not canthaxanthin or astaxanthin, as in other carotenoproteins. This purple salp pigment is completely different from all other known animal carotenoproteins and clearly merits further detailed study.

The Rhynchosciara americana pigment.
Carotenoproteins are usually considered characteristic pigments of marine invertebrate animals, but they have also been found in terrestrial animals, including insects. A recent paper reports the isolation and characterisation of a violet carotenoprotein from the haemolymph of a fly Rhynchosciara americana (Ref. 25). This pigment has molecular weight 157000 and consists of four apparently identical subunits. Three molecules of echinenone (β,β-caroten-4-one) and one of canthaxanthin are present per molecule of protein. The absorption spectrum is complicated but has been analysed as a superimposition of two spectra, λ_{max} 465 and 545 nm respectively. The complex exhibits circular dichroism in the

visible region, which must be induced by the protein conformation since the free carotenoids are optically inactive. Two sites of carotenoid-protein interaction are indicated, one unrestricted and the other distorted.

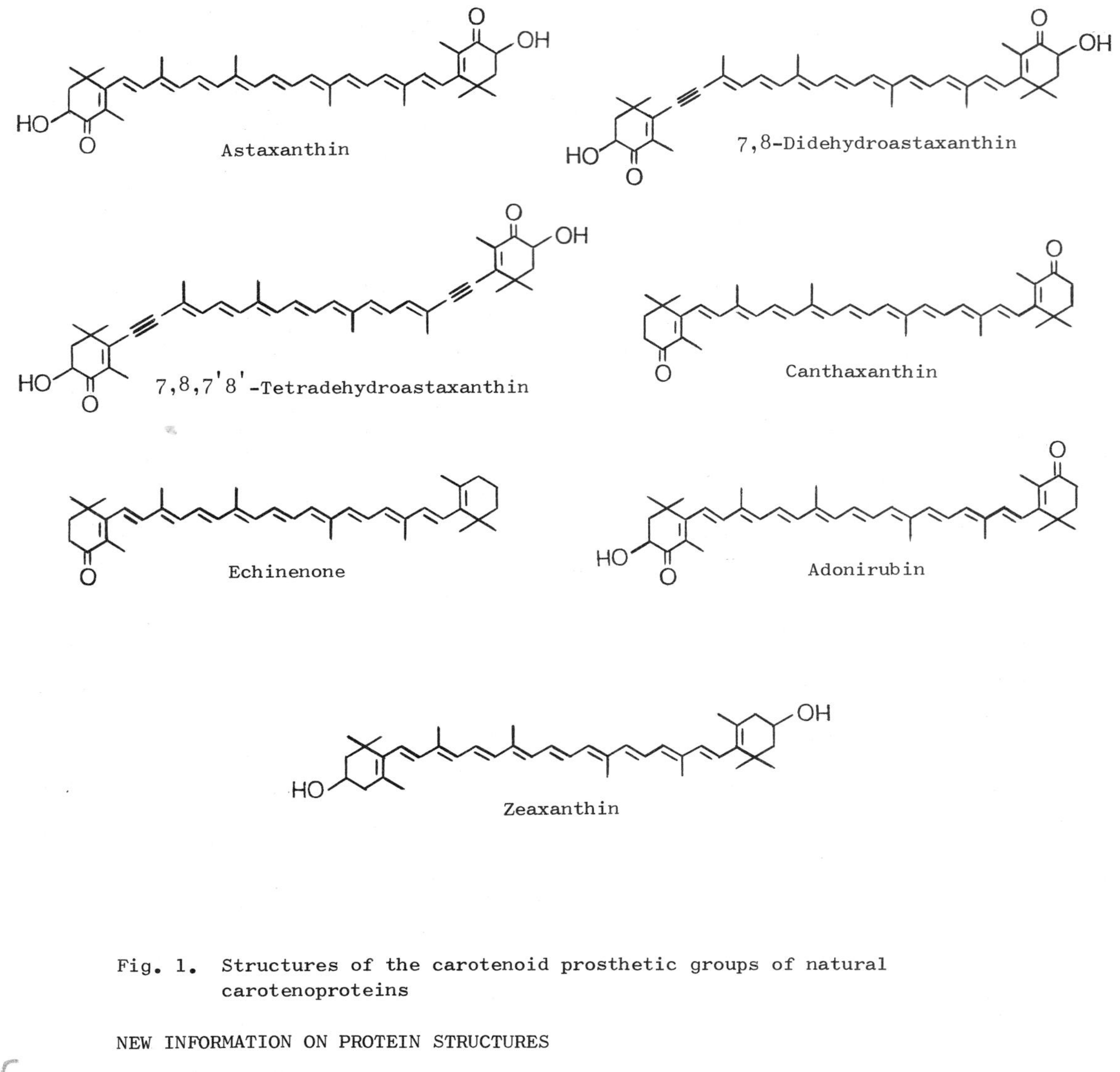

Fig. 1. Structures of the carotenoid prosthetic groups of natural carotenoproteins

NEW INFORMATION ON PROTEIN STRUCTURES

Quaternary structures.

Crustacyanin. The native blue lobster protein α-crustacyanin, λ_{max} 628 nm, dissociates reversibly at low ionic strength to give the purple α'-crustacyanin which on standing changes irreversibly into β-crustacyanin (λ_{max} 585 nm) which is electrophoretically heterogeneous (ref. 26, 27). It was known that each α-crustacyanin molecule yields eight β-crustacyanin units each binding two molecules of astaxanthin, and that, on removal of the carotenoid, the β-crustacyanin dissociates into the colourless apoprotein, which is about half its size (ca. 20000 daltons). Details have now been published (Ref. 28) of studies of the quaternary structure of crustacyanin, as summarised by Zagalsky (Ref. 1). The apoprotein, apocrustacyanin, was separated into five electrophoretically distinct components which seemed to fall into two sets, A_1, C_1 and C_2 (22000 daltons) and A_2 and A_3 (19000 daltons). The amino acid compositions were similar, but some small though real differences were found between the sets. Combinations of two of the five components are used to form the various β-crustacyanins. The preference seems to be for a β-crustacyanin to be made from one protein from each of the two apoprotein sets. Table 2 shows the apoprotein composition of the six β-crustacyanins that have been detected. α-Crustacyanin is an octameric form of β-crustacyanin, and the contribution of the different β-forms to the octamer structure differs depending on the method of dissociation used. Thus α-crustacyanin dissociated by dialysis contains approximately five $\beta_{1\ a+1\ b}$, two β_2 a and one β_4 crustacyanins, whereas treatment with KCNS or urea gives increasing amounts of β_3-crustacyanin.

The overall picture that emerges is of α-crustacyanin as a composite octameric structure, with different contributions from the various β-crustacyanin units, which are themselves composed of different combinations of apoprotein subunits. Astaxanthin (one molecule per apoprotein) is thought to effect the dimerisation to form β-crustacyanin by altering the tertiary structure of the subunits rather than by acting as a direct cross link.

TABLE 2. Apoprotein subunit composition of the six β-crustacyanin components separable by DEAE-cellulose chromatography

β-Crustacyanin	Subunits
β_1 a	$A_2 + C_2$
β_1 b	$A_2 + C_1$
β_2 a	$A_3 + C_1$
β_2 b	$A_3 + C_2$
β_3	$A_2 + A_1$
β_4	$A_3 + A_1$

The quaternary structures of α-crustacyanin and the Velella pigment (see below) have now been examined by electron microscopy (Ref. 29). In the electron micrograph of α-crustacyanin several different structures consistent in size with the Stokes radius of the protein (73Å) were distinguished, including diffuse rings and four and five-sided structures composed of four to six or an indefinite number of subunits. The individual subunits appeared spherical and were of β-crustacyanin size. Double-lined structures were also seen. Two models were suggested to account for the observed electron microscope patterns (Fig. 2).

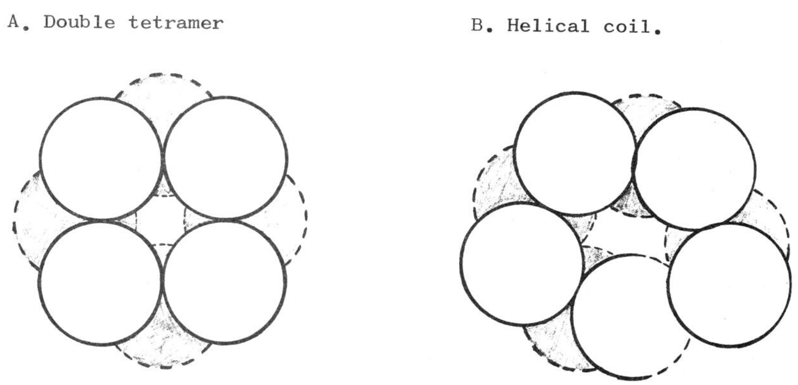

Fig. 2. Proposed model for the quaternary structure of α-crustacyanin (after Zagalsky).

The Velella carotenoprotein. Velella velella is a surface-living oceanic chondrophore and its blue mantle tissue is pigmented by an astaxanthin-protein. The complicated subunit structure of this pigment, and theimportance of anion-binding sites in determining the quaternary structure have been investigated in detail (Ref. 6). What appears to be the native blue pigment, V_{620} (designated from its λ_{max}, 620 nm) is a polymeric form, most likely a tetramer, of the V_{600}, which in turn appears to be an octamer of the purple V_{570}. Pigment V_{570} can be separated by electrophoresis into six components, each of which appears to be a dimer of apoprotein or pigment form V_{545} units (23000 daltons). Two astaxanthin molecules are present per apoprotein subunit. The apparent heterogeneity of the apoprotein, V_{545} and V_{570} may arise artificially due to the easy deamidation of some acidic amino acid residues.

Pigments V_{620} and V_{600} have specific anion (Cl^-)-binding sites which influence the spectroscopic properties and the quaternary structures. In the absence of halide ions the pigments dissociate reversibly to give V_{600}-size and V_{570}-size products with λ_{max} 583 and 565 nm respectively. It was proposed that the anion-binding sites consist of clusters of basic amino acid residues which impose stereospecific restrictions on the binding. V_{600} may have three such sites per apoprotein subunit. However, V_{570} and the apoprotein do not possess high affinity halide ion binding sites.

Like crustacyanin, the *Velella* pigments have recently been examined by electron microscopy (Ref. 29). Chloride-containing solutions of V_{600} exhibited two types of structure, parallel rows of particles, tramline in appearance and of variable length, together with apparently hexagonal diffuse ring structures. A double hexagon structure is suggested with the linear arrays arising because of unravelling of the hexagons. The individual particles which make up the hexagons correlate with the size of V_{570}. Pigment V_{620} in Cl^--containing solution gave particles of various sizes but suggesting a cylinder structure viewed from different angles. Parallel arrays of subunits, presumed to arise by unravelling of the cylindrical structures, were also seen. A model was proposed (Fig. 3) which considers V_{620} to be a cylindrical assembly formed by helical coiling of the double chains of subunits. Conversion of V_{620} into V_{600} would involve unwinding of the helical chains followed by re-coiling into double hexagons, or dissociation to form V_{570} subunits.

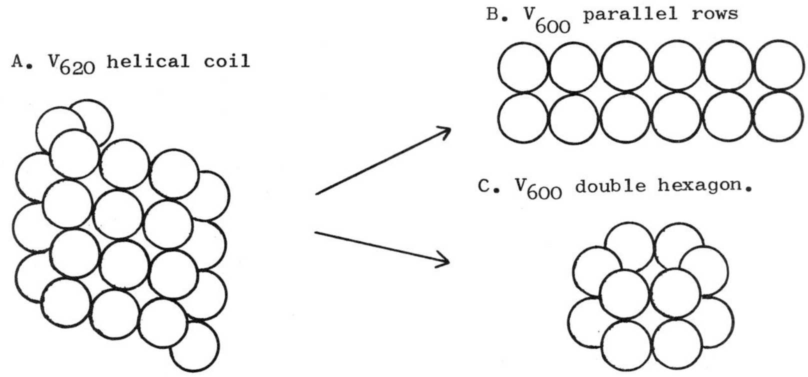

Fig. 3. Proposed models for the quaternary structure of the carotenoprotein of *Velella velella* (after Zagalsky).

Primary Structure: The *Asterias rubens* carotenoprotein. The purple carotenoprotein of *Asterias rubens*, being a relatively simple structure with molecular weight 43000 and four 11000 dalton subunits, appears to be the most suitable of the carotenoproteins yet described for amino acid sequence determination. This is currently being undertaken in our laboratory by manual, automatic and mass spectrometric procedures. The protein has been digested with trypsin, chymotrypsin, thermolysin and cyanogen bromide, and by partial acid hydrolysis, to give a large number of smaller peptides which have been separated and purified, often with difficulty because of their hydrophobic nature. N-terminal degradation by the modified dansyl-Edman procedure and sequential C-terminal analysis by a carboxypeptidase method have been performed on many of these peptides. Although the complete sequence is not yet known, substantial progress has been made, and the following conclusions may be drawn:

i). 129 amino acid residues are present per subunit

ii). Only one N-terminal amino acid was detected, aspartic acid. This and the relatively small number of large peptides obtained by partial digestion, provides strong evidence in support of the identity of the four subunits.

iii). The first 28 amino acids from the N-terminal end of the protein have been sequenced by an automatic method (Fig. 4).

iv). Hydrophobic groups of leucine, isoleucine and phenylalanine residues together appear to occur frequently.

v). Performic acid oxidation indicates the presence of 2-3 disulphide bridges.

In spite of the progress made to date, much work remains before the complete sequence can be constructed.

Asp - Thr - Gly - Glu - Met - Ala - Ala - Glu - Val -
- X - Thr - Cys - Asp - X - Thr - Val - Tyr - X -
- Thr - Cys - Leu - Arg - Thr - Ile - X - Ile - Phe/Lys - Asp.......

Fig. 4. Amino acid sequence of the N-terminal end of the *Asterias rubens* carotenoprotein.

SPECTROSCOPIC STUDIES

The light absorption spectra of carotenoproteins are used as a first means of characterisation. Not only is the shift in the carotenoid absorption spectrum that occurs on binding to protein striking and diagnostically useful, but variations in the vibrational fine structure may give information about the rigidity that binding imposes on the molecule. More on this topic will be included below when the properties of reconstituted carotenoproteins are discussed. In addition to u.v./visible light absorption spectroscopy, several other techniques can be expected to give useful information about carotenoproteins. The use of two of these methods, circular dichroism (c.d.) and resonance Raman spectroscopy has been increasing recently, and a novel method, photoacoustic spectroscopy, has also been proved capable of yielding valuable data.

Resonance Raman Spectroscopy

This technique is especially useful for probing protein-chromophore interactions. When incident light is scattered by a sample, a small energy difference may be observed between the incident and the scattered light. This energy difference represents changes in the vibrational energy of the molecule in the electronic ground state. When the wavelength of the incident or exciting light is close to an absorption maximum of the sample, the induced dipole becomes very large and the scattering of light is greatly enhanced. This enhanced or resonance condition gives rise to Raman lines of greatly increased intensity. The value of the resonance Raman technique for carotenoprotein work lies in the fact that greatly enhanced Raman lines are obtained for the light-absorbing chromophore (carotenoid molecule) but not for the non-absorbing protein. Information can thus be obtained selectively about the chromophore, more particularly about the electronic ground state of the chromophore and the way this is affected by binding to protein. Several examples of the use of the resonance Raman method in carotenoprotein work have recently been reported.

Lobster carotenoproteins. Three main lobster carotenoprotein pigments have been characterised, crustacyanin and 'yellow pigment' from the carapace and ovoverdin from the eggs and ovaries. All three of these have been studied by resonance Raman spectroscopy. α-Crustacyanin (λ_{max} 628 nm), β-crustacyanin (λ_{max} 585 nm) and γ-crustacyanin (λ_{max} 610 nm) were examined with 647.1 nm excitation (Ref. 30). Each spectrum was characterised by a strong C=C double bond stretching band near 1500cm^{-1} which contrasts with the ν c=c band in free astaxanthin, which occurs at around 1520cm^{-1}. Thermal denaturation of α-,β- and γ-crustacyanin causes this band to shift from 1494, 1498 and 1497 cm^{-1} respectively to 1520cm^{-1} as the protein-carotenoid interactions are broken. The shift in the Raman ν c=c band shows that the protein binding has resulted in a large change in the electronic configuration of the ground state of the astaxanthin molecule. A reciprocal correlation has been made between ν c=c and the light absorption maximum, which holds for the crustacyanins and other purple or blue proteins.

Ovoverdin has two λ_{max}, at 460 and 640 nm. The resonance Raman spectrum (Ref. 30) shows two distinct C=C stretching vibrations at 1500 and 1525cm^{-1} obtained by excitation at 647.1 and 488.0 nm respectively, thus confirming the presence of two distinct astaxanthin chromophores in quite different environments. The 640 nm - absorbing chromophore is similar to that of α-crustacyanin, whereas the 460nm-absorbing species is electronically similar to free astaxanthin.

The lobster shell 'yellow pigment' behaves differently (Ref. 8). Its light absorption spectrum shows a hypsochromic shift of about 70nm and λ_{max} at 409 nm, but the resonance Raman spectrum differs little from that of free astaxanthin in acetone. From this it was concluded that the electronic ground state of astaxanthin is unchanged on binding, so the hypsochromic shift must be a result of a destabilised excited state. The conclusion reached was that the astaxanthin molecules are stacked one on top of another, giving rise to exciton interactions between the chromophores.

The *Asterias rubens* carotenoprotein. (Ref. 24). The carotenoprotein of *A. rubens* is purple with λ_{max} 555-570 nm and a mixture of three similar carotenoids, astaxanthin, 7,8-didehydroastaxanthin and 7,8,7',8'-tetradehydroastaxanthin as prosthetic group. The natural carotenoprotein, and a reconstitution product with 7,8-didehydroastaxanthin both gave two Raman bands in the C=C vibration region at 1523 and 1505cm^{-1}. The 1505cm^{-1} band obeys the ν versus $^1/\lambda$ correlation. The reason for the splitting has not yet been explained satisfactorily. Also significant was the fact that no acetylenic fundamental band was observed in the 2100-2200cm^{-1} region, which may be tentative evidence against extensive electron delocalisation beyond the triple bond(s) of the bound carotenoid.

Ovorubin and the astaxanthin-proteins of *Velella velella* and *Pomacea insularum*. (Ref. 31). Resonance Raman spectra have been recorded for these astaxanthin proteins, and a detailed study presented of the spectrum of ovorubin (a red protein from the snail *Pomacea canaliculata*) resulting from excitation at 530.8nm, within the contour of the main absorption band (λ_{max} 508nm). The spectra contained many more vibrational bands in the 300-1600cm^{-1} region than did that of free astaxanthin, and the extra bands were all attributable to the astaxanthin part of the complexes. A great deal of similarity was found in the vibrational band wave numbers of the various complexes, suggesting a high degree of similarity in the astaxanthin conformations of them all. Differences were seen, however, in the 'fingerprint' region, 1100-1400cm^{-1}. The reciprocal correlation between $\nu_{c=c}$ and light absorption maximum appeared to hold for all the astaxanthin complexes examined.

Deductions about the spectral shift mechanism, from the resonance Raman results. In the light of their resonance Raman results for crustacyanin and ovoverdin, Salares, Carey and coworkers (Ref. 30) considered various possible mechanisms for the shift in absorption spectra seen in the blue pigments. In particular, they rejected the 'distortion hypothesis', i.e. the idea that twisting about one or more double bonds may be responsible. They concluded that the shift could best be explained by a polarisation mechanism in which charged groups (amino acid sidechains) near the polyene chain of astaxanthin cause a rearrangement of the π-electrons, resulting in a permanent induced dipole and increased π-electron delocalisation in the ground state, and thus a smaller energy difference between this and the excited state. The other workers whose results have been outlined above (Ref. 24, 31) also consider such a charge polarization mechanism most likely, but Clark *et al.* (Ref. 31) argue that the resonance Raman results do not rule out completely a distortion mechanism as wholly or partially responsible for the shift.

Resonance Raman spectra of pigments *in situ*. An important application of the resonance Raman technique is to obtain spectra of samples *in situ*, e.g. α-crustacyanin in the lobster shell. The spectra obtained have all been similar to those of samples in solution, proving that the pigments have not been adversely affected by the isolation and purification procedures used.

Circular Dichroism

No systematic c.d. study has been undertaken, but c.d. spectra have been reported for a small number of carotenoproteins. Some useful information has been obtained, which emphasises the potential of the method for carotenoprotein studies.

Exciton interactions. The visible region c.d. spectra of α- and β-crustacyanins (Ref. 27), the *Velella* V_{620} pigment (Ref. 6) and the yellow pigment of lobster carapace (Ref. 27) all show evidence of exciton splitting, due to electronic interactions between different chromophore molecules in close proximity. It was concluded that the degenerate exciton interactions responsible for the splitting in the c.d. spectrum of the *Velella* V_{620} pigment is between pairs of carotenoid molecules either within apoprotein units or between adjacent apoprotein units. Dissociation of the V_{620} pigment, e.g. by desaturation of the Cl^- binding sites abolishes the interactions, and no exciton splitting is seen in the c.d. spectra of V_{600} or smaller pigments. The excition splitting thus arises either because of interactions between carotenoid chromophores on adjacent V_{600}-size fragments when these are associated in V_{620}, or because occupation of the halide ion binding sites alters the relative orientation of the prosthetic groups or their distance apart. The c.d. spectrum of V_{600} was slightly affected by the presence or absence of halide ions, that of V_{570} not affected at all.

Induced circular dichroism. The violet carotenoprotein isolated from the haemolymph of the fly *Rhynchosciara americana* exhibits c.d. in the visible region, even though the carotenoid prosthetic groups canthaxanthin and echinenone are optically inactive (Ref. 25). This c.d. must be induced due to asymmetry imposed upon the chromophore by binding to protein. The c.d. spectra were affected by alterations in the pH of the solution, and showed evidence of two distinct sites of carotenoid-protein interactions. Work with alloporin (Ref. 32) and the starfish carotenoproteins (Ref. 33) shows that complexes prepared by recombination of the apoprotein with the different optical isomers of astaxanthin (3R,3'R; 3R,3'S; 3S,3'S) give approximately identical c.d. spectra. This is further evidence that the asymmetry or distortion imposed on the chromophore by the protein is more important than the intrinsic chirality of the carotenoid molecule in determining the c.d. properties of the complex.

Protein c.d. C.d. in the ultra-violet region gives a good indication of the extent of helical structure in a protein. In the case of the carotenoproteins so far examined (crustacyanin and the *Velella* pigment) the helix content is very low.

Photoacoustic Spectroscopy.
This new technique has been used to investigate the distribution of carotenoproteins as a function of depth within the lobster carapace (Ref. 9). When a pigment molecule absorbs light of an appropriate wavelength, the excitation energy has to be lost from the excited state produced. In particular this energy may be lost as heat by non-radiative pathways. In photoacoustic spectroscopy the heat so generated is detected and measured as a function of exciting light wavelength, and since the heat generated depends on the intensity of absorption at any wavelength, the method gives a spectrum similar to a light absorption spectrum, but has the advantage that the spectrum can be obtained from different depths within the sample. This technique applied to lobster shell revealed a near-continuum of astaxanthin absorption energies or wavelengths spanning the visible region. The pigments were shown to be in an anisotropic distribution, showing a gradual progression from blue-absorbing to red-absorbing species from the outside to the inside of the endocuticle. It was proposed that this progressive and essentially continuous shift in the absorption maximum is due to gradually changing but highly specific pigment-pigment and pigment-protein interactions, which may be part of the ultrastructure of the endocuticle. It may well, therefore, be impossible to isolate discrete chemical species corresponding to each absorption, but denaturation or the isolation procedure give rise to a small number of species such as α-crustacyanin and the 'yellow pigment'.

CAROTENOID-PROTEIN RECOMBINATION STUDIES

TABLE 3. Yields and absorption spectra of complexes obtained by recombination of the apoproteins of crustacyanin, ovorubin and the *Asterias rubens* pigment with a range of carotenoids.

Carotenoid Name	λ_{max} (nm)[a]	Crustacyanin Yield[b]	λ_{max}	Ovorubin Yield	λ_{max}	Asterias Yield	λ_{max}
Astaxanthin	490	+++	630	+++	517[c,e]	+++	585
7,8-Didehydroastaxanthin	493	++	611	+++	500[c]	+++	565
7,8,7',8'-Tetradehydroastaxanthin	495	+	580	++	490[c]	+++	545
15,15'-Didehydroastaxanthin	465	++	528	++	484[c]	+++	535
Astacene	497	+++	620	++	517[c]	+++	585
Actinioerythrol	520	+	ca620	+++	523	+++	575
Adonirubin	490	+++	626	+++	512[c]	++	ca540
Adonixanthin	480	X		+++	509	+	495
3-Hydroxyechinenone	480	-		+	510[c]	+	n.d.
Canthaxanthin	490	++	618	++	512[c]	+	ca580
Echinenone	480	+	n.d.	X		X	
Crustaxanthin	460	X		+	493[d]	X	
Zeaxanthin	460	X		++	484[d]	+	460
Isozeaxanthin	460	X		-		(+)	460
β-Cryptoxanthin	460	X		X		X	
β-Carotene	460	X		X		X	
[Natural carotenoprotein]			631		(484)512(545)		560

a. Carotenoid λ_{max} in aqueous media
b. Yields:- +++>30%, ++ 10-30%, + 0-10%, X no complex formed, - not tested, n.d. not determined
c. Spectrum showing increased fine structure
d. Spectrum showing decreased fine structure
e. (3S,3'S)-Astaxanthin. (3R,3'S)-Astaxanthin gave λ_{max} 513 nm, (3R,3'R)-astaxanthin 517 nm

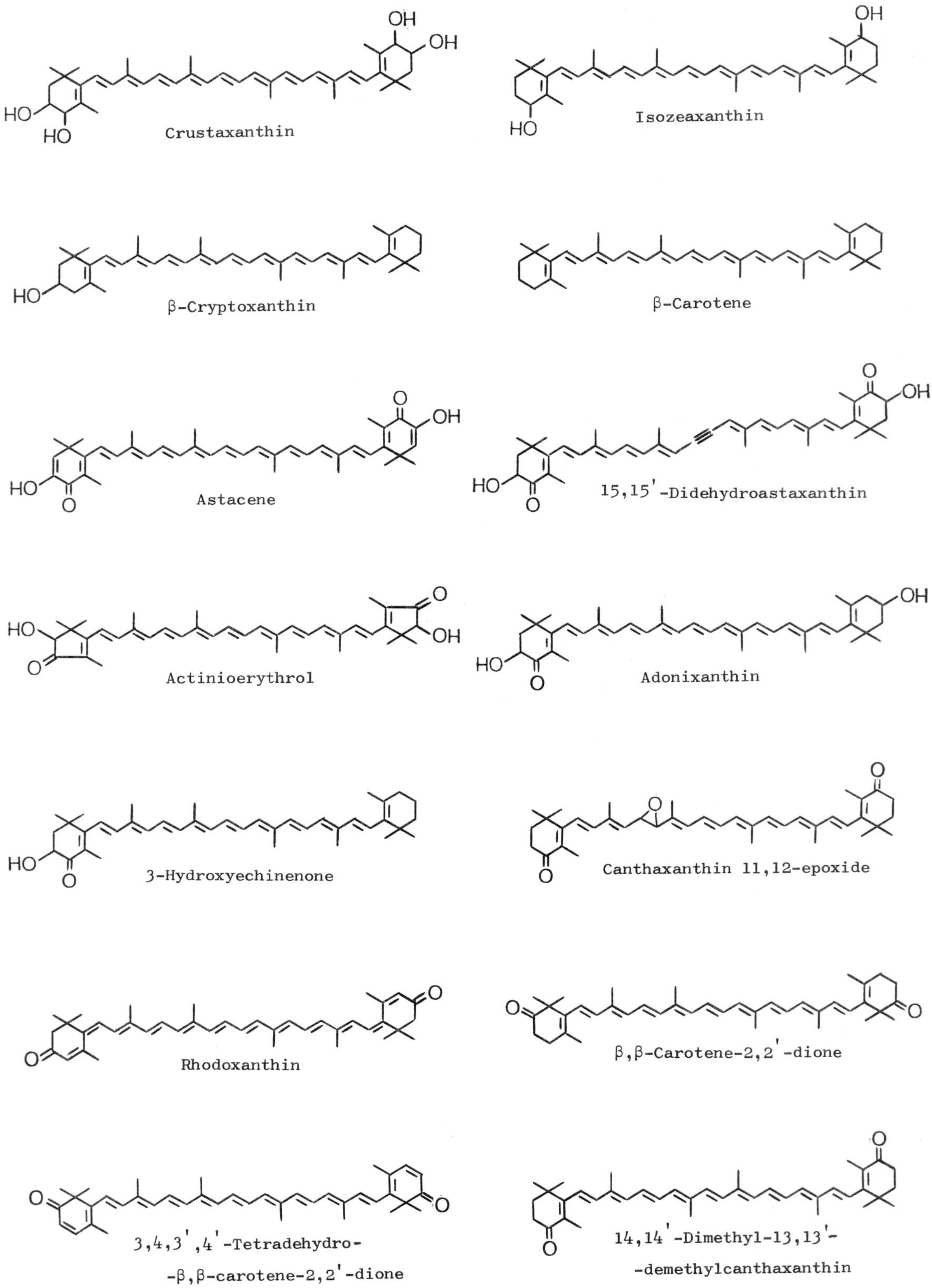

Fig. 5. Structures of carotenoids used in recombination studies with carotenoprotein apoproteins.

In his review (Ref. 1), Zagalsky included tables listing the yields and absorption spectra of carotenoid-proteins obtained by incubation of the apoproteins from five natural carotenoproteins (crustacyanin, ovorubin and the pigments of Velella velella, Aristeus antennatus and Anomalocera patersoni) with a range of carotenoids. Conclusions were drawn from this about the specificity of binding and, in particular, the structural requirements of the carotenoid to produce the most efficient binding, subunit association and spectral shift. We have now obtained a wider range of carotenoids and have thus been able to extend the work of Zagalsky not just with crustacyanin and ovorubin but also the carotenoproteins of the starfish Asterias rubens and Marthasterias glacialis. Table 3 lists the yields of carotenoid-protein complexes obtained from various carotenoids and the apoproteins of crustacyanin, ovorubin, and the Asterias pigment. The structures of the carotenoids used are given in Fig. 1 and 5. It is intended that full details of this work will be published shortly, but the main findings and conclusions are outlined below.

The Asterias rubens carotenoprotein.

The natural purple carotenoprotein of A. rubens contains a mixture of three carotenoids, astaxanthin, 7,8-didehydroastaxanthin and 7,8,7',8'-tetradehydroastaxanthin. The carotenoid composition is variable, depending on the geographical origin of the animals and presumably reflecting dietary availability of the respective carotenoids. The binding causes a shift in λ_{max} from around 490 nm to up to 570 nm. Although considerable difficulty has been encountered - factors such as ionic strength, pH and the organic solvent used are critical - it has proved possible to recombine the apoprotein with a range of carotenoids (Table 3).

The best yields of recombination complexes were obtained with astaxanthin and related compounds with hydroxy-groups at both C-3 and C-3' and oxo-groups at both C-4 and C-4'. The three optical isomers of astaxanthin, (3R,3'R), (3R,3'S), and (3S,3'S) formed complexes equally well. The presence of acetylene groups in the chromophore did not adversely affect the ability to bind, as might be expected in view of the constitution of the natural pigment. The protein also accepted the five-membered ring carotenoid actinioerythrol and the oxidised product astacene as readily as astaxanthin. Complexes were formed, albeit in poorer yield, with carotenoids having either the two (C-4,C-4') oxo-groups but no or one C-3 hydroxy-group or the two (C-3, C-3') hydroxy-groups but no or one C-4 oxo-group. Carotenoids with oxygen function on only one ring did not bind to the protein. For the maximum spectral shift the two oxo-groups and at least one hydroxy-group were required. The spectral shifts observed with the acetylenic analogues were considerably smaller than with astaxanthin itself, though the chromatographic and electrophoretic properties of the respective complexes were indistinguishable. This phenomenon is considered further below, when the mechanism of the spectral shift is discussed.

Ovorubin

In the case of ovorubin, the red astaxanthin-protein of Pomacea canaliculata, binding of the carotenoid to protein results in a much smaller spectral shift of only 20-25 nm, but also causes a pronounced increase in the vibrational fine structure of the absorption spectrum (Fig.6). There are thus three parameters to be considered for recombination of apoovorubin and various carotenoids, the yield of complex formed and the spectral shift as before, and also the effect on the spectral fine structure. Zagalsky successfully achieved recombination of apoovorubin with astaxanthin and several related carotenoids. We have now obtained products with a much larger number of carotenoids (Table 3). The three optical isomers of astaxanthin, 7,8- and 15,15'-didehydroastaxanthins, adonixanthin, adonirubin and actinioerythrol all formed complexes in good yield (30-60%). Rather lower yields (10-25%) were obtained with astacene, canthaxanthin, zeaxanthin and 7,8,7',8'-tetradehydroastaxanthin, but only traces of complexes with 3-hydroxyechinenone, crustaxanthin and 9,9'-dicis-7,8,7',8'-tetradehydroastaxanthin, and no complex was formed at all with β-carotene. Three or four ring oxygen functions are thus required for most efficient binding, though one oxo-group or one hydroxy-group on each ring (e.g. canthaxanthin, zeaxanthin) is sufficient to allow complex formation in moderate yield. Astacene binds much less efficiently than astaxanthin, an effect that is presumably due to the different chemical nature of the C-3,3' oxygen functions in the two structures. The presence of an acetylene group at C-7,8 or C-15,15' had no effect on the efficency of binding, but 7,8,7',8'-tetradehydroastaxanthin, with two acetylene groups, bound in lower yield.

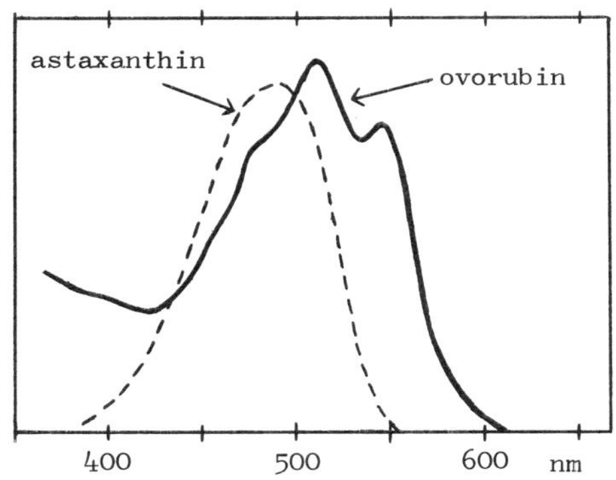

Fig. 6. Light absorption spectra of ovorubin and astaxanthin.

Spectral shifts of about 20-30 nm, i.e. comparable to that in the natural carotenoprotein, were exhibited by the recombination products from astaxanthin, astacene, canthaxanthin, adonirubin, adonixanthin, zeaxanthin, 3-hydroxyechinenone and crustaxanthin. Of the acetylenic derivatives, 15,15'-didehydroastaxanthin gave a 'normal' bathochromic shift of 19 nm, but the shift obtained with 7,8-didehydroastaxanthin was only 7nm and the low yield 7,8,7',8'-tetradehydroastaxanthin complex showed a hypsochromic shift of 5 nm. The bathochromic shift obtained with actinioerythrol was very small (3 nm). With virtually all other carotenoproteins that have been studied, e.g. crustacyanin and the Asterias rubens pigment, C-4 oxo-functions in both rings are essential for production of the large bathochromic spectral shift. This is not the case with ovorubin, in which some of the largest shifts were seen with adonixanthin and 3-hydroxyechinenone (only one oxo-group) and even zeaxanthin and crustaxanthin which have no oxo-groups at all. Another interesting observation was that although the three optical isomers of astaxanthin bound to give complexes in approximately equal yields, the spectral shifts observed were different; (3S,3'S)-isomer, 22 nm; (3'R,3'S), 23 nm; (3R,3'R), 27 nm. This phenomenon has not been observed with any other carotenoprotein.

Spectral fine structure. Except at low temperature, astaxanthin and other oxocarotenoids exhibit broad featureless absorption spectra with virtually no vibrational fine structure. When astaxanthin is bound in ovorubin, not only does the absorption spectrum shift bathochromically but fine structure is observed (Fig. 6). This is taken to indicate that constraints are placed on the conformation of the astaxanthin by binding to the protein. The recombination studies indicated that all the carotenoids with two 4-oxo-β-rings showed a considerable increase in spectral fine structure on binding. The cyclopentenone carotenoid actinioerythrol showed only a very small increase in fine structure. In the case of carotenoids with only one C-4 oxo-group the increase in fine structure was also very small. Binding of zeaxanthin (two hydroxy-groups and no oxo- functions) caused almost complete loss of vibronic structure seen in the spectrum of free zeaxanthin. It thus appears that binding through the C-4 and C-4' oxo-groups is responsible for holding the carotenoid molecule in a relatively rigid environment, probably controlling the angle of twist of the ring with respect to the main polyene chain. This effect is quite distinct from the spectral shift. Zeaxanthin shows a relatively large shift but the spectrum loses rather than gains fine structure on binding. In many ways, therefore, the carotenoid-protein binding in ovorubin is quite different from that in the other complexes, and detailed comparative investigations, including an extensive spectroscopic study of recombination complexes, should be fruitful.

Crustacyanin.
Zagalsky (Ref. 1) investigated the ability of apocrustacyanin to combine with a wide range of carotenoids. He concluded that oxo-groups at C-4 of both β-rings were essential for binding to occur with association of apoprotein units to give a β-crustacyanin structure, whereas compounds with only one C-4 oxo-group may bind, with low affinity, but give only apoprotein-sized complexes, i.e. the protein conformational changes necessary for dimerisation of β-crustacyanin did not occur. Our work has confirmed these findings. Our results also showed that the best yields of recombination products were obtained with carotenoids with two C-4 oxo-groups, especially when one or two C-3 hydroxy-groups were also present. Acetylenic astaxanthin analogues and the cyclopentenone actinioerythrol did not bind as efficiently as the normal 4,4'-dioxo-β,β-carotene derivatives. The three optical isomers of astaxanthin bound equally well and gave products with identical absorption spectra. This is perhaps to be expected in view of the recent report of Rønneberg et al. (Ref. 32) that natural crustacyanin contains all three isomers in its prosthetic group.

The most useful of our findings was that, under our conditions, canthaxanthin was bound efficiently; the yields obtained by Zagalsky with canthaxanthin were low. This has allowed us to examine selected canthaxanthin analogues and derivatives which have given information which may be relevant to the mechanism of the spectral shift, and will be discussed below.

Deductions about the spectral shift in blue and purple carotenoproteins from recombination studies.
In general, covalent bonds are not involved in carotenoid-protein associations or in producing the spectral shift. Oxo-groups in the carotenoid are important. At least one such group is essential, and two preferred for the most efficient binding and for production of the spectral shift. This has led to suggestions that the carbonyl groups are vital for both binding and the spectral shift through enolisation, Schiff base formation or hydrogen bonding to protein amino acid sidechains. However, the two effects, binding and the spectral shift, may be separable. Thus if a polarisation mechanism is considered, the oxo-group(s) conjugated with the polyene chain may be involved directly in the polarisation and hence the spectral shift as well as binding. Alternatively the oxo-groups may simply hold the molecule in position for other charged protein groups to interact with the polyene and affect the electronic configuration. If the distortion hypothesis is considered, binding through the carbonyl groups is likely to be an extremely important factor in controlling

twisting of the entire molecule or chromophore about double bonds. Some information that may be relevant has been provided by the recombination work.

Dehydroastaxanthins. Although in most cases the acetylenic analogues 7,8-didehydroastaxanthin and 7,8,7',8'-tetradehydroastaxanthin are bound by carotenoprotein apoproteins almost as well as astaxanthin itself, the spectral shifts produced are considerably smaller. When models are used to compare astaxanthin and its acetylenic derivatives two alternatives are indicated (Fig. 7):-

1). If the polyene chain is maintained in the same position, the ring oxygen functions in the acetylenic compounds must be a considerable distance away from their normal position in astaxanthin. This would be expected to reduce the binding efficiency and any polarising effect of protein groups on the C-4 oxo-functions.

2). If the oxygen functions in the different molecules are maintained in similar positions so that the efficiency of their interactions should not be diminished greatly, the polyene chain is then forced to adopt a different position or angle with respect to the rings. If a distortion mechanism is operating, the twisting of the chromophore must be different so the spectral shift would be different, probably smaller. If polarisation is responsible for the shift, the polyene chain is held out of its normal position so there would be reduced interaction with charged groups on the protein

A. With superimposition of the polyene chains.

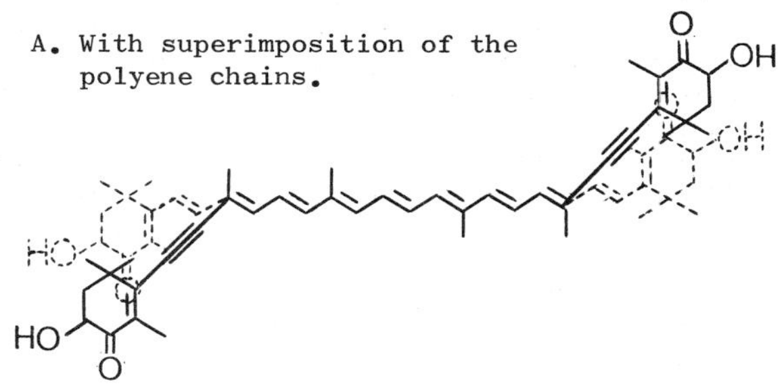

B. If the oxygen functions adopt similar positions.

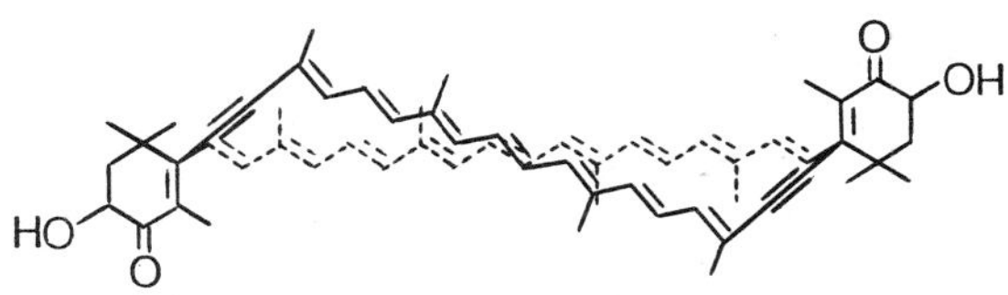

Fig. 7. Comparison of the orientation of astaxanthin and 7,8,7',8'-tetradehydroastaxanthin.

TABLE 4. Recombination of apocrustacyanin with canthaxanthin derivatives and analogues

Carotenoid	λ_{max} (nm)	Recombination product Yield[a]	Recombination product λ_{max}	Spectral shift $\Delta\lambda_{max}$
Canthaxanthin	481	++	618	+137
Canthaxanthin-11,12-epoxide	373	+	446	+73
Rhodoxanthin	495	+	485	-10
β,β-Carotene-2,2'-dione	459	+	447	-12
3,4,3',4'-Tetradehydro-β,β-carotene-2,2'-dione	490	+++	647	+157
14,14'-Dimethyl-13,13'-demethyl-canthaxanthin	466	+	465	-1

[a] See Table 3.

Canthaxanthin analogues. Several dioxocarotenoids, analogues of canthaxanthin, were obtained and their recombination with apocrustacyanin was examined. The structures of these compounds are given in Fig. 5 and the results of the recombination experiments in Table 4. The main findings are summarised below.

1). Rhodoxanthin with oxo-groups at C-3 and C-3' and the retro arrangement of double bonds did not bind with apocrustacyanin. Whether this is due to the oxo-groups being out of position or to the different stereochemistry of the retro structure about the C-6,7 double bond is not known.

2). Compounds with the oxo-groups at position 2 and 2' of the two β-rings were bound by apocrustacyanin. Models show that by suitable rotation about the C-6,7 bond the 2-oxo group can readily occupy approximately the same spatial position as a 4-oxo group (Fig. 8). The fact that such compounds are bound shows that the orientation of the C-1 and C-5 methyl groups is not of crucial importance.

3). 3,4,3',4'-Tetradehydro-β,β-carotene-2,2'-dione bound to give a blue complex, λ_{max} 647 nm, but binding of β,β-carotene-2,2'-dione resulted in no bathochromic shift. From this the tentative conclusion may be drawn that although the isolated oxo-groups can bind, conjugation of these with the main polyene system is necessary to bring about the large bathochromic spectral shift. An electronic or partial polarisation effect extending through the conjugated carbonyl groups is therefore suggested to be necessary for the spectral shift.

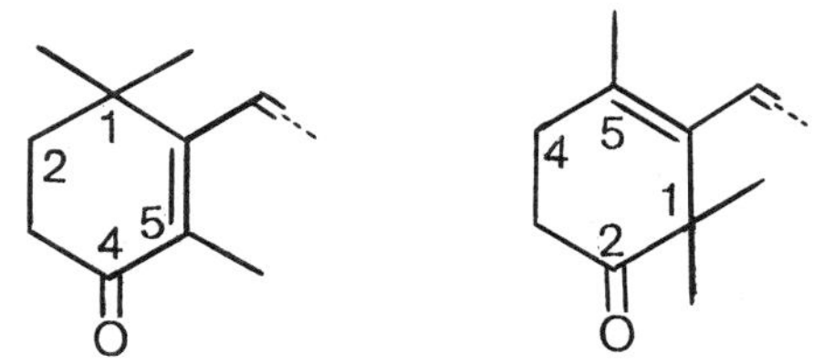

Fig. 8. Comparison of possible orientations of the rings of 2-oxo-β- and 4-oxo-β-carotenoids.

4). Canthaxanthin-11,12-epoxide. In this deserivative the epoxy-group imposes a break in conjugation in the polyene chain. The compound bound relatively efficiently and also gave a bathochromic shift of 73 nm. It thus appears that as long as the ring carbonyl group is conjugated with a sizeable part of the polyene chain a break in the conjugation towards the centre of the chromophore does not prevent binding or the spectral shift.

5). 13,13'-Demethyl-14,14'- dimethylcanthaxanthin is a synthetic derivative with the central methyl substituents at C-14,14' instead of the normal C-13,13' positions. It was bound by apocrustacyanin in good yield but no spectral shift was obtained. The different arrangement and hence different spatial orientation of these methyl substituents prevented the spectral shift, presumably either by preventing close access of the chromophore to the amino acid sidechain responsible for the partial polarisation or, if the distortion mechanism is important, by preventing the normal twisting about the C=C double bonds.

Overall it can be seen that there are two major factors which affect the spectral shift, binding through the ring carbonyl groups which must be in conjugation with a substantial amount of the polyene system, and then a further effect on the central part of the polyene chromophore itself.

FINAL CONCLUSIONS

Progress can be expected in the next few years on several fronts. Enormous numbers of carotenoproteins remain to be described, isolated and characterised. The Salpa pigment shows that new carotenoprotein types differing fundamentally from the astaxanthin-proteins may be expected. Further work on primary structures should lead to the determination of the full amino acid sequence of at least one carotenoprotein in the near future, and more details can be expected about quaternary structures, especially in view of recent success in crystallising the Velella pigments V_{620} and V_{600} (Ref. 34).

As a wider variety of carotenoids becomes available, recombination studies with apoproteins should allow the structural requirements for binding and the spectral shift to be worked out, and should give valuable information about the geometry of the binding sites. Detailed and systematic application of spectroscopic techniques, especially circular dichroism, resonance Raman and n.m.r. spectroscopy, to such model recombination and natural complexes should give much information about the mechanism of binding and the spectral shift.

Acknowledgements. - We are extremely grateful to Dr. Peter Zagalsky, Bedford College, London, for samples of ovorubin, crustacyanin and the Velella velella pigments, and for providing pre-publication manuscripts of his recent work, to Dr. H. Kayser, University of Ulm, Dr. G. P. Moss, Queen Mary College, London and F. Hoffmann-La Roche and Co. Ltd., Basel, for supplying carotenoid samples, and to Dr. J. Van Beeumen, University of Gent, for help and advice on peptide sequencing. We thank the Science Research Council and Hoffmann-La Roche for financial support.

REFERENCES

1. P. F. Zagalsky, Pure Appl. Chem. 47, 103-120 (1976).
2. R. Powls and G. Britton, Biochim. Biophys. Acta 453, 270-276 (1976).
3. P.-S. Song, P. Koka, B. B. Prézelin and F. T. Haxo, Biochemistry 15, 4422-4427 (1976).
4. D. F. Cheesman, W. L. Lee and P. F. Zagalsky, Biol. Rev. 42, 131-160 (1967).
5. W. L. Lee (ed.), Carotenoproteins in Animal Coloration, Dowden, Hutchinson and Ross, Stroudsberg, Pennsylvania (1977).
6. P. F. Zagalsky and P. J. Herring, Phil Trans. Roy. Soc. London, B, 279, 289-326 (1977).
7. P. F. Zagalsky and B. M. Gilchrist, Comp. Biochem. Physiol. 55B, 195-200 (1976).
8. V. R. Salares, N. M. Young, H. J. Bernstein and P. R. Carey, Biochemistry 16, 4751-4756 (1977).
9. M. L. Mackenthun, R. D. Tom and T. A. Moore, Nature 279, 265-266 (1979).
10. P. F. Zagalsky, Comp. Biochem. Physiol. (in press)
11. H. von Euler and H. Hellström, Hoppe-Seyler's Z. Physiol. Chem. 28, 77-89 (1934).
12. G. W. Francis, R. R. Upadhyay and S. Liaaen-Jensen, Acta Chem. Scand. 24, 3050-3052 (1970).
13. C. C. Shone, G. Britton and T. W. Goodwin, Comp. Biochem. Physiol. 62B, 507-513 (1979).
14. A. Elgsaeter, J. D. Tauber and S. Liaaen-Jensen, Biochim. Biophys. Acta 530, 402-411 (1978).
15. B. Renstrøm, J. D. Tauber, A. Elgsaeter and S. Liaaen-Jensen, Biochem. Syst. Ecol. 7, 147-148 (1979).
16. H. M. Fox and G. Vevers, The Nature of Animal Colours, Sidgwick and Jackson, London (1960).
17. G. M. Armittand G. Britton, Absts. 6th Int. Symp. Carotenoids, Liverpool (1981).
18. G. M. Armitt, Ph.D. Thesis, University of Liverpool (1981).
19. D. L. Fox and D. W. Wilkie, Comp. Biochem. Physiol. 36, 49-60 (1970).
20. H. Rønneberg, G. Borch, D. L. Fox and S. Liaaen-Jensen, Comp. Biochem. Physiol. 62B, 309-312 (1979).
21. H. Rønneberg, D. L. Fox and S. Liaaen-Jensen, Comp. Biochem. Physiol. 64B, 407-408 (1979).
22. B. Czeczuga, Comp. Biochem. Physiol. 68B, 339-343 (1981).
23. P. J. Herring, Comp. Biochem. Physiol. 61B, 391-393 (1978).
24. C. C. Shone, G. Britton and E. M. Thomas, unpublished results.
25. W. R. Terra, C. Ferreira, A. G. de Bianchi and K. Zinner, Comp. Biochem. Physiol 68B, 89-93 (1981).
26. D. F. Cheesman, P. F. Zagalsky and H. J. Ceccaldi, Proc. Roy. Soc. London B164, 130-151 (1966).
27. M. Buchwald and W. P. Jencks, Biochemistry 7, 844-859 (1968).
28. R. Quarmby, D. A. Norden, P. F. Zagalsky, H. J. Ceccaldi and R. Daumas, Comp. Biochem. Physiol. 56B, 55-61 (1977).
29. P. F. Zagalsky and R. Jones, Comp. Biochem. Physiol. (in press).
30. V. R. Salares, N. M. Young, H. J. Bernstein and P. R. Carey, Biochim. Biophys. Acta 576 176-191 (1979).
31. R. J. H. Clark, N. R. D'Urso and P. F. Zagalsky, J. Am. Chem. Soc. 102, 6693-6698 (1980).
32. H. Rønneberg, H. Berger, B. Renstrøm, G. Borch and S. Liaaen-Jensen, Absts. 6th Int. Symp. Carotenoids, Liverpool (1981).
33. G. M. Armitt, S. Y. M. Lau, G. Britton, B. Maudinas, J. Lemâtre unpublished results.
34. P. F. Zagalsky, Comp. Biochem. Physiol. (in press).

SYNTHETIC AND STRUCTURAL STUDIES OF VISUAL PIGMENTS

Robert S. H. Liu

Department of Chemistry, 2545 The Mall, University of Hawaii,
Honolulu, Hawaii 96822, USA

Abstract - Properties of synthetic visual pigments prepared from isomers of retinal, aromatic retinals and fluorinated retinals are described together with discussions of structural information on rhodopsin derived from such analogue studies.

INTRODUCTION

The isolation of "retinene" from a photobleached sample of frog rhodopsin by Wald in the late thirties (Ref. 1) and the subsequent characterization of its structure by Morton and coworkers at Liverpool (Ref. 2) were perhaps the two most important results that opened the way for studies of visual pigments at the molecular level. It is therefore most appropriate for the organizing committee to include the subject of visual pigments in this symposium, held at one of the birth places of the field.

The exact way this retinene (which Morton subsequently renamed retinal) interacted with opsin, the glycoprotein in the retina and the role it played in the visual process were the central concern of George Wald and the small research group he assembled at Harvard (Ref. 3). The remarkable insight of this group has become more apparent in recent years when many of their conclusions were verified by new experimental evidence obtained from elaborate equipment that has since appeared on the scene (Ref. 4).

Refinements of the early conclusions by more recent theoretical and experimental studies have led to the following general picture of the visual pigment rhodopsin, and the events following the photo-excitation process. The chromophore (11-*cis*-retinal) is bound to a lysine residue in the glycoprotein opsin linked by a Schiff base in its protonated form. Other secondary interactions, probably an anion from the protein pointing toward a specific position along the polyene chain, contributes to the red shift of the visual pigment (Ref. 5, 6). The visual cycle is initiated by a photochemical process producing a red shifted primary photo-product (the bathorhodopsin). Its formation is rapid (within a few pico seconds) (Ref. 7) and it is stable at temperatures below the boiling point of liquid nitrogen (Ref. 8). Reaction of the thermally labile intermediate proceeds in a stepwise manner. All intermediates have been detected by fast kinetic methods at physiological temperatures as well as by low temperature spectroscopy. The exact nature of the primary photochemical event is still of some controversy. The fast rise time of bathorhodopsin raised some doubt (Ref. 7) to the original postulate of the process being geometric isomerization (Ref. 5). Other processes involving relatively small changes of relative positions of atoms (such as hydrogen migration) were postulated (Ref. 9, 10). However, more recent experimental evidence appears to reaffirm the earlier conclusion that the primary process involves the isomerization of the 11-cis chromophore to a distorted trans-like geometry (see below).

The structure of the protein however is still not well understood. In spite of the recent significant findings by Hargrave and coworkers (Ref. 11), only approximately 25% of the primary structure of the difficult protein is known (M.W. approximately 38,000). The protein has yet to be crystallized for X-ray diffraction studies. Hence, its tertiary structure is still highly speculative. In the absence of such direct information of the protein, we along with others have pursued an indirect method using modified retinals to probe for structural information of the binding site of opsin. Especially helpful are the recent advances in methods of synthesis, separation and characterization of polyenes and their isomers which make the preparation of the "keys" relatively routine. In this report this approach will be discussed; in particular many of the retinal analogues prepared in our laboratory for probing structural information of the "lock" will be described. Selected results from other groups will also be mentioned.

Stereospecificity of the binding site

The early work of rhodopsin analogue studies was that of Wald and coworkers (Ref. 12). Six geometric isomers of retinal were available to them: all-trans; 9-cis; 11-cis; 13-cis; 9-cis,13-cis and 11-cis,13-cis. Rhodopsin was formed upon mixing 11-*cis*-retinal with opsin and a pigment absorbing at a slightly different wavelength was formed with 9-*cis*-retinal (Note a). The remaining four were thought not to be reactive with opsin. (The pigments detected from the two dicis isomers were believed to be due to prior isomerization of the retinal to the reactive monocis isomers.) That only 9-*cis*-retinal, which structurally resembles 11-*cis*-retinal, appeared to form a pigment analogue led to the common belief of the high stereospecificity of the binding site of opsin. However, two recent events appear to cast doubt on this specificity.

First Nakanishi, Ebrey and coworkers (Ref. 13) reinvestigated the 9-*cis*,13-*cis*-retinal system. They concluded by comparison of CD spectra that the pigment derived from interaction with opsin is different from rhodopsin and 9-*cis*-rhodopsin. Furthermore they were successful in recovering the retinal from the pigment by first denaturing the protein in the dark with an organic solvent. Analyses by high pressure liquid chromatography revealed that the geometry was unchanged from the original 9-cis,13-cis. Hence the doubly bent dicis isomer was shown conclusively to form a pigment analogue as well.

Secondly a group of new geometric isomers has since been prepared allowing the testing of the stereospecificity of the binding site on a broader base. Of the six new geometric isomers (7-cis; 7-cis,9-cis; 7-cis,11-cis; 7-cis,13-cis; 9-cis,11-cis and 7-cis,9-cis,13-cis) we have prepared so far (Ref. 14-16) five contain the sterically crowded 7-cis geometry. It was introduced by selective sensitized irradiation (Ref. 17). The preparation for 7-*cis*, 11-*cis*-retinal is shown in Fig. 1 as a representative example. The retinonitrile of the

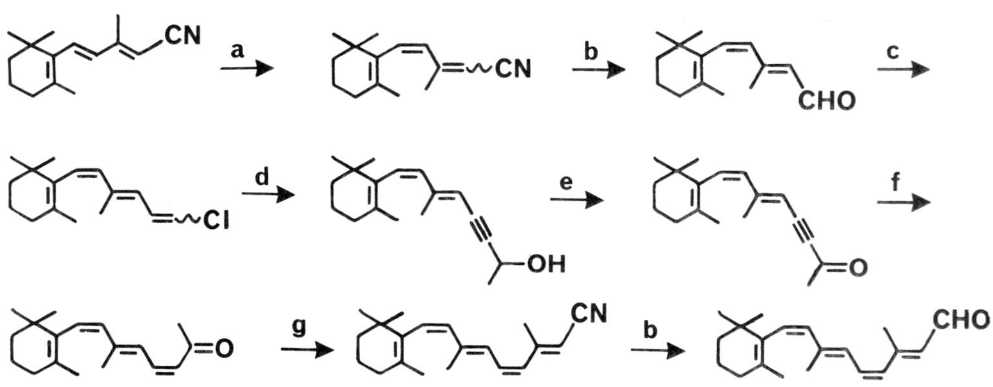

Fig. 1. A synthetic sequence to 7-*cis*,11-*cis*-retinal. a. hν/sen. b. DIBAH. c. $(C_6H_5)_3PCHClBr$/BuLi. d. (1) 2 BuLi; (2) CH_3CHO. e. MnO_2. f. H_2/Lindlar. g. $(EtO)_2POCH_2CN$/NaH-C_6H_6.

7-cis,11-cis,13-cis isomer was also prepared but the aldehyde form was found thermally unstable (Ref. 15). Additionally, Okamura and coworkers (Ref. 18) reported the synthesis of 9-*cis*,11-*cis*,13-*cis*-retinal which was also found to be stable at low temperatures only. Therefore, among the sixteen possible geometric isomers of retinal (Fig. 2), only two have not been reported in the literature. Recently in a preliminary experiment using a reaction sequence similar to that for 7-*cis*,11-*cis*-retinal, Dr. Kini isolated two new isomers of retinonitrile. The ^{1}H-NMR spectra were consistent with those of the missing 7-cis,9-cis, 11-cis and all-cis isomers (Ref. 19). In a separate experiment a fluorinated retinal with the missing tricis geometry has been prepared by Dr. Asato (see below).

The results of reaction of these isomers with cattle opsin (Ref. 15, 16, 19, 20) are summarized in Table 1. From the viewpoint whether for a given isomer a pigment was formed or not (third column), the conclusion that the opsin binding site exhibits little stereospecificity

---

Note a: "Isorhodopsin" was the common name given to the pigment. However, with the current knowledge of the existence of many more isomeric rhodopsins of known geometry, it appears unwise to continue the use of such non-descriptive common names. In this paper, when not specified otherwise, "rhodopsin" implies the 11-cis geometry. All modifications of the chromophore (including those other than geometrical isomerism) are specified with the proper prefixes. When preceded by a prefix indicating the geometry, "rhodopsin" becomes a generic name with no implied geometry. Hence, "isorhodopsin" is referred to as 9-*cis*-rhodopsin and "isoporphyropsin" as 9-*cis*-3-dehydrorhodopsin.

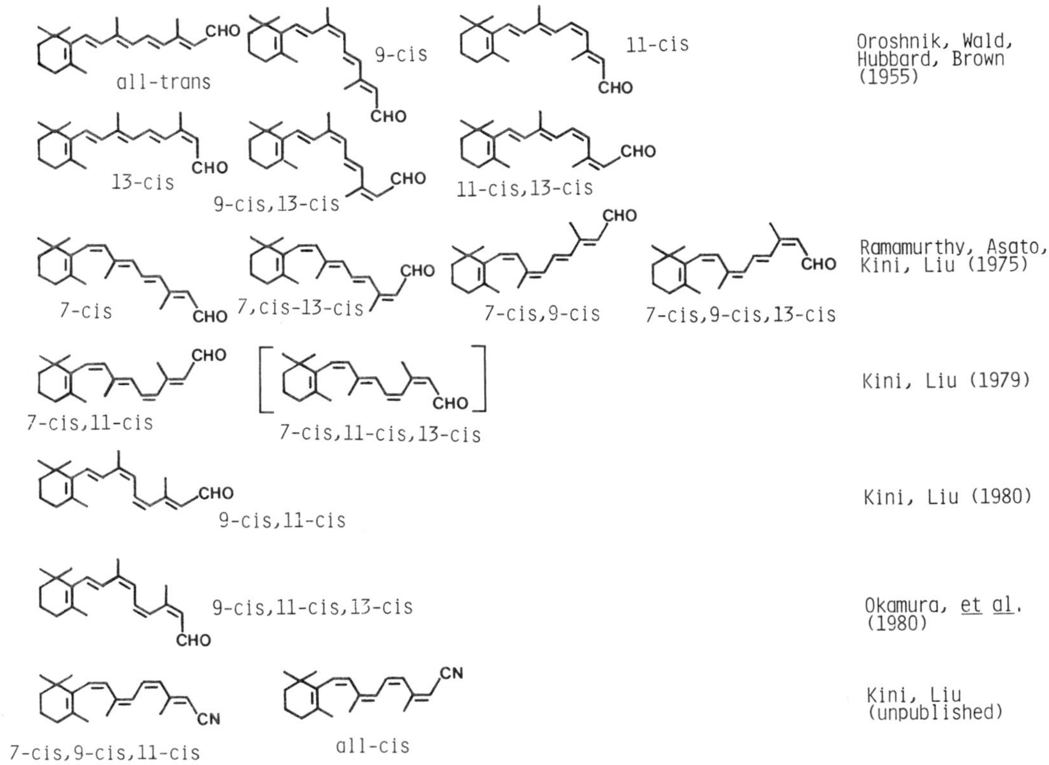

Fig. 2. Sixteen possible geometric isomers of retinal and their preparation in chronological order. The aldehydes of the last two are still unknown. 7-*cis*,11-*cis*,13-*cis*-Retinal is unstable.

is inevitable because among all the isomers tested only two (13-cis and all-trans) did not form pigments. (The ambiguous results on the 11-cis,13-cis isomer will have to be resolved). However before one discards the notion of stereospecificity of opsin, the rate of pigment formation must be considered. Results in the fourth column show (only qualitatively meaningful because they were extracted from papers published by several laboratories based on

TABLE 1. Properties of stable isomers of retinal and rhodopsin

Isomer	Retinal[a] λ_{max}, nm	Pigment Analogue	$\tau_{1/2}$[c]	Rhodopsin λ_{max}, nm	Yield	Ref.
All-trans	383	-		None	0	12, 41
7-cis	377	+	>4h	450	~40%	20
9-cis	373	+	7.5m	483	>90%	12, 41
11-cis	379.5	+	<5m	498	100%	12, 41
13-cis	375	-		None	0	12, 41
7-cis,9-cis	351[b]	+	>4h	460	~40%	20
7-cis,11-cis	374	+	>4h	455	~40%	15
7-cis,13-cis	357[b]	+	>4h	455	~40%	19, 20
9-cis,11-cis	368	+	2h	480	~20%	16
9-cis,13-cis	368	+	30m	481	>90%	13
11-cis,13-cis	373	+	?	498(?)	<10%	d
7-cis,9-cis,13-cis	346[b]	+	>4h	455	~40%	20
9-cis,11-cis,13-cis	302	e				18

a. In ethanol, unless otherwise specified. b. In hexane. c. Approximate time required for 50% pigment formation when a limiting quantity of opsin reacted with a retinal isomer in digitonin at room temperature. d. Its formation was considered a result of prior isomerization to 11-*cis*-retinal (R. Hubbard and G. Wald, J. Gen. Physiol., 36, 269-315 (1952-3)). However only 13-*cis*-retinal was later isolated (Ref. 12). e. Not tested.

experiments conducted under slightly different conditions) that the 11-cis isomer and the structurally similar 9-cis isomer reacted with opsin at a rate much faster than other isomers. Also, the yields of pigment formation from most of the isomers did not approach that of 11-*cis*-retinal (column six in Table 1). Therefore, it appears that the stereospecificity of opsin derived from early results of Wald still holds provided that the criteria is not limited to the binding ability of protein.

<u>Longitudinal restrictions of the binding site</u>

Failure of the all-trans and the 13-cis isomers to react with opsin can be rationalized by the presence of a longitudinal restriction of the binding site, a concept first advanced by Matsumoto and Yoshizawa (Ref. 21), subsequently refined by us (Ref. 22). From a much simplified model by assuming that all C-C bonds were of equal length, all C-C-C angles were 120° and all molecules were planar, Matsumoto and Yoshizawa (Ref. 21) reached the conclusion that of the sixteen possible geometric isomers, the all-trans isomer had the longest distance between the carbonyl carbon and the center of the cyclohexenyl ring (the critical distance). The 13-cis isomer fell into the next group along with the 7-cis,9-cis, 9-cis,11-cis and 11-cis,13-cis isomers. All remaining isomers had much shorter critical distances. Therefore, it was suggested that the failure of the all-trans and the 13-cis isomers to react with opsin was due to the existence of a longitudinal restriction in the binding site to accommodate these isomers. However, this model failed to account for the positive result with 7-*cis*,9-*cis*-retinal and the more recently prepared 9-cis,11-cis isomer.

The X-ray crystal structures of 13-*cis*-retinal (Ref. 23) and methyl 7-*cis*,9-*cis*-retinoate (Ref. 24) have recently been determined (the retinal of the latter is an oil). Their stereoviews are shown in Fig. 3 and 4. (Note that the 13-cis isomer exists in two different conformations about the 6,7 single bond with each unit cell containing one of each conformer.) From these and from the crystal structure published for 11-*cis*-retinal (Ref. 25), the critical distances were calculated.

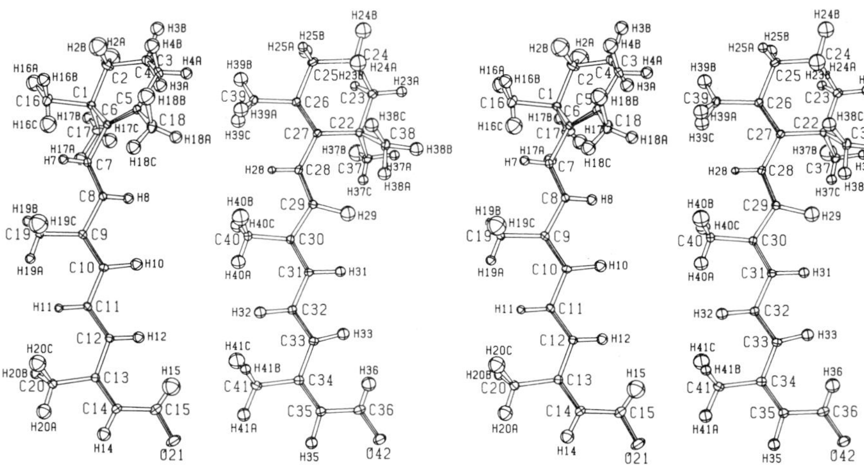

Fig. 3. A stereoview of 13-*cis*-retinal showing the 6-*s*-cis and 6-*s*-trans conformers which coexist in the crystal structure.

The critical distance for 11-*cis*-retinal, the native chromophore, is 9.6-10.9A when allowing rotation of the relatively flexible 12,13 single bond (Fig. 5). The critical distance of either one of the two conformers of 13-*cis*-retinal is 11.2A. Rotation of the 6,7 bond, the most flexible single bond, has a negligible effect on this critical distance. Therefore, the molecule remains too long to fit into the binding site. On the other hand, while the critical distance of the 7-cis,9-cis isomer directly from the crystal structure (11.1A) is also outside the limits of the binding zone, because of steric hindrance the molecules is not planar at carbons 7-10 (twisted 27° from planarity). A further rotation about the 8,9 bond rapidly shortens the critical distance so that it readily falls within the preferred binding distance (Fig. 5). Therefore, it is not surprising that 7-*cis*,9-*cis*-retinal forms a pigment analogue with opsin, albeit at a reduced rate. Incidentally because of failure of all-*trans*-C_{17}-aldehyde to react with opsin, we can raise the lower limit of the binding site to 10.1A.

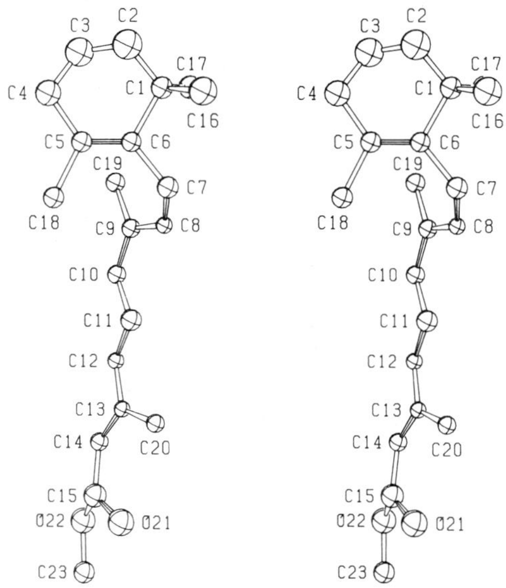

Fig. 4. A stereoview of methyl 7-*cis*,9-*cis*-retinoate.

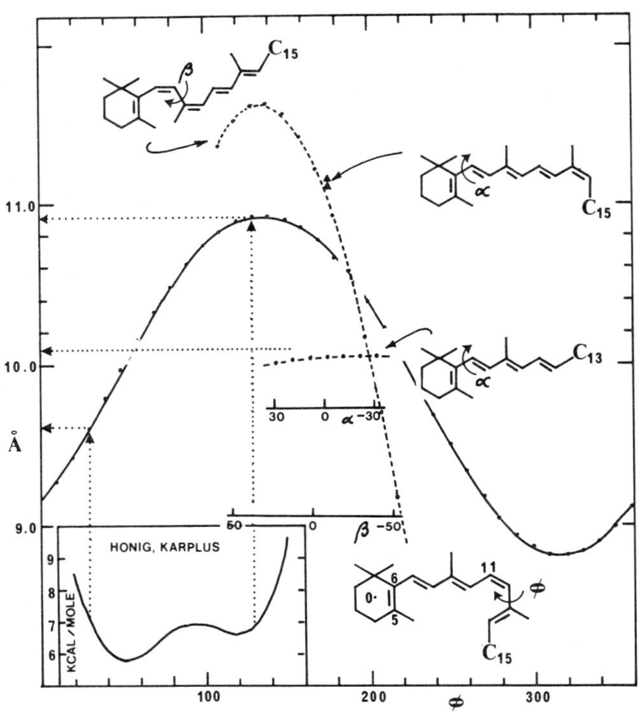

Fig. 5. The critical distances for binding based on crystal structures of retinal isomers and derivatives. Solid line (——) represents the distance by rotating the flexible 12,13-single bond. The insert shows the most likely conformation based on calculations by B. Honig and M. Karplus, Nature (London) 229, 558-560 (1971). ▲, the critical distance for the two conformers of 13-*cis*-retinal. The dashed lines (---) are for the C_{17}-aldehyde, which shows the insignificant changes in the critical distance by rotating the 6,7-single bond, and for the 7-*cis*,9-*cis*-retinal which shows a large change in the critical distance by rotating the now flexible 8,9-single bond.

The photobleaching process of 7-*cis*-rhodopsin

A reasonable question one might ask is whether the interaction of opsin with these isomers of retinal (or other analogues) involved the same portion of the protein chain. The answer is found in a study of photobleaching of 7-*cis*-rhodopsin by low temperature spectroscopy (Ref. 26). A sample of the pigment analogue in a suspension in 75% glycerol was irradiated with 437 nm light at -190°C. The disappearance of the 450 nm absorption band was accompanied by the appearance of a much red shifted band centered at 510 nm (Fig. 6a). The end absorption curve (no. 14) was found to be identical to that obtained from irradiation of rhodopsin. The composition was earlier (Ref. 8) identified as a mixture of bathorhodopsin (540 nm), rhodopsin (498 nm) and 9-*cis*-rhodopsin (486 nm). Interconversions of these three species were achieved by further irradiating the mixture with light of different wavelengths (Fig. 6b-d). The absorption spectrum of the batho-intermediate from 7-*cis*-rhodopsin was

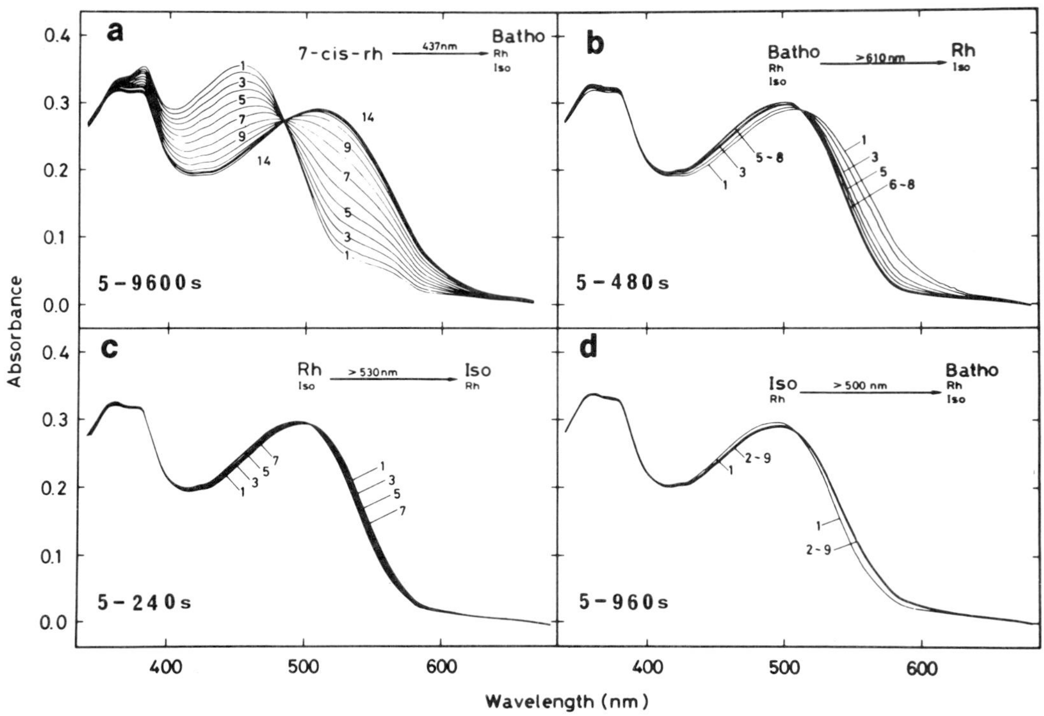

Fig. 6. Photoreaction of 7-*cis*-rhodopsin at liquid nitrogen temperature (a) 7-*cis*-rhodopsin (curve 1) irradiated at 437 nm (curves 2-14). (b) Irradiation of above to remove bathorhodopsin. (c) Irradiation of b to enhance formation of 9-*cis*-rhodopsin. (d) Irradiation of c to form an equilibrium mixture of batho-, 9-*cis*-rhodopsin and rhodopsin.

obtained by taking the difference spectra of the sample before and after long wavelength irradiation. It was found identical to that from rhodopsin. Furthermore, upon warming, the batho-intermediate underwent transitions to two consecutive intermediates at temperatures and with absorption spectra identical to those of lumi-rhodopsin and meta-I-rhodopsin. This appeared to be compelling evidence that an identical primary photo-product was formed from 7-*cis*-rhodopsin and rhodopsin, which could have happened only if the two chromophores occupied an identical binding site. Furthermore, from the structurally different 7-cis and 11-cis isomers, the only logical structure for the common primary photo-product appeared to be the all-trans isomer. This new evidence for the geometric isomerization model for the primary photochemical process is in agreement with the not isomerizable, hence non-bleachable pigments recently prepared by the Columbia group (Ref. 27, 28).

Wavelength attenuated visual pigments

With the exception of 3-dehydrorhodopsin (Ref. 29, 30), absorptions of all other synthetic visual pigments are blue shifted from that of rhodopsin. In an attempt to prepare other red shifted pigments, we synthesized a series of aromatic retinals shown in Fig. 7 (Ref. 31). It should be mentioned that the possibility of preparing wavelength attenuated pigments has added significance following the recent demonstration by Pepperberg *et al.* (Ref. 32) and by Crouch *et al.* (Ref. 33) that retinal analogues can be incorporated into living systems.

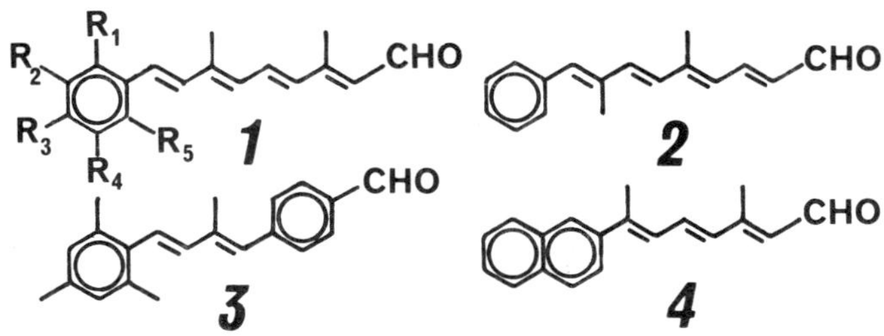

	R_1	R_2	R_3	R_4	R_5
a	H	H	H	H	H
b	Me	H	H	H	H
c	Me	H	Me	H	Me
d	Cl	H	F	H	H
e	H	OMe	OMe	OMe	H
f	H	$-OCH_2O-$		H	H

Fig. 7. Structures of aromatic retinal analogues.

The all-trans isomers of aromatic retinals were synthesized via sequences similar to those reported by Weedon (Ref. 34). The mono-cis isomers were obtained by photoisomerization of the trans followed by separation by preparative high pressure liquid chromatography (HPLC). Results of incubation of these analogues with cattle opsin are shown in Table 2.

TABLE 2. Absorption properties of aromatic rhodopsin analogues and 3-dehydrorhodopsin from 3-dehydroretinal (*5*)

Compound	Absorption maximum (nm) of pigments, if formed[a]					
	All-trans	7-cis	9-cis	11-cis	13-cis	9-cis,13-cis
1a	None	--	485[b]	494	None	--
1b	None	--	482	496	None	None
1c	None	--	470	480	None	--
1d	None	--	470	460	None	--
1e	--	--	None	--	--	--
1f[c]	None	--	None	--	--	--
2	None	--	--	None	--	--
3	None	--	None	--	--	--
4[c]	None	--	470[d]	470[d]	None	--
5	None	464[e]	498[e,f]	517[f]	None	498[g]

a. All data from Ref. 31, unless specified otherwise. b. M. G. Motto, M. Sheves, K. Tsujimoto, V. Balogh-Nair and K. Nakanishi, J. Am. Chem. Soc. 102, 7947-7949 (1980). c. M. Denny and A. E. Asato, unpublished results. d. The test sample was a 1:1 mixture of the 9-cis and 11-cis isomers. e. Ref. 30. f. Ref. 29. g. H. Matsumoto, A. E. Asato and R. S. H. Liu, unpublished results.

That the phenyl, *o*-tolyl, mesityl and β-naphthyl analogues can form pigment analogues first indicates some flexibility of the hydrophobic pocket of the binding site. This is substantiated by the adamantyl analogue recently reported by Nakanishi and coworkers (Ref. 35). The negative results on the *m*- and *p*-substituted compounds point out a limit to this flexibility. The phenyl, *o*-tolyl, mesityl and naphthyl pigment analogues have absorption maxima quite similar to those of rhodopsin. This is perhaps not surprising in view of the fact that the corresponding retinals also have quite similar absorption properties. The absorption maxima of the retinals with electron donating substituents (*1e, f*) are much red shifted. Their failure to form pigments with opsin unfortunately precluded possible formation of red shifted pigments. Other appropriately substituted aromatic retinals should be examined.

Fluorine labelled visual pigments

Because of the wealth of structural information that one can usually obtain from nuclear magnetic resonance (NMR) spectroscopy, the possibility of applying this method to study properties of visual pigments is of high interest. However, because of the size of the protein and the need of a detergent for its solubilization, the use of ^{1}H-NMR to examine the chromophore of the pigment appears to be out of question. The use of ^{13}C-NMR was recently demonstrated (Ref. 36). A ^{13}C-labelled rhodopsin was prepared with the label located at C-14 of the retinal. The signal was weak relative to those of the detergent. Although the assignment of the weak signal to the unprotonated Schiff base is not of general acceptance (Ref. 6, 37), the experimental accomplishment remains a significant achievement.

For several years we have been interested in exploring the possibility of using fluorine labels to examine visual pigments (Ref. 38). The advantages of such a label are its sensitivity and the absence of any background signals. Furthermore fluorine is not much larger than hydrogen, thus not likely to exert any unusual steric effect. On the other hand, the high electronegativity of the fluorine atom introduces the risk that the electronic properties of the pigments could be changed, even to an extent that the fluorinated pigments might not retain properties characteristic of the pigments. Therefore, it is first necessary to establish the existence of stable fluorinated visual pigments and to compare their properties with rhodopsin before a systematic ^{19}F-NMR study can be conducted.

The procedures of Machleidt (Ref. 39) were adopted in our preparation of the fluorinated retinals. As a representative example, the synthesis of 12-fluororetinal is illustrated below (Ref. 40). The unique feature in this sequence is the fact that the Horner reaction

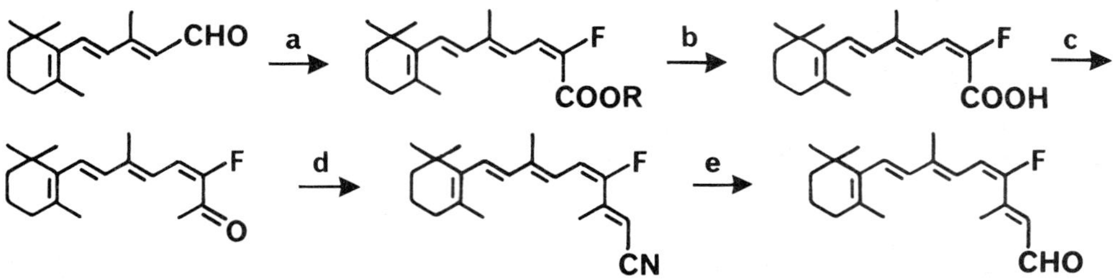

Fig. 8. A synthetic sequence to 11-*cis*-12-fluororetinal. a. $(EtO)_2POCHFCO_2R$/LDA. b. KOH/H_2O-MeOH. c. Excess MeLi. d. $(EtO)_2POCH_2CN$/LDA. e. DIBAH.

at the C-15 stage gave predominantly the 11-cis (11*E*) isomer representing one of the few cases of a stabilized Wittig reagent giving the thermodynamically less stable cis isomer. The preparation of other fluorinated retinals (10-, 14-fluororetinal; 10,14-difluororetinal) followed similar routes. 11-Fluororetinal was also prepared but it was found to be much less stable. Photoisomerization and separation by preparative HPLC gave most of the cis isomers of interest. (Two representative chromatograms are shown in Fig. 9).

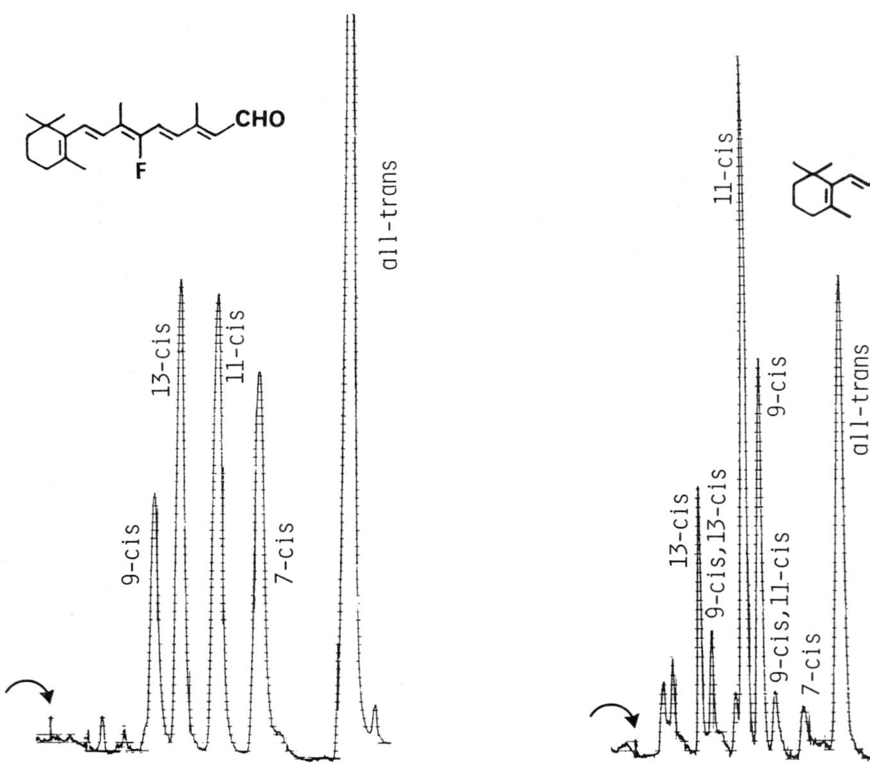

Fig. 9. Chromatograms of irradiated mixtures of two fluorinated retinals. Lichrosorb SI-60 column; solvent 4-6% ether in hexane. Left, 10-fluororetinal; Right, 14-fluororetinal.

Results of incubation of these isomers of fluorinated retinals with extracts of cattle opsin are shown in Table 3. Clearly stable pigments can be obtained from these modified retinals; and the same selectivity of opsin is noticed in these series: i.e., the 13-cis and the trans isomers do not form pigments while those of 11-cis and 9-cis geometry form pigments readily. Interestingly, several of the pigment analogues exhibit absorption much red-shifted from

TABLE 3. Absorption maxima (nm) of isomers of 10-fluoro-, 12-fluoro-, 14-fluoro- and 10,14-difluororetinal[a] (in parentheses) and the rhodopsin analogues

Isomer	10F-Rhodopsin[b]	12F-Rhodopsin[c]	14F-Rhodopsin[b]	10F,14F-Rhodopsin[d]
all-trans	None (369)	None (368)	None (379)	None (375)
7-cis	484 (347)	None (363)[d]	None (369)	--
9-cis	486 (356)	485 (362)	511 (372)	e (360)
11-cis	502 (340)	505 (363)	527 (370)	f
13-cis	None (359)	None (355)	None (375)	None (360)
7-cis,9-cis	464 (347)	--	--	--
7-cis,11-cis	--	500 (353)[d]	--	--
9-cis,13-cis	484 (355)	--	513 (368)	510 (362)
7-cis,9-cis,11-cis	--	None (357)[d]	--	--
7-cis,9-cis,13-cis	460 (340)	--	--	--

a. In hexane. b. Ref. 38. c. Ref. 40. d. H. Matsumoto, A. E. Asato, M. Denny and R. S. H. Liu, unpublished results. e. Not tested. f. Retinal unstable under HPLC conditions.

that of rhodopsin. The objective of the previous project was therefore partially achieved in an accidental way.

There were, however, clear differences between these pigments and rhodopsin. The most obvious one was the thermal stability. While similar to rhodopsin 12-fluororhodopsin solubilized in digitonin was stable at room temperature in the dark and even in the presence of a high concentration of hydroxylamine (a reagent used to remove any unreacted retinal and random Schiff bases involving amino groups outside the binding site of opsin) (Ref. 41), all other fluorinated pigments degraded slowly at room temperature with the rate further accelerated after the addition of hydroxylamine. Therefore, we found it necessary to examine further whether these pigment analogues still retained all characteristic properties of rhodopsin. The photobleaching sequences of two pigment analogues were examined by low temperature spectroscopy (Ref. 40, 42).

Inthesame manner as described before, a sample of 12-fluororhodopsin was irradiated at low temperature and the subsequent photochemical and thermal changes were monitored by its UV-VIS absorption spectra. The formation of a batho-product (λ_{max} = 572 nm) along with 9-*cis*-12-fluororhodopsin during the irradiation process was detected. Its similarity to the parent rhodopsin system was further reflected in its ability to convert to a lumi (λ_{max} = 517 nm) and a meta-I (λ_{max} = 495 nm) intermediate at temperatures greater than -140°C and -50°C respectively. On the other hand, when a sample of 9-*cis*-10-fluororhodopsin was irradiated under the same conditions only reversible formation of its 11-cis isomer was detected. No long wavelength absorptions, attributable to a batho-intermediate, were detected (not even at liquid helium temperature). Clearly, the batho-intermediate was not formed in this system. It was therefore concluded that positioning the fluorine substituent at C-10 has substantially changed the protein-substrate interaction so that the latter system is no longer a satisfactory model for the visual pigment (Ref. 42). Since 12-fluororhodopsin appeared to be an acceptable substitute for rhodopsin, we first examined this system by ^{19}F-NMR spectroscopy. The results are still of preliminary nature. However, they successfully demonstrate feasibility of the method and will be described below.

The NMR sample was prepared in the following manner. Opsin extract from 200 cattle retinae was incubated with a slight excess of 11-*cis*-12-fluororetinal. The resultant pigment was purified by low temperature (4°C) column chromatography on a hydroxyapatite column. The chromatogram and conditions for the chromatography are shown in Fig. 10. The early fractions contained either unreacted retinal or degraded protein. The fractions corresponding to the pigment were collected and concentrated. The end concentration was approximately 0.4 mM.

The ^{19}F-NMR spectrum of the pigment with 2000 transients is shown in Fig. 11a, b (the expanded spectrum in 11c) with the chemical shift relative to that of trifluoroacetic acid. The sample was subsequently bleached by light (>400 nm) at 0°C, the spectrum again recorded (11d, e). A large chemical shift change associated with the bleaching process is evident, and that of the product is consistent with that of a retinal, released from the photobleaching process.

The most striking feature of the absorption signal of the pigment is its width. The half-height width is slightly above 100 Hz which unfortunately obscured any coupling constant data ($^3J_{H,F}$ ≈ 22-35 Hz) which are so useful for configurational and conformational information. It is not immediately clear whether the width is due to chemical shift anisotropy or from dipolar contributions. If for the former it will be of great interest to record the spectrum at a lower magnetic field.

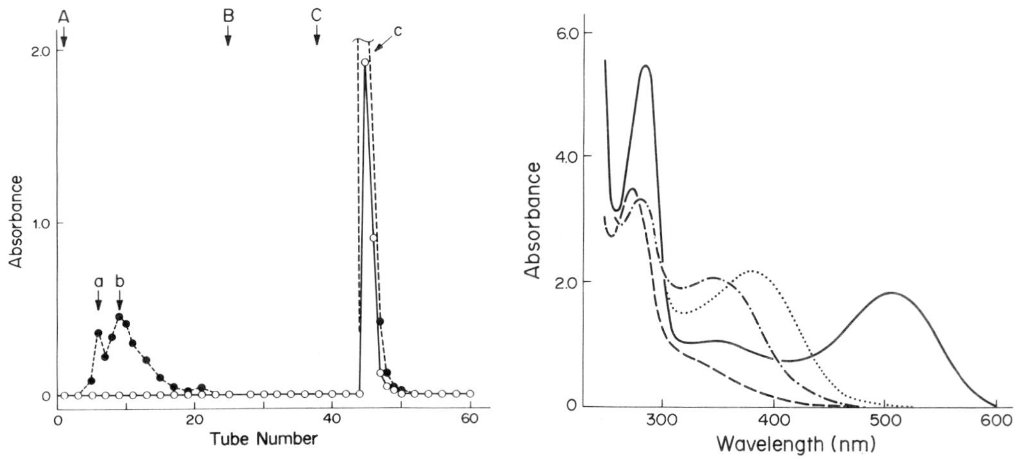

Fig. 10. Chromatographic purification of 12-fluororhodopsin. Left: elution profile of 12-fluororhodopsin on a hydroxylapatite column (Bio-Gel HTP). Eluants: A, 1% Ammonyx LO-Hepes; B, 0.25 M sodium phosphate and 1% Ammonyx LO-Hepes; C, 0.15 M sodium phosphate and 1% Ammonyx LO-Hepes. o——o, A_{500}; ●——●, A_{280}. Right: absorption spectra of peak a (---), peak b (—·—), peak c (——) and photobleached c (···).

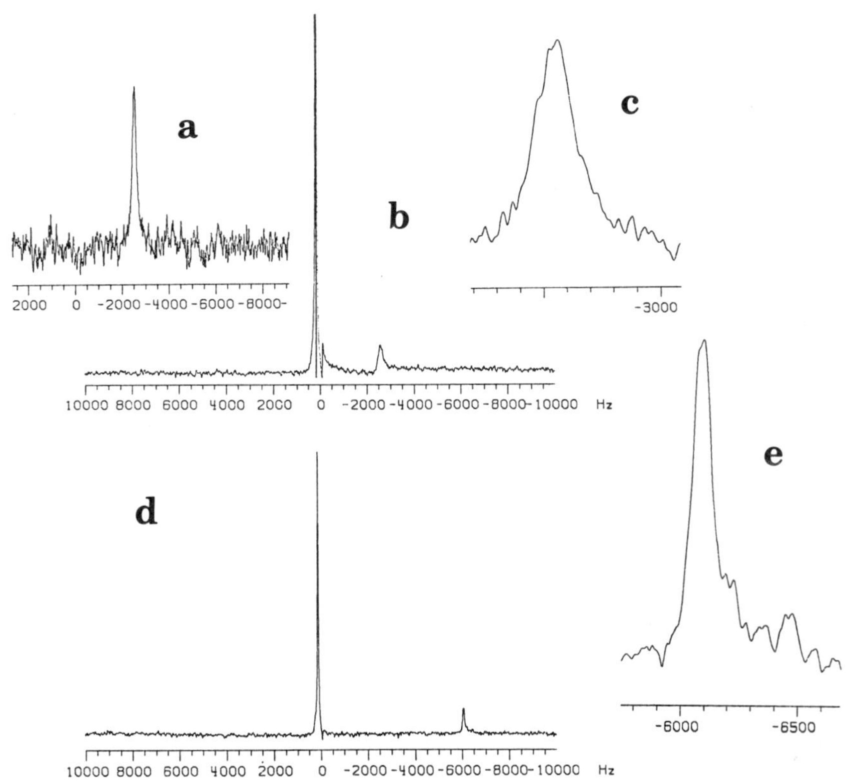

Fig. 11. ^{19}F-NMR spectra of 12-fluororhodopsin (approx. 0.4mM) solubilized in 10% Ammonyx LO with phosphate buffer (pH 7.0) recorded on a Nicolet NT-150 spectrometer at 141.182 MHz with a 12 mm sample tube. Deuterium oxide (5%) was added for locking. Probe temperature: 4°C. a. 12-Fluororhodopsin in the dark. Number of scans: 2000; acquisition time: 204.8 msec. b. Sample a after addition of a small amount of CF_3CO_2H. c. Partial expansion of a. d. Sample b after photobleaching with >440 nm light at 0°C. e. Partial expansion of d.

In the absence of other detailed ^{19}F-NMR data, including a comprehensive collection of chemical shifts and coupling constants of all retinal isomers, the Schiff bases and the protonated Schiff bases under different conditions, it is premature to extract other structural information. All these and other fluorinated retinals are being actively examined in our laboratory.

Acknowledgement - The work described above was possible only through the participation of the following associates and students at the University of Hawaii: A. E. Asato, M. Denny, A. Kini, H. Matsumoto, V. Ramamurthy and C. Simmons, and fruitful collaboration with the following scientists: F. W. Dahlquist, W. J. deGrip, K. Seff and T. Yoshizawa. The work done at UH was generously supported by the U.S. Public Health Services (AM-17806), and partly by the UH Biomedical Program. Fig. 3, 4 and 6 were reprinted with permission from Ref. 22, 26. Copyright (1980) American Chemical Society.

REFERENCES

1. G. Wald, Nature 134, 65 (1934); J. Gen. Physiol. 19, 351-371 (1935-36).
2. R. A. Morton, Nature 153, 69-71 (1944); S. Ball, T. W. Goodwin and R. A. Morton, Biochem. J. 42, 516-523 (1948).
3. Summarized in: G. Wald, Science 162, 230-239 (1968).
4. For a recent review on the subject see: M. Ottolenghi, Adv. Photochem. 12, 97-200 (1980).
5. A. Kropf and R. Hubbard, Ann. N.Y. Acad. Sci. 74, 266-280 (1958).
6. B. Honig, U. Dinur, K. Nakanishi, V. Balogh-Nair, M. A. Gawinowicz, M. Arnaboldi and M. G. Motto, J. Am. Chem. Soc. 101, 7086-7088 (1979).
7. G. E. Busch, M. L. Applebury, P. M. Rentzepis, Proc. Natl. Acad. Sci., USA 69, 2802-2806 (1972).
8. T. Yoshizawa and G. Wald, Nature 197, 1279-1286 (1963).
9. K. van der Meer, J. J. C. Mulder and J. Lugtenberg, Photochem. Photobiol. 24, 363-367 (1976).
10. K. Peters, M. L. Applebury and P. M. Rentzepis, Proc. Natl. Acad. Sci., USA 74, 3119-3123 (1977).
11. P. A. Hargrave, S.-L. Fong, J. H. McDowell, M. T. Mas, D. R. Curtis, J. K. Wang, E. Juşzczak and D. P. Smith, Neurochem. 1, 231-244 (1980); J. K. Wang, J. H. McDowell and P. A. Hargrave, Biochem. 19, 5111-5117 (1980).
12. G. Wald, P. K. Brown, R. Hubbard and W. Oroshnik, Proc. Natl. Acad. Sci., USA 41, 438-450 (1955); 42, 578-580 (1956).
13. R. Crouch, V. Purvin, K. Nakanishi and T. Ebrey, Proc. Natl. Acad. Sci., USA 72, 1538-1542 (1975).
14. V. Ramamurthy and R. S. H. Liu, Tetrahedron 31, 201-206 (1975); A. E. Asato and R. S. H. Liu, J. Am. Chem. Soc. 97, 4128-4130 (1975).
15. A. Kini, H. Matsumoto and R. S. H. Liu, J. Am. Chem. Soc. 101, 5078-5079 (1979).
16. A. Kini, H. Matsumoto and R. S. H. Liu, Bioorg. Chem. 9, 406-410 (1980); M. Denny, M. Chun and R. S. H. Liu, Photochem. Photobiol. 33, 267-269 (1981).
17. V. Ramamurthy and R. S. H. Liu, J. Am. Chem. Soc. 98, 2935-2942 (1976).
18. C. G. Knudsen, S. C. Carey and W. H. Okamura, J. Am. Chem. Soc. 102, 6355-6356 (1980).
19. A. Kini, H. Matsumoto and R. S. H. Liu, unpublished results.
20. W. J. DeGrip, R. S. H. Liu, V. Ramamurthy and A. E. Asato, Nature 262, 416-418 (1976).
21. H. Matsumoto and T. Yoshizawa, Vision Res. 18, 607-609 (1978).
22. H. Matsumoto, R. S. H. Liu, C. Simmons and K. Seff, J. Am. Chem. Soc. 102, 4259-4262 (1980).
23. C. Simmons, R. S. H. Liu, M. Denny and K. Seff, Acta Crystallogr., in press.
24. C. Simmons, A. E. Asato, R. S. H. Liu and K. Seff, unpublished results.
25. R. D. Gilardi, I. L. Karle and J. Karle, Acta Crystallogr. Sect. B, 28, 2605-2612 (1972).
26. S. Kawamura, S. Miyatani, H. Matsumoto, T. Yoshizawa and R. S. H. Liu, Biochem. 19, 1549-1553 (1980).
27. M. A. Gawinowicz, V. Balogh-Nair, J. S. Sabol and K. Nakanishi, J. Am. Chem. Soc. 99, 7720-7721 (1977).
28. H. Akita, S. P. Tanis, M. Adams, V. Balogh-Nair and K. Nakanishi, J. Am. Chem. Soc. 102, 6370-6372 (1980).
29. M. Azuma, K. Azuma and Y. Kito, Biochim. Biophys. Acta 295, 520-527 (1973).
30. H. Matsumoto, A. E. Asato and R. S. H. Liu, Photochem. Photobiol. 29, 695-698 (1979).
31. H. Matsumoto, A. E. Asato, M. Denny, B. Baretz, Y.-P. Yen, D. Tong and R. S. H. Liu, Biochem. 19, 4589-4593 (1980).
32. D. R. Pepperberg, P. K. Brown, M. Lurie and J. E. Dowling, J. Gen. Physiol. 71, 369-396 (1978); R. Crouch and D. R. Pepperberg, Invest. Ophthalmol. 17, 1024-1029 (1978).
33. R. Crouch, S. Katz, K. Nakanishi, M. A. Gawinowicz and V. Balogh-Nair, Photochem. Photobiol. 33, 91-95 (1981).

34. K. R. Bharucha and B. C. L. Weedon, J. Chem. Soc. 1571-1577 (1953).
35. R. A. Blatchly, J. D. Carriker, V. Balogh-Nair and K. Nakanishi, J. Am. Chem. Soc. 102, 2495-2497 (1980).
36. J. Shriver, G. Mateescu, R. Fager, D. Torchia and E. W. Abrahamson, Nature 270, 273-274 (1977).
37. A. Yamaguchi, T. Unemoto and A. Ikegami, Photochem. Photobiol. 33, 511-516 (1981).
38. A. E. Asato, H. Matsumoto, M. Denny and R. S. H. Liu, J. Am. Chem. Soc. 100, 5957-5960 (1978).
39. H. Machleidt and R. Wessendorf, Liebigs Ann. Chem. 679, 20-25 (1964); 681, 21-29 (1965).
40. R. S. H. Liu, H. Matsumoto, A. E. Asato, M. Denny, Y. Shichida, T. Yoshizawa and F. W. Dahlquist, submitted to J. Am. Chem. Soc.
41. R. Hubbard, P. K. Brown and D. Bownds, Methods Enzymol. 18, 615-653 (1971).
42. Y. Shichida and T. Yoshizawa, unpublished results.

RETINOL-BINDING PROTEINS AND THEIR FUNCTIONS

John Glover

Department of Biochemistry, University of Liverpool, Liverpool L69 3BX

Abstract - Retinol is transported from the liver to its functional tissues via plasma retinol-binding protein which binds to specific receptors on their outer cell-membranes. Only the retinol is transferred across the membranes, and this then encounters a cellular retinol-binding protein, which can carry it the remaining short distance to the nucleus, where the vitamin is believed to act. The properties of the two proteins are compared in relation to their respective functions and their particular importance in controlling the supply of retinol for reproductive tissues is discussed.

INTRODUCTION

The fat-soluble retinol, like the carotenoids from which it is derived, functions in a predominantly aqueous environment and needs the assistance of protein for its transport. Following the discovery that it occurred in plasma mainly in the alcohol form, it was considered likely that a special carrier was involved and the specific retinol-binding protein (RBP) was first isolated in a pure state from human plasma by Kanai, Raz and Goodman (Ref. 1) and later crystallised as long thin needles by Haupt and Heidi (Ref. 2). Since then many of its properties have been determined in a number of laboratories and more recently, its amino acid sequence elucidated by Rask, Arundi and Peterson (Ref. 3).

Following the isolation of a specific carrier protein for retinol from plasma, the possibility was considered by analogy with the transport of steroid hormones, that retinol might also be associated with protein within the cytoplasm of its target cells. This was demonstrated by Bashor, Toft and Chytil (Ref. 4) who detected such a protein initially in the cytosol of testicular tissue using sucrose gradient ultracentrifugation and later in most other tissues except muscle. The protein has now been purified by Ong and Chytil (Ref. 5) and shown to be a single polypeptide chain of 14,600 daltons. These two proteins are responsible for the transport of retinol from the liver stores to its target within the functional cells. Their properties and functions are described and compared. This transport system is quite separate from the non-specific low density lipoprotein system, which is responsible for transferring freshly absorbed retinol in the ester form from the intestine to the liver.

PLASMA RETINOL-BINDING PROTEIN

Plasma RBP is synthesised in the liver as a single polypeptide of 21,000 daltons and it has one binding site for retinol which is not attached covalently but is probably held by hydrophobic forces within a fold of the protein. In plasma it associates with thyroxine-binding prealbumin (TBPA) to form a 1:1 complex of approximately 75,000 daltons (Ref. 6) and this is considered to be of physiological importance in preventing rapid loss of the vitamin through the kidney. It is interesting that RBP has a relatively high content of 22 aromatic amino acids out of the total 182 residues (Ref. 3) and like prealbumin is also unusual in that it does not contain any carbohydrate moiety as do most other plasma proteins secreted by the liver.

Optical rotatory dispersion and circular dichroism studies reveal that the protein has a largely unordered structure with little or no α-helix but 20% of β-conformation (Ref. 7). The folds of the protein are held together by 3 dithio-bonds and H-bonds.

The main physical properties of the molecule are summarised in Table 1. It possesses three key sites related to its function namely the binding sites for retinol and prealbumin as well as the one responsible for linking to its membrane receptors in functional tissues.

Binding site

Information regarding the nature of the binding site is as yet limited and has been obtained indirectly from studies on ultraviolet absorption, on fluorescence and on the capacity of the protein to bind analogues. Some work, however, has also been done to examine the effects of chemically blocking particular amino acid groups on the capacity of the molecule to bind either retinol or prealbumin (Ref. 8).

TABLE 1. Properties of plasma retinol-binding protein

Molecular weight	21,000	Retinol binding site	1
Amino acids	182	Association cons't	$5.6 \times 10^6 M^{-1}$
N-terminal	Glutamic acid	Isoelectric point	pH 4.5
COOH-terminal	Leucine	Mobility	α_2
U V absorption $\lambda\lambda$ max	278; 329 nm	$E^{1\%}_{1cm}$	= 17.5
Fluorescence : Excitation	289; 332 nm	Emission	342 nm; 456 nm

Among the earliest observations, it was noted that the protein on isolation from plasma was heterogeneous, in that it could be resolved into several components by electrophoresis or isoelectric focussing. Two of these exhibited fluorescence and still carried retinol but other higher mobility ones did not bind retinol and were devoid of fluorescence (Refs. 6,9).

This heterogeneity does not arise through losses of amino acids because the amino acid composition of the apoprotein, incapable of binding retinol, is the same as that of the holoprotein (Ref. 10). It occurs through increases in the negative charge of the protein in two ways. The primary one appears to be due to the loss of one or more amide groups, which do not affect retinol binding. A further increase in net negative charge occurs when the ligand retinol is removed from its binding site. It is not known, however, whether this second one arises simply from a change in conformation of the molecule or from some interaction of a charged group directly with retinol. The ultraviolet transmission scan of the purified protein fraction at 280 nm and 330 nm (for retinol) after separation of its components by electrophoresis on a polyacrylamide gel illustrates this heterogeneity (Fig. 1).

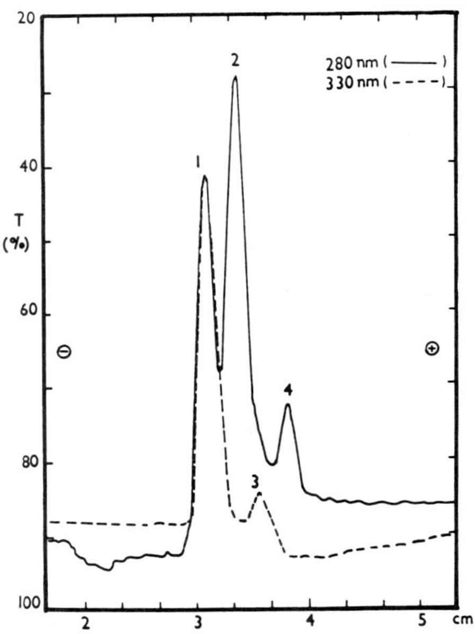

Fig. 1. Ultraviolet transmittance scan of a polyacrylamide gel electrophoretogram of human plasma RBP at 280 nm (——) and 330 nm (····) Peaks 1 and 3 in the 330 nm trace are due to slow and fast moving components of holoRBP, whereas peaks 2 and 4 in the 280 nm trace show the presence of their respective apoproteins.

The ultraviolet absorption of the protein shows that the retinol is lying in a hydrophobic environment since λ max at 329 nm is similar to that for the vitamin in hydrocarbon solvents. Its fluorescence in the bound form is, however, 14 times stronger than that for retinol in solution indicative that energy transfer can occur from adjacent amino acids. Peaks in the excitation spectrum at 278 nm and in the emission spectrum at 342 nm in addition to those for retinol indicate that some energy transfer can arise from one or more of the 4 tryptophanes present in the protein. Modification of two of the tryptophanes with 2 hydroxy-5 nitrobenzyl bromide does not affect retinol binding, but changes in the remaining two destroy it (Ref. 8). It seems likely that retinol lies close to at least one tryptophane residue. Again, acetylation of all the lysines and up to 3 tyrosyl residues with N-acetylimidazole did not affect the binding of retinol to the protein, but prevented the latter from binding to prealbumin (Ref. 11). Attempts either to esterify retinol bound to RBP or to oxidise it with alcohol dehydrogenase have been unsuccessful and suggest that the carbinol group is well protected or sterically hindered from access to these enzymes (Ref. 12).

Attachment of analogues. Further information has been gleaned from studies on the capacity of the protein to bind analogues to the most physiologically active or β-form of retinol. The interaction of the native apoprotein with a variety of analogues has been examined in several laboratories (Refs. 13, 14, 15, 16).

Some compounds examined in our own laboratory were chosen to show up variations in binding which might arise through changing (a) the β-ionone ring; (b) the terminal C-15 group and (c) the length of the side chain. Others have examined the effects of changing some of the double bonds in the side chain from *trans* to *cis*-conformations (Refs. 13, 14). The native purified holoprotein is first extracted with solvent to remove the retinol and then incubated immediately with a tenfold molar excess of the new ligand under test for binding. In relation to the first group (a) it has been found that altering the double bond in retinol from the 5, 6 position to 4, 5 as in α-retinol prevents the molecule from fitting into the binding site. Again, opening up the ring structure, typified by γ-retinol, does not lead to any successful linking of the molecule to the protein. The insertion of an additional double bond in the 3, 4 position, as in vitamin A_2 however, inhibits but does not prevent a successful complex from being made as can be seen from Fig. 2 which shows the absorption spectra of the 3-dehydroretinol complex. However, the half saturation time of the apoprotein by retinol is only 1 min. compared with 17 min. for 3-dehydroretinol.

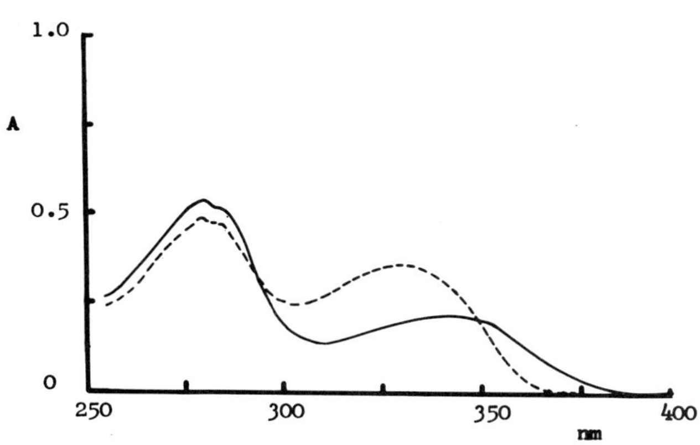

Fig. 2. Absorption spectra of the complexes formed between apoRBP and retinol (......) and 3 dehydroretinol (______).

With regard to group (b) both retinal and retinoic acid bind to the apoprotein to yield complexes with uv absorption maxima at 392 nm and 335 nm respectively due to the chromophores of the ligands (15). The bathochromic shift of λmax for retinal from 367 nm in hexane to 392 nm is indicative that the aldehyde group is lying adjacent to a basic group on the protein. The half saturation times for these ligands are 8 min. and 16 min. respectively (15). It has also been shown that the oxime and some Schiff base derivatives of the aldehyde bind to the protein (Ref. 16). Thus, it is possible to modify the terminal carbinol and still achieve some binding. Similarly, it is possible to bend the side chain as in 9-*cis*, 11-*cis* and 13-*cis* retinols and still achieve some complex formation with the protein (Refs. 13, 14). However, if the chain is lengthened as in β-apo-10'-carotenal or esterified by palmitate then the ligand will not become attached. Retinylacetate, however, can bind to the protein but very slowly. However, this would be of little use to the animal since retinol *in vivo* is esterified mainly with palmitate.

Although several analogues like the above metabolites of retinol can form complexes with RBP *in vitro*, these do not appear to be formed *in vivo*, e.g. when vitamin-deficient rats are maintained on retinoic acid, none of the latter appears to be associated with RBP (Ref. 17). The inability of α-retinol to bind to the protein can be readily explained when its structural model is compared with that of β-retinol. The β-ionone ring is planar with the all-*trans* side chain in β-retinol, but in α-retinol the ring is distorted with the gem dimethyl group and part of the ring projecting well above the horizontal plane of the side chain to make a much more bulky head group, which presumably cannot fit the cleft in RBP capable of binding the flatter β-retinol. Consequently α-retinol, which is known to be absorbed from the intestine and stored in the liver (Ref. 18) and is biologically active *in vitro* when applied directlytotissues (Ref. 19), cannot express that activity *in vivo* due to its inability to bind to the specific carrier protein. Retinoic acid, however, which is partially water soluble and can bind to albumin bypasses the normal retinol transport system to reach the various target cells where it can carry out some of the functions of vitamin A.

UPTAKE OF RETINOL FROM RETINOL-BINDING HOLOPROTEIN BY TISSUE CELLS

It has been demonstrated that holoRBP binds to specific receptors on plasma membranes of functional tissues such as the pigment epithelium of the eye (Ref. 20), the intestinal mucosae (Ref. 21) and the interstitial cells of the testes (Ref. 22). The link is through the polypeptide and the affinity constant for the receptor is of the order of $2 \times 10^{11} M^{-1}$ (Ref. 20) in the rat and $4.8 \times 10^{9} M^{-1}$ in the chick (Ref. 23). The mechanism of the release of retinol from this complex is not yet understood. Clearly a change occurs in the protein to enable retinol to leave the complex quickly and the apoprotein is then released back into circulation. It seems to be incapable of taking up a second load of retinol (e.g. from material freshly absorbed from the intestine (Ref. 24). Since apoprotein formed from RBP has a greater net-negative charge, the change may simply involve the loss of an amide group to open up the conformation of the active site. Retinol once released could quickly penetrate the lipid phase of the cell membrane, but may need another protein to collect it on the inside.

CELLULAR RETINOL-BINDING PROTEIN

The above role is fulfilled by cellular RBP (M.W. 14,600) which is much smaller than the plasma carrier and differs from it in amino acid composition and immunologically. Again, the cellular protein possesses only one binding site for the vitamin. Following the detection and purification of the protein, its capacity for binding analogues of retinol was also examined in competitive binding studies by Ong and Chytil (Ref. 25). They found that α-retinol successfully competed with β-retinol for the binding site, but analogues such as retinal and retinoic acid where the terminal carbinol group was altered could not compete. When the cytosol from chick retinas was exposed to N-ethylmaleimide, the binding of retinol to cellular RBP was unaffected (Ref. 26) and similarly the addition of dithiothreitol did not prevent retinol from binding, hence it appears that the attachment of the vitamin is not dependent on the presence of intact dithio-groups as is the case for the plasma protein. The binding capacities of the two proteins for various ligands are compared in Table 2.

It is clear that the cellular RBP expresses higher specificity for the terminal carbinol group whereas the plasma protein needs to have the correct ring moiety. Cellular RBP has a different electrophoretic mobility from the corresponding plasma protein and possesses a different antigenicity (Ref. 27). The ultraviolet absorption spectrum of pure cellular RBP (Ref. 28) as shown in Fig. 3 is quite different from that of its plasma counterpart.

The λmax has undergone a bathochromic shift to 350 nm and the absorption band shows more fine structure, suggesting a change in the orientation of the double bonds or strong interaction between them and the protein. The dissociation constant at 1.6×10^{-8} means, however, that the binding of retinol is only about tenfold stronger than that for plasma RBP and so favours the transfer of retinol into the cell.

FUNCTIONS OF PLASMA AND CELLULAR RETINOL-BINDING PROTEINS

At present a little more is known about plasma RBP than the cellular protein because it has been easier to obtain and analyse in animal plasma. In the normal vitamin-A replete animal it was soon found that the plasma concentration was variable from day to day and even at various times of the day, clearly depending on the rate of synthesis of the protein which has a half life of only 7.5h in the rat (Ref. 29) and 6.6h in a primate (*Macaca* irus) (Ref. 30).

TABLE 2. Differences in the binding of analogues of retinol to plasma and cellular retinol-binding proteins

Analogue	Binding capability	
	Plasma RBP[a] (M.W. 21,000)	Cellular RBP[b] (M.W. 14,600)
All-*trans* β-retinol	+	+
Cis-isomers		
9-*Cis* β-retinol	+[c]	+
13-*Cis* β-retinol	+	+
Ring isomers		
α-retinol	-	+
γ-retinol	-	
3-dehydroretinol	+(6)[d]	+(100)
C-15 modifications		
Retinaldehyde	+	-
Retinoic acid	+	-
Retinyl acetate	+	-
Retinyl palmitate	-	-

Notes: a, b and c. Details compiled from Ref. 15, 24 & 14 respectively.
Note d. Figures in parentheses refer to relative rates of binding compared to that for β-retinol taken as 100.

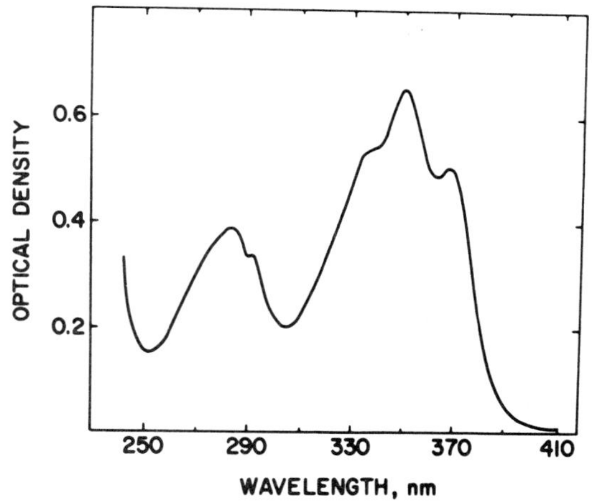

Fig. 3. Absorption spectrum of the complex between cellular RBP and retinol (from Chytil & Ong, Ref. 28).

In conducting studies over longer periods, it was observed that the plasma level in seasonal breeding animals increased during the breeding season when the gonads were growing and declined again as their regression set in (Refs. 31, 32). These changes are illustrated in Figs. 4 and 5 for sheep and birds (Japanese quail) respectively.

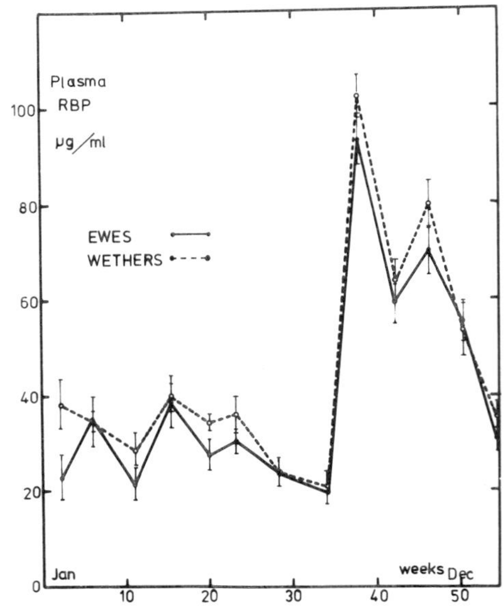

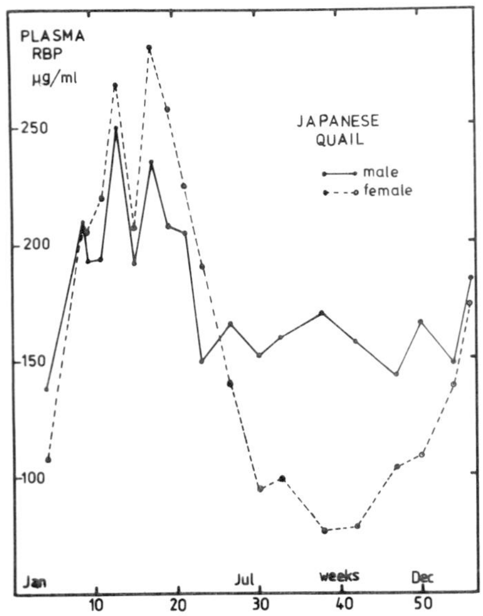

Fig. 4. Seasonal changes in concentration of plasma holoRBP in ewes and wethers (castrated rams).

Fig. 5. Seasonal changes in concentration of plasma holoRBP in Japanese quail (Coturnix coturnix japonica).

Similar changes occur in the polyoestrous rat (Ref. 33), (see Fig. 6) and in children (Ref.21) as they pass through puberty, in that the plasma concentration increases about twofold but in these instances remains at the higher adult level.

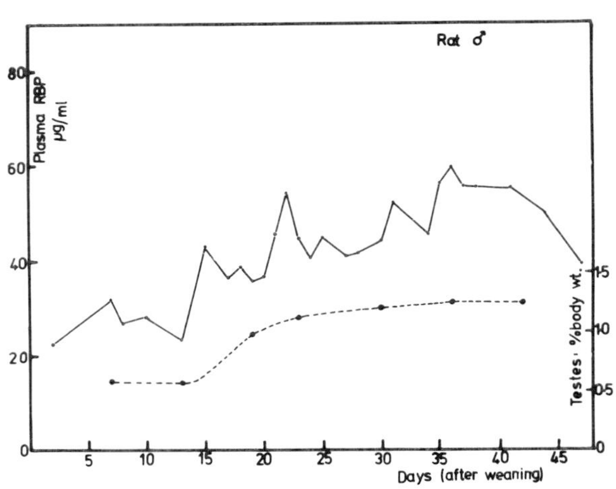

Fig. 6. Increase in concentration of plasma holoRBP (——) in groups of young immature male rats during their development into adults. The parallel increase in testicular weights expressed as a percentage of body weight (•••••) is also shown.

Thus a greater supply of retinol is maintained for the growth and maintenance of the gonads, which had previously been shown to have a specific requirement for retinol rather than retinoic acid (Ref. 34).

The observed changes which are cyclic in seasonal breeding animals are clearly under the control of hormones related in some way to the pineal-hypothalamus-pituitary system, which can be influenced by light. It has been demonstrated that the glucocorticords, corticosterone and hydrocortisone can stimulate the synthesis of RBP in primary liver cell cultures (Ref. 35), but whether this hormone is responsible for the cyclic change in RBP is not yet clear. It is interesting too that TBPA, which is also associated with RBP in the transport of retinol is also subject to cyclic fluctuations in seasonal breeding animals (Ref. 36) but in the opposite manner to that of RBP as shown in Fig. 7, where they are plotted together to show their relative concentration in molar terms and in relation to gonadal development.

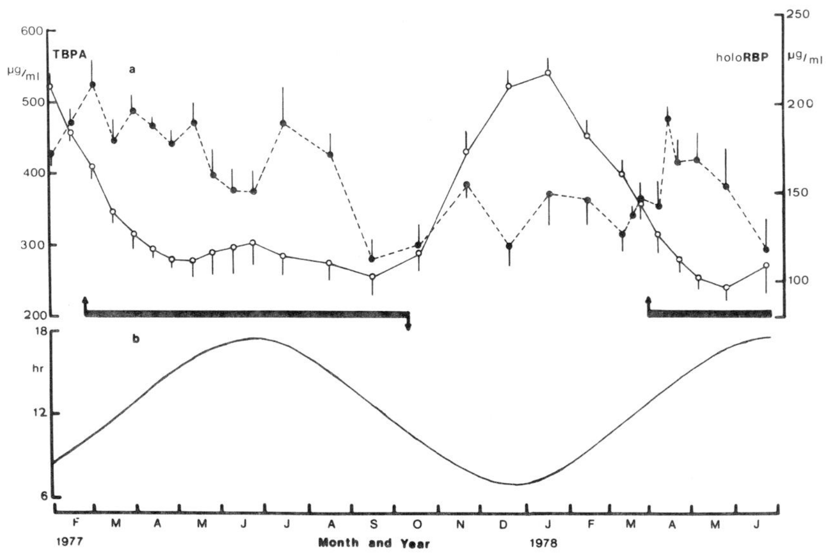

Fig. 7. (a) Seasonal changes in plasma TBPA (—o—o) in relation to those of holoRBP (··•··•·) and to (b) variations in photo period. The bars indicate the period of gonadal activity from development (↑) to regression (↓). The concentration scales used are in the ratio of their respective molecular weights (i.e., 2.5:1) so that points where the graphs cross indicate the times when the two proteins are present in equimolar amounts.

Prealbumin seems to be of particular importance in thyroxine as well as vitamin A transport. It can be seen that when the gonadal development is initiated the ratio of RBP to TBPA is in excess of 1:1 and when the regression occurs, TBPA is in excess (Refs. 37, 38). This could possibly mean that more holoRBP is available in the free form (not complexed with TBPA) for easier penetration to the interstitial cells which carry its receptors so enabling a greater supply of retinol to become available for promoting growth of the gonadal cells.

At all events it would appear that the plasma RBP is much more than a simple carrier for the vitamin. It is highly involved in controlling the supply of retinol to the functional tissues. Some of the known functions of the two proteins may be summarised as in Table 3.

From this it can be seen that animals use specific proteins for retinol distribution in a manner very similar to those for steroid hormones , vitamin D_3 and biologically active derivatives. Specific carriers for either retinaldehyde or retinoic acid have not been detected in plasma and perhaps since metabolites can be readily formed from retinol in all tissues, there is no physiological requirement for such proteins in extracellular fluids. Furthermore, both these forms of vitamin A have reactive groups which can enable them to become readily attached non-specifically to proteins generally. β-Carotene and other non-polar provitamins A on the other hand, are transported like retinyl esters in body fluids in association with other lipids attached to low density lipoproteins synthesised in the intestine and liver. These lipids are less toxic and consequently have much less requirement for transport in plasma under such strict control as the biologically-active retinol molecule.

TABLE 3. Functions of plasma and cellular retinol-binding proteins

Plasma RBP

1. Shows high specificity for β-ionone ring type analogues of retinol.

2. Controls retinol secretion from the liver.

3. Limits transport of retinol to target tissues.

4. Protects retinol against oxidative or enzymic attack.

5. Binds to specific cell receptors in target tissues for retinol transfer.

6. Forms 1:1 complex with prealbumin to prevent rapid loss of vitamin through the kidney.

Cellular RBP

1. Shows high specificity for terminal carbinol of retinol.

2. Assists with uptake of retinol into tissue cells.

3. Is widely distributed in epithelial tissues but absent from muscle.

4. Transports retinol from plasma membrane to nucleus.

REFERENCES

1. M. Kanai, A. Raz and DeW.S. Goodman, J. Clin. Invest. 47, 2025 (1968)
2. V.H. Haupt and K. Heidi, Blut 24, 94 (1972)
3. L. Rask, H. Arundi and P.A. Peterson, Febs Lett 104, 55-58 (1979)
4. M.M. Bashor, D.O. Toft and F. Chytil, Proc. Natn. Acad. Sci U.S.A., 70, 3483-3487 (1973)
5. D.E. Ong and F. Chytil, J. Biol. Chem. 253, 828 (1978)
6. A. Raz, T.T. Shiratori and DeW.S. Goodman, J. Biol. Chem. 245, 1903 (1970)
7. A.M. Gotto, S.E. Lux and DeW.S. Goodman, Biochim. Biophys. Acta 271, 429-435 (1972)
8. J. Horwitz and J. Heller, J. Biol. Chem. 249, 7181-7185 (1974)
9. J. Glover, Vitam. and Horm. (New York) 31, 1-42 (1973)
10. W. Kirby, Ph.D. Thesis, Univ. of Liverpool (1971)
11. J. Heller and J. Horwitz, J. Biol. Chem. 250, 3019-3023 (1975)
12. S. Weston and J. Glover, (Unpublished observations)
13. DeW. S. Goodman and A. Raz, J. Lipid Res. 13, 338-346 (1972)
14. J. Horwitz and J. Heller J. Biol. Chem. 248, 6308-6316 (1973)
15. H. Muhilal and J. Glover, Biochem. Trans. 3, 744-746 (1975)
16. J. Horwitz and J. Heller, J. Biol. Chem. 249, 4712-4719 (1974)
17. J.E. Smith, P.O. Milch, Y. Muto and DeW.S. Goodman, Biochem J. 132, 821-827 (1973)
18. S.R. Ames, W.J. Swanson and P.L. Harris, J. Am. Chem. Soc. 77, 4136 (1955)
19. M.B. Sporn, N.M. Dunlop, D.L. Newton and W.R. Henderson, Nature 263, 110-113 (1976)
20. J. Heller, J. Biol. Chem. 250, 3613-3619 (1975)
21. P.A. Peterson, S.F. Nilsson, L. Östberg, L. Rask and A. Vahlquist, Vitam. Horm. (New York) 32, 181-214 (1974). L. Rask and P.A. Peterson, J. Biol. Chem. 251, 6360-6366 (1976)
22. B.W. McGuire, M.C. Orgebin-Crist and F. Chytil, Endocrinology 108, 658-667 (1981)
23. M.K. Bhat and H.R. Cama, Biochim. Biophys. Acta 587, 273-281 (1979)
24. J. Glover, L. Moxley, H. Muhilal and S. Weston, Clin. Chim. Acta. 50, 371-380 (1974)
25. D.E. Ong and F. Chytil, J. Biol. Chem 250, 6113-6117 (1975)
26. B. Wiggert and G.J. Chader, Exp. Eye. Res. 21, 143 (1975)
27. T. Abe, B. Wiggert, D.R. Bergsma and G.J. Chader, Biochim. Biophys. Acta. 498, 355 (1977)
28. F. Chytil and D.E. Ong, Vitam. and Horm (New York) 36, 1-32 (1975)
29. H. Muhilal and J. Glover, Br. J. Nutr. 32, 549-558 (1974)
30. A. Vahlquist, Scand. J. Clin. Lab. Invest. 30, 349-362 (1972)
31. J. Glover, C. Jay, R.C. Kershaw and P.E.B. Reilly, Br. J. Nutr. 36, 137-141 (1976)
32. J. Glover, D.J. Heaf and S. Large, Br. J. Nutr. 43, 357-366 (1980)
33. R.C. Kershaw, Ph.D. Thesis, University of Liverpool (1978)
34. J. N. Thompson, J.McC. Howell and G.A.J. Pitt, Proc. R. Soc. (Biol) 159, 510-535 (1964)
35. J.E. Smith, C. Borek, and DeW.S. Goodman, Ann. N.Y. Acad. Sci 359, 171-181 (1981)
36. M. El-Sayed, D.J. Heaf and J. Glover, Gen. Comp. Endocrinol. 41, 539-545 (1980)
37. J. Glover and D.J. Heaf, Discussion in "Biological Clocks in Seasonal Reproductive Cycles" (Eds B.K. and D.E. Follett) p.198-201 Bristol Scientechnica (1981)
38. D.J. Heaf, M. El-Sayed, B. Phythian, J. Carroll and J. Glover, J. Endocr. (in press) (1981)

GENETIC ANALYSIS OF CAROTENOGENESIS IN RHODOPSEUDOMONAS CAPSULATA

Barry L. Marrs

Department of Biochemistry, Saint Louis University School of Medicine, Saint Louis, MO 63104, USA

Abstract - Seven genes specifically affecting carotenogenesis have been identified in the photosynthetic bacterium *Rhodopseudomonas capsulata*. A metabolic grid for carotenogenesis is consistent with the accumulation pattern of intermediates in these mutants. Mutants that accumulate no carotenoids have been isolated, and their light-harvesting polypeptides examined. These observations are consistent with a role for uncomplexed polypeptides in regulation of carotenogenesis. Two genetic exchange systems suitable for mapping are available in *R. capsulata*: capsduction and conjugation. Capsduction is mediated by the gene transfer agent of this species, and it is an excellent tool for fine structure mapping. Conjugation is mediated by a promiscuous plasmid with enhanced chromosome mobilizing ability, pBLM2. R-prime derivatives of pBLM2 have been isolated that incorporate a 40 megadalton block of DNA carrying the genes for photopigments and photopigment-binding proteins. The *R. capsulata* DNA carried on the R-prime has been cloned using recombinant DNA techniques, and the restriction fragments bearing the genes for carotenogenesis have been identified.

INTRODUCTION

The photosynthetic bacterium *Rhodopseudomonas capsulata* accumulates the carotenoid spheroidene while growing by either fermentation or photosynthesis in the absence of oxygen. The presence of oxygen has various effects upon the accumulation of spheroidene, depending upon the concentration of the gas. In the range below about one percent of atmospheric oxygen tension the amount of carotenoid synthesized is not affected, but a mixture of spheroidene and a 2-oxo-derivative, spheroidenone, is accumulated (Ref. 1). At higher pO_2's pigment synthesis is progressively inhibited. The inhibition of carotenoid synthesis is accompanied by inhibition of synthesis of both bacteriochlorophyll and the photosynthetic membrane structure that normally binds those pigments (Ref. 2).

Carotenoids and bacteriochlorophyll are normally found complexed with light-harvesting and reaction center polypeptides in intracytoplasmic membrane structures (Ref. 3). Since some carotenoids continue to be synthesized at oxygen tensions high enough to repress the other components of the photosynthetic apparatus, carotenoids would seem capable of associating with other cellular entities as well. As in other photosynthetic organisms, the carotenoids serve dual roles in *R. capsulata*: they harvest radiant energy and transmit it to bacteriochlorophyll so that chemical energy may eventually be stored, and they protect the organism from photooxidative damage by quenching bacteriochlorophyll triplets and other excited molecules before they can react with oxygen to form highly reactive singlet oxygen (Ref. 4). We have employed a biochemical genetics approach to study carotenogenesis and photosynthetic membrane formation and their regulation by oxygen.

MUTANTS WITH ALTERED CAROTENOID METABOLISM

Mutations may affect carotenoid metabolism in two distinctly different ways: by altering or inactivating the structure of an enzyme directly involved in carotenoid biosynthesis, or by altering another cellular component with regulatory interactions with carotenogenesis.

Biosynthetic mutants

Examples of the first of these categories are listed in Table 1.

TABLE 1. Mutants that accumulate atypical carotenoids

Phenotype	Genotype	Carotenoids Accumulated	Biosynthetic Step Affected
Blue-green	crtB or crtE	None	Unknown
Blue-green	crtH	Phytoene	Dehydrogenase
Green	crtC	Neurosporene	Hydratase
Green	crtD	Neurosporene, Hydroxyneurosporene, Methoxyneurosporene	3-4,dehydrogenase
Muddy-brown	crtF	Demethylspheroidene and Demethylspheroidenone	O-methylase
Yellow-brown	crtA	Spheroidene	Oxygenase

The phenotypes of mutants blocked in carotenoid biosynthesis are described in part by the colors of photosynthetic cultures of each mutant. Such description is possible because the carotenoids are not essential for photosynthesis. Blue-green mutants have no colored carotenoids, and thus are sensitive to photooxidative damage (Ref. 5). Furthermore, all known blue-green mutants lack an antenna complex known variously as light-harvesting II or B800-850 (Ref. 6). Mutants which contain any colored carotenoid (i.e., contain carotenoids with nine or more conjugated double bonds) appear to be resistant to photooxidative damage. Indeed, aside from the color, it is difficult to find any differences among green, yellow-brown and wild type strains. This raises questions about why spheroidene is accumulated by wild type strains instead of neurosporene. It is possible that color is the key, if the amount of radiant energy available on the average in nature favors the longer wavelength absorption maxima of spheroidene and spheroidenone.

Mutants lacking O-methylase activity (muddy) have one unusual phenotypic trait. Cultures of these strains accumulate high levels of secondary mutants with additional alterations in carotenoid or bacteriochlorophyll synthesis. Revertants that have regained wild type carotenoid synthesis are also found. It appears as if one of the demethylated compounds accumulated by muddy-brown mutants has a deleterious affect on growth, and any additional mutation that decreases the accumulation of the demethylated compounds confers a growth advantage. The secondary carotenoid mutation may block directly the biosynthetic pathway at a stage before demethylspheroidene, and green and blue-green mutants are common. Mutants blocked in bacteriochlorophyll synthesis all accumulate reduced amounts of carotenoids, independent of the chemical nature of the carotenoids, and thus a wide variety of mutants unable to synthesize mature bacteriochlorophyll are found. Muddy-brown strains are thus very useful for generating additional mutations of interest.

Metabolic grid for carotenoid biosynthesis

It is possible to propose a biosynthetic pathway for the carotenoids of R. capsulata, based upon the compounds accumulated in mutants (Ref. 7). This sort of exercise has been done in the past (Ref. 8), and this updated version should also be regarded as sheer speculation until the appropriate reactions can be demonstrated biochemically. The observation of phytoene accumulators, but no mutant strain of R. capsulata that accumulates a pentaene or heptaene carotenoid, suggests that one enzyme may carry out the successive oxidation to convert phytoene to neurosporene. Neurosporene is normally hydrated across the 1-2 double bond to form hydroxyneurosporene. From this point the order of reactions appears to be branched, hence a metabolic grid best describes the reactions. Hydroxyneurosporene may be methylated to methoxyneurosporene, or it may be oxidized to demethylspheroidene. Demethylspheroidene can then be methylated, and methoxyneurosporene can be oxidized, to give spheroidene. Hydration at the opposite end of the molecule across the 1'-2' double bond is also possible. An oxo-function can be added to the 2-carbon in any of the decaene molecules in the presence of O_2.

Regulatory mutants

An example of a second type of mutation that may affect carotenoid metabolism has already been given above. It is clear that any mutation that interferes with normal bacteriochlorophyll synthesis greatly diminishes carotenoid synthesis. The mechanism for this effect is unknown, but it probably involves a normal regulatory interaction that serves to coordinate pigment syntheses in the wild type. For example, a particular bacteriochlorophyll -protein complex might activate transcription of the genes for carotenoid biosynthesis, or the uncomplexed protein might inhibit that transcription. The same effects might be brought about through activation or inhibition of enzyme activities without changes in the amounts of enzyme present. Opportunities for distinguishing among these alternatives will be discussed below, but it should be clear that carotenoid and bacteriochlorophyll syntheses are intimately related, and other similar relationships could exist.

Another sort of mutation that might affect carotenoid metabolism is more speculative. Mutations in crtB and crtE block carotenoid synthesis before the accumulation of any forty carbon carotenoid. Several possible functions might be suggested for these genes. They might code for a regulatory region like a promotor, or for an enzyme that synthesizes phytoene from twenty carbon precursors, or for a carotenoid binding protein. If free carotenoids feedback inhibit their own synthesis, the absence or alteration of a binding protein could lead to the cessation of synthesis at very low levels of carotenoid. Since all blue-green mutants accumulate light-harvesting I complex which can bind carotenoids (Ref. 9), this idea is not appealing. The light-harvesting II polypeptide composition of blue-green mutants is of interest in this connection, since mutants of the crtB, crtE and crtH types each synthesize one of the light-harvesting II polypeptides (10 kd), although no mature light-harvesting II complex is made. None of these mutants accumulates significant amounts of the 14 kd light-harvesting II polypeptide, and some have the 8 kd light-harvesting II polypeptide and some do not. One carotenoidless strain, which contained the 10 kd light-harvesting II polypeptides, reverted to regain carotenoid synthesis and simultaneously lost the 10 kd polypeptide. This is consistent with the hypothesis that the 10 kd polypeptide, if not properly integrated in a light-harvesting II complex, might mediate the inhibition of carotenoid synthesis.

MAPPING MUTATIONS AFFECTING CAROTENOGENESIS

It is of interest to map mutations affecting carotenogenesis so that the number of genes involved may be defined, and the arrangement of those genes be determined. This information permits construction of strains with new combinations of mutations, isolation of the genes in question, and it also suggests mechanisms of regulation at the transcriptional level.

Genetic exchange mechanisms

Two mechanisms of genetic exchange are known in R. capsulata. The first, capsduction, is apparently unique to R. capsulata (Ref. 10). It involves the production of DNA-containing particles (gene transfer agents or GTA) by a donor, and the absorption of the particles and utilization of the DNA by a recipient. Capsduction effects the transfer of small DNA segments (2.8 megadaltons), and as a consequence it is useful for mapping mutations that are separated by less than 2.8 megadaltons on the chromosome--this amounts to about five average sized genes (Ref. 11). The second genetic exchange mechanism for R. capsulata is conjugation. Conjugation in this species has been shown to be mediated by the plasmid pBLM2, a derivative of RP1, which is a promiscuous, antibiotic-resistance plasmid (Ref. 12). In this process cell-cell contact is established and large tracts of chromosomal DNA may be transferred from the pBLM2-bearing donor to the recipient. This enables linkage relationships between widely separated genes to be established, but genes relatively close to each other are not easily resolved.

Mapping with GTA

Carotenoid biosynthetic genes have been mapped by two basic paradigms using capsduction (Ref. 13). The distance between any mutation conferring the blue-green phenotype and any other mutation causing the accumulation of colored spheroidene precursors may be determined by treating the blue-green parent with a cell-free GTA preparation from the carotenoid accumulator and then performing photooxidative killing on the population. Blue-green cells that have not acquired a good copy of the gene allowing colored carotenoid synthesis are killed by illuminating in the presence of O_2. Most survivors have incorporated a piece of the donor chromosome in place of their mutated DNA, and a fraction of them also acquire the mutation from the donor that blocks carotenoid synthesis at a later step. The frequency of transfer of the donor phenotype can be used to calculate the distance between the two mutations in question. The other type of cross that has been used in GTA-based mapping of the photopigment region involves a recipient that cannot photosynthesize, for example, because it cannot synthesize bacteriochlorophyll. Non-photosynthetic recipient cells are treated with GTA from a photosynthetically competent donor with a mutation affecting carotenoid color. The cells that can form colonies photosynthetically are then counted, and the fraction with the donor phenotype again gives the cotransfer frequency from which the distance between the mutations can be calculated. From these types of crosses the gene order crtA, crtB, crtC, crtD, crtE, crtF was established. crtH could not be shown to be linked to this gene cluster.

Mapping with pBLM2 and the isolation of R-prime derivatives
As expected, conjugational crosses involving markers that mapped in the photopigment region (established by GTA crosses) resulted in a high degree of cotransfer, and new linkages among markers were established. New mutations blocking bacteriochlorophyll synthesis at a variety of steps were almost as tightly linked to carotenoid markers as were those bacteriochlorophyll biosynthetic genes that had shown linkage in GTA-based mapping (Ref. 13). A mutation affecting photosynthetic reaction center synthesis was also found to be nearby, and markers for tryptophan auxotrophy and rifampicin resistance were more weakly linked to the photopigment genes.

An important discovery was made while we were carrying out crosses to determine the arrangement of these markers. We crossed a donor bearing crtD and reaction center (rxc) mutations times a recipient that was bchA (bacteriochlorophyll minus) and crtB, and we selected for photosynthetic progeny. Because we already knew the map order crtB - crtD - bchA, and knew that rxc was somewhere outside that cluster, we were surprised to find that a large fraction of photosynthetic progeny had wild type carotenoids. Since it was unlikely that recombination could account for that result, we correctly deduced that R-prime-bearing progeny were being produced. R-prime plasmids are formed when a section of chromosomal DNA is covalently integrated into the circle of R-factor DNA. The integrated chromosomal DNA then is transferred and replicates with the plasmid DNA, and it represents a second copy of each of the chromosomal genes it carries, when it is present in R. capsulata. The wild type colonies in this cross were the result of complementation between the plasmid-borne and resident chromosomal markers. It is important to appreciate that working with pigmentation markers in a well mapped genetic region greatly facilitated the observation and isolation of R-prime plasmids.

R-prime plasmids were isolated from the colonies with wild type pigmentation in crosses like that described above by conjugation with Escherichia coli. This is possible because of the promiscuous nature of the R-primes, and because they still carry the original antibiotic resistance determinants of the R-factor from which they were derived. The R-primes are unstable in R. capsulata, presumably because they carry a duplicated piece of chromosome and thus can pair and recombine with the chromosome. The R-primes are stable in E. coli, and we store them there. From their E. coli repository strains the R-primes may be physically isolated, or they may be crossed into R. capsulata mutants to test for complementation. If the R-prime carries functional R. capsulata DNA that is homologous to the mutated gene of the recipient, complementation will occur. It turns out that all of the R-primes isolated to date will complement all of the mutations in our collection that alter photosynthetic membrane formation. Mutations that block photosynthesis because they interrupt electron transport are not complemented. It thus seems that all the genes specific for photosynthetic membrane and photopigment synthesis are carried by the 40 megadalton (average) piece of chromosome picked up by the R-primes. This represents only about 2% of the chromosome, so it would seem that the genes for photosynthesis are tightly clustered.

Cis-trans tests
The ability to introduce R-primes and thereby create partial diploids in R. capsulata enables cis-trans tests to be performed. Cis-trans tests define the limits of genes, and enable one to determine the number of cistrons (genes) to which a cluster of mutations belong. For example, it was believed that the two clusters of mutations leading to inactivation of the 3-4,dehydrogenase were actually two genes, and they were named crtD and crtG. We have since shown that all of these mutations are part of the same cistron, and thus the evidence so far is for one polypeptide, not two, needed for that reaction.

CLONING THE GENES FOR CAROTENOGENESIS

R-prime DNA is a natural cloning vehicle for the genes for photosynthesis. This DNA is easily isolated and may be subsequently subdivided by restriction endonucleases to give smaller fragments that may be cloned individually by recombinant DNA techniques. We have identified four fragments of DNA produced by the restriction endonuclease BamHI which carry the genes for carotenogenesis, crtA-crtF. We have not yet isolated the piece of DNA carrying the crtH gene. The identification of which fragments bear which genes involves the return of the individual cloned fragments to R. capsulata mutants. A system to accomplish this genetic exchange was developed in collaboration with Stanley Cohen's group at Stanford University. A plasmid that would cause the mobilization of the cloning vehicle from E. coli to R. capsulata was constructed from plasmid R751 and a ColE1 derivative RSF2233. It was also necessary to isolate mutants of R. capsulata that were more receptive to foreign DNA than was wild type. A restriction-minus R. capsulata mutant was isolated, and a crtF mutation was moved into it, so that mutations affecting carotenogenesis and bacteriochlorophyll synthesis could be quickly isolated by the technique described earlier.

These developments have led to our current capability to test some of the existing hypotheses concerning carotenogenesis. We can use the isolated DNA fragments as probes to study the pattern of transcription of mRNA for carotenogenesis. For example, how does oxygen tension affect the transcription of those genes? Once the basic *in vivo* pattern of transcription has been established, we can use the R-primes as a source of template DNA to study its transcription *in vitro*. Hypotheses about regulation of transcription could then be rigorously tested.

The cloned genes will also provide the possibility of producing large quantities of any of the carotenoid biosynthesis enzymes desired. It should also be possible to engineer *R. capsulata* to devote more of its energy to carotenoid synthesis, and if that carotenoid were a relatively reduced molecule like phytoene, it might provide a useful source of fuel.

Acknowledgement - This work was supported by grants from the Public Health Service, GM20173 and GM00098 and by grant PCM78-27038 from the National Science Foundation.

REFERENCES

1. K. Schmidt, *The Photosynthetic Bacteria*, Ch. 39, Plenum Press, New York (1978).
2. S. Kaplan, *The Photosynthetic Bacteria*, Ch. 43, Plenum Press, New York (1978).
3. R.J. Cogdell and J.P. Thornber, *FEBS Lett.* 122, 1-8 (1980).
4. R.J. Cogdell, M.F. Hipkins, W. MacDonald and T.G. Truscott, *Biochim. Biophys. Acta* 634, 191-202 (1981).
5. W.R. Sistrom, M. Griffiths and R.Y. Stanier, *J. Cell. Comp. Physiol.* 48, 473-515 (1956).
6. W.R. Sistrom, *The Photosynthetic Bacteria*, Ch. 44, Plenum Press, New York (1978).
7. P.A. Scolnik, M.A. Walker and B.L. Marrs, *J. Biol. Chem.* 255, 2427-2432 (1980).
8. S. Liaaen Jensen, G. Cohen-Bazire and R.Y. Stanier, *Nature* 192, 1168-1172 (1961).
9. P.A. Scolnik, D. Zannoni and B.L. Marrs, *Biochim. Biophys. Acta* 593, 230-240 (1980).
10. J.D. Wall, P.F. Weaver and H. Gest, *Arch. Microbiol.* 105, 217-224 (1975).
11. H.C. Yen, N.T. Hu and B.L. Marrs, *J. Mol. Biol.* 131, 157-168 (1979).
12. B.L. Marrs, *J. Bacteriol.* in press (1981).
13. H.C. Yen and B. Marrs, *J. Bacteriol.* 126, 619-629 (1976).

STEREOCHEMICAL ASPECTS OF CAROTENOID BIOSYNTHESIS

B.V. Milborrow

School of Biochemistry, University of New South Wales, P.O. Box 1,
Kensington, N.S.W. 2033, Australia.

Abstract - The stereochemistry of cyclisation or quasi-cyclisation in the C_{50}-carotenoids is compared with that in the C_{40}-carotenoids: the chiral and prochiral sites involved show mirror-image symmetry in the two series. The absolute configuration at C-2, in the cyclic and acyclic C_{50} compounds, the inhibition of the enzymes by diphenylamine, and its antagonism by thiamin, suggest that the enzyme that forms the acyclic carotenoids may represent an ancestral form of the cyclase.

The 4-pro-R hydrogen atom of mevalonate is retained in lycopene and at C-2, and C-6 of ε and γ C_{50}-carotenoids and at C-2 of β C_{50}-carotenoids; both C-2 hydrogen atoms of mevalonate are retained at C-4 of the β and γ isomers. This excludes the possibility that β, γ and ε-rings are interconverted.

The elaboration of C_{40}-carotenoids by the marine dinoflagellate *Amphidinium carterae* has been followed by feeding [^{14}C]lycopene, [^{14}C] zeaxanthin and ^{14}C and ^{3}H labelled mevalonates. Zeaxanthin is converted into neoxanthin and then into diadinoxanthin or peridinin. The allene group retains a hydrogen atom at C-8 derived from C-2 of mevalonate. This shows that the allene is converted into an acetylene, rather than the reverse. The labelling pattern of peridinin shows that it is formed by the deletion of C-13, C-14 and C-20 (C-13Me) from neoxanthin.

The absolute configuration at C-3' of the ε-ring of lutein was originally deduced to be the same as that at C-3 of the β-ring from the apparent retention of the 5-pro-S hydrogen atom of mevalonate. The ^{14}C:^{3}H ratios of lutein formed from [2-^{14}C,5R-5-$^{3}H_1$] and [2-^{14}C,5S-5-$^{3}H_1$]mevalonate, and those of 3'-monooxolutein formed by oxidation, show that the 5-pro-R hydrogen atom is retained at C-3'.

Other recent advances in carotenoid biosynthesis will be reviewed.

INTRODUCTION

Over the last 30 to 40 years we have witnessed the triumphal progress of comparative biochemistry; give or take a few amino acid residues, many enzymes are the same in plants, animals and bacteria. So accustomed have we become to study one enzyme from one organism and a second from another that it came as quite a surprise to find that there are two quite different enzymes which operate with mirror-image stereochemistry to form the rings of carotenoids. A considerable effort has been devoted to the elucidation of the mechanisms of cyclisation and other aspects have received less attention. The biosynthesis of the

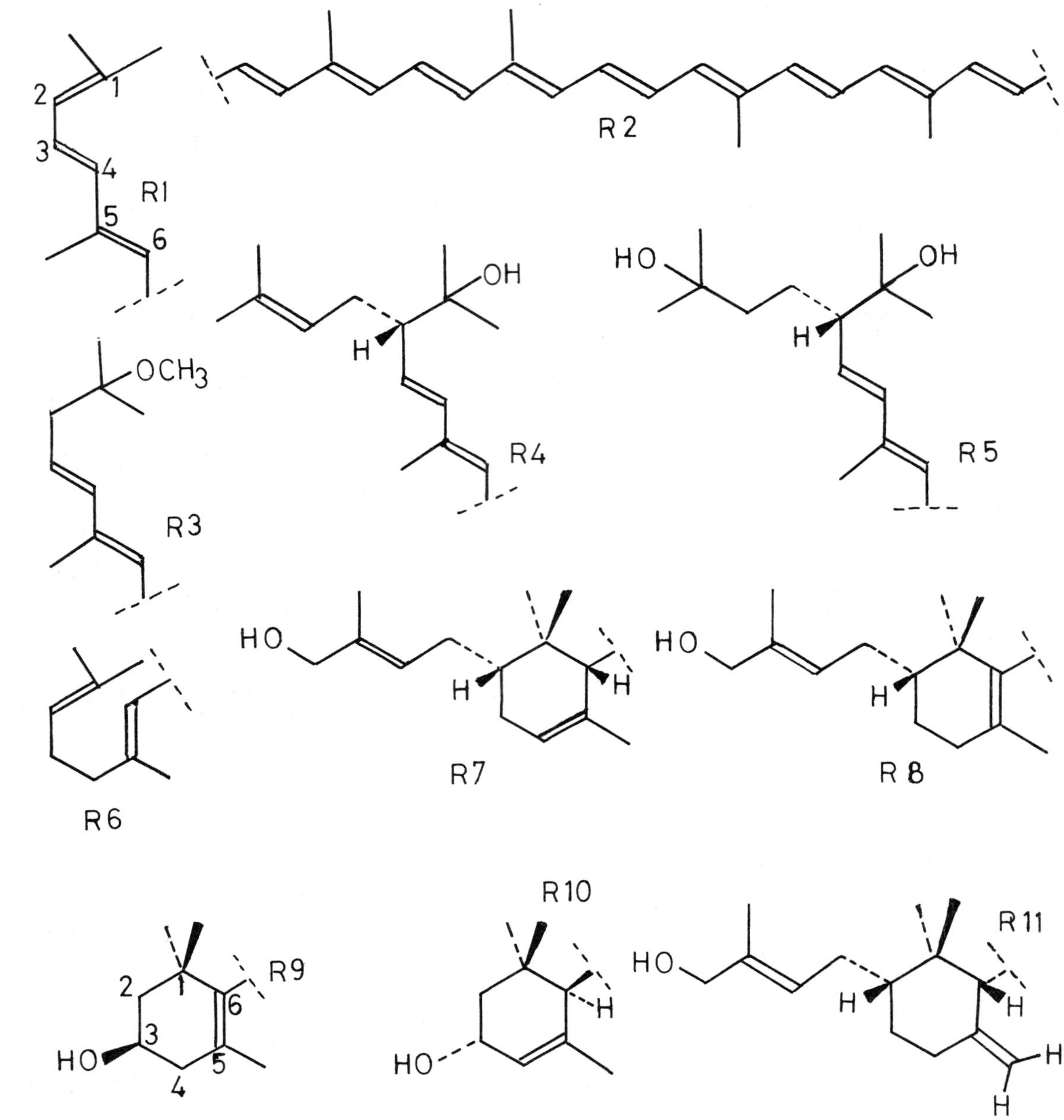

Structure

1.	Dehydrolycopene	R1,R2,R1	6.	Decaprenoxanthin	R7,R2,R7
2.	Spirilloxanthin	R3,R2,R3	7.	C.p.450(symmetrical)	R8,R2,R8
3.	Bisanhydrobacterioruberin	R4,R2,R4	8.	Zeaxanthin	R9,R2,R9
4.	Bacterioruberin	R5,R2,R5	9.	Lutein	R10,R2,R9
5.	Lycopene	R6,R2,R6	10.	Sarcinaxanthin	R11,R2,R11

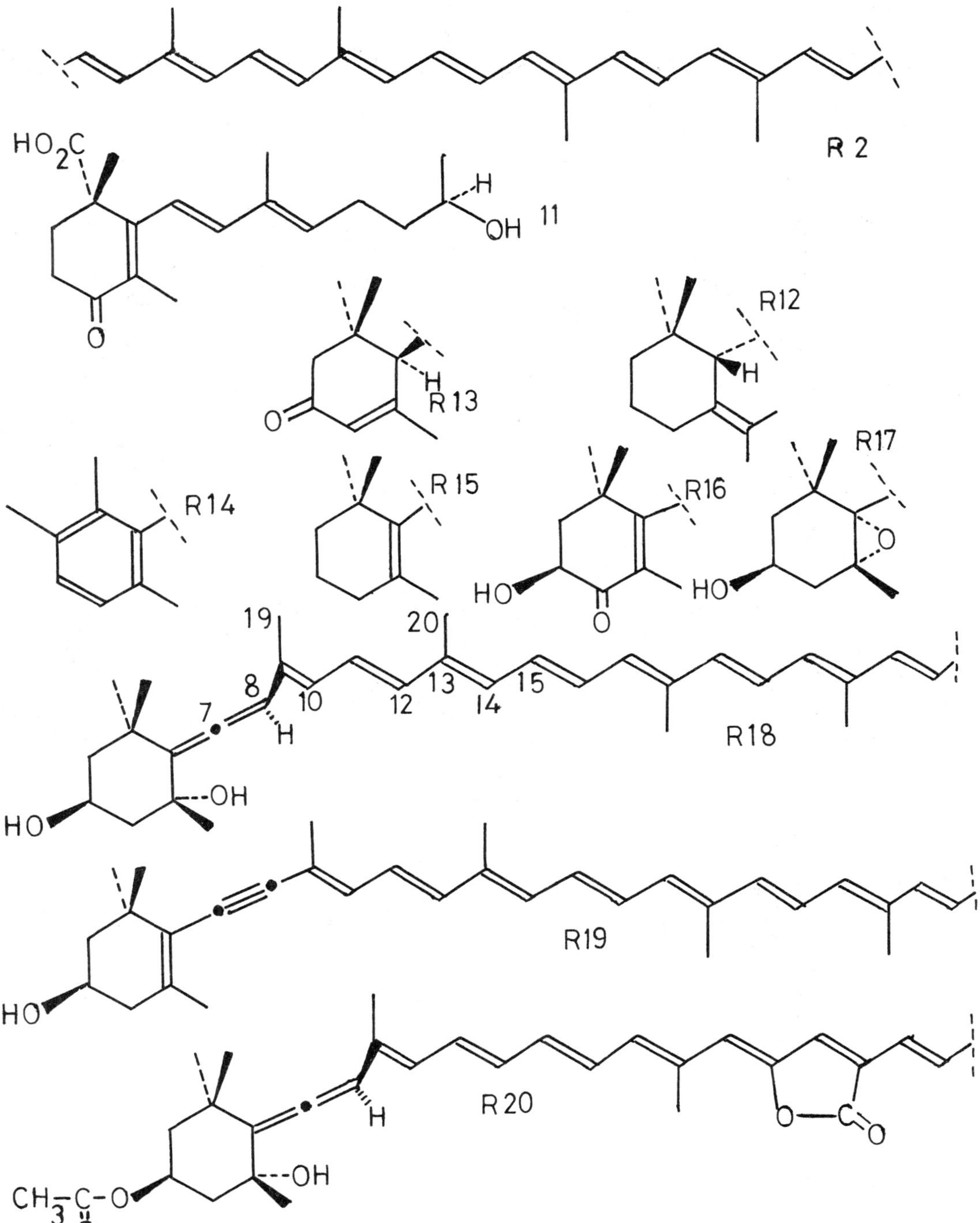

Structure

11. Trisporic acid			16. Astaxanthin	R16,R2,R16
12. γ,γ-Carotene	R12,R2,R12		17. Neoxanthin	R17,R18
13. Monooxolutein	R13,R2,R9		18. Diadinoxanthin	R17,R19
14. Chlorobactene	R14,R2,R6		19. Peridinin	R17,R20
15. β,ψ-Carotene	R15,R2,R6			

carotenoids can be divided into 3 phases: (i) From the head to head condensation of two geranyl geranyl pyrophosphate molecules to lycopene or dehydrolycopene. (ii) Cyclisation or quasi-cyclisation reactions. (iii) Elaboration. The reactions of the first phase have been reviewed recently (Ref. 1) and will not be discussed separately here. Most of the stereochemical features of the cyclisation reactions involved in C_{40} carotenoid formation were worked out by Professor Goodwin and his colleagues some time ago. More recently they have elucidated the prochirality at C-1 and C-2 of β-rings (Ref. 2 & 3). The investigation of the stereochemistry of the C_{50} carotenoids is now in hand. Quasi-cyclisation is the term we have used to refer to reactions involving C-1 and C-2 of lycopene which appear analogous to cyclisation. These reactions include the hydration of dehydrolycopene leading to (1) spirilloxanthin (2) or bisanhydrobacterioruberin (3) to bacterioruberin (4) and the isoprenylation of lycopene (5) and dehydrolycopene (1) to bisanhydrobacterioruberin (3). Phase (iii) comprises reactions such as hydroxylation to more exotic ones which give rise to allenes, acetylenes, aromatic rings or shortened polyene chains. Strangely, these reactions have been little studied.

We started our work on the C_{50} bacterial carotenoids because knowledge of the stereochemistry of cyclisation in the C_{40} series was then incomplete. We thought that it would be simple to define all the stereochemical features in the C_{50} series and so we set out to do this. It was a Pandora's box of scientific interest, frustration and fascination, laced with serendipity.

Methods for determining ^{14}C:^{3}H ratios in carotenoids

Most of our recent work has made use of the ^{14}C:^{3}H ratios of the carotenoids, formed from labelled mevalonates, to probe features of the biosynthesis of the various structures. The accuracy of the technique has been improved by the use of HPLC to purify the carotenoids with the minimum of destruction. Furthermore, the mevalonate samples have been chromatographed on reverse-phase HPLC as ion pairs with P.I.C. reagents (Ref. 4). The precision with which the radioactivity is measured has also been improved by the use of a series of quenched standards for scintillation counting. The intense colour of carotenoids interferes with scintillation counting and samples are usually decolourised before the radioactivity is measured. Provided the bleaching reaction is carried out in butanol solution in a sealed vessel any ^{3}H lost from the carotenoid as water is exchanged into the butanol. However, as even colourless solutions may quench the scintillant, the solutions are spiked with, successively, standard ^{3}H- and ^{14}C-containing compounds. Correction is then made for quenching in the two channels. Unfortunately, this procedure is inadequate because the true ^{3}H counts in the ^{3}H channel are quenched to a different degree from the ^{14}C disintegrations which "cross over" and are recorded as counts in the ^{3}H channel. This effect becomes more important as the proportion of ^{14}C to ^{3}H increases. We overcome the problem by supplying precursors with relatively high ^{3}H contents and preparing a 3-dimensional array of varying proportions of ^{3}H and ^{14}C in standards quenched with differing amounts of β-carotene. The samples of labelled carotenoids were not decolourised, this treatment was omitted in order to avoid loss of ^{3}H. They were counted, with spiking, over a range of concentrations and the amounts of ^{14}C and ^{3}H present were determined by interpolation from the standard quenching curves. This procedure gives a precise measure of their ^{14}C:^{3}H ratios (Ref. 5).

CYCLISATION IN THE C_{50} CAROTENOIDS

Our interest in carotenoids arose from work on the phytohormone abscisic acid. We hoped to compare its biosynthesis with that of carotenes because of similarities in structures between the two. At the time several stereochemical features of the C_{40} carotenoids had not been defined and we considered that it would be relatively easy to investigate all the stereochemical features of cyclisation in the C_{50} ε,ε-carotenoid decaprenoxanthin (6) so that it could be used as a basis for comparison. An advantage the C_{50} carotenoids have over their C_{40} counterparts is that the extra isoprene unit defines the absolute configuration of the group added to C-2 (Ref. 6). In the β,β compound C.p.450 (7) the configuration of the group added is the reverse of that of the hydrogen atom added to C-2 during the formation of the C_{40} β,β-carotenoid zeaxanthin (8)(Ref.2). The configuration at C-6' of the ε-ring of C_{40} β,ε-carotene is the mirror-image of that at C-6 of the ε,ε C_{50} decaprenoxanthin.

The cells of Flavobacterium dehydrogenans which produce decaprenoxanthin did not incorporate more than 5 dpm from 5 x 10^6 dpm of [^{14}C]mevalonate (10 μCi/μmol) using a wide range of procedures to assist penetration. Eventually it was found that the cell walls of F. dehydrogenans cells could be weakened with lysozyme, stressed by washing and suspending in water, and then ruptured by mild sonication. This procedure gave a cell-free preparation that incorporated 70000 dpm of [^{14}C]mevalonate into decaprenoxanthin (Ref.7). The same method has since been used successfully with other bacteria to investigate the fate of various prochiral hydrogen atoms of mevalonate at C-2, C-4 and C-6 of the β, γ- and ε-rings of the C_{50} bacterial carotenoids.

^{14}C:^{3}H ratios of decaprenoxanthin, incorporating [2-^{14}C,4*R*-4-^{3}H$_1$]mevalonate showed that 4-*pro-R* hydrogen atoms of mevalonate were retained at C-2 and C-6 (Table 1). On the other hand, the 2-*pro-S* hydrogen atom of mevalonate was retained at C-4 (Ref. 7) whereas the 2-*pro-R* was retained at C-4 in the ε-ring (Ref. 8) of carotene from higher plants.

TABLE 1. Incorporation of [2-^{14}C,4*R*-4-^{3}H$_1$]mevalonate into decaprenoxanthin

	^{14}C dpm	^{3}H dpm	^{14}C:^{3}H ratio normalised to mevalonate	^{14}C:^{3}H ratio normalised to lycopene*	Expected ^{14}C:^{3}H ratio
Mevalonate	120612	61349	(1:1)	-	-
Lycopene	5961	2882	8:7.54	(8:8)	-
Deshydroxy-decapreno-xanthin	6761	3412	10:9.80	10:10.41	10:10
Decapreno-xanthin	75063	37801	10:9.80	10:10.41	10:10

* The ^{14}C:^{3}H ratio observed is close to that expected if all the 4-*pro-R* hydrogen atoms were retained.

TABLE 2. Incorporation of [2-^{14}C,2<u>R</u>-2-$^{3}H_1$]- and [2-^{14}C,2<u>S</u>-2-$^{3}H_1$]mevalonate into decaprenoxanthin

	^{14}C dpm	^{3}H dpm	$^{14}C:^{3}H$ ratio normalised to mevalonate	$^{14}C:^{3}H$ ratio normalised to lycopene	Expected $^{14}C:^{3}H$ ratio: if 2-pro-S retained at C-4	if 2-pro-R retained at C-4
Mevalonate (2R-$^{3}H_1$)	22248	67588	(1:1)	-	-	-
Lycopene	102114	257862	8:6.64	8:8	-	-
Monocyclic carotenoids (C_{45})	7755	17405	9:6.64	9:7.98	9:7.67min 9:8.0 max	9:8.67min 9:9.90max
Decapreno-xanthin	11566	23322	10:6.65	10:8.00	10:7.33min 10:8.0 max	10:9.33min 10:10.0max
Mevalonate (2S-$^{3}H_1$)	375726	2317582	(1:1)	-	-	-
Lycopene	9903	44668	8:5.84	(8:4)	-	-
Decapreno-xanthin	15335	82624	10:8.70	10:5.98	10:5.33min 10:6.0 max	10:3.3min 10:4.0max

We have recently been able to show that the 4-<u>pro-R</u> hydrogen atom of mevalonate is also retained at C-2,2' of the β,β C_{50} carotenoid C.p.450 (Ref. 9) (7) and at C-2,2' and C-6,6' of the C_{50} γ,γ-carotenoid sarcinaxanthin (10) produced by <u>Micrococcus luteus</u> (formerly <u>Sarcina lutea</u> (Table 3).

TABLE 3. Incorporation of [2-^{14}C,4<u>R</u>-$^{3}H_1$]mevalonate into sarcinaxanthin and C.p.450.

	^{14}C dpm	^{3}H dpm	$^{14}C:^{3}H$ ratio normalised to mevalonate	$^{14}C:^{3}H$ ratio normalised to lycopene	Expected $^{14}C:^{3}H$ ratio if 4-pro-R were retained at C-6
Mevalonate	27064	141815	(1:1)	-	-
Lycopene	17421	92506	8:8.11	(8:8)	-
Sarcina-xanthin	9849	52985	10:10.27	10:10.13	10:10
Mevalonate	28320	133954	(1:1)	-	-
Lycopene	4709	22462	8:8.07	(8:8)	-
C.p.450	13685	52550	10:8.12	10:8.05	10:10

Further experiments showed that two hydrogen atoms from C-2 of mevalonate are retained at C-4 of C.p.450 and at C-4 of sarcinaxanthin (Ref. 9) (Table 4). This shows that in the C_{40} series the β, γ and ε-rings are not interconverted (the evidence does not exclude γ to β and γ to ε conversions) and is in accord with the formation of a carbonium ion at C-5 which then gives rise to β, γ or ε-rings. This parallels the scheme originally proposed for the β and ε-rings of C_{40} carotenoids by Goodwin (Ref. 8).

TABLE 4. Incorporation of [2-^{14}C,2RS-2-$^{3}H_2$]mevalonate into sarcinaxanthin and C.p.450.

	^{14}C dpm	^{3}H dpm	^{14}C:^{3}H ratio normalised to mevalonate	^{14}C:^{3}H ratio normalised to lycopene	Expected ^{14}C:^{3}H ratio if both ^{3}H atoms retained at C-4
Mevalonate	5817	60264	(1:2)	-	-
Lycopene	8878	70758	8:12.31	8:12	-
Sarcina-xanthin	8042	67549	10:16.22	10:15.81	10:16
Mevalonate	7913	60534	(1:2)	-	-
Lycopene	2269	13274	8:12.24	(8:12)	-
C.p.450	7870	49580	10:16.47	10:16.15	10:16

All these data are consistent with a model for the cyclisation of C_{50} carotenoids in which lycopene is folded with β-face of the future ring (β in the nomenclature of Rose _et al_) (Ref.10) against the enzyme. In other words, it is proposed that the face of the C_{50} carotenoid towards the observer, as the ring conventionally drawn, is the one held by the enzyme. C-6 is presumed to be close to the enzyme while C-1 is slightly further away. This arrangement (Scheme 1) leaves space for the incoming isoprene unit to join to C-2 from the α-side. Significantly, the hydrogen atom at C-4 that is lost (the 2-_pro-R_ of mevalonate) projects from the α-face of the ring, away from the enzyme and into the medium. This, we consider, is a significant feature and accounts for the selection of which hydrogen atom is lost from C-4, rather than its being the result of a conformational difference.

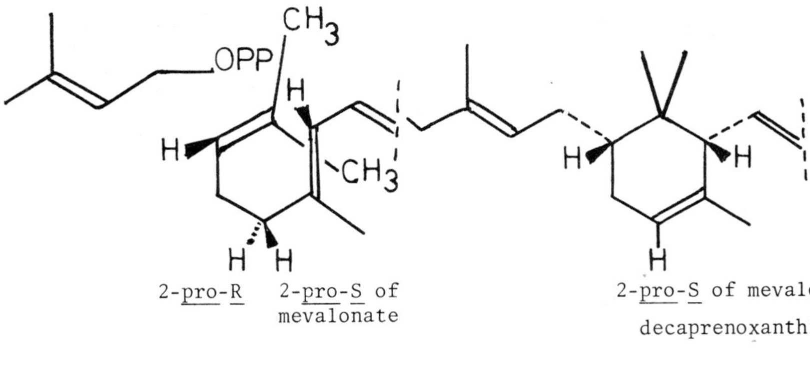

Scheme 1. Isoprenylation of lycopene to form an ε-ring of decaprenoxanthin. The postulated intermediate is viewed from the β-face which, it is suggested, is the side against the enzyme.

The mirror-image model, of course, would apply to the C_{40} carotenoids where the presumptive α-face would be held by the enzyme and the incoming group (H^+) would attach to C-2 from the β-face and the 4-_pro-S_ hydrogen atom of lycopene (2-_pro-S_ of mevalonate) is lost to the medium. Thus cyclisation appeared to have been carried out by mirror-image mechanisms in the C_{40} and C_{50} series although the stereochemistry of previous reactions of biosynthesis were the same as in higher plants.

In the first experiment in which a cell-free preparation of _M.luteus_ was incubated at pH 7.8

with [2-^{14}C,2RS-2-$^{3}H_2$]mevalonate the major labelled carotenoid was identified as decaprenoxanthin (6) and it had lost two tritium atoms per molecule that were expected to have been retained in sarcinaxanthin (10). The experiment was repeated at pH 7.0 and yielded sarcinaxanthin with the expected ^{14}C:^{3}H ratio. The isomerisation was investigated by incubating sarcinaxanthin sample (200μg), from either [2RS-2-$^{3}H_2$]- or [4R-4-$^{3}H_1$]mevalonate, in ether (300μl) and 0.1 M potassium hydroxide (500μl) for 48h. The major product was identified as decaprenoxanthin in 85% yield and the distinctive infra red absorption at 888 cm^{-1} of sarcinaxanthin, attributed to the exocyclic methylene group at C-5 (Ref.11), was absent in the products. A minor component, present in 3% yield amongst the isomerisation products, was identified as symmetrical, C.p.450. Sarcinaxanthin, prepared from [2-^{14}C, 4R-4-$^{3}H_1$]mevalonate, gave C.p.450 with a ^{14}C:^{3}H ratio of 10:7.86 which was close to the ratio of 10:8 expected for the loss of ^{3}H atoms from C-6 and C-6'. Sarcinaxanthin derived from [2-^{14}C,2RS-2-$^{3}H_2$]mevalonate gave decaprenoxanthin with a ^{14}C:^{3}H ratio of 10:13.73, close to the expected value of 10:14 for the loss of a ^{3}H atom from C-4 and C-4'. There was no significant change in the ratio of the alternative product (Ref.9).

Isomerisation of the γ-ring would be expected to yield the β-ring as the major product because the wholly conjugated polyene system is more stable than that with two isolated double bonds. Models show that, during isomerisation to an ε-ring, there need be no steric interaction between the hydrogen atom at C-8 and the methyl group at C-5 whereas interaction between these groups would be expected if the presumptive β-ring occupied the same plane as the polyene chain. It appears, therefore, that steric effects rather than relative stabilities, could determine the proportions in which the products are formed.

UNCYCLISED C_{50} CAROTENOIDS

We also examined the biosynthesis of the uncyclised C_{50} bacterioruberin (4) from the primitive, halophilic Halobacterium halobium (Ref.5). It has the same configuration at C-2 as the other C_{50} compounds and not only is the 4-pro-R hydrogen atom of mevalonate retained at C-2 (Table 5) but the enzyme that isoprenylates 3,4-dehydrolycopene (2) is inhibited by diphenylamine and the inhibition is antagonised by thiamin (Table 6). The product is bisanhydrobacterioruberin (3).

TABLE 5. Incorporation of [2-^{14}C,4R-4-$^{3}H_1$]mevalonate into bacterioruberin by Halobacterium halobium cells

	^{14}C dpm	^{3}H dpm	^{14}C:^{3}H ratio normalised to mevalonate	^{14}C:^{3}H ratio normalised to neurosporene	Expected ratio if 4R,$^{3}H_1$ of mevalonate retained at all positions
Mevalonate	30671	264077	(1:1)	-	-
Neurosporene	2280	18856	8:7.68	8:8	8:8
Bacterioruberin	16275	131665	10:9.40	10:9.78	10:10

TABLE 6. Inhibition of bacterioruberin production in H.halobium cells by diphenylamine and its antagonism by thiamin 1mg/l.

Diphenylamine concentration 10^{-6} M	Bacterioruberin µg/g cells No thiamin added	Bacterioruberin formed in the presence of thiamin (1mg/l)
0	39	56
5	17	24
25	<1	16

The isoprenylation occurs with hydroxylation at C-1 and we have suggested that the enzyme that carries out the isoprenylation reaction evolved into the cyclase. This would occur if the original enzyme mutated to accept lycopene (1) rather than dehydrolycopene (2) and the hydroxyl group adding to C-1 came to be replaced by C-6.

The next reaction in the formation of bacterioruberin is the hydration of the double bond of the added isoprenyl group and, like hydroxylation at C-1 and isoprenylation at C-2, the reaction is inhibited by diphenylamine and stimulated by thiamin. This reaction could be analogous to the hydration of the terminal double bonds during the formation of spirillo-xanthin (2). It seems possible that the enzyme responsible for this latter reaction in the anaerobic, photosynthetic bacteria could have evolved into the C_{40} cyclase of the aerobic cyanobacteria (blue-green algae) by the same processes of replacement of dehydrolycopene by lycopene and the hydroxyl by C-6. If this had occurred then the prochirality of the geminal methyl groups at C-1 of spirilloxanthin can be predicted to be the opposite to that of those at C-1 of bacterioruberin. A further possibility is that the enzyme that carries out the hydration reaction to form spirilloxanthin operates with the same chirality as that which hydrates the dimethylallyl residue to form bacterioruberin. This leads to the prediction that the methyl groups, derived from C-2 and C-3Me of mevalonate, of the two hydroxylated centres of bacterioruberin have opposite chirality.

Cultures of H. halobium contain traces of β-carotene and Corynebacterium poinsettiae forms traces of bacterioruberin (Ref.12,13) when suffering thiamin deficiency. These occurrences suggest that under unfavourable conditions the enzyme of H. halobium that normally hydrates the double bond of the dimethyl allyl group may accept and cyclise lycopene. Similarly, the cyclase that normally forms the β,β C_{50} C.p.450 may hydroxylate C-1 of lycopene during the addition reaction instead of forming a bond between C-1 and C-6.

CYCLISATION OF C_{40} CAROTENOIDS

Goodwin, Britton and colleagues have defined the origin of the prochiral hydrogen atoms at C-2 of the C_{40} β-carotenoid zeaxanthin (9) produced by a Flavobacterium sp. (Ref.2). They prevented cyclisation by incubating the cells with nicotine and then washed out the inhibitor and replaced the medium with D_2O. This procedure caused zeaxanthin to be made in which the hydrogen atom derived from the 4-*pro-R* position of mevalonate at C-4 was protium and the hydrogen atom derived from the medium was deuterium (Scheme 2). NMR spectrometry was then used to relate the configuration at C-2 to the chiral centre at C-3. They also defined the arrangement of the geminal methyl groups at C-1 of zeaxanthin by feeding [2-^{13}C]mevalonate to the Flavobacterium sp. and were again able to relate the configuration of the ^{13}C enriched prochiral methyl group at C-1 to the chiral centre at C-3 (Ref.3).

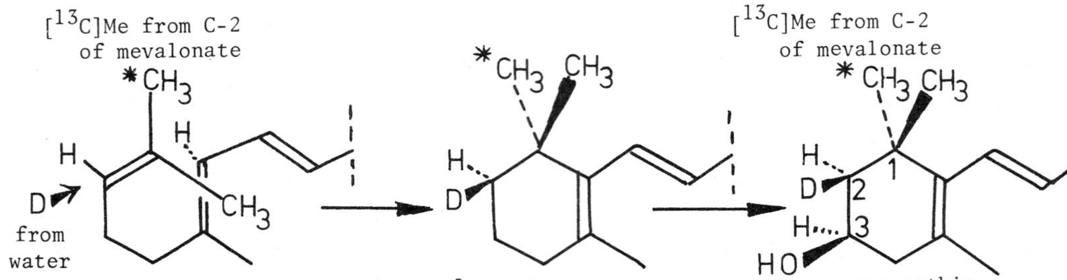

β-carotene zeaxanthin

Scheme 2. Stereochemistry of cyclisation to form the β-rings of zeaxanthin (Ref.2,3). Lycopene cyclised in D_2O gave C-2S zeaxanthin while [C-1EMe-^{13}C]lycopene, derived from [C-2-^{13}C]mevalonate, gave C-1S zeaxanthin.

The fungus Phycomyces blakesleeanus converts β-carotene into trisporic acid (12) (Ref.14) and its labelling pattern and chirality at C-1 (carotene numbering) indicate that the 1-pro-R methyl group of the β-carotene was derived from the C-3 methyl group of mevalonate. This is the reverse of the pattern in zeaxanthin formed by the Flavobacterium sp. Either one determination is in error or a different mechanism of cyclisation occurs in the bacterium and the fungus. There are two variants of the second alternative: the mechanisms may be a perfect mirror-image, concerted reactions, for example with the 6re face attacking the 2si face of lycopene in the Flavobacterium system with lycopene in an almost planar conformation (as in Scheme 2). On the other hand the fungal cyclase could utilise a 2si to 6re addition in a boat folded lycopene intermediate.

There is as yet no direct observation to discriminate between these alternatives but circumstantial evidence suggests that fungi may utilise a mirror-image C_{40} cyclase mechanism. The fungus Caloscypha fulgens forms β,γ-carotene (12) in which C-6' has the opposite absolute configuration to that at C-6 of the ε-rings formed by higher plants (Ref.15). These rings, therefore, must be made by a mirror-image mechanism because boat or chair folding could reverse the arrangement of the C-1 geminal methyl groups but would not affect the absolute configuration at C-6.

STEREOCHEMISTRY OF HYDROXYLATION OF LUTEIN

The β,ε-carotenoid lutein (9) is unusual in that the 3'-hydroxyl group of the ε-ring has the opposite arrangement in space to the 3-hydroxyl group commonly present in β-rings. It was originally proposed (Ref.16) that the 3'-hydroxyl group had the same absolute configuration as it does in the β-rings of zeaxanthin (8). This was based on the apparent retention of a tritium atom from the 5-pro-S position of mevalonate at C-3'. Insertion of a 3'R-hydroxyl group at this position, with retention of configuration, would give this result. The demonstration by Buchecker et al (Ref.17) and Andrewes et al (Ref.18) that the hydroxyl group at C-3' was S meant that either the $^{14}C:^{3}H$ ratios were aberrant or that the chiral centre at C-3' was inverted after the 5-pro-S hydrogen atom of mevalonate had been replaced by the hydroxyl group.

We have recently re-investigated this problem (Ref.19) by feeding 5S- and 5R-tritiated mevalonate samples to opening flower buds of Marigold (Calendula officinalis). The $^{14}C:^{3}H$ ratios of lutein and other carotenoids were obtained and showed, quite clearly, that the 5-pro-R hydrogen atom of mevalonate was retained at C-3' of lutein and the 5-pro-S hydrogen atom of mevalonate at C-3 of the β-ring (Table 7). This result is the reverse of that obtained previously and the data from samples derived from both 5R- and 5S-tritiated mevalonates agree.

The labelled lutein samples were subjected to oxidation by the nickel peroxide method described by Liaaen-Jensen *et al* (Ref.11) to confirm that the 5*R*-tritium of mevalonate was at C-3' and thereby to avoid reliance on overall $^{14}C:^{3}H$ ratios. The reported yields of 20% 3'-monooxolutein (13) were obtained with 20 mg samples whereas we could not obtain more than 2-3% yields when working at the 10-20μg scale although a range of conditions were tested in some 40 experiments. Oxidation removed the equivalent of one tritium atom per molecule from the sample derived from [5*R*-5-$^{3}H_1$]mevalonate while the sample derived from [5*S*-5-$^{3}H_1$]mevalonate was virtually unaffected (Table 7).

This result established that a hydrogen atom from the 5-*pro-R* position in mevalonic acid is retained at C-3' of lutein and this, together with the known configuration of the hydrogen atoms in the precursors and the absolute configuration at C-3' of lutein, shows that hydroxylation occurs at C-3' with retention of configuration.

TABLE 7. $^{14}C:^{3}H$ ratios of carotenoids formed in *Calendula officinalis* flower heads from [2-^{14}C,5*S*-5-$^{3}H_1$]- and [2-^{14}C,5*R*-5-$^{3}H_1$]mevalonic acids

Compound	^{14}C dpm	^{3}H dpm	$^{14}C:^{3}H$ ratio normalised to mevalonate	$^{14}C:^{3}H$ ratio normalised to Neurosporene	Expected ratio if 5*R*-^{3}H of mevalonate retained at C-3'
5*R*-5-$^{3}H_1$					
Mevalonate	5421	38869	(1:1)	-	-
Neuro-sporene	1204	5297	8:4.91	(8:5)	-
β-Carotene	8500	30175	8:3.96	8:4.03	-
Zeaxanthin	5890	21321	8:4.04	8:4.11	-
Lutein	9707	26210	8:3.01	8:3.07	8:3
			$^{14}C:^{3}H$ ratio normalised to mevalonate	$^{14}C:^{3}H$ ratio normalised to phytoene	Expected ratio if 5*R*-^{3}H of mevalonate retained at C-3'.
5*S*-5-$^{3}H_1$					
Mevalonate	13619	83076	1:1	-	-
Phytoene	2108	9296	8:5.78	8:6	-
β-Carotene	12096	52132	8:5.65	8:5.87	-
Zeaxanthin	3977	11652	8:3.84	8:3.98	-
Lutein	6262	23170	8:4.85	8:5.03	8:5
Lutein from [5*R*-5-$^{3}H_1$]mevalonate	^{14}C dpm	^{3}H dpm		$^{14}C:^{3}H$ ratio normalised to original lutein	Expected ratio if 5*R*-^{3}H of mevalonate retained at C-3'.
Recovered	6311	10476		8:3.04	8:3
Monooxo-lutein	932	1081		8:2.12	8:2
Lutein from [5*S*-5-$^{3}H_1$]mevalonate					
Recovered	5463	14750		8:5.03	8:5
Monooxo-lutein	761	2024		8:4.95	8:5

ARYL CAROTENOIDS

The biosynthesis of the aryl carotenoids has not been explored beyond the initial work of Moshier and Chapman (Ref.20). These authors found that chlorobactene (14), formed by Chloropseudomonas ethylica from [2-^{14}C]mevalonate, carried a methyl group derived from C-2 of mevalonate at C-1 and an unlabelled methyl group, presumably derived from C-3Me of mevalonate, at C-2. The occurrence together of β,ψ-carotene (15) and chlorobactene (Ref.21) and of β,β-carotene, isorenieratene, renieratene and renierapurpurin (Ref.22) is consistent with the hypothesis that β,ψ- and β-carotenes are the precursors of monocyclic and bicyclic aryl carotenoids respectively. However, the occurrence together does not exclude the possibility that the shift of a methyl from C-1 to C-2 of lycopene does not occur during the cyclisation reaction. A β-ring carotene may not be liberated from the cyclase as a free intermediate.

Although we know that the C-2 of mevalonic acid remains at C-1 while the methyl group derived from C-3Me moves to C-2 we do not know the stereochemistry of the reaction. Aryl carotenoids are formed in fungi and until the question of the stereochemistry of the cyclases in fungi is resolved the stereochemistry of the methyl migration cannot be taken as established.

FROM β-CAROTENE TO ASTAXANTHIN

Two lines of research have shed some light on the pathway of astaxanthin (16) biosynthesis, these are: characterisation of carotenoid structures in crustaceans and other invertebrates and investigation of [15,15'-$^{3}H_{2}$]β-carotene metabolism in prawns and lobsters by Katayama and colleagues (Ref. 23 & 24). These crustaceans contained a range of labelled 3-hydroxy and 4-oxo carotenoids after being supplied with tritiated β-carotene in a synthetic diet. In contrast to this, red sea bream (Evyanis japonica) were not able to carry out the metabolism but did accumulate [^{3}H]astaxanthin in their skin when fed prawns from the earlier experiments that contained the labelled material (Ref.25).

The prawns (Penaeus japonicus) and lobsters (Panulirus japonicus) which had fed on the synthetic diet were extracted after 14 days and the guts and carapaces were analysed separately. A different set of ^{3}H carotenoids were found in the two parts and Katayama et al (Ref. 23 & 24) concluded that some reactions occur in the gut while others occur in the carapace. This may be so, but the duration of the experiment leaves time for a thorough partitioning of the products. Indeed, it is not certain that lobster or prawn enzymes do carry out the metabolism, the intestinal microflora could be responsible. However, the failure of the red sea bream to metabolise [^{3}H]β-carotene makes this unlikely.

The presence of label in a number of intermediates cannot be used to construct a pathway in experiments of two weeks duration and in the absence of specific activity data. The results could be used to argue the opposite; namely that the unmetabolised by-products remain while the active, true intermediates disappear.

It would be unwise, at present, to consider that there is just one pathway from β-carotene to astaxanthin but rather that an oxygen atom has to be introduced at C-3 and C-4 of each ring and, if the C-4 oxygen is inserted as a hydroxyl group, it then has to undergo oxidation to a 4-ketone. The oxidation reactions may occur in a grid pattern, according to enzyme specificity and activity, rather than in a single sequence of reactions in a conventional pathway (Scheme 3). The occurrence of several of the required intermediates in prawns and lobsters can be taken to lend support to this suggestion. If this is confirmed then the presence of any particular compound may reflect a slow rate of metabolism rather than its being an important intermediate.

Scheme 3. Occurrence of Carotenoids related to astaxanthin

Conversion of β-carotene into astaxanthin could proceed via compounds at any position on the grid and a rapid turnover and low concentrations of the components of the most active route could lead to their being overlooked.

Ring 1	Substituents of Ring 2					
	0	3-OH	4-OH	4-oxo	3,4-OH	3OH,4-oxo
0	β-carotene	β-crypto xanthin	isocrypto* xanthin	echinenone*	3,4-dihydroxy-β-carotene	3-hydroxy-echinenone
3-OH	β-crypto-xanthin	zeaxanthin				dorada-xanthin
4-OH	isocrypto* -xanthin		isozea-xanthin	4'-hydroxy-** -echinenone		
4-oxo	echinenone*		4'-hydroxy-** echinenone	cantha-xanthin		phoenico-xanthin**
3,4-OH	3,4-dihydroxy -β-carotene				crustaxanthin	idoxanthin
3-OH, -4-oxo	3-hydroxy-echinenone	dorada-xanthin		phoenico-xanthin**	idoxanthin	asta-xanthin**

Because of symmetry some compounds appear twice

* Formed from [^{3}H]β-carotene by lobsters and present in internal organs.

** Formed from [^{3}H]β-carotene by lobsters and present in carapace. Data from Katayama *et al*, (1973a,b).

Hsu, Rodriguez and Chichester (Ref.26) also fed labelled lutein (9) to goldfish and found that it was converted into astaxanthin (16). Presumably an enzyme is present that can isomerize the ε-ring to a β-ring at some stage of the oxidation process. The 3'-hydroxyl group of ε-ring of lutein has the opposite absolute configuration to that of the 3,3'-hydroxyl groups of zeaxanthin and even to that of the 3-hydroxyl group of its β-ring (Ref.17 & 18). Isomerisation and oxidation of lutein to astaxanthin, therefore, would be expected to give 3,3'-*S*,*R* astaxanthin, partially enantiomeric to that (3,3'-*S*,*S*) formed from zeaxanthin. Rønneberg *et al* (Ref.27) have chromatographed samples of astaxanthin from lobster shells and found 3,3'-*R*,*R*, *RS*, and *SS* forms were present and the conditions of isolation did not cause any epimerisation. The biosynthetic source of these three forms of astaxanthin has not yet been established but it is quite likely that they arise from carotenoids with one or two ε-rings. The ratios of *S*,*S*:*R*,*S*:*R*,*R* were in the approximate ratio of 4:2:1. If partial epimerisation had occurred then the amount of *S*,*R* (meso) should exceed the amount of *R*,*R*, as was observed. These carotenoids in lobsters may be second or third hand; absorbed from a plant source, oxidised, and passed along a food chain at any step of which there may be selection for one precursor or one epimer over another.

There is, however, another possible explanation of the origin of *RS*- and *RR*-astaxanthin, namely that during the formation of the blue caroteno-protein conjugate some derivative of the 4-keto group is formed, possibly with the generation of a 3,4 double bond. The conjugate is so weak that it is cleaved by some organic solvents and heating and the astaxanthin is regenerated. Partial racemisation could occur during such a process while the chirality at C-3 was still in the presence and under the influence of the protein.

CAROTENOIDS OF MARINE ALGAE

Marine algae contain a variety of extensively modified carotenoids whose biosynthesis has been neglected. We have recently used various labelled mevalonates, and carotenoids formed from them, to follow the course of biosynthesis of some of these compounds.

The dinoflagellate *Amphidinium carterae*, maintained in axenic culture, gives cell-free systems which form neoxanthin (17), diadinoxanthin (18) and peridinin (19) from [^{14}C]zeaxanthin (8) (Ref.28). [2-^{14}C,2*RS*-2-$^{3}H_2$]mevalonate was incorporated into neoxanthin and the ^{14}C:^{3}H ratio showed that the hydrogen of C-8 in the allene of neoxanthin is derived from C-2 of mevalonate (Table 8); this result excludes the acetylene as a precursor (Ref.29) and supports the mechanism (Scheme 4) proposed by Goodwin (Ref.30).

Labelled neoxanthin was fed to the cell-free system and was converted into diadinoxanthin so the allene group is isomerised to the acetylene, as proposed by Britton (Ref.31). The mechanism can be drawn, as in Scheme 5, with an almost identical arrangement in space of the interacting parts. As the enzyme that forms the allene must have evolved before the one that forms the acetylene, it is possible, therefore, that the acetylene-forming enzyme could have evolved by modification of the allene-forming one.

TABLE 8. Incorporation of [2-^{14}C,2*RS*-2-$^{3}H_2$]- and [2-^{14}C,4*R*-4-$^{3}H_1$]mevalonic acids into carotenoids by cell-free preparations of *Amphidinium carterae*

Compound	^{14}C dpm	^{3}H dpm	^{14}C:^{3}H ratio normalised to mevalonate	^{14}C:^{3}H ratio normalised to lycopene
Mevalonate	4637	43634	(1:2)	-
Lycopene	5473	37381	8:11.62	(8:12)
β-Carotene	5989	40426	8:11.48	8:11.86
Zeaxanthin	3910	26353	8:11.46	8:11.84
Neoxanthin	6231	41935	8:11.44	8:11.82
Diadinoxanthin	3247	20002	8:10.47	8:10.84
Peridinin	8910	59964	8:11.44	8:11.82
Mevalonate	4917	40074	(1:1)	-
Lycopene	3124	25179	8:7.91	(8:8)
β-Carotene	6125	36811	8:5.90	8:5.97
Zeaxanthin	6731	40319	8:5.88	8:5.95
Neoxanthin	4800	28752	8:5.88	8:5.95
Diadinoxanthin	3621	21473	8:5.82	8:5.89
Peridinin	8527	43232	8:4.98	8:5.03

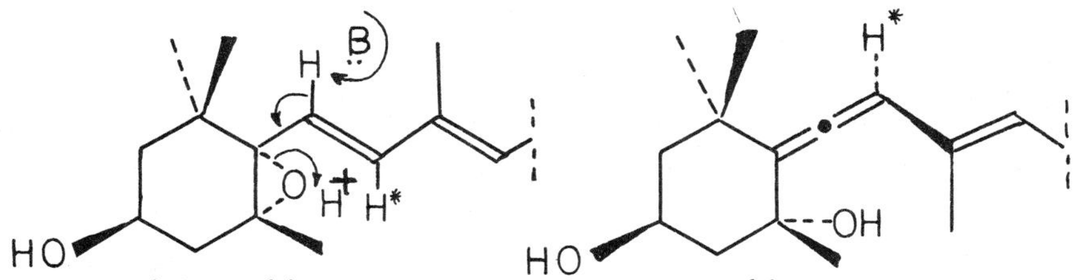

violaxanthin neoxanthin

Scheme 4. Proposed mechanism for the formation of an allene group from the ring of violaxanthin (modified from Ref.30). In our experiments, zeaxanthin (8) was fed to <u>A. carterae</u> so that involvement of a 5,6-peroxide or epoxide still remains to be demonstrated.

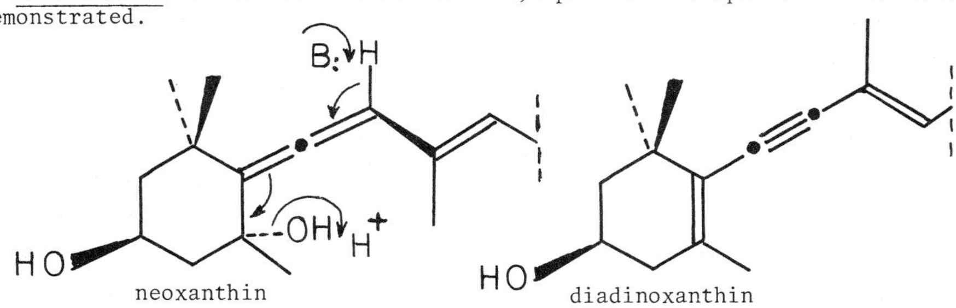

neoxanthin diadinoxanthin

Scheme 5. Proposed scheme for the formation of an acetylene group from the allene of neoxanthin (modified from Ref.31).

The other major product formed from lycopene, zeaxanthin or neoxanthin was peridinin (19). This is an unusual carotenoid in that it comprises 37 carbon atoms and appears to have lost a methyl group and two other carbons from the polyene chain. The demonstration that [^{14}C] zeaxanthin and [^{14}C]neoxanthin were converted into peridinin established that it was indeed formed by the deletion of three carbon atoms from a C_{40} carotenoid and not by assembly from C_{10}, C_{15} and C_2 moieties (Ref.28). The absence in peridinin of the C-20 (C-13 methyl) of neoxanthin suggests that it is this methyl group, and the carbon atom to which it was attached, that were removed. The question to be answered was which other carbon atom is removed: C-12 derived from C-2 of mevalonate or C-14, derived from C-4 of mevalonate? [2<u>RS</u>-2-$^3H_2$]- and [4<u>R</u>-4-$^3H_1$]mevalonates were then fed to cell-free systems of <u>A. carterae</u> and the peridinin was found to have lost one 4<u>R</u>-^{3}H present in neoxanthin but retained the 2-^{3}H. This suggested that C-14 of neoxanthin was lost (Ref.29) (Table 8).

The molecule of peridinin has another unique feature, namely a lactone ring, apparently formed by hydroxylation of C-11' and oxidation of the C-9' methyl (C-19') to a carboxyl group. It was thought that this could provide a model for the excision reaction, having the advantage that the lactone ring could hold the two ends of the molecule together while the C-14:C-15 bond was broken and reformed as a C-12:C-15 bond. An inherent, testable consequence of this proposal is that the hydrogen atom at C-15, derived from the 5-<u>pro-S</u> of mevalonate, would be lost on hydroxylation of C-15. Experiments with [5<u>RS</u>-5-$^3H_2$]mevalonate showed that it was retained, so the hypothesis has to be discarded.

The nature of the excised fragment is crucial to an understanding of the mechanism of chain shortening and the obvious, but unlikely, possibility of propine being liberated was readily discounted when air bubbled through the preparation failed to trap significant radioactivity in a nujol trap after lycopene, derived from [3-^{14}C]mevalonate, had been fed. Lycopene derived from [4<u>R</u>-4-$^3H_1$]mevalonate gave [^{3}H]peridinin and 70% of the label calculated to have been present at C-14 of neoxanthin was recovered in the water, so it appeared probable that C-14 was oxidised to a carboxyl group. The aqueous residue contained an acidic compound that was extracted into acid ethyl acetate and found to be lactate by HPLC (ref.32). Further work to define the source of the oxygen atoms and the chirality is in hand but there are now enough constraints for us to be able to put forward a working hypothesis that can account for the chain-shortening reaction. It is known that lipoxygenase can cleave carotenoids (Ref.33 & 34) and consequently it is proposed that the reaction is initiated by such an enzyme.

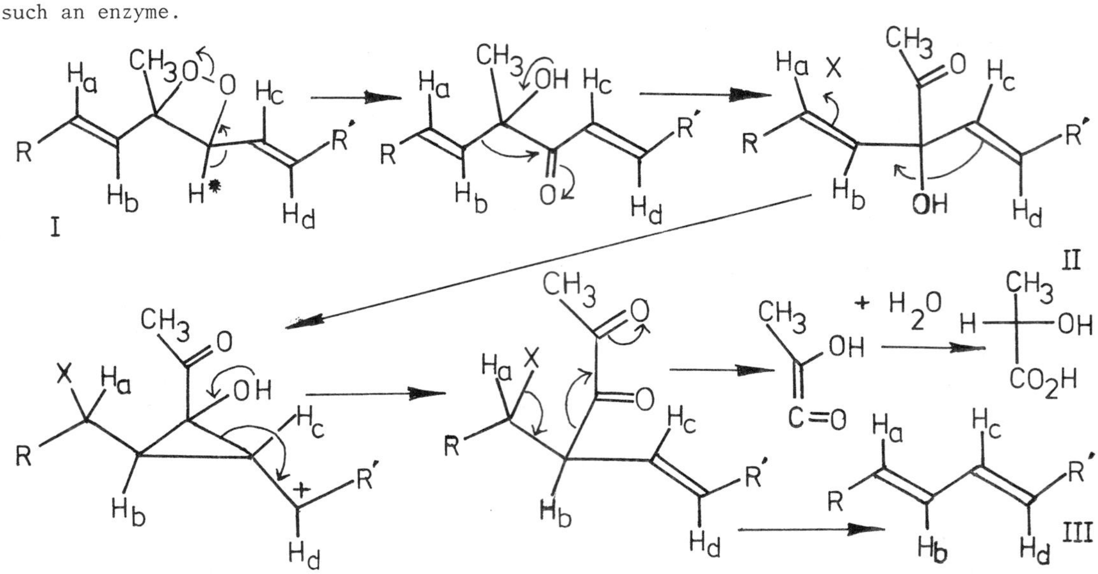

Scheme 6. Suggested mechanism for the chain-shortening reaction during peridinin biosynthesis. Neoxanthin is assumed to be oxidised to the stable intermediate I. Re-arrangement and hydration gives lactic acid II and peridinin III.

The mechansim is speculative and more information is needed before other alternatives can be eliminated, however, the proposal enables us to formulate experiments by which various features can be tested.

New enzymic reactions in eukaryotic, evolutionary times have probably evolved by the modification of pre-existing enzyme proteins. The mechanism proposed for the formation of peridinin, for example, could have evolved from a lipoxygenase type of enzyme. So we have come full circle to a reconsideration of comparative biochemistry but in a subtly different way. Carotenoid research provides several examples of reactions that make us consider not only the proteins that carry out the same catalytic activity in different organisms but how the various reactions have evolved. The biosynthetic pathways of carotenoids may show the footprints of evolutionary change.

Acknowledgement - Thanks are due to Mrs. Dale Fahey and Mr. I.E. Swift for their considerable contributions to the research on carotenoid stereochemistry. Dr.A.M. Duffield of the Biomedical Mass Spectrometry Unit of the University of N.S.W. obtained the mass spectra, Mrs. Betty Netting helped with the production of bacterial cultures and Dr. S.W. Jeffrey of C.S.I.R.O. Fisheries and Oceanography Research Institute, Cronulla N.S.W. provided the *A. carterae* cells. The work was supported, in part, by the Australian Research Grants Committee.

REFERENCES

1. J.W. Porter and S.L. Spurgeon, Pure Appl. Chem. 51, 609-622 (1979).
2. G. Britton, W.J.S. Lockley, N.J. Patel, T.W. Goodwin and G. Englert, J. Chem. Soc. Chem. Commun. 655-656, (1977).
3. G. Britton, T.W. Goodwin, W.J.S. Lockley, A.P. Mundy and N.J. Patel, J. Chem. Soc. Chem. Commun. 27-28, (1979).
4. B.A. Bidlingmeyer, J. Chromatog. Sci. 18, 525-539 (1980).

5. I.E. Swift and B.V. Milborrow, Biochem. J. 187, 261-264 (1980).
6. A.G. Andrewes, S. Liaaen-Jensen and O.B. Weeks, Acta Chem. Scand. Ser.B, 29, 884-886 (1975).
7. D. Fahey and B.V. Milborrow, Phytochem. 17, 2077-2082 (1978).
8. T.W. Goodwin, Biochem. J. 123, 293-329 (1971).
9. I.E. Swift and B.V. Milborrow, (unpublished results).
10. I.A. Rose, K.R. Hanson, K.D. Wilkinson and M.J. Wimmer, Proc. Natl. Acad. Sci. USA, 77, 2439-2441 (1980).
11. S. Liaaen-Jensen, S. Hertzberg, O.B. Weeks and U. Schwieter, Acta Chem. Scand. Ser.B, 22, 1171-1186 (1968).
12. M.P. Starr and S. Saperstein, Arch. Biochem. Biophys. 43, 157-168 (1953).
13. S.C. Kushwaha, M.B. Gochnauer, D.J. Kushner and M. Kates, Can. J. Microbiol. 20, 241-245 (1974).
14. J.D. Bu'Lock, D.J. Austin, G. Snatzke and L. Hruban, J. Chem. Soc. Chem. Commun. 255-256 (1970).
15. M. Hallenstvet, R. Buchecker, G. Borch and S. Liaaen-Jensen, Phytochem. 16, 583-585 (1977).
16. T.J. Walton, G. Britton and T.W. Goodwin, Biochem. J. 112, 383-385 (1969).
17. R. Buchecker, P. Hamm and C.H. Eugster, Helv. Chim. Acta. 57, 631-633 (1972).
18. A.G. Andrewes, G. Borch and S. Liaaen-Jensen, Acta Chem. Scand. Ser.B, 28, 139-140 (1974)
19. B.V. Milborrow, I.E. Swift and A.G. Netting (in press).
20. S.E. Moshier and D.J. Chapman, Biochem. J. 136, 395-404 (1973).
21. S. Liaaen-Jensen, E. Hegge and L.M. Jackman, Acta Chem. Scand. Ser.B, 18, 1703-1718 (1964).
22. M. Yamaguchi, Bull. Chem. Soc. Jap. 31, 739-742 (1958).
23. T. Katayama, M. Shimaya, M. Sameshima and C.O. Chichester, Int. J. Biochem. 4, 223-226 (1973).
24. T. Katayama, Y. Kunisaki, M. Shimaya, K.L. Simpson and C.O. Chichester, Comp. Biochem. Physiol. 46B, 269-272 (1973).
25. T. Katayama, T.Miyahara, Y. Tanaka, M. Sameshima, K.L. Simpson and C.O. Chichester, Bull. Jap. Soc. Sci. Fisheries 40, 97-103 (1974).
26. W.J. Hsu, D.B. Rodriguez and C.O. Chichester, Int. J. Biochem. 3, 333-338 (1972).
27. H. Rønneberg, B. Renstrøm, K. Aareskjold, S. Liaaen-Jensen, M. Vecchi, F.J. Leuenberger, R.K. Müller and H. Mayer, Helv. Chim. Acta 63, 711-715 (1980).
28. I.E. Swift, B.V. Milborrow and S.W. Jeffrey (in press).
29. I.E. Swift and B.V. Milborrow (in press).
30. T.W. Goodwin, In: Carotenoids, Ed. O. Isler, 577-636, Birkhaüser Verlag, Basel (1971)
31. G. Britton, Comp. Org. Chem. Ed. E. Haslam 5, 1025-1042 (1979).
32. I.E. Swift and Milborrow, B.V. (unpublished data).
33. R.D. Firn and J. Friend, Planta 103, 263 (1972).
34. J.A. Olson, Vitam. Horm. 26, 1-63 (1968).

MEDICAL APPLICATIONS AND USES OF CAROTENOIDS

Micheline M. Mathews-Roth

Channing Laboratory, Department of Medicine, Harvard Medical School, and Brigham and Women's Hospital, 180 Longwood Avenue, Boston, Mass., 02115, USA.

Abstract - In spite of the availability of synthetic vitamin A, the principal medical use of carotenoid pigments remains as a dietary source of vitamin A. In addition, colored carotenoids, because of their photoprotective function in green plants and photosynthetic bacteria, are administered to patients with certain dermatologic diseases, to alleviate the photosensitivity associated with these conditions. Recently, vitamin A and its derivatives have been shown to have anti-tumor activity. In addition, animal experiments suggest that carotenoid pigments, irrespective of their vitamin A activity, may have anti-tumor activity for light-induced (UV-B) tumors of the skin. All these various aspects of carotenoid use are discussed.

INTRODUCTION

The primary use in man of carotenoid pigments, whether taken in as carotenoid-containing foods or administered as dietary supplements, is the prevention or correction of vitamin A deficiency. The discovery that the carotenoid pigments ubiquitously present in the plant kingdom played an important role as protective agents against photosensitization by the plants' own chlorophyll has led to another medical use for carotenoids in man: their use as protective agents in certain skin diseases aggravated by light. Very recently, carotenoids have become of interest as possible tumor-preventative agents, especially those pigments with vitamin A activity. We will examine these various uses of carotenoid pigments, and also briefly discuss the studies which led to the use of carotenoids in the treatment of human photosensitivity.

USE OF CAROTENOIDS IN NUTRITION

Man, like other animals, cannot synthesize vitamin A. Hence, dietary carotenoids are man's main source of this vitamin. In spite of the current availability and use of synthetic vitamin A for the nutrification of food, or in single or multiple vitamin supplements, carotenoid vitamin A precursor-containing foods are still a very significant source of this vitamin in the diets of humans. Diets in various parts of the world vary greatly in their content of vitamin A, either available directly in meat, fish, eggs or dairy foods, or as the various pro-vitamins A in vegetable sources. Beta-carotene is the most important pro-vitamin A, mainly because of its presence in plants widely consumed by man and livestock, and because it is the pro-vitamin A with the greatest activity (Ref. 1).

In addition to availability in the diet, several factors such as protein intake, the amount, nature and dispersion of dietary fat, and the digestibility of the carotenoid-containing food may influence the absorption and utilization of beta-carotene and other pro-vitamins. The transformation of beta-carotene to vitamin A (retinol) in the animal (plants do not contain vitamin A as such) is thought to occur by cleavage of the carotenoid molecule at the central double bond (Ref. 2 & 3), or to a much lesser degree, by cleavage of the conjugated chain adjacent to one beta-ionone ring followed by sequential oxidative removal of fragments containing 2 to 5 carbon atoms (Ref. 4 & 5). Many studies have shown that the main point of conversion of ingested carotenoids is the intestinal mucosa. Conversion may also occur in the liver.

Carotenoids have been found in human milk (Ref. 6 & 7). There are at least two reported instances of breast-fed infants becoming carotenemic on their carotenemic mothers' milk (Ref. 8 & 9). Carotenoids also play some role in the coloration of human skin (Ref. 10 & 11). This property made feasible the use of carotenoids in man as light-protective agents in human photosensitivity diseases.

The manner in which carotenoids are excreted is not clear. They do not seem to be excreted as such in the urine. For a more detailed discussion of carotenoid metabolism, the reader is referred to the book by Bauernfeind (Ref. 12).

DEVELOPMENT OF THE IDEA TO USE CAROTENOIDS FOR THE TREATMENT OF PHOTOSENSITIVITY

It is now well-documented that carotenoid pigments function to protect green plants and photosynthetic as well as non-photosynthetic bacteria against photosensitization, particularly by endogenous photosensitizers, such as porphyrins and chlorophyll (Ref. 13 & 14).

Lethal photosensitization can be induced in laboratory animals by the administration of hematoporphyrin and exposure to strong light (Ref. 15). Because of the striking protective action of carotenoids in bacteria and in plants, it seemed possible that carotenoids might prevent this lethal effect also. To test this possibility, mice were given 1 mg. of hematoporphyrin intraperitoneally before exposure to strong visible light. Half of the animals had received 3 mg. of beta-carotene intraperitoneally 18 to 24 hours before receiving the injection of hematoporphyrin and being exposed to light. It was found that significantly more animals that received the beta-carotene survived the treatment with hematoporphyrin and light than did those mice that had not received the beta-carotene (Table 1). Controls showed that the vehicle in which the beta-carotene was suspended, a mixture of Tween-80 and saline, offered no protection against photosensitization, and that control animals given either beta-carotene or hematoporphyrin survived well if kept in the dark. Thus, beta-carotene was effective in preventing the lethal photosensitization of mice induced by the injection of hematoporphyrin and exposure to visible light (Ref. 16).

TABLE 1. Protective effect of beta-carotene on photosensitization of mice by hematoporphyrin and visible light.

Group	Light Exposure	Number Animals	Number Dead	Number Alive
Hematoporphyrin*	yes	27	21	6
Hematoporphyrin* and carotene #	yes	27	9	18
Hematoporphyrin* and Tween 80-saline	yes	8	7	1
Hematoporphyrin*	no	8	0	8
Carotene#	no	8	0	8

* Animals received 1 mg. intraperitoneally before exposure to light.
\# Carotene was suspended in Tween 80-saline. Animals received 3 mg. of this mixture intraperitoneally 18 to 24 hours before exposure to light.
Data in this table taken from Ref. 16.

In view of the results of the studies in bacteria and in animals, it now seemed feasible, because of the lack of toxicity of carotenoids in man, to administer beta-carotene to patients with photosensitivity. The disease chosen for study was erythropoietic protoporphyria (EPP). Patients with this abnormality of porphyrin metabolism complain of itching, burning, redness and swelling of the skin exposed to the sun (Ref. 17). Erythrocyte, plasma and stool protoporphyrin levels are increased, but urine porphyrin levels are within normal limits. Typical lesions may be induced by exposing the patients' skin to sunlight, or to strong artificial light (e.g. xenon arc, filtered to transmit light from 380 to 600 nm) under controlled conditions in the laboratory.

Could carotenoid pigments, which can protect against the photosensitization induced by the porphyrin group of chlorophyll also protect against the photosensitization induced by the porphyrin group of protoporphyrin? In a collaborative study, we treated with beta-carotene (15-90 mg./day p.o.) 3 patients with EPP, each of whom had elevated erythrocyte, plasma and stool protoporphyrin levels. All 3 patients, a 10-year old girl, her 39-year old father, and an unrelated 35-year old man, showed marked improvement in their ability to tolerate exposure to sunlight, as well as an increased ability to tolerate exposure to xenon arc lamp (phototesting) after they had taken beta-carotene for 4 to 6 weeks. Protection continued for as long as beta-carotene was taken; when the medication was stopped, photosensitivity returned.

Since publication of the report of these three patients in 1970 (Ref. 18), we treated with beta-carotene 130 additional patients, in collaboration with their personal physicians (Ref. 19 & 20). As a result of our experience with this larger number of patients, we have found that in many cases we have had to use higher doses of beta-carotene (up to 180 mg./day) than we used with the first 3 patients: the dosage needs to be individualized for each patient (Ref. 19 & 20). Of the 133 patients treated with these individualized doses, 22 have reported little or no improvement, and the remaining 111 have reported significant improvement in their ability to tolerate sunlight without developing symptoms of photosensitivity

(Table 2). Over 75% report a four-fold or more increase in tolerance to sunlight. The majority now engage in outdoor activities from which they excluded themselves before carotene treatment started. The great majority of the children can now play outdoors in daylight. Some patients still get reactions when they expose themselves for a long time to the sun. Others can spend all day outdoors with no trouble, and some only an hour or two before developing symptoms, although in general the treated patients report that they can tolerate sunlight better than before treatment.

TABLE 2. Effect of beta-carotene on tolerance to sunlight of patients with EPP

Number of Patients	%	Protection Index*
10		1#
	16	
12		2#
27		3 - 5
39		6 - 10
15	84	11 - 15
6		16 - 20
24		>21
Total: 133	100%	

* Protection index is defined as the number of minutes of summer sunlight tolerated without the development of symptoms after therapy, divided by the number of minutes of summer sunlight tolerated without the development of symptoms before therapy. An index of less than 3 represents no improvement.

\# Patients showed little or no improvement despite blood carotene levels of at least 400 μg.% following intake of highest dose appropriate for their ages.

In addition to the patients' subjective reactions of improved tolerance to sunlight, we used phototesting with xenon arc light before and during beta-carotene therapy as an objective method of evaluating the effects of this treatment (Ref. 19 & 21). Tolerance to this light increased in those patients who reported benefit from carotene therapy. No increased tolerance was found in those patients reporting no improvement (Table 3).

In the six year period of the study (1969-1975), no toxic side-effects (other than occasional transient loose stools) from the ingestion of these high doses of beta-carotene were found. These doses are the equivalent of up to four pounds of carrots a day. The carotenodermia which usually develops has not bothered most of the patients. Although we found in another study that beta-carotene had no effect in preventing sunburn (Ref. 22), it appears to have a small effect in increasing tanning as opposed to burning. Many of our patients report that for the first time in their lives they were able to develop a suntan.

Treatment with beta-carotene has had no effect on the abnormalities of porphyrin metabolism which are characteristic of EPP. All of the 133 patients had elevated erythrocyte, plasma and stool porphyrins at the time they entered the study, and their porphyrins have remained elevated in spite of beta-carotene treatment.

In 22 reports of the successful use of beta-carotene for the treatment of photosensitivity in EPP, over 75% of the patients treated reported a significant improvement in their ability to tolerate light exposure, and no side effects from the use of beta-carotene were observed (Ref. 23 to 44). One study reporting little or no improvement has also appeared (Ref. 45); however, these workers used a much lower dose of beta-carotene than that recommended by us (Ref. 19 & 20). Later, some of the patients from the unsuccessfully treated group were given higher doses of beta-carotene by another investigator and the patients seemed to have noted some increased tolerance to light while taking the higher doses (Ref. 44). These results emphasize the importance, as we have mentioned (Ref. 19 & 20), of individualizing the dose to each patient, and increasing the dose until the patient reports some improvement.

The problem of individualizing treatment is also important in the conduct of a controlled trial and makes double blind designs almost impossible. At a minimum, such trials should use a dose of beta-carotene large enough to produce amelioration of symptoms in the majority of patients; a minimum period of 3 months' treatment at doses giving blood levels of at least 800 μg% - for adults at least 180 mg./day should be given (Ref. 19).

From our results, and those of other workers listed above, it can be concluded that beta-carotene, when administered in sufficiently high doses, can be an effective therapy for ameliorating photosensitivity in most patients with EPP.

TABLE 3. Tolerance to xenon arc light; minutes to develop minimal erythema.

Patient	Before therapy*	During therapy#
1	13.33	36.67
2	20.00	40.00
3	.75	5.64
4	18.33	25.71
5	8.00	16.67
7	5.20	12.00
8	6.00	9.33
9	23.33	38.30
10	8.33	31.67
11	3.67	31.67
12	5.00	14.00
13	10.00	41.67
14	6.25	13.75
15	6.25	13.33
16	10.00	15.56
34	3.75	8.75
35	6.67	20.00
37	4.00	15.00
38	12.50	25.00
39	2.00	10.00
42	5.00	15.00

* Average for each patient of all phototests before therapy started, when patient first entered study, as well as tests done before therapy started in subsequent years of the study, when patient had not taken beta-carotene during winter (serum carotene level <250 μg%) in all years patient was in study.

\# Average for each patient of all phototests in which serum carotene level exceeded 400 μg% in all years patient was in the study.

Paired t-test on data in this Table; $p<.001$. Data taken from Ref. 21.

However, it must be pointed out that there are limits to the protective ability of carotenoids. As can be seen from our data, some patients receive little or no benefit from beta-carotene treatment. In general, these are patients who have very high levels of red cell and/or plasma porphyrins. Carotenoid administration seems also to offer a slight degree of protection in patients given intravenous hematoporphyrin derivative for cancer investigation, but this protection is not sufficient to allow unrestricted activity (Ref. 46). Thus it is important to realize that even when carotene doses are increased to the highest achievable levels, significant protection may not occur in the presence of extremely high levels of porphyrins.

Since beta-carotene administration seemed to be effective in protecting against photosensitization in EPP, it seemed logical to see if it could prevent photosensitization in other photosensitivity diseases.

There have been 7 reports on the use of carotenoids in the treatment of congenital porphyria (Gunther's disease) (Ref. 35 & 47 to 52). Five report some decrease in the number of new lesions produced, in some cases allowing the patient fairly normal exposure to light. Seip et al. reported phototesting one patient using a xenon arc lamp (Ref. 47). Before treatment he reacted with marked erythema after 10 minutes' exposure to this light, and during treatment he developed only mild erythema after forty minutes of exposure. These authors stressed, as we do, the importance of maintaining high levels of carotene in the blood. Here, as in EPP, carotenoids do not correct the biochemical defect, so it is important that whatever hematologic treatment the patient is receiving must be continued during carotenoid therapy. Carotene treatment will not heal old scars - hence the best cosmetic effects will occur if therapy is started when patients are very young.

Several groups of workers have reported the use of carotenoids (usually a mixture of beta-carotene and canthaxanthin) in the treatment of polymorphous light eruption (PMLE) with varying degrees of success (Ref. 42 and 53 to 57). Jansen treated 66 patients, 51 of whom responded favorably (Ref. 53). Wennersten and Swanbeck treated 8 patients, all of whom showed improvements in the minimal erythema dose tested with an appropriately filtered xenon arc lamp (Ref. 54). Thune treated 17 patients, only 5 of whom showed a more than 3-fold increase in tolerance to sunlight (Ref. 55). On phototesting, he found "a significant increase in minimal erythema dose for unfiltered light (xenon arc) at the 5% level of probability". Some of the patients also needed a sunscreen to achieve maximal therapeutic effect. Haeger-Aronsen et al. found improvement in 15 out of 18 patients with PMLE (Ref. 42). Parrish et al. found complete remission in only 6 out of 19 patients, and got much better results using PUVA treatment (Ref. 56). In our collaborative study, only 9 out of 27 patients reported improvement with carotene treatment, most also needing the concurrent application of a sunscreen, though sunscreen alone was not beneficial (Ref. 20).

Fusaro and Johnson reported success in treating with high doses of beta-carotene the hereditary form of PMLE found in American Indians (Ref. 57). They treated 5 patients and stated that each patient was able to perform normal activities outdoors without avoiding the sun and without showing symptoms of photosensitivity, and reappearance of skin lesions.

Although some workers have shown objective evidence by phototest of improved light tolerance in PMLE with carotene treatment, it is obvious from these various reports that carotenoids are not as effective in the treatment of PMLE as they are in the treatment of EPP. It would seem sensible to use carotenoids in the therapy of PMLE only when the usual modes of therapy are ineffective, impractical or contraindicated.

Carotenoids have been found by other workers as well as by our group to be ineffective in the treatment of actinic reticuloid (Ref. 20 & 58), porphyria cutanea tarda (Ref. 20, 59 & 60), solar urticaria (Ref. 20, 35 & 58) and hydroa aestivale (Ref. 20). Two groups of workers have found a beneficial effect of carotenoid treatment in lupus erythematosus, but another group had success in only 1 out of 26 patients (Ref. 42, 61 & 62). Bickers et al. suggest that beta-carotene may be effective in ameliorating the photosensitivity in hydroa vacciniforme (Ref. 63), and Husquinet et al. (Ref. 64) have reported some success in a patient with porphyria variegata, who developed no lesions for 2 years while taking carotene, in spite of elevated stool and urine porphyrins. Eales reported also some success in treating this disease (Ref. 39). Pietzcker reports successfully using carotenoids to ameliorate the appearance of certain patients with vitelligo (Ref. 65).

Since the number of patients with these various diseases who have been treated with carotenoids is small, we still do not really know the extent of the pigments' effectiveness in these conditions: clearly more work needs to be done. However, since the above-described studies have also reported no significant toxicity from carotenoid ingestion, it is probably sensible to give a trial of beta-carotene (or a mixture of beta-carotene and canthaxanthin, as used in Europe) to patients with any kind of photosensitivity disease, who have not responded to other forms of therapy. In EPP, carotenoids seem to be the treatment of choice.

Other therapeutic uses have also been reported for carotenoids. Karagezyan (Ref. 66) and Shabykin (Ref. 67) have used carotene in various skin diseases other than photosensitivity diseases, with some success. Some authors have suggested a role for carotenoids in olfaction. However, Moulton conclusively demonstrated that carotenoids are not involved in the olfactory machanism (Ref. 68). On the somewhat more speculative side, some work has been done suggesting that carotenoids may have some role in "oxidations". Karnaukhov has done a series of studies in which he suggests that carotenoids and myoglobin function as an "intracellular oxygen stock" in lipofuschin granules in ageing tissues and in mollusc neurons (Ref. 69 to 72). Campbell, and Nelson et al. suggest that a diet rich in carrots protects rats against acute anoxia (Ref. 73 to 75). Gainer suggests that the water-soluble carotene crocetin increases oxygen diffusion in atherosclerosis, increases fermentation yields and growth of tissue culture cells (Ref. 76 to 78). Perhaps in view of these interesting preliminary observations, the possible role of the involvement of carotenoids in oxidative metabolism ought to be thoroughly investigated.

Stanier has pointed out the ecological importance of carotenoids to photosynthetic organisms (Ref. 79), and we found a similar ecological value of these pigments for non-photosynthetic bacteria (Ref. 80). It is interesting to note that even for those bacteria which normally colonise the human skin, the presence of carotenoids may be of some value. We surveyed the bacteria colonizing the surface of the skin of a group of frequent sunbathers and a group of infrequent sunbathers. We found that although frequent sunbathing does not greatly affect the total number of bacteria on the skin, it does increase the proportion of bacteria containing carotenoid pigments to a statistically significant degree (Ref. 81).

At the last Carotenoid Symposium, Boutwell discussed the anti-tumor effects of vitamin A (Ref. 82). Since that time, evidence in animal experiments as well as in human epidemiological studies suggest rather strongly that vitamin A and/or its derivatives have a protective effect against tumors arising in epithelial tissues. Recently Peto et al. have comprehensively reviewed this subject (Ref. 83). Several studies in animals have shown that a similar protective effect can be achieved in chemically induced and in ultraviolet light (UV-B; 290-320 nm) induced skin tumors, by administering beta-carotene instead of vitamin A. In addition, a suggestion of protection against cancer by the ingestion of carotenoid-containing vegetables can be found in human cancer epidemiology studies (Ref. 83). The animal studies using beta-carotene raised the question of whether the protective effect was due to vitamin A to which beta-carotene can be readily converted in the animals used in the studies, or whether it was due to an effect of the carotenoid molecule itself. To effect a separation of carotenoid molecule action from vitamin A action, we repeated the experiments with beta-carotene, and in parallel experiments tested the effects on tumor formation of canthaxanthin (4,4' diketo beta-carotene), a carotenoid pigment which cannot be converted to vitamin A in the animal body, but which has been found to act as a protective agent against photosensitization (Ref. 84), and of phytoene (7,8,11,12, 7',8',11',12' octahydro $-\psi,\psi$-carotene), the beta-carotene precursor which has no vitamin A activity, but has some protective activity against sunburn in experimental animals (Ref. 85).

As our test-animal, we used female hairless mice of the Philadelphia Skin and Cancer Hospital strain. The mice were divided into 5 goups. Each group received either beta-carotene, canthaxanthin, or their placebo incorporated into food bricks, or phytoene or its placebo by injection. Descriptions of preparation of the carotenoid-containing foods and injections have been given elsewhere (Ref. 86 & 87). Three methods of tumor induction were used on mice from each of the pigment and placebo groups; 1) application of dimethyl-benz-a-anthracene (DMBA) followed by thrice-weekly applications of croton oil, 2) application of DMBA followed by twice-weekly irradiation with low doses of UV-B, and 3) high doses of UV-B alone (7.2 kJ/m^2). Details of these methods are given elsewhere (Ref. 88 & 89).

We found that administration of beta-carotene caused a delay in the appearance of and a decrease in the number of skin tumors in hairless mice in each of the three methods of tumor induction used. Canthaxanthin, and phytoene, the pigments with no vitamin A activity, caused a delay in appearance and decreased the number of skin tumors induced by UV-B radiation alone but these latter two pigments had no inhibitory effect on tumors induced by DMBA and croton oil application. In addition, phytoene had no effect on inhibiting tumors by DMBA and low-dose UV-B irradiation, whereas canthaxanthin had some effect (Fig. 1).

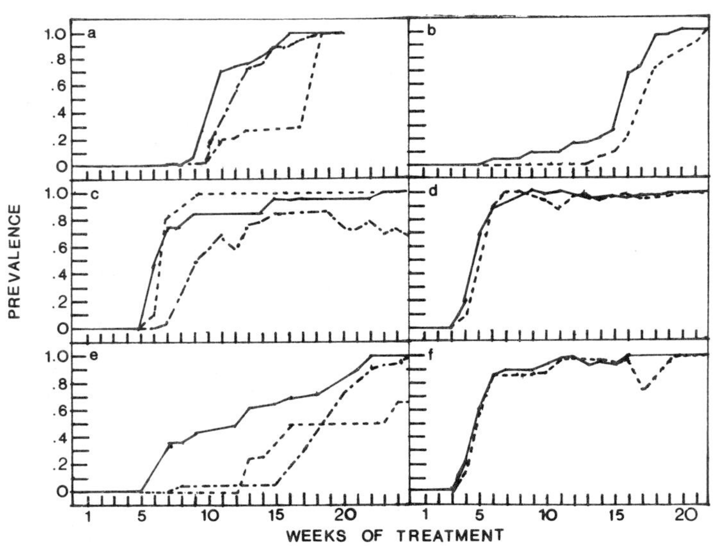

Fig. 1. Prevalence of tumors (ratio of number of mice with tumors to number of survivors) in mice treated with beta-carotene or with canthaxanthin, phytoene, or their respective placebos with the three methods of tumor induction. a) Mice treated with beta-carotene (-●-), canthaxanthin (- - -), or placebo (——); tumors induced by UV-B irradiation alone. b) Mice treated with phytoene (- - -) or placebo (——); tumors induced by UV-B irradiation alone. c) Mice treated with beta-carotene, canthaxanthin or placebo (symbols as in a); tumors induced by DMBA-croton oil applications. d) Mice treated with phytoene or placebo (symbols as in b)); tumors induced by DMBA-croton oil applications. e) Mice treated with beta-carotene, canthaxanthin or placebo (symbols as in a)); tumors induced by DMBA and low-dose UV-B irradiation. f) Mice treated with phytoene and placebo (symbols as in b)); tumors induced by DMBA and low-dose UV-B irradiation.

These studies suggest that carotenoid pigments, irrespective of their vitamin A activity, can prevent or slow down the growth of skin tumors induced by UV-B alone, but those pigments with no vitamin A activity have no effect on tumor induction by DMBA and croton oil. As to tumors induced by DMBA and low-dose UV-B, the finding that canthaxanthin has some activity and that phytoene has not may not be surprising. In this case, UV-B could be acting as a promoter, or as a co-carcinogen. Phytoene may be able to have an effect on the initiator activities of UV-B, but it has no effect in a system initiated by DMBA. Canthaxanthin, because of differences in molecular structure which make it more effective in quenching excited species, may not be able to affect initiation by DMBA, but may have an effect on promotion or co-carcinogenicity by UV-B.

LACK OF TOXICITY OF CAROTENOIDS

Studies performed by ourselves and others on patients with EPP as well as on normal volunteers have confirmed reports in the literature that the ingestion of large amounts of pure beta-carotene has not led to serious side-effects. (Ref. 90 & 91). We detected no abnormalities in blood sugar, blood urea nitrogen, total bilirubin or serum glutamate-oxaloacetate transaminase in either EPP patients or normal volunteers during carotenoid treatment (Ref. 19, 20 & 22).

The complete blood count was not affected by carotene intake. Many of the patients with EPP had a mild anemia (Ref. 92). This was not worsened or improved by carotene intake. Leucopenia has been reported in patients who ingested large amounts of carrots (Ref. 93 & 94). This phenomenon was found to reverse itself when the patient stops eating the abnormal amount of carrots. We found no evidence of leucopenia in any of our patients or volunteers. The absence of this finding in our study strengthens the suggestion of other workers that the leucopenia was probably due to substances other than beta-carotene present in the carrots (Ref. 90 & 91). Indeed they reported that the administration of pure beta-carotene did not induce leucopenia in a patient who had experienced leucopenia after eating large amounts of carrots (Ref. 90 & 91). Methemoglobinemia has recently been shown to result from the consumption of large amounts of carrot juice (Ref. 94): this is another example of the toxicity of large amounts of vegetables and their products.

None of our patients was found to develop abnormally high levels of serum vitamin A. This confirms what has been reported in the literature, that individuals ingesting large amounts of beta-carotene do not develop hypervitaminosis A (Ref. 90, 91 & 96).

We also found that, as in animal studies (Ref. 97), abnormal amounts of beta-carotene and vitamin A do not accumulate in the liver or the brain as a result of the ingestion of crystalline beta-carotene (Ref. 98). In addition, it would appear that no pathological structural changes have occurred in liver as a result of high levels of beta-carotene intake. Again, the same is probably also true of brain.

From the results of our studies and from the data found in the literature, it would seem that there is no marked direct toxicity from the ingestion of large quantities of pure beta-carotene. On the other hand, those individuals developing carotenemia and carotenodermia by means of increased intake of carotenoid-containing foods are at some risk for the development of some hematological abnormality. They also may encounter other difficulties because of the accompanying usually inadequate diet, and occasionally because of the misdiagnosis of their "jaundice" by a physician unaware of their dietary indiscretions, and unfamiliar with carotenemia. Thus, because of the potential dangers associated with excessive ingestion of carotenoid-containing foods, we do not recommend that photosensitive patients obtain relief from their photosensitivity by increasing the intake of such foods. Pure beta-carotene, either in the beadlet (water-dispersible) formulation, or as crystalline beta-carotene for those rare individuals allergic to the non-carotenoid beadlet components, is indeed the preparation to be recommended.

MECHANISMS OF THE CAROTENOIDS' PROTECTIVE FUNCTION

How carotenoids might be exerting their photoprotective function is being actively investigated at this time. Studies to date suggest that the high levels of protoporphyrin present in the erythrocytes, plasma, or extracellular fluid, or intracellular organelles (e.g. lysosomes) of the skin of patients with EPP can be stimulated to an excited state (triplet state) by visible light, which can penetrate skin to the level of the dermal capillaries (Ref. 99). The excited protoporphyrin may either destroy cell components directly, or may react with molecular oxygen to form singlet oxygen, a moiety that can be highly damaging to cellular components. Direct cell damage, or damage to cells or cellular organelles such as lysosomes, with release of chemical mediators that in turn damage other cells or organelles, would then cause the manifestations of itching, burning, erythema and edema experienced by the patient with EPP.

Beta-carotene can quench singlet oxygen and inhibit free radical formation *in vitro* (Ref. 100 & 101), and the ability of carotenoids to confer protection is correlated with the ability of the carotenoids to quench singlet oxygen *in vitro* (Ref. 102). However, some degree of free radical inhibition by carotenoids is a possible alternative mechanism of action. Mechanisms of carotenoid protection in EPP have not yet been studied in an animal model. Further work should elucidate the definitive mode of action of the carotenoids' protective effect in animal models, and eventually in patients with EPP.

In non-porphyric photosensitivity diseases, the chromophore responsible for the abnormal reactions is not known, and is in all likelihood different from that in EPP: the mechanisms responsible for the induction of abnormal responses may not have the same molecular basis. Thus it is not surprising to see that for some diseases, carotenoids may not be as effective a photoprotector as they are in EPP. Here also, much work needs to be done on the mechanisms of photosensitization in these diseases.

How carotenoid pigments exert their protective function against tumor development is also unknown. As mentioned above, beta-carotene as well as canthaxanthin and phytoene can inhibit the formation of free radicals, which have been implicated in UV-B induced tumors. Beta-carotene and canthaxanthin are also able to quench singlet excited oxygen (Ref. 102). Although phytoene absorbs light in the UV-B range, unpublished calculations by Lamola (personal communication) suggest that physical shading would be an unlikely mechanism of action.

Weight for weight, beta-carotene and canthaxanthin have an equal effect in preventing photosensitivity to visible light. Anderson and Krinsky found that beta-carotene and canthaxanthin are equally effective in protecting liposomes against dye-sensitized photooxidation (Ref. 84). As we mentioned, the administration to photosensitive patients of a mixture of beta-carotene and canthaxanthin appears to give as good protection against photosensitization by visible light in EPP as does beta-carotene alone (Ref. 35 & 42).

Some aspects of the accumulation of carotenoids in skin are intriguing from a mechanistic point of view. Clinical observation of patients with carotenodermia has long demonstrated that this coloration is most obvious in those areas of the body with a prominent horny layer, such as the palms of the hands, soles of the feet, knees, and other areas of skin that are subject to mechanical irritation. Gandy (Ref. 103 & 104) also suggested that in addition to areas subject to mechanical irritation, carotenoids are deposited in greater amounts in areas subject to irritation by physical factors, including light. The observation that light may play a part in regulating the intensity of carotenodermia was suggested by Klose (Ref. 105), who observed that carotenodermia was confined to areas exposed to light in infants fed carrots, and suggested that this might be due to the influence of light. He found that in a group of infants given the same food, carotenodermia developed only in those infants whose cribs were kept near the window. Interestingly the findings of Edwards and Duntley on the distribution of carotenoids in the skin of the whole body fairly well parallels those areas of the body exposed to light (Ref. 10). These findings are interesting in view of the protective function of carotenoids. They might suggest a function of the carotenoid pigments normally present in skin; that is, a certain level of protective pigments is always present to "balance" the potential photosensitizing pigments such as cytochromes and other porphyrin pigments, flavins, etc., which are also always present. Thus, in conditions of increased light exposure, the body might increase the deposition of carotenoids in light-exposed areas: if there was sufficient carotenoid present in the diet, this would be seen as some carotenodermia in the light-exposed areas, explaining the findings of Klose, and possibly also of Gandy. Visible light has been measured to penetrate skin through the epidermis into the dermal layer (Ref. 106). As skin contains potential photosensitizers as we pointed out above, it would indeed seem important that exposed skin have some kind of protective mechanism to guard against photosensitization. I suggest that such a protective mechanism exists, and that the carotenoids in skin play an integral role in its function. Thus in diseases such as the porphyrias, the normal balance of photosensitizers and photoprotectors is altered by the presence of increased amounts of porphyrins. With carotenoid therapy, we seek to re-establish the balance; this can usually be done, except in the case of large amounts of photosensitizers where not enough carotenoids can be absorbed to restore the balance.

It is intriguing to think that there might be some increase of carotenoid pigments in light-exposed areas in view of the protective function of the carotenoids. However, other than the observations of Klose (Ref. 105), there is no data to suggest that light really does play a role in increasing the deposition of carotenoids in the skin of man. Interestingly, in certain bacteria and fungi, light indeed does play a role in the deposition of carotenoids (Ref. 107). The possibility remains that carotenoids are more prevalent in light exposed areas simply because there is more horny layer in these areas. In addition, those areas of the body exposed to light are also usually exposed to mechanical irritation, resulting in increased formation of horny layer, so it is hard to say which factor could be more important. It would seem that certain physical and probably also anatomical factors influence the development of the horny layer. Because of the affinity of carotenoids for the horny layer, the pigments are predominant in those areas of marked horny layer deposit. If the diet is high in carotenoids, carotenodermia becomes most marked in those areas. Grof et al. suggest a histamine-mediated mechanism to explain the deposit of carotene in these areas (Ref. 108). I suggest that perhaps such a mechanism is not necessary since the carotenoids naturally accumulate in skin cells. When physical irritation occurs there is a more rapid division of cells and resultant formation of horny layer, and thus accumulation of carotenoids in the area, the degree again being related to the amount of carotenoid intake. However, the Grof suggestion is appealing if there were some mechanism in the skin for the regulation of the level of photoprotector; then some mechanism would be necessary to get more carotenoids into the area susceptible to photosensitization. As there is the suggestion that the first damages in porphyrin photosensitization may be at the level of the dermal capillary, it is clear that much more work needs to be done to study the factors involved in the development of carotenodermia and its possible role in the protection of skin cells against photosensitization.

REFERENCES

1. S.Y. Thompson, Proc. Nutr. Soc. 24, 136-146 (1965).
2. D.S. Goodman and H.S. Huang, Science 149, 879-880 (1966).
3. J.A. Olsen, Amer. Jour. Clin. Nutr. 9, No. 4, part 2, 1-12 (1961).
4. J. Glover and E.R. Redfearn, Biochem. Jour. 58, xv (1954).
5. J. Glover and E.R. Redfearn, Vit. and Hormones 18, 371-386 (1960).
6. S. Kon and N.E. Mawson, Spec. Report Ser., Med. Res. Council, London, No. 269 (1950).
7. M. Lesher, J.K. Brody, H.H. Williams and I.G. May, Amer. Jour. Dis. Child. 70, 182-192 (1945).
8. S. Almond and R.F.L. Logan, Brit. Med. J. II, 235-241 (1942).
9. M.L. Thomson, Arch. Dis. Child. 18, 112 (1973).
10. E.A. Edwards and S.Q. Duntly, Amer. Jour. Anat. 63, 1-33 (1939).
11. E.A. Edwards, J.B. Hamilton, S.Q. Duntley and G. Hubut, Endocrinology 28, 119-123 (1941).
12. J.G. Bauernfeind, Carotenoids as Colorants and Vitamin A Precursors, Academic Press, New York, (1981).
13. O. Isler, Carotenoids, p. 669, Birkhauser, Basel (1971).
14. M.M. Mathews and W.R. Sistrom, Arch. fur Mikrobiol. 35, 139-146 (1960).
15. R.L. Lipson and E.J. Baldes, Arch. Dermatol. 82, 508-516 (1960).
16. M.M. Mathews, Nature 203, 1092 (1964).
17. J.B. Stanbury, J.D. Wyngaarden and D.S. Fredrickson, The Metabolic Basis of Inherited Disease, p. 1166, McGraw-Hill, New York (1978).
18. M.M. Mathews-Roth, M.A. Pathak, T.B. Fitzpatrick, L.C. Harber and E.H. Kass, New Engl. Jour. Med. 282, 1231-1234 (1970).
19. M.M. Mathews-Roth, M.A. Pathak, T.B. Fitzpatrick, L.C. Harber and E.H. Kass, Jour. Amer. Med. Assoc. 228, 1004-1008 (1974).
20. M.M. Mathews-Roth, M.A. Pathak, T.B. Fitzpatrick, L.C. Harber and E.H. Kass, Arch. Dermatol. 113, 1229-1232 (1977).
21. M.M. Mathews-Roth, E.H. Kass, T.B. Fitzpatrick, M.A. Pathak, and L.C. Harber, Arch. Dermatol. 115, 1381-1382 (1979).
22. M.M. Mathews-Roth, M.A. Pathak, J.A. Parrish, T.B. Fitzpatrick, E.H. Kass, K. Toda and W. Clemons, Jour. Invest. Dermatol. 59, 349-353 (1972).
23. H. Baart de la Faille, D. Suurmond, L.N. Went, J. van Steveninck and A.A. Schothorst, Dermatologica 145, 389-394 (1972).
24. M.B. Lewis, Austr. Jour. Dermatol. 13, 75-78 (1972).
25. T.A. Chapel, R.H. Stewart and S.B. Webster, Arch. Dermatol. 105, 572-573 (1972).
26. C.R. Anderson, Arch. Dermatol. 106, 412-413 (1972).
27. I. Wurker, Zeit. Haut. Geschch. 47, 1006-1007 (1972).
28. V.K. Hopsu-Havu, P.E. Terho, T. Hollmen, Ann. Clin. Res. 5, 111-185 (1973).
29. E.J. Moynahan, and B. Leppard, Proc. Roy. Soc. Med. 66, 1085-1086 (1973).
30. F. Gschnait and K. Wolff, Hautarzt 25, 72-80 (1974).
31. G.H. Grupper, G. Girard and C. Davatchy, Bull. Soc. Fr. Dermatol. et Syph. 82, 249-250 (1975).
32. E. Beckert and J. Metz, Hautarzt 25, 195-196 (1974).
33. R.A. Marsden and R.P.R. Dawber, Proc. Roy. Soc. Med. 70, 572-574 (1977).
34. S.T. Zaynoun, J.A.A. Hunter, F.J. Darby, P. Zarembski, B.E. Johnson and W. Frain-Bell, Brit. Jour. Dermatol. 97, 663-668 (1977).
35. G. Goerz and H. Ippen, Dtch. Med. Wschr. 102, 1051-1055 (1977).
36. S. Nonaka, T. Hirowatari, T. Honda, T. Shimoyana, M. Hori, H. Yamaura, N. Fujiwara, I. Takahashi, K. Nishimoto and M. Nogita, Jap. Jour. Dermatol. 87, 7-32 (1977).
37. J. Barth, Dermatol. Monatschr. 160, 601 (1978).
38. W.L. Weston, Jour. Allergy Clin. Immunol. 61, 408 (1978).
39. L. Eales, South Afr. Med. Jour. 54, 1050-1052 (1978).
40. E. Rossi, D.H. Curnow and H. Schenberg, Pathology 10, 17-26 (1978).
41. G. Niebauer, P. Mischer, and I. Formanek, Mod. Prob. Ped. 20, 86-101 (1978).
42. B. Haeger-Aronsen, G. Krock and M. Abdulla, Internat. Jour. Dermatol. 18, 73-82 (1979).
43. K. Thomsen, H. Schmidt and A. Fischer, Dermatologica 159, 82-86 (1979).
44. A. Shafrir, Proc. Roy. Soc. Med. 70, 574 (1977).

45. M.F. Corbett, A. Herxheimer, I.A. Magnus, C.A. Ramsay and A. Kobza-Black, Brit. Jour. Dermatol. 97, 655-662 (1977).
46. G.L. Zalar, M.B. Poh-Fitzpatrick, D.L. Krohn, R. Jacobs and L.C. Harber, Arch. Dermatol. 113, 1392-1397 (1977).
47. M. Seip, P.O. Thune and L. Eriksen, Acta Dermatovener, 54, 239-240 (1974).
48. I.B. Sneddon, Proc. Roy. Soc. Med. 67, 593-594 (1974).
49. E.C. Jung, Dtsch. Med. Wschr. 102, 279-280 (1977).
50. M.M. Mathews-Roth, R.G. Haining and T.R. Kinney Amer. Jour. Dis. Child. 131, 366 (1977).
51. G.S. Stretcher, Arch. Dermatol. 114, 1242-1243 (1978).
52. H. Storck and J. Kaufmann, Dermatologica 157, 323-333 (1978).
53. C.T. Jansen, Dermatologica, 149, 363-373 (1974).
54. G. Wennesten and G. Swanbeck, Acta Dermatovener. 54, 491-499 (1974).
55. P. Thune, Acta Dermatovener. 56, 127-133 (1976).
56. J.A. Parrish, M.J. Levine, W.L. Morrison, E. Gonzalez, and T.B. Fitzpatrick, Brit. Jour. Dermatol. 100, 187-193 (1979).
57. R.M. Fusaro and J.A. Johnson, Jour. Amer. Med. Assoc. 243, 231 (1980).
58. A. Kobza, C.A. Ramsay, and I.A. Magnus, Brit. Jour. Dermatol. 88, 157-166 (1973).
59. H. Ippen, Dtsch. Med. Wschr. 86, 127-133 (1961).
60. M.A. Pathak, Sunlight and Man, p. 655, Univ. of Tokyo Press, Tokyo (1974).
61. C.H. Newbold, Brit. Jour. Dermatol. 95, 100-101 (1976).
62. E.L. Dubois and C. Patterson, Jour. Amer. Med. Assoc. 236, 138 (1976).
63. D.R. Bickers, L.K. Demar, V. DeLeo, M.B. Poh-Fitzpatrick, J.M. Aronberg and L.C. Harber, Arch. Dermatol. 114, 1193-1196 (1978).
64. H. Husquinet, A. Noirfalise and M.T. Parent, Jour. Genet. Hum. 26, 367-383 (1978).
65. F. Pietzcker and V. Kuner-Beck, Hautarzt 30, 308-311 (1979).
66. M.A. Karagezyan, N.N. Antonik and I.A. Ulitina, Vestn. Dermatol. Vener. 36, 30-33 (1962).
67. G.P. Shabykin and A.I. Godorazhy, Vestn. Dermatol. Vener. 41, 71-73 (1967).
68. D.G. Moulton, Nature 195, 1312-1313 (1962).
69. V.N. Karnaukhov, Exptl. Cell Res. 64, 301-306 (1971).
70. V.N. Karnaukhov, Exptl. Cell Res. 80, 479-483 (1973).
71. V.N. Karnaukhov, Tsitologiia 15, 538-542 (1973).
72. V.N. Karnaukhov, T.R. Taturyunas and V.V. Petrunyaka, Mech. Ageing and Dev. 2, 201-210 (1972).
73. J.A. Campbell, Quart. Jour. Exptl. Physiol. 28, 231-241 (1938).
74. J.A. Campbell, Quart. Jour. Exptl. Physiol. 29, 259-275 (1939).
75. D. Nelson, S. Goetzel, S. Robins and A.C. Ivy, Proc. Soc. Exptl. Biol. and Med. 52, 1-2 (1943).
76. M.J. King and J.L. Gainer, Amer. Inst. Chem. Engin. Symp. Ser. 73, No. 167, p. 1-5 (1967).
77. E.S. Wilkins, J.L. Gainer and M.G. Wilkins, Experientia 33, 1028 (1977).
78. J.L. Gainer and G.M. Chisholm, III, Atherosclerosis 19, 135-138 (1974).
79. R.E.O. Williams and C.C. Spicer, Microbial Ecology, 7th Symposium of the Society of General Microbiology, p. 56, Cambridge Univ. Press. Cambridge (1957).
80. M.M. Mathews and W.R. Sistrom Nature 184, 1892 (1959).
81. D. Gerber, M. Mathews-Roth, C. Fahlund, D. Hummell and B. Rosner, Internat. Jour. Dermatol. 18, 571-574 (1979).
82. R.K. Boutwell and A.K. Verma, Pure and Appl. Chem. 51, 857-866 (1979).
83. R. Peto, R. Doll, J.E. Buckley and M.B. Sporn, Nature 290, 201-208 (1981).
84. S.M. Anderson and N.I. Krinsky, Photochem. Photobiol. 18, 403-408 (1973).
85. M.M. Mathews-Roth and M.A. Pathak, Photochem. Photobiol. 21, 261-263 (1975).
86. M.M. Mathews-Roth, D. Hummell and C. Crean, Nutr. Rep. Internat. 16, 419-423 (1977).
87. M.M. Mathews-Roth, C. Crean and M. Clancy, Nutr. Rep. Internat. 17, 581-584 (1978).
88. J.D. Nelson and C. Grassi, Current Chemotherapy and Infectious Disease, p. 1503, American Society for Microbiology, Washington, D.C., (1980).
89. M.M. Mathews-Roth, Oncology in press, (1981).
90. C. Niemann and H.J. Klein Obbink, Vitam. Horm. 12, 69-99 (1954).
91. R. Ostwald and G. M. Briggs, Toxicants Naturally Occurring in Foods, p. 183, Food Protection Commission, Nat. Sci. Found., Washington, D.C. (1967).
92. M.M. Mathews-Roth, Jour. Amer. Med. Assoc. 230, 824 (1974).
93. J. Gjerlow, Tidj. Norske. Legeforen. 86, 33-34 (1966).
94. H.W. Josephs, Amer. Jour. Dis. Child. 67, 33-43 (1944).
95. J.P. Keating, M.E. Lell, A.W. Strauss, H. Zarkowsky and G.E. Smith, New Eng. Jour. Med. 288, 824-826 (1973).
96. H. Hoch, Biochem. Jour. 37, 430-433 (1943).
97. R.E. Bagden, G. Zbinden and A. Studer, Toxicol. Appl. Pharmacol. 2, 225-236 (1960).
98. M.M. Mathews-Roth, A. Abraham and T. Gabuzda, Clin. Chem. 22, 922-923 (1976).
99. V.A. DeLeo, M.B. Poh-Fitzpatrick, M.M. Mathews-Roth, and L.C. Harber, Amer. Jour. Med. 60, 8-22 (1976).
100. E. Fugimori and M. Tavla, Photochem. Photobiol. 5, 877-887 (1966).
101. C.S. Foote and R.W. Denny, Jour. Amer. Chem. Soc. 90, 6233-6235 (1968).

102. M.M. Mathews-Roth, T. Wilson, E. Fujimori and N.I. Krinsky, Photochem. Photobiol. 19, 217-222 (1974).
103. D.T. Gandy, Southern Med. Jour. 8, 444-446 (1935).
104. D.T. Gandy, Med. Rec. and Annals (Houston) 47, 274-275 (1964).
105. E. Klose, Munch. Med. Wschr. 66, 419-420 (1919).
106. M.A. Everett, E. Yeargers, R.M. Sayre and R.L. Olsen, Photochem. Photobiol. 5, 533-542, (1966).
107. A.C. Giese, Photophysiology, Vol. 6, p. 47, Academic Press, New York (1971).
108. P. Grof, J. Bodzay, and A. Kovaks, Acta Med. Acad. Sci. Hung. 24, 129-139 (1967).

INDUSTRIAL AND COMMERCIAL USES OF CAROTENOIDS

Dr. H. Kläui

F. Hoffmann-La Roche & Co., Limited Company,
Vitamin and Fine Chemical Division, 4002 Basle, Switzerland

...ght absorbing ability of carotenoids is their most important charac-...ic, biologically as well as technologically.

...efore, the use of carotenoids as food colours and as pigmenters in ani-... feeds will primarily be considered in this paper. The use of carotenoids ... pharmaceuticals and cosmetics will be mentioned only briefly, as well as ...he photoconductive properties, although these latter have not yet reached any practical importance in technology.

The use of carotenoids as food colours is particularly interesting not only because the colouration of food is currently under discussion, but also because the relationship between Man and colour has always played an important role. The more important aspects of this relationship include the basic biological function of certain colour substances, the informative value of colours, and the non-utilitarian, and often emotional effect of colours.

Why is the relatively small visual part of the whole electromagnetic spectrum so important for life on earth?

The visual part offers optimum conditions for life:

- about 30% of solar energy lies within the visual frequencies which correspond to the wavelengths between 400 and 750 nm;
- the light rays which penetrate the atmosphere and spread linearly are ideal biological sensory signals over long distances;
- these wavelengths are poorly absorbed by the biologically most important liquid, water, and therefore suffer only small losses;
- the effect of these rays making up the visual spectrum is the least harmful for living organisms;
- the absorption energy of these wavelengths between ultraviolet and infrared has the best photochemical effect on molecular processes, namely photosynthesis in plants and photoreceptors in animals.

Almost all organisms have developed their light-sensitive organs within these spectrum frequencies.

Colour is the common basic factor for the practical and industrial uses of carotenoids, and these may further be influenced by the metabolite functions, and particularly provitamin A activity, of some of the carotenoids. The vital role of vitamin A and its isomers for most visual systems is well-known, but this and other nutritional contributions of the vitamin A active carotenoids are considered to be outside the scope of this presentation.

A wide variety of foods, namely vegetables, tomatoes, mushrooms, apricots, oranges, berries, egg yolk, butter, chicken, shrimps, lobsters, salmon, trout etc. owe their characteristic red, orange or yellow colour principally to carotenoid colouring agents, as do certain food extracts from natural sources such as palm oil, paprika, annatto and saffron.

Carotenoids occur widely and are abundantly distributed throughout nature, and the total natural carotenoid production has been estimated at about 100 million tons per year (1). Most of this output is in the form of four major carotenoids: fucoxanthin, the pigment of many marine algae and the three main carotenoids in green leaves, lutein, violaxanthin and neoxanthin. By comparison, all other carotenoids are produced in quite small amounts, though some like beta-carotene and zeaxanthin occur very widely and others such as lycopene, bixin, astaxanthin, crocetin and capsanthin constitute the principal pigment in a particular organism. A detailed review of the occurrence of carotenoids is given by Weedon (2).

The most important use of carotenoids as colouring agents is connected with the colouration of food products.

The addition of colour to foods dates back to the time before written records were kept. Colours and foods are inseparable. Colour has always played a significant role in determining the acceptability of foods. We expect to see food in its "natural colour", a natural appearance is appetizing, and we become cautious when a food shows an unexpected colour, interpreting it as a possible sign of spoilage, poor processing or even as an indication of adulteration.

Colour is thus an indication and early signal of the inherent qualities of a food such as freshness, wholesomeness and readiness for consumption, and the proper colour of a food when served arouses one's interest in anticipation of food ingestion and in recollection of past satisfaction.

The association of colour and acceptability of foods is universal, although there may be significant differences depending on geographical location, ethnic background, religious and social factors, past history and personal habits. What may be attractive to one individual or group may be unappetizing or even repulsive to another (3).

The interesting relationship between colours and odours has been examined by Déribéré (4). The author generalizes about certain correlations and sets forth certain well defined tendencies. He also provides spectra of colour-odour relationships and associations with their combined influence on taste perception. Schultz (5) has examined colour-taste preferences and similarly illustrated the interrelationship between taste and colour in food preferences. Cynthia et al. (6) report on the effects of colourants and flavourants on identification, perceived flavour intensity and hedonic quality of fruit-flavoured beverages and cakes. Results showed that colour masking dramatically decreased flavour identification of fruit-flavoured beverages, while atypical colours induced incorrect flavour responses that were characteristically associated with the atypical colour. In addition, the colour level of beverages had significant effects on their overall acceptability, acceptability of colour and of flavour, as well as on flavour intensity. The same results were shown with cake samples, whereby a significant interaction of colour and flavour level was observed on overall acceptability.

In general terms, colour is an extremely important attribute or property of most food products because

- it usually influences the customer's first judgement of the product and
- it provides sensory information and plays an important role in taste recognition and taste intensity, and these factors influence the overall acceptability of the product, and thus not only make a pleasing contribution to the human food supply, but also improve safety.

This last factor is one of the most important reasons also for the use of colourants in drug preparations: colours aid significantly the problems of identification of drugs and therefore ensure a protection against confusion in the use of medicaments. This is of particular importance not only in hospital pharmacies when medicaments are given to patients by nurses, but also in bulk warehouses and in the packaging halls of the pharmaceutical industry.

Another reason for colouring drugs is connected with the appearance of a drug preparation which should always remain constant. In those cases where a preparation is naturally discolouring during the period of storage, a more uniform appearance of the dosage form may be achieved by initial colouration.

Partly associated with the appearance is the use of added colour to achieve a desirable cosmetic effect. Preparations for the treatment of skin conditions such as acne may, in addition to their therapeutic ingredients, also contain a skin-tone colour to conceal the blemishes caused by the primary condition (7).

For these reasons, the colouring of drugs is today recommended by pharmaceutical manufacturers, pharmacists and physicians. However, colour was always closely associated with diseases and their specific treatment, and the use of colouring agents to improve the appearance and other characteristics of pharmaceuticals and in the treatment of illness in general has been reported in early documents.

After this side glance on some aspects of colour in cosmetics and pharmaceuticals, let us revert to the practically much more important use in food and feeds.

The main groups of natural colouring substances in food are carotenoids, anthocyanins, porphyrins and chlorophylls.

Within nature's own food colours, carotenoids play a particularly interesting role due to their varied biological functions which include the following:

- they are accessory pigments in energy transference in the photosynthetic process,

- in simple and higher plant forms they show photo-responses such as phototropism,

- they play a photo-protective role in some bacteria and also in man under certain circumstances,

- they have a functional role in the oxygen cycle such as quenching singlet-oxygen,

- certain structures can be physiologically converted to vitamin A.

Another biological effect of carotenoids is connected with reproduction. It is known that many animals when kept in captivity will cease to reproduce. This applies to flamingos kept in zoos: after a short time the bird's feathers become colourless and the flamingos will not display and mate. Dr. Wackernagel in Basle's zoo found that addition of canthaxanthin to the feed restored the birds' colour which was followed by displaying, mating and reproduction. In another case there are indications that the hatchability of trout eggs is diminished in the absence of carotenoid pigments. A similar effect has been observed recently with the dairy cow, where beta-carotene was found to improve the fertility.

The great variety of carotenoids - more than 350 compounds have been found in nature - and the fact that they are probably the most widespread natural pigments - although their colour is often masked by chlorophyll - may be interpreted as an indication for the presence of a common specific function. A hypothesis that carotenoids may have played an important double role in the evolution of aerobic life was presented by Krinsky (8). According to the author, those organisms which gradually developed the biosynthetic mechanism to manufacture carotenoid pigments enjoyed a selective environmental advantage in the competition for the utilization of visible radiation. As biological evolution proceeded, oxygen evolved as a result of photosynthetic processes. In the presence of the widespread phytin-pigments, this could be converted to singlet oxygen which starts photo-oxygenation reactions more quickly than normal oxygen. Carotenoids can quench singlet oxygen and de-activate it back to ground-state molecular oxygen, thus playing another major role in the oxygen evolutionary process.

In this connection one could ask, did the aerobic multicellular organisms develop predominantly because they comprised a much better energy conversion system - the respiration process based on the oxidation of carbon to carbon dioxide and hydrogen to water yields 19 times more energy than the anaerobic fermentation process -, or because oxygen - in its gaseous state - proved to be the ideal transportation and diffusion form of the main component required for the energy-producing oxidation?

It is assumed that the evolution of aerobic life goes back to some three and a half thousand million years, and that this development was probably only made possible by the early production of various complementary protective measures which guarded against the toxic effects of oxygen-based peroxidation. In addition to the singlet oxygen quenching carotenoids, antioxidants such as ascorbic acid for aqueous and tocopherol for lipid systems, which scavenge singlet oxygen, developed.

Since I devoted most of my professional time and efforts during the last decades to the practical applications of the antioxidant vitamins C and E and to the colouring properties of carotenoids, you will understand why I particularly like Krinsky's hypothesis which imparts to these compounds such a vital role in the development and survival of aerobic life forms.

The chemical and physical properties of carotenoids are the most important factors for their practical application.

The following table summarizes some chemical and physical properties of four carotenoids produced by synthesis in commercial quantities and developed for use in foods and feeds:

Beta-Carotene

Apocarotenal

Apocarotenoic ester and

Canthaxanthin

The carotenoids astaxanthin and zeaxanthin are not yet commercially available, but are under development in our research laboratories.

PHYSICO-CHEMICAL DATA AND BIOLOGICAL PROPERTIES OF CAROTENOIDS *)

	β-Carotene	Apocarotenal	Apocarotenoic ester	Canthaxanthin
Colour of oily solution (different concentrations)	yellow to orange	orange to orange-red	yellow to orange	red
Melting point of crystalline compound	176 - 182° C	136 - 140° C	134 - 138° C	approx. 210° C
Vitamin A activity	yes	yes	yes	no
Solubility (g/100 ml solution, 20° C)				
- Fats, oils	0.05 - 0.08	0.7 - 1.5	approx. 0.7	approx. 0.005
- Orange oil	0.2 - 1.0	approx. 3.1	3.4 - 4.4	approx. 0.04
- Water	insoluble	insoluble	insoluble	insoluble
- Glycerol	insoluble	insoluble	insoluble	insoluble
- Ethanol	below 0.01	approx. 0.1	below 0.1	below 0.01
- Cyclohexane	approx. 0.1	approx. 0.8	approx. 2	below 0.01
- Ether	approx. 0.1	approx. 1.5	approx. 2.5	approx. 0.03
- Chloroform	approx. 3	approx. 20	approx. 30	approx. 10
- Acetone	approx. 0.1	approx. 1.8	approx. 1.2	approx. 0.03
Spectrophotometric data **)				
λ max. (in cyclohexane)	455 - 456 nm	460 - 462 nm	448 - 450 nm	468 - 472 nm
$E_{1\,cm}^{1\,\%}$ (in cyclohexane)	{ 456 nm > 2400 485 nm > 2030	461 nm > 2530 388 nm > 2030	449 nm > 2440 475 nm > 2000	470 nm > 2110

*) H. Kläui, Carotenoids as Food Colours, in J. Solms Ed., Functional Properties of Fats in Foods, Publ. Forster Verlag, 133-169 (1973), Zürich

**) The carotenoids isomerize in solution during storage or on heating; the predominant isomer in the equilibrium mixture is the trans compound. The values given correspond to the trans isomer.

The application of carotenoids to the colouration of foods is in most cases rather more difficult than the use of artificial colouring agents: the handling of the practically water-insoluble carotenoids depends on the conversion of these compounds into water-dispersible application forms. Furthermore, carotenoids require a good quality of the other food ingredients or carrier substances present, since partially oxidized essential oils, for example, lead to oxidation of the carotenoids and thus to bleaching. In these cases, carotenoids act as indicators of the quality of a food product.

The carotenoids available on the market yield yellow to red tints. Vegetable extracts containing crocin from saffron give a bright yellow and are - as glucosides - water-soluble and very stable. The synthetically produced carotenoids are available in pure form and in practically unlimited quantities, whereas most natural extracts are available only in restricted quantities, or only seasonally, and in varying quality.

Special application forms have been developed for the different applications, and special processes are also offered. As fat-soluble compounds, carotenoids lend themselves to the colouration of fat based foods. Very fine dispersions in a gelatin-sugar matrix or in other carriers, or emulsions of oily solutions are used in water based foods. The stability of carotenoids is excellent when air can be excluded, e.g. in carbonated beverages, and they are not unduly sensitive to heat and pH. Carotenoids have in general a very high colouring strength, and due to this fact they may in some cases be competitive with azo-dyes.

An aspect which may be quite important for the practical application of carotenoids in beverages is the fact that carotenoids are stabilized by ascorbic acid, whereas azo dyes show rapid fading, especially in the presence of ascorbic acid and light. This factor is particularly relevant in citrus drinks which are commonly expected to be a good source of vitamin C.

There is a general trend, today, towards natural food and natural food ingredients. However, the extraction of the colour from a food product may devaluate this and may not be desirable from a worldwide economical point of view. Therefore, extracts of non-food products, e.g. of flower and other plant material appeared on the market as "natural colours".

Here, however, the author feels that a certain differentiation would be appropriate: he must point out that products derived from natural sources, or "natural products", are not necessarily safe. They may not even be assumed to be any safer than synthetic products (9).

It is not the mere occurrence in nature which decides the harmlessness of a natural substance, but its presence in food products known from experience to be edible and harmless. Nature produces not only edible products, but also many of the strongest poisons, remember, e.g. the many mycotoxins, botulinus and other bacterial toxins, marine toxins, solanine, strychnine, cyanides and many others. Some may even be associated with beautiful colours, as in the well known cases of the toadstool (Amanita muscaria) or the deadly night-shade (Atropa belladonna).

Natural food products, on the other hand, and their ingredients, which have proven to be innocuous for Man over very long periods of time do justify in the author's opinion the donation of a preferential status over new products whose tolerance or toxicity is usually examined only in animal tests. This would not mean that any colouring agent which occurs naturally in foods should be admitted as colour additive more or less routinely and without any toxicological testing. Furthermore, due regard must be paid to the fact that the exclusive use of any single food colour as a colouring agent in the food industry will increase its overall consumption, e.g. the use of betanine as a colouring agent in yoghourts and other dairy products, ice creams and others would probably increase the amount ingested significantly compared to that consumed when occasionally beetroot is eaten alone as a vegetable. Consequently, a toxicological evaluation is essential for natural products also.

Specifications and constant quality of the pure carotenoids available by synthesis and their identity with nature's food colours made their extensive toxicological study possible. Based on the specifications and toxicological evaluation presented, the Joint FAO/WHO Expert Committee on Food Additives has classified these carotenoids in List A (I), which contains those additives which have been fully evaluated by the experts and which have either been given an acceptable daily intake (ADI) value or have not been limited toxicologically.

Thus, carotenoids combine in an ideal way practical long term use by Man with scientific evaluation under experimental conditions.

Future safety-testing will become increasingly sophisticated, since

- when administered in large enough quantities or according to extraordinary experimental conditions, all substances, natural or artificial, can be injurious to life forms

- on the other hand, modern analytical methods today allow the detection of parts per trillion of a substance.

Consequently, the toxicological evaluation should be adapted individually: factors such as the relation between the amount normally consumed, and the amount the consumer is exposed to when expanding its use as a colouring agent, the amount and nature of accompanying substances (in extracts e.g.), the possibility to characterize the product and to fix chemical specifications, biological and metabolic data already available and - last but not least - practical experience in Man should be considered.

And this situation clearly indicates that absolute assurance of safety for natural food constitutents is an illusory objective. It also indicates, however, that practical experience in Man is a particularly valuable factor in safety evaluation. Through experience Man has learned to avoid food with conspicious toxic effects, and special food processing methods were developed to eliminate or inactivate toxic ingredients, and carotenoids, so far, seem to be safe.

Some food products of animal origin, e.g. the egg yolks and the skin and shanks of poultry, owe their yellow colour to the absorption of carotenoid pigments, predominantly zeaxanthin and lutein, present in their diet.

Therefore, the content of carotenoids of these products is considered as a sign of quality. The addition of suitable carotenoids to animal feed may be used as an indirect method of colouring food (10).

In many parts of the world a well-pigmented broiler is preferred and it is, therefore, important for the broiler grower to be able to produce birds with the degree of pigmentation desired by the market. In other areas of the world the very opposite tendency is observed when the consumer demands broilers with absolutely white meat.

Previously, when poultry were kept on free-range, the problem of skin and yolk pigmentation did not exist because lower physiological response (slower growth and fewer eggs) and ample feeding of green grass and yellow corn resulted in adequately pigmented eggs and birds. Today, however, without grass feeding and with modern methods of large volume poultry raising, such as the use of low fibre, high-energy feeds, and birds with high physiological capacity, the production of well-pigmented birds and highly pigmented eggs has become difficult to achieve.

In modern commercial feeds the pigmenting burden falls on yellow corn (Maize) which does not always produce adequate results without the aid of some alfalfa.

Within the past few years, milo, wheat and barley have become recognized as high-energy and economical cereal grains for poultry. When these grains replace yellow corn the natural carotenoids in the feed are further depressed (11).

In order to overcome all the difficulties described above, the poultry industry now uses extracts from natural sources of carotenoids or concentrated, dry, stabilized synthetic carotenoids which are readily transferred to the poultry product and can be mixed into the feed without major alteration of the feed formula.

The most important of the first type of pigmenters are lucerne extracts and maize gluten meal (12). Extracts of lucerne, rich in lutein, are sold under various brand names, as are also those of the Tagetes plant, which confer a pure yellow colour. Reddish concentrates are prepared from extracts of red pepper (13, 14, 15).

The most important of the second type of pigmenters are the ethyl ester of β-apo-8'-carotenoic acid and canthaxanthin, which have a wide application in poultry layer and fattener rations, whereas two other carotenoids, which are also available in stabilized form as commercial commodities, namely β-apo-8'-carotenal and citranaxanthin, contribute only to the colour of eggs but are not deposited in the skin of broilers.

The main source of the red and yellow colouration of birds exhibited in zoos or kept for pleasure are the carotenoids contained in their food. Since, however, the feed which they receive in captivity in general differs fundamentally from that which they find in their natural environment, the birds often tend to lose their natural colours. The feed of zoo- and cage-birds should, therefore, be reinforced with carotenoids of natural or synthetic origin (16).

The natural food of fish contains carotenes and carotenoids which can be deposited in the flesh, as such, or metabolized, giving the flesh an attractive pink colour. T. Kanemitsu and H. Aoe (17) reported the presence of astaxanthin in the flesh of five species of pacific salmon. In addition to this pigment, H. Thommen and U. Gloor (18) found canthaxanthin and β-carotene in the flesh of the lake trout (Salmo trutta). Since the most notable differences between wild types of fish and those bred in ponds lies in the colouration of the flesh, many attempts are made to correct this sign of inferior quality by feeding carotenoid-rich feed. One of the most promising ways consists of feeding synthetic canthaxanthin in stabilized form (19, 20, 21).

The use of carotenoids for the colouration of pharmaceutical preparations has already been mentioned briefly. Water-dispersible carotenoids have been found suitable for colouring sugar-coated tablets (22, 23, 24).

It has been found that embedding the carotenoids in a sugar coating helps to maintain good stability of colour: at normal as well as at higher temperatures and during prolonged storage excellent stability of colour was achieved.

In a sugar syrup the stability of canthaxanthin proved to be only limited (25).

The fat-soluble carotenoids were also tested in suppositories, in order to characterize, distinguish or identify them. This might be of particular interest for hospital pharmacies. The microcrystalline carotenoids can be added direct to the molten suppository base, whereby the compatibility with the drug used has to be established in every case (26).

Before concluding, a few words should be said about carotenoids as photoconductors. Although not really an industrial application, β-carotene and other carotenoids show promising properties as photo-conductors. The semiconductivity in carotenoids is another subject under study, as well as carotenoids in bilayer systems and carotenoids as photo-detectors and colour-discriminators.

These studies were aiming at the possible discovery of "tailor-made" highly conducting materials of technological importance and the solution of hitherto unexplained phenomena occurring in certain biophysical processes, such as photosynthesis and vision. At the forefront of these studies have been the carotenoids, known to be present as such or in combination with proteins in certain vital places of animal and human organisms. In vertebrates it is known that the visual pigments rhodopsins, porphyropsins and cyanopsins, all complexes of retinal or vitamin A aldehyde with the protein opsin, are located in the outer segments of the rods and cones. The attachment of the 11-cis-retinal to opsin in rhodopsin is to a primary amino group of either lysine or phosphatidyl ethanolamine, and retinal results from β-carotene - or provitamin A - in a biological cleavage reaction and subsequent oxidation of retinol to retinal. J.O. Williams (27) considers in his chapter "Carotenoids as Photoconductors" the essential theoretical background relevant to any discussion of the role of carotenoids as photoconductors, and he assesses critically the experimental evidence so far available and suggests possible areas where further effort is needed either to see further clarification on physical or biophysical points or in an effort to develop "carotenoid photoconductive technology".

REFERENCES

1. L. Zechmeister, quoted by W. Karrer, Konstitution und Vorkommen der organischen Pflanzenstoffe, p. 716, Birkhäuser, Basle (1958).
2. B.C.L. Weedon, in Carotenoids,(O. Isler, Ed.) p. 29-59, Birkhäuser, Basle (1971).
3. H. Kläui, Some Aspects of Colour and Man, IUFOST-Symposium, Einsiedeln (1979).
4. M. Dériběré, Parfümerie Kosmetik 52, 369-377 (1971).
5. H.G. Schultz, Symposium on Colour in Foods (H.G. Farrell, J.R. Wagner and M.S. Peterson, eds.) p. 16-23, Quartermaster Food and Container Institute, Chicago/Illinois (1954).
6. N. Cynthia Du Bose et al., J. Food Sci. 45, 1393-1399 (1980).
7. C.J. Swartz and J. Cooper, J. Pharm. Science 51, 89 (1962).
8. N.I. Krinsky, Pure and Applied Chem. 51, 649-660 (1979).
9. H. Kläui, Haltbarkeit von Fruchtsaftgetränke-Pulvern in: Neue Erkenntnisse auf dem Gebiete der Frucht- und Gemüsesäfte, Symposium, Bled (1980).
10. J.C. Bauernfeind et al.,Use of Carotenoids, in Carotenoids, p. 743-770, Birkhäuser, Basle (1971).
11. S. Borenstein and I. Bartov, Brit. Poultry Sci. 8, 213-221 (1967a).
12. R.G. Ratcliff, E.J. Day et al., Poultry Sci. 41, 1529-1532 (1962).
13. S. Scholtyssek, R. Kirsammer et al., Arch. Geflügelk. 29, 249-262 (1965).
14. W.P. Williams, R.E. Davies et al., Poultry Sci. 42, 691-699 (1963).
15. S. Poppe, Arch. Geflügelz. und Kleintierkunde 13, 137 (1965).
16. H. Wackernagel, Internat. Z. Vitaminforsch. 34, 141-143 (1964).
17. T. Kanemitsu and H. Aoe, Bull. Japan Soc. Sci. Fish 24, 209-215 (1958).
18. H. Thommen and U. Gloor, Naturwissenschaften 52, 161-162 (1965).
19. J. Deufel, Arch. Fischereiwissenschaft 16, 125 (1965).
20. P.J. Schmidt and E.G. Baker, J. Fish Res. Bd. Canada 26, 357-360 (1969).
21. E.T. Savolainen Jouko and H.G. Gyllenberg, Lebensm.-Wiss. u. Technol. 3, 18-20 (1970).
22. H. Kläui, A. Capeder et al., Pharm. Ind. 25, 173 (1963).
23. H. Kläui and K. Münzel, Pharm. Acta Helv. 40, 153 (1965).
24. K. Münzel, Deutsche Apotheker Zeitung 9, 277 (1967).
25. F. Hoffmann-La Roche & Co. AG, internal communication (1978).
26. K. Münzel and W. Füller, Pharm. Acta Helv. 44, 2081 (1969).
27. J.O. Williams, Carotenoid Color Technology (I.C. Bauernfeind, Ed.), Academic Press, New York (1981).

ADDITIONAL READING

1) GENERAL FOOD APPLICATIONS AND REVIEWS

J.C. Bauernfeind, Carotenoids: A Class of Natural Pigments in Food, in: Encyclopaedia of Food Science, Avi Publ., 113-126 (1978).

J.C. Bauernfeind, Carotenoids and Food Technology, in: Encyclopaedia of Food Technology, Avi Publ., 163-173 (1978).

E. Baumgartner, Carotenoids and Foodstuffs, Alimenta 15, (2) 31 (1976).

A. Corral, Carotenoids in Food, Afinidad 288, 747-749 (1971).

J. Coulson, Prospects for the Use of Natural Colouring Materials in the Food Industry, International Flavours and Food Additives 9, (5) 207-208, 210, 216 (1978).

J.N. Counsell, The Flavour Industry 2, (9) 519-524 (1971).

J.J.P. Drake, Food Colours - Harmless Aesthetics or Epicurean Luxuries? Toxicology 5, 3-42 (1975).

A. Emodi, Carotenoids, Properties and Applications, Food Technology 32, (5) 38-40, 42, 79 (1978).

C. Engel, Natural Colours. Their Stability and Application in Food, Scientific and Techn. Surveys, No. 117, Nov. 1979.

FDA / USA, Synthetic Carotenoids Safely Recreate Nature's own Colours, Snack Food 65, (10) 24-25 (1976).

T. Fujii, Food Colouring Agents. Use of Carotenoids, Shokuhin Kogyo 15, (14) 60-66 (1972)

H.T. Gordon, The Carotenoids - Current Status as Food Colourants/Chapter 4 in: Current Aspects of Food Colourants, T.E. Furia, Ed. p. 41-48 (1977) Publ. CRC (West Palm Beach).

D. Hicks, Benefits of Added Colourings in Food and Drinks, Int. Flavours and Food Additives 10, 31-32 (1979).

G. Jeffries, Natural Colours, Food Processing Ind. 48,(576) 33, 35 (1979).

O. Isler, History and Industrial Application of Carotenoids and Vitamin A, Pure & Appl. Chem. 51, 447-462 (1979).

H. Kläui, W. Hausheer et al., Fat Soluble Vitamins (International Encyclopaedia of Food and Nutrition, Vol 9), R.A. Morton Ed. (Pergamon Press, Oxford) p. 113-159 (1970).

H. Kläui, Carotenoids as Food Colours, in: Functional Properties of Fats in Foods. J. Solms, Ed. (Forster Verlag, Zürich) p. 133-169 (1971).

H. Kläui, Tocopherol, Carotene and Ascorbyl Palmitate, Int. Flavours and Food Addit. 7, (4) 165-172 (1976).

H. Kläui and O. Raunhardt, Colouring of Foods with Carotenoids, Alimenta 15, 37-45 (1976).

H. Kläui, Färben mit Naturfarbstoffen in: Probleme der Ernährungs- und Lebensmittelwissenschaft 5, 331-351 (1978) (W. Maudrich Verlag, Wien, München, Bern).

H. Kläui and O. Isler, Warum und womit färbt man Lebensmittel? Chemie in unserer Zeit 15, (1)(1981).

H. Kläui and J.C. Bauernfeind, Carotenoids as Food Colours in: Carotenoid Colour Technology, J.C. Bauernfeind, Ed. (Academic Press, New York) (1981).

K. Kojima, Kinds and Source of Natural Food Colours, Their Acceptability, Safety Evaluation and Points Requiring Further Elucidation, e.g. Safety Evaluation of Polynuclear Hydrocarbons in Carbon Black. Beturia Caused by Betanin (Red Beet Pigments), Hypervitaminosis A due to Carotenes, and Mutagenicity of Flavone Pigments. The Toxicological Assessment of Natural Food Colourants. In: Chemical Toxicology of Food (FSTA (1979) 11, 100579), 319-327 (1978).

S. Liaaen-Jensen, Carotenoids - useful Pigments from Nature's Palette, Naturen 101, (2) 75-80 (1977).

L. Lipparini and L. Laghi, Considerations on the Use of Natural Dyestuffs. Review Includes Data on: Natural Colourants, Canthaxanthin, β-Apo-8'-Carotenal and β-Carotene. Industrie Alimentari 16, (11) 81-88 (1977).

H. Mikkelsen, J.C. Larsen et al., Hypersensitivity Reactions to Food Colours with Special Reference to the Natural Colour Annatto Extract. Archives of Toxicology, Suppl. 1, 141-143 (1978).

H. Pfander, Carotenoid Glycosides, Carotenoids 4, Pure and Appl. Chem. 47, 121-128 (1976).

M. Philip , How will we Colour Soft Drinks of the Future? Food Prod. Dev. 12, (8) 24-25 (1978).

R. Rajalakshmi, K.V. Chari et al., Comparative Availability of β-Carotene in Different Vegetables as Compared to that of Pure β-Carotene and Vitamin A, Baroda J. Nutr. 2, (2) 103-119 (1975).

J. Walford, Synthetic Colourings for Food, International Flavours and Food Additives 9, (5) 215-216 (1978).

B.C.L. Weedon, Occurrence, in: Carotenoids, O. Isler, Ed. (Birkhäuser, Basel) p. 29-60 (1971).

2) SPECIAL FOOD APPLICATIONS

2.1 Fat and Oils, Margarine, Dairy Products

G.A. Allman, Colouring For Fat Based Foods, Internat. Flavours and Food Addit. 7, (3) 111-115 (1976).

J.B. Davis, J.M. Robinson, Studies on an Alleged Toxic Hazard of Heat-Bleached Palm Oil, J. Food Technology 14, 253-264 (1979).

H. Kroschel, S. Grunnert, On the Significance of the Carotenoid and Chlorophyll Colouring Agents for the Fat Industry, Lebensmittelindustrie 20, (7) 317-321 (1973).

H. Lueck, Problems Encountered with the Colouring of Cheese by Means of Water-soluble β-Carotene Preparations, S. Afr. J. Dairy Technol. 5, (4) 181-185 (1973).

H. Lueck et al., Animal & Dairy Sci. Res. Inst ., Irene. Colour Measurements of Edible Fats, Fette-Seifen-Anstrichmittel 77, (4) 131-135 (1975).

M.L. Meara, G.S.D. Weir, The Effect of β-Carotene on the Stability of Palm Oil, RIV. IT. Sostanze Grasse 53, (7) 178-180 (1976).

Miami Margarine Co., Yogo-Light Spread Low Calorie Margarine / Butter Substitute / USA, Food Product Development 12, (5) 50 (1978).

A.L. Protsenko et al., Carotene Butter Colouring, Annatto Butter Colouring, Molochn. Prom-st 1, 31 (1978).

- Talignani, L. Caloz et al., Use of Natural and Synthetic Natural Colours in Ice Cream Products, Zucker- und Süsswarenwirtschaft 31, (12) 448, 450-451 (1978).

A.S. Vecher, A.N. Kulikova, USSR, Patent No. 380302 (19.7.1971) A 23c, A 231 (Assignee: Institute of Experimental Botany, Academy of Sciences Belorussian S.S.R.). Cheese Colouring Material Carotene.

Yamada, Koichi et al., Japan, Patent No. 76147532, Applic. No. 75/71657 (13.6.1975) (Assignee: Lion Fat and Oil Co., Ltd.). Palm Oil Carotene Conc.

M. Yver, F.M. Luquet, Food Additives. Problems of Butter Colouration (β-Carotene), Industries Aliment. Agric. 90, (1) 23-25 (1973).

2.2 Bakery and Pasta Products

Anon., Synthetic Nature-Identical β-Carotene May Replace Existing Yellow Colourings in Bakery Goods, Food Product Development 11, 57 (1977).

L.A. Burov, N.G. Nazarenko, Carotenoids in Gluten and Colour of Pasta Products, Khlebopekarnaya i Konditerskaya, No. 8, 30-31 (1975).

L.A. Burov et al., Yellow Colourants are used in Pasta from Soft Wheat Flour with Concurrent Improvement of Nutritional Value: They are Riboflavin, β-Carotene Preparation, Extract of Wine Yeasts, and Sweet Whey Proteins. Khlebopekarnaya i Konditerskaya Promyshlennost No. 6, 33-34 (1979).

R. Drapron et al., Lipoxygenase Action During Bread Making. Destruction of Essential Fatty Acids. Carotenoids and Tocopherols, Deterioration of the Flavour of the Bread. Ann. Technol. Agric. 23, (3) 353-365 (1974).

V.I. Drobot et al., Effect of Carotene Preparation on Quality of Bread. Promislovist Zbirnik, No. 6, 31-33 (1975).

KK Kyowa Hakko Kogyo, Bread Prodn. Using Flour Containing Carotene and/or Vitamin A and Oil and Fat, Japanese Patent 5-4143-539 (1979).

A. Marine Font and M. Alvarez Reverter, Pasta Products. Their Natural Colouring and Additives in Relation to their Quality, Circ. Farm. 31, (240) 383-402 (1973).

S.T. McCready et al., Palatability and Colorimetric Characteristics of Sponge Cakes Prepared with Egg Yolks of Varying Colour Intensities and Hues, Cereal Sci. Today 18, (7) 202-205 (1973).

A.A. Metzner, Colouring Short Shelf Life Bakery Products with β-Carotene, Cereal Foods World 23, (3) 120-123 (1978).

S.S. Mkhitaryan, L.A. Burov et al., Carotenoid Changes During the Production of Pasta Products, Izvestiya Vysshikh Tekhnologiya, Moskovskii 4, 56-58 (1975).

I.M. Roiter et al., Effect of Carotene Containing Preparation on Biochemical Processes in Dough, Izvestiya Vysshikh Zavedenii Tekhnologiya 2, 38-41 (1976).

2.3 Beverages

R.R. Cruese et al., Pigmentation and Colour Comparison of Ruby and Star Ruby Grapefruit Juice, J. Agric. Food Chem. 27, (3) 641-642 (1979).

S. Gherardi et al., Storage Stability of Natural Colourants which could be Used in Fruit Sirups and Refreshment Drinks, Industria Conserve 53, 163-167 (1978).

H. Kläui, U. Manz, The Colouring of Fruit Juices and Carbonated Beverages with Carotenoids, Beverages 8, (1) 16 (1967).

V.A. Papanov, Industrial Treatment of Squash with Carotene Preparations, Tr. Vitam. Prir. Syr'ya. Vses. Nauch.-Tekh. Soveshch, 173-179 (1971).

V. Philip, How will we Colour Soft Drinks of the Future?, Food Product Development 12, (8) 24-25 (1978).

G. Saldana et al., Carrot Beverages, J. Animal Sci. 41, (5) 1243-1244 (1976).

H. Kläui, Haltbarkeit von Fruchtsaftgetränke-Pulvern in: Neue Erkenntnisse auf dem Gebiete der Frucht- und Gemüsesäfte" Symposium, Bled (1980). (Internat. Fruchtsaftunion)

2.4 Fruits, Vegetables

H. Iriyama, Carotenoid Food Colouring from Tomato, Jap. Patent No. 80 01311, Applic. No. 77/88850, (26.7.1977) (Assignee: Kagome Co., Ltd.).

H. Yokoyama et al., Colouring Fruits and Vegetables. USA, Patent No. 3911148, Applic. No. 404.980 (10.10.1973) (Assignee: United States Dept. of Agriculture) (Grapefruit Carotene Lycopene).

2.5 Meat and Meat Substitutes

CO. Armour, Colour Treatment for Soybean Food Products used as Meat Substitutes and Extenders. Gives Red Colouration which Alters Suitably on Cooking / Canthaxanthin - Betanin. U.S. Pat. 3958019 / 1976, Applic. No. 492 619 (29.7.1974).

F.L. Billings, The Pigmentation of Canned Salmon with Canthaxanthin, Canadian Proc. 1-6 (1971).

D.D. Boon, Colouration in Bivalves (Sea Food), J. Food Sci. 42, (4) 1008-1012, 1015 (1977).

D. Klein, The Problem of Declaring the Presence of Paprika in "Brühwurst" Products, Fleischwirtschaft 58, (2) 227-228, 239 (1978).

J.E. McNeal, Qualitative Tests for Added Colouring Matter in Meat Products, (Beet Powder, Saffron, Paprika, Turmeric, Annatto, Cochineal, Carotenoids) J. Assoc. of Anal. Chem. 59, (3) 570-577 (1976).

2.6 Stability in Foods: Effect of Heat, Radiation etc.

F.M. Basiouny, R.H. Biggs, Effects of UV B Radiation on Pigment Changes and Quality of Citrus Fruits, Proc. FLA State Hortic Soc. 87, 281-289 (1974).

E. Bancher et al., Influence of Cobalt-60. Gamma-Irradiation of β-Carotene Solutions. I. Qualitative and Quantitative Investigations of Irradiated Petroleum Ether and N-Heptane Solutions, Int. J. Vitam. Nutr. Res. 42, (3) 355-61 (1972).

E. Bancher et al., Influence of Cobalt-60. Gamma Irradiation of β-Carotene Solutions. II. Qualitative and Quantitative Investigations of Irradiated Tributyrin Solutions, Int. J. Vitam. Nutr. Res. 42, (3) 362-67 (1972).

M. Beyers et al., Gamma-Irradiation of Subtropical Fruits. I: Compositional Tables of Mango, Papaya, Strawberry, and Litchi Fruits at the Edible-Ripe Stage. J. Agr. Food Chem. 27, (1) 37-42 (1979).

M. Beyers, A.C. Thomas, Gamma-Irradiation of Subtropical Fruits. 4. Changes in Certain Nutrients Present in Mangoes, Papayas and Litchis during Canning, Freezing, and Gamma-Irradiation. J. Agr. Food Chem. 27, (1) 48-51 (1979).

B. Bhushan et al., Effect of Polar Radiation Degradation Products of β-Carotene and Vitamin A on Rat Liver Lysosomes, Agric. Biol. Chem. 41, (1) 125-130 (1977).

J. Carnevale et al., Fluorescent Light Catalyzed Autoxidation of β-Carotene, J. Agric. Food Chem. 27, (2) 462-463 (1979).

W. Grosch et al., Co-oxidation of β-Carotene and Canthaxanthin by Purified Lipoxygenases from Soya Beans, Zeitschr. Lebensm.-Unters. und Forschung 165, (2) 77-81 (1977).

A. Hussain, E.C. Maxie, Effect of Gamma Rays on Shelf Life and Quality of Orange Juice, Int. Biodentn. Bull. 10, (3) 81-86 (1974).

T. Inal et al., Sterilisation of Spices by Means of Gamma Rays, Fleischwirtschaft 55, (5) 675-677 (1975).

W.G. Lee, Carotene Stereoisomerization in Sweet Potatoes as Affected by Rotating and still Retort Canning Processes, J. Food Sci. 39, (6) 1188-1190 (1974).

K. Lorenz, Microwave Heating of Foods Changes in Nutrient and Chemical Composition, Crit. Rev. Food Sci. Nutr. 7, (4) 339-370 (1976).

L.B. Mabesa, R.E. Baldwin, Flavour and Colour of Peas and Carrots Cooked by Microwaves, J. Of Microwave Power 13, (4) 321-326 (1978).

S. Mirza, I.D. Morton, Effect of Different Types of Blanching on the Colour of Sliced Carrots, J. of the Science of Food and Agr. 28, (11) 1035-1039 (1977).

T.V. Ramakrishnan, F.J. Francis, Stability of Carotenoids in Model Aqueous Systems, J. of Food Quality 2, (3) 177-189 (1979).

M.R.R. Rao, A.F. Novak, Thermal and Microwave Energy for Shrimp Processing, Marine Fisheries Review 37, (12) 25-30 (1975).

U.H. Renqvist et al., The Effect of Traditional Cooking Methods on Carotene Content in Tropical Leafy Vegetables, Ind. J. Nutr. Dietet. 15, 154-158 (1978).

F. Snauwaert et al., Studies on the Carotenoids and Carotenoproteins of the Crustacean "Cragnon Vulgaris Fabr.", in Relation to their Stability upon Gamma Irradiation, Proc. IV Int. Congress Food Sci. & Technol. IV, 115-123 (1974).

A.C. Thomas, M. Beyers, Gamma Irradiation of Subtropical Fruits. 3. A Comparison of the Chemical Changes Occurring During Normal Ripening of Mangoes and Papayas with Changes Produced by Gamma-Irradiation, J. Agr. Food Chem. 27, (1) 157-163 (1979).

P. Thomas, M. Janave, Effects of Gamma Irradiation and Storage Temperature on Carotenoids and Ascorbic Acid Content of Mangoes on Ripening, J. Sci. Food Agr. 26, 1503-1512 (1975).

3) FEED APPLICATIONS

N. Abdul Malak et al., Pigmentation of Rainbow Trout by Canthaxanthin, Ann. Inst. Michel Pacha 7, 30-40 (1975).

M. Bonsembiante, G.M. Chiericato, Experimental Results Concerning Use of Some Natural and Synthetic Pigmenting Agents in Diets for Broilers, Rivista di Zootecnia e Veterinaria, (1) 7-17 (1978).

C.B. Chawan, R.W. Gerry, Shrimp Waste as a Pigment Source in Broiler Diets, Poultry Sci. 53, (2) 671-676 (1974).

G. Choubert, P. Luquet, Effects of Pelleting and Storage of Compounded Fish Feeds on their Canthaxanthin Content: Effects on digestibility and Muscle Pigmentation in the Rainbow Trout, Annales of Zootechnie 28, (2) 145-157 (1979).

J.N. Ellis, The Use of Natural and Synthetic Carotenoids in the Diet to Colour the Flesh of Salmonids, J.E. Halver and K. Tiews. Finnish Nutrition and Fishfeed Technol. Vol. 2. Proceedings of a World Symposium, Hamburg, West Germany. June 20-23 (1978) (Heenemann Verlagsgesellschaft: Berlin West Germany).

D.L. Fletcher et al., A Model System for Predicting Egg Yolk Colour Using β-Apo-8 Carotenal and Canthaxanthin, Poult. Sci. 56, (5) 1714 (1977).

M. Halaj et al., Effect on Egg Yolk Colour of Paprika in Feed for Laying Hens, Acta Zootech. 32, 123-130 (1976).

G.M. Herrick et al., Apocarotenoate Skin Pigmentation, Broiler, Poult. Sci. 51, (2) 428-435 (1972).

T.C. Lee et al., Stability of Vitamin A and Provitamin A (Carotenoids) in Extrusion Cooking Processing, Aiche Symposium Series 74, (172) 192-195 (1978).

W.L. Marusich et al., Zeaxanthin as a Broiler Pigmenter, Poult. Sci. 55, (4) 1486-1494 (1976).

T. Matsuno et al., Intensification of Colour of Fancy Red Carp with Zeaxanthin, Nippon Suisan Gakkaishi 45, (5) 627-632 (1979).

G. Neamtu et al., Researches on the Utilization of Carotenoid Pigments. I. Rev. Roum. Biochim.13, (3) 209-217 (1976).

G. Neamtu et al., Researches on the Utilization of Carotenoid Pigments. II. Pigmentation of Egg Yolk, Rev. Roum. Biochim. 14, (2) 109-115 (1977).

G. Neamtu et al., Studies on the Use of Carotenoid Pigments. III. Egg Yolk, Stud. Cercet. Biochim. 20, (1) 63-69 (1977).

G. Neamtu et al., Effect of Carotenoid Pigments on the Pigmentation of Egg Yolk, Rev. Roum. Biochim. 15, (2) 143-149 (1978).

G.M. Norman et al., Deposition of Orally Administered β-Carotene, β-Apo-8'-Carotenoic Acid Ethyl Ester, and Zeaxanthin in the Egg Yolk by Laying Hens, Brit. Poult. Sci. 14, (5) 507-519 (1973).

G.M. Norman et al., Effect of Dietary and Parenteral β-Apo-8'-Carotenoic Acid Ethyl Ester and Zeaxanthin on Tissue and Blood Pigment Levels in the Laying Hen, Brit. Poult. Sci. 14, (5) 521-530 (1973).

A.G. Panetsos et al., Study on the Yolk Pigments of Chicken Eggs and the Improvement of Yolk Colour, Proc. World Vet. Congr., 20th. 2, 1037-1043 (1975).

C.C. Ruffini, A.M. De Giovanni, Diet and Pigmentation in Aviculture, Riv. Zootec. Vet. 2, 143-154 (1975).

J.J.N. Silveira, R.N. Kronka, Effect of Cortegg on Egg Yolk Pigmentation, Bol. Ind. Anim. 29, (2) 393-400 (1972).

P.W. Waldroup et al., An Estimation of the Time Required to Develop Adequate Pigmentation for Broilers, Nutr. Rep. Int. 20, (4) 567-572 (1979).

4) PHARMACEUTICALS

D. François et al., Canthaxanthin to Colour Hard Gelatin Capsules, Manuf. Chem. Aerosol News 50, (4) 48, 51, 76 (1979).

H. Hirsing, Injectable Carotenoid Emulsions, Ger. Patent No. 2236899, Applic. No. P 22 36 899.6, 27.7.1972 (Assignee: Philips Patentverwaltung GmbH).

H. Hirsing, Carotenoid Emulsions,Ger. Patent No. 2254105, Applic. No. P 22 54 105.5, 4.11.1972 (Assignee: Philips Patentverwaltung GmbH).

H. Kläui et al., Wasserlösliche Carotinoidpräparate als Dragierfarbstoffe, Pharm. Ind. 25, p. 173 (1963).

H. Kläui, K. Münzel, Dragéefärbung mit Carotinoidfarbstoffen, Pharm. Acta Helv. 40, p. 153 (1965).

H. Kläui, W.F. Koerner, Sunburn Preventing Pharmaceuticals for Oral Use, Ger. Patent No. 2129653, Applic. No. 70/10.481, 10.7.1970 (Assignee: F. Hoffmann-La Roche & Co. AG).

K. Münzel, Färbung von Zuckerdragées mit einigen Naturfarbstoffen, Deutsche Apotheker Zeitung 9, p. 277 (1967).

K. Münzel, W. Füller, Färbung von Suppositorien, Pharm. Acta Helv. 44, p. 208 (1969).

T. Shiio, T. Yoshihama, Anti-tumor Composition, Jap. Patent No. 1509587, Applic. No. 75/34459, 19.8.1975 (Assignee: Ajinomoto Co.).

5) COSMETIC APPLICATIONS

Anon., β-Carotene, (F.D.A.) Washington D.C., Fed. Regist. 42, (127) p. 33722-3 (1.7.1977).

Z. Baclawska-Krzeminska, J. Kulesza, Biologically Active Compounds in Cosmetics, Tluszcze, Srodki Piorace, Kosmet. 15, (3) 29-43 (1971).

E. Boudonis, Carotene Sun Tanning Compn., French Patent No. 2384500, Applic. No. 77/8619, 21.3.1977.

E. Boudonis, Canthaxanthin, Carotene Sunburn Compn.,French Patent No. 2392673 Applic. No. 77/16812, 31.5.1977.

Yu.A. Fedorov et al., Carotene, U.S.S.R. Patent No. 347063, 23.12.1970.

C. Navarro, M.J. Navarro, Product Containing Carotene Used for Skin Colouring, French Patent No. 2430765, Applic. No. 78/21618, 13.7.1978.

J. Pelechova et al., Cosmetic and Dermatological Preparation, Czech. Patent No. 153635, Applic. No. 3223/71, 4.5.1971.

P. Rovesti, S.B. Curri, Cutaneous Bioactivating Effect of Carotenoids Conjugated with Permeable Molecules, Riv. Ital. Essenze. Profumi, Piante Off., 60, (6) 360-364 (1978).

C. Ruiz Alonso, Cosmetics or Drugs, Rev. Fac. Farm., 39, p. 21-33 (1977).

M.C. Seguin, Composition Containing Carotenoids and Xanthophylls Administered Orally to Colour the Skin without Exposure to the Sun, French Patent No. 2339403, Applic. No. 76/2515, 30.1.1976.

E.A. Shaftan et al., Use of Extracts from Fructus Rosae for Cosmetic Purposes, Rastit. Resur. 14, (2) 208-211 (1978).

A.R. Tedgui-Zagame, Bronzing Agents Absorbable by Mouth,French Patent No. 2320732, Applic. No. 75/24391, 14.8.1975.

A.R. Tedgui-Zagame, Pharmaceutical, Cosmetic, and Food Compositions Containing Tanning Agents, French Patent No. 2328454, Applic. No. 75/32263, 22.10.1975.

A.R. Tedgui-Zagame, Oral Suntanning Compositions, French Patent No. 2338038, Applic. No. 75/25391, 14.8.1975

N.N. Tikhomirova, N.A. Asanova, Deodorant, U.S.S.R. Patent No. 504539, Applic. No. 1,989,807, 14.1.1974 (Assignee: All-Union Scientific-Research Institute of the Chem. Industry, Sverdlovsk).

E. Uus, E. Siirde et al., Chlorophyll - Carotene Paste, U.S.S.R. Patent No. 342628, 6.1.1971 (Assignee: Tallin Polytechnic Institute).

6) APPLICATION FORMS / FORMULATIONS

Anon., Preparation of New Application Forms of Carotenoid Dyes by Ultramicronization, Res. Discl. 170, p. 51 (1978).

Anon., Preparation and Application of Chlorophyll Preparations, Res. Discl. 173, p. 8 (1978).

T.W. Antoshkiw et al., Water-dispersible, Carotenoid-containing Powder Mixtures, Ger. Patent No. 2534091, Applic. No. 497.025, 13.8.1974 (Assignee: F. Hoffmann-La Roche & Co. AG).

H. Ashida et al., Carotenoid Solubilization for Use as Food Dyes, Jap. Patent No. 72 25220, Applic. No. 71 16,311, 22.3.1971 (Assignee: Soda Aromatic Co., Ltd.).

Kokai Tokkyo Koho, Food Colour Canthaxanthin Prepn., Jap. Patent No. 78 78229, Applic. No. 2657477, 18.12.1976 (Assignee: BASF, AG).

A. Emodi et al., Water-dispersible, Optically-clear Carotenoid Colours, Food Technol (Chicago) 30, (7) 58-60 (1976).

T. Fujita et al., Red Food Colouring Agent from Euphausia, Jap. Patent No. 77 48191, Applic. No. 74/148571, 27.12.1974 (Assignee: Nippon Suisan Kaisha Ltd., Kyowa Hakko Kogyo Co. Ltd.).

T. Hirose, H. Iriyama, Carotenoids for Food Colouring,Jap. Patent No. 77 18218, Applic. No. 70/87850, 8.10.1970 (Assignee: Kagome Co., Ltd.).

- Carotenoid Colouring Agent (A Powdered, Water-dispersible Carotenoid, Comprising 2 - 15% Carotenoid of Particle Size less than 0.01 my m. 1 - 6% Sodium Lauryl Sulphate. 75 - 90% Water-soluble Carrier,

0.01 - 0.5% Preservative. 0.05 - 0.3% Stabilizing Agent and 1 - 10% Antioxidant. Product giving Excellent Clarity and Colour , Brit.Patent (1978) 1 502 895) (Assignee: Hoffmann-La Roche AG).

R. Josse, H. Kläui, Colouring Preparation for Beverages (Apocarotenal, Carotenoid), Ger. Patent No. 2901071, Applic. No. 78/372, 13.1.1978 (Assignee: F. Hoffmann-La Roche & Co. AG).

Y. Ikawa et al., Water-Dispersible Carotenoid Colouring Agents, Jap. Patent No. 75 75215, Applic. No. 73 124.124, 5.11.1973 (Assignee: Sanei Chemical Ind. Ltd.).

Y. Ikawa, H. Kagimoto, Carotenoid Food-Colouring Agents, Jap. Patent No. 75 104230, Applic. No. 74 10.825, 24.1.1974 (Assignee: Sanei Chemical Ind. Ltd.).

Y. Ikawa, H. Kagimoto, Carotenoid Colourants, Jap. Patent No. 75 104231, Applic. No. 74 10.826, 24.1.1974 (Assignee: Sanei Chemical Ind. Ltd.).

- Carotenoid Food Colouring Agents are Prepared by Homogenizing Bixin in an Oil Medium Containing a Surfactant, Jap. Patent (1977) 5 224 535 (Assignee: Sanei Chemical Ind. Ltd.).

H. Iriyama, Carotenoid Food-Colouring Agent from Tomato Waste, Jap. Patent No. 79 24940, Applic. No. 77/88850, 26.7.1977 (Assignee: Kagome Co., Ltd.).

- Carotenoid Colouring Agent (Alkali is added to Pressed Carrot Juice, Heated to 60 - 80° and Acidified), Jap. Patent (1977) 5 218 218 (Assignee: Kagome Co. Ltd.).

H. Kläui et al., in Fat Soluble Vitamins (International Encyclopaedia of Food and Nutrition, Vol 9), R.A. Morton, Ed., (Pergamon Press, Oxford) p. 113-159 (1979).

F.K. Marcus, Natural Carotenoid Food Colourings, Especially Lycopene, Ger. Patent No. 2554924, Applic. No. 2554924, 6.12.1975 (Assignee: Marcus, Dr. Friedrich Karl, Chemische Fabrik K.G.).

R.P. Nikolaev, L.K. Brzhezina, Stable β-Carotene Preparation for the Colouring and Vitamin Supplementation of Edible Fats, Maslo-Zhir. Prom-st. 7, 24-25 (1979).

G. Rovesti, Hydrodispersible Natural Colour, Extracted by Means of Orange Oil from Citrus Waste Materials, Riv. It. Ess. Profumi. Piante Offic. Aromi. Saponi. Cosmetici. Aerosol. 60, (2) 66-68 (1978).

- Storage Stable Water-Dispersible Powder of Oil-Soluble Substances, such as Vitamins A, D and E, Dyes, Essential Oils and Medicaments / β-Carotene Watersoluble 10%, Derwent Basic. Abstr. 3545X Patent (1970) (Assignee: Riken-Vitamin-Oil).

- Water-Dispersible Carotenoid Colouring Agents, Cent. Patents Index Week W50, 103 (1976) (Assignee: Sanei Chem. Ind. KK).

- Stable Water-Dispersible Carotenoid Colourants Prepn. - Carotenoid Soln. (in Weakly-Polar Solvent), Homogeneously Dispersed in Oil-Water System, Jap. Patent 0104-231 (1975) (Assignee: Sanei Chem.).

T. Suyama et al., Carotenoid Colouring Agent, Jap. Patent No. 77 12207, Applic. No. 70/57999, 2.7.1970 (Assignee: Sankyo Co. Ltd.).

I. Watanabe et al., Powdered Water-Soluble Food Colouring Agent, Jap. Patent No. 76 36223, Applic. No. 74/109148, 21.9.1974 (Assignee: Fuji Seito Co. Ltd.).

Y. Yamamoto, F. Ueda, β-Carotene Food-Colouring Agent, Jap. Patent No. 79135822, Applic. No. 78/43296, 14.4.1978 (Assignee: Kawai Seiyaku Co.Ltd.)

7) MISCELLANEOUS

7.1 Microbial Pigments / Natural Carotenoids

Anon., Microbial Pigments are Subject of Study that Assesses use as Food Colourants, Food Prod. Development 13,(5) p. 12 (1979).

G. Choubert, Jr., Tentative Utilization of Spirulin Algae as a Source of Carotenoid Pigments for Rainbow Trout, Aquaculture 18, (2) 135-143 (1979).

P. Dupaigne, Red Colouring Matter of Natural Origin, Fruits 29, (12) 797-814 (1974).

Hadarim Hod Hasharon Ltd., On the Analysis of Tagetes Extract, Deut. Getränke-Industrie 31, (6) 132 (1976).

E.A. Johnson et al., The Yeast Phaffia Rhodozyma as a Dietary Pigment Source for Salmonids and Crustaceans, J. Fish Res. Board Can. 34, (12) 2417-2421 (1977).

T. Philip, Utilization of Plant Pigments as Food Colourants, Food Prod. Development 9, (3) 50-56 (1975).

A.A. Shmidt et al., Use of Microbiological β-Carotene for Colouring Margarine, Maslo-Zhir. Prom-st. 2, 23-26 (1977).

V. Silerio, Filiberto, C. Mendoza de Flores et al., Evaluation of Spiruline (Spirulina Geitleri) as a Dietary Pigment Source for Fattening Chickens, Tec. Pecu. Mex. 31, 47-54 (1976).

T.P. Slyusarenko et al., The Characteristics of Some β-Carotene Producing Yeast Isolated from Commercial Media, Pishchevaya Promyshlennost' Republik 20, 96-98 (1975).

7.2 Carotenoids as Antioxidants and Inhibitor of Photooxidation

D. Bellus, Physical Quenchers of Singlet Molecular Oxygen, Adv. Photochem. 11, 105-205 (1979).

H. Berger et al., Base Oil Compositions Having Improved Light Stability, U.S. Patent No. 4031016, Applic. No. 641052, 15.12.1975 (Assignee: SHELL Oil, Co.).

R.S. Davidson, K.R. Trethewey, The Role of the Excited Singlet State of Dyes in Dye Sensitized Photooxygenation Reactions, J. Am. Chem. Soc. 98, (13) 4008-4009 (1976).

K. Enmanji et al., Fluorescent Dyes with Improved Fading Resistance, Jap. Patent No. 78 33224, Applic. No. 76/107473, 7.9.1976 (Assignee: Mitsubishi Electric Corp.).

K. Enmanji et al., Nontoxic Light Stabilizers for Transparent Polymers, Jap. Patent No. 78 127583, Applic. No. 77/42269, 12.4.1977 (Assignee: Mitsubishi Electric Corp.).

A. Farmilo, F. Wilkinson, Mechanism of Quenching of Singlet Oxygen in Solution, Photochem. Photobiol. 18, (6) 447-450 (1973).

R.A. Larson, L.L. Hunt, Photooxidation of a Refined Petroleum Oil: Inhibition by β-Carotene and Role of Singlet Oxygen, Photochem. Photobiol. 28, (4-5) 553-555 (1978).

M. Nowakowska, The Use of β-Carotene for the Evaluation of the Role of Singlet Oxygen in Longwave UV Photooxidation of Polystyrene, Singlet Oxygen React. Org. Compd. Polym. (Pap. EUCHEM Conf.) (1978) 254-263 (Publ. Wiley, Chichester England).

M. Nowakowska, β-Carotene inhibited photooxidation of polystyrene. 2., Makromol. Chem. 181, (5) 1021-1027 (1980).

J.F. Rabek, D. Lala, Carotenoids as Effective Stabilizers Against Photooxidation of cis-1,4-polybutadiene, J. Polym. Sci. 18, (6) 427-437 (1980).

7.3 Carotenoids in Polymers

T. Chappat et al., Photooxidation of β-Carotene in a Poly(vinyl chloride) Matrix, C.R. Hebd. Seances Acad. Sci. 287, (5) 175-178 (1978).

K. Fujimoto et al., Polymerization of Conjugated Dienes Using a Photosensitizer, Brit. Patent No. 129 0020, Applic. No. 35,948/69, 17.7.1969 (Assignee: Dunlop Holdings Ltd.).

H. Kamogawa, Preparation of Polyene Polymer Containing Carotene Derivative as Polyene Unit, J. Polym. Sci. 10, (12) 929-934 (1972).

H. Kamogawa, Vinyl Polymer with Conjugated Double Bond Side Chains, Jap. Patent No. 74 18192, Applic. No. 72 57.869, 10.6.1972 (Assignee: Agency of Industrial Sciences and Technology).

M. Kitano, Polypropylene Film, Jap. Patent No. 72 32290, Applic. No. 69 98.065, 5.12.1969 (Assignee: Matsushita Electric Industrial Co., Ltd.).

H. Kitano, Material Resistant to an Insulating Oil, Jap. Patent No. 73 44194, Applic. No. 69 98.811 (Assignee: Matsushita Electric Industrial Co., Ltd.).

M. Kitano, Insulating Material, Jap. Patent No. 75 04039, Applic. No. 69 98.812, 8.12.1969 (Assignee: Matsushita Electric Industrial Co., Ltd.).

K. Riistama, O. Harva, Effect of Some Conjugated Polyenes on the Radical Polymerization of Styrene, Finn. Chem. Lett. 4-5, 149-152 (1977).

7.4 Miscellaneous Uses and Properties

M. Aizawa et al., Photoelectrochemical Energy Conversion System Modeled on the Photosynthetic Process, Electrochim. Acta 23, (11) 1185-1190 (1978).

H. Asai, Odour System, Kotai Butsuri 10, (7) 369-373 (1975).

G.S. Beddard, R.S. Davidson, Quenching of Chlorophyll Fluorescence by β-Carotene, Nature 267, No. 5609, 373-374 (1977).

L. Brehmer, H. Haensel, Study on the Effect of the Surrounding Gas Atmosphere on the Electrical Surface Conductivity of all-trans-β-Carotene, Z. Phys. Chem.(Leipzig) 258, (5) 926-937 (1977).

D.K. Das Gupta, K.V.I.S. Kaler, Charge Transport in Semi-conducting Biopolymers, Amorphous Liq. Semicond. Proc. Int. Conf. 7th, 780-784 (1977).

M. De Mets, Relation between Cathodoluminescence and Molecular Structure of Organic Compounds, Microsc. Acta 76, (5) 405-414 (1975).

D. Den Engelsen, B. De Koning, Ellipsometry of Spread Monolayers. 2. Coloured Systems, J. Chem. Soc. 70, (11) 2100-2112 (1974).

K. Enmanji et al., Liquid Crystal Display Devices, Jap. Patent No. 78 57186, Applic. No. 76/132806, 4.11.1976 (Assignee: Mitsubishi Electric Corp.).

A. Ghosh, B. Mallik et al., Effect of Adsorption of Vapors on the Electrical Conductivity of some Polyene Semi-conductors, Proc. - Indian Acad. Sci. 89, (2) 209-217 (1980).

D. Hayward, R. Pething, Frequency Dependence of the Conductivity of Molecular Solids, Phys. Status Solidi A 32, (2) p. K177-K180 (1975).

Y. Hoshino, K. Tateishi, Charge Carrier Mobility Measurements in β-Carotene Glass by Transient Photoconductivity, J. Phys. Soc. Jap. 41, (5) 1625-29 (1976).

Y. Hoshino, K. Tateishi, Photoconductivity Mechanism in β-Carotene Glass, J. Phys. Soc. Jap. 46, (1) 72-76 (1979).

R.L. Jelfo, Photoelectrophoretic Imaging Composition Containing β-Carotene, U.S. Patent No. 3616398, 24.12.1969.

H. Kamogawa, Polymers Containing Conjugated Polyenes, Jap. Patent No. 74 22500, Applic. No. 72 62.135, 21.6.1972 (Assignee: Agency of Ind. Sci. and Technology).

T. Kawaguchi et al., Photoconductive Properties of Zinc Oxide Chemisorbed Natural Dye, Tokyo Gakugei Daigaku Kiyo, Dai-4-bumon 31, 119-122 (1979).

J. Lafferty et al., Electron-Transfer Reactions Involving Chlorophyll A and Carotenoids, Chem. Communication 2, 70-71 (1976).

B. Mallik et al., Compensation Temperature in Some Semi-conducting Polyenes, Jpn. J. Appl. Phys. 19, (1) 207-208 (1980).

T. Miwa, Flash Photolysis Intermediate of β-Carotene, Chiba Daigaku Kogakubu Kenkyu Hokoku 21, (39) 37-46 (1970).

M. Nanasawa, H. Kamogawa, Preparation of Model Polymers for Visual Pigment and Spectral Changes, Bull. Chem. Soc. Jpn. 52, (6) 1727-1730 (1979).

E.P. Raynes, I.A. Shanks, Liquid Crystal Devices, Brit. Patent No. 1459046, Applic. No. 74/11607, 15.3.1974 (Assignee: Secretary of State for Defence, London).

R. Reich, K.-U. Sewe, The Effect of Molecular Polarization on the Electrochromism of Carotenoids. I. Photochem. Photobiol. 26, (1) 11-17 (1977).

T. Saito, K. Tatsuishi, Electrophotographic Photoconductor Layer, Jap. Patent No. 78 31137, Applic. No. 76/104984, 3.9.1976 (Assignee: Nippon Telegraph and Telephone Public. Corp.).

K. Sauer, Photosynthetic Membranes, Acc. Chem. Res. 11, (7) 257-264 (1978).

F. Takahashi, Photoelectrolysis Using Chlorophyll Electrodes, Elektrohimiya 13, (11) 1674-78 (1977).

K. Tatsuishi et al., Photoconductive Materials for Electrophotography, Jap. Patent No. 78 27431, Applic. No. 76/101121, 26.8.1976 (Assignee: Nippon Telegraph and Telephone Public Corp.).

T. Ohnishi et al., Electrical and Spectroscopic Investigations of molecular Layers of Fatty Acids Including Carotene, Bull. Chem. Soc. Jpn. 51, (6) 1714-1716 (1978).

N. Yamamoto et al., Electrical Properties of Langmuir films of fatty acid salts and carotenoic acid, Bull. Chem. Soc. Jpn. 51, (12) 3462-65 (1978).

CAROTENOIDS IN RELATION TO CHLOROPLASTS AND OTHER ORGANELLES

Jerome A. Schiff, Francis X. Cunningham, Jr. and Michael S. Green

Institute for Photobiology of Cells and Organelles, Brandeis University
Waltham, Mass. 02254, USA

Abstract - During light-induced chloroplast development in dark-grown non-dividing cells of *Euglena gracilis* var. *bacillaris* carotenoids rise concomitantly with other plastid thylakoid constituents. When carotenoid biosynthesis is selectively blocked at phytoene with SAN 9789, the synthesis of chlorophyll, sulfolipid and thylakoid polypeptides is also inhibited indicating a tight co-control of membrane constituents during thylakoid assembly. This insures that the membranes are assembled correctly and that potential sensitizers of deleterious photoreactions such as chlorophyll are not synthesized in the absence of protecting carotenoids. In higher plants this co-control is far less stringent and normal proplastids and prothylakoids are made in the absence of carotenoid biosynthesis. Growth of etiolated beans on SAN 9789, however, produces in darkness all of the familiar deetiolation phenomena normally seen after exposure to red light; the effect is not directly on phytochrome since far-red light does not reverse the effect of SAN. Abscisic acid is related to carotenoids and its level may be changed by SAN treatment leading to the deetiolation responses in darkness. In certain bleached mutants such as W_3BUL, *cis* ζ-carotene accumulates and is photoisomerized to *trans* by blue light. This activity is associated with a cell fraction of very low density. The action spectrum, which is somewhat different from the ζ-carotene absorption spectrum, may result from various photostationary states between *cis* and *trans* ζ-carotene at each wavelength. Wild-type cells make *trans* carotenoids in darkness and must have a means of isomerization that does not involve light. The normal development of the stigma (but not the paraflagellar body) in *Euglena* requires light and carotenoids; the structure, composition and biosynthesis of hematochrome remain to be determined in this species.

INTRODUCTION

Carotenoid pigments perform several functions in cells. They protect photosynthetic and non-photosynthetic cells from deleterious photoreactions, serve as antennas that absorb light and transfer it to the photosynthetic reaction centers and play a role in light perception. In non-photosynthetic cells carotenoids are contained in organelles other than chloroplasts. In photosynthetic cells this is also true, but the large concentrations of carotenoids in chloroplast thylakoid membranes often makes it difficult to localize and define the carotenoids in other cellular locations. It has now become apparent that even the outer envelope of chloroplasts has a carotenoid constitution somewhat different from that of the thylakoids and may serve as a biosynthetic reservoir for carotenoids passing to the thylakoids (Ref.1). The overall literature concerning the subjects to be discussed in this review has been surveyed (Ref. 2); our objective will be to discuss several aspects related to our current research.

CAROTENOIDS AND CHLOROPLAST DEVELOPMENT

Photosynthetic cells in darkness generally contain carotenoid pigments associated to a large extent with the prothylakoids of proplastids and etioplasts (Ref.3 & 4). During light-induced chloroplast development in various systems carotenoids increase. In *Euglena gracilis* var. *bacillaris* (Ref.3 & 5) carotenoids rise concomitantly with other plastid thylakoid constituents (Fig.1) and with the increase in the amount of thylakoid membranes (Ref.6 & 7). β-Carotene, diatoxanthin and diadinoxanthin are already present in dark-grown cells and increase during chloroplast development. Neoxanthin appears for the first time at about 4 hrs. of development (Ref.5), the time when photosynthetic oxygen evolution is first measurable (Ref.3), suggesting that this pigment may play an important role in photosynthesis apart from absorption of light and energy transfer to chlorophyll. Preillumination eliminates the 12 hr. lag in chlorophyll synthesis in *Euglena* but not the lag in carotenoid formation (Ref.8), probably because there are sufficient carotenoids in the dark-grown cells for the first 12 hrs. of development (apart from neoxanthin). Illuminated seedlings of etiolated higher plants must

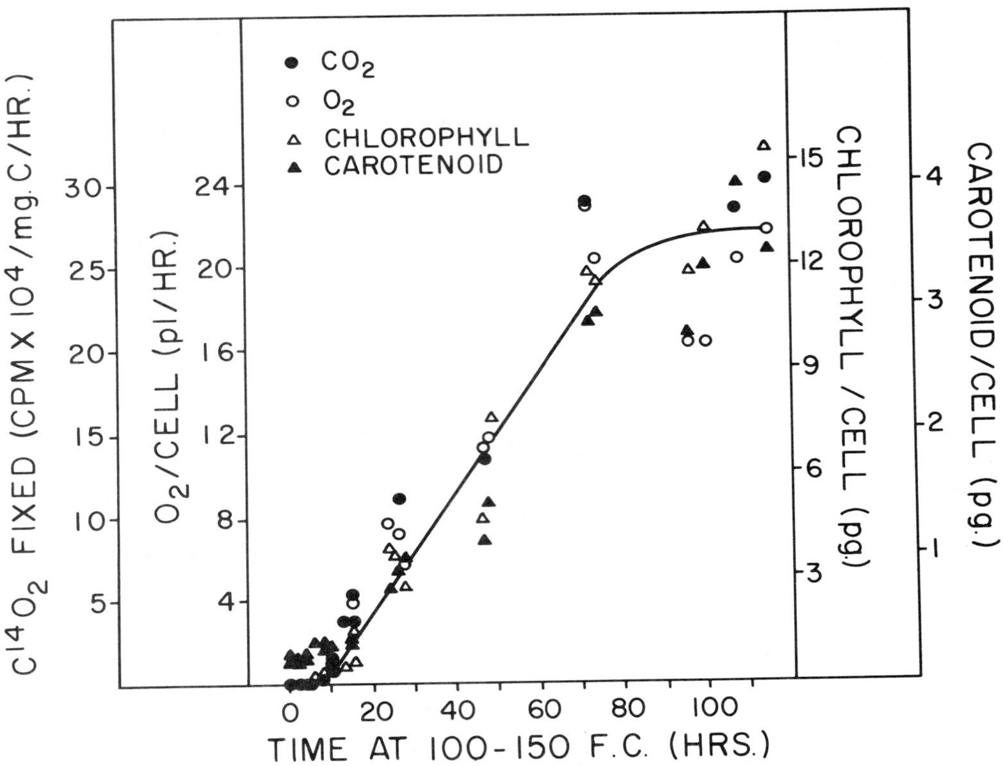

Fig. 1. Appearance of photosynthesis, chlorophyll and carotenoids when dark-grown non-dividing cells of *Euglena gracilis* var. *bacillaris* are placed in the light (Ref. 6). Although obscured by the overlap of points, there is a twelve hr. lag in the rise of these constituents; net photosynthesis is first detectable at about 4 hrs. of development. Note that carotenoids start at a higher level than the other parameters in the dark-grown cells but rise concomitantly with the others during the period of major development.

reach a certain stage of plastid development before energy transfer from carotenoids to chlorophyll can be detected (Ref.9). Other plastid thylakoid constituents such as sulfolipid and thylakoid polypeptides also increase concomitantly with chlorophyll and carotenoid pigments (Ref.10 & 11).

The formation of thylakoid constituents in *Euglena* is under extremely tight control. Thus when carotenoid synthesis is selectively blocked at the phytoene stage by the herbicide norfluorazon (SAN 9789), the synthesis of chlorophyll, sulfolipid and thylakoid polypeptides is also inhibited (Ref.10, 11 & 12). This serves to insure that the membrane is assembled correctly and that potential sensitizers of deleterious photoreactions such as chlorophyll and other pigmented molecules are not synthesized in the absence of protecting carotenoids. It is a curious fact that many molecules selected by evolution to serve as electron transport carriers are colored and, therefore, absorb light in the visible region of the spectrum. The same molecular constitution that provides a favorable redox potential for electron transport also seems to provide electronic energy levels that allow phototransitions to take place with the photon energies available in the visible region of the spectrum. Evolution would have to cope with these light reactions and their products, particularly in photosynthetic organisms that are exposed to high light fluxes. The flavins are particularly troublesome in this respect but in intact cells these molecules may be bound or sequestered in such a manner as to lower their capacity to undergo deleterious photoreactions. In the case of the cytochromes, the presence of iron largely quenches the photochemical activities of these pigments. However, the evolution of molecules such as carotenoids which, through various mechanisms, can prevent the consequences of such damaging reactions would be a most important factor in curbing unwanted photoreactions (Ref.13). For this reason, there would have been a strong selection for the control mechanisms seen in *Euglena* that insure the concomitant formation of carotenoids during thylakoid biosynthesis.

Possibly because the early development of leaves of higher plants following seed germination can occur in the absence of light or in dim light, a tight regulation of prothylakoid membrane synthesis by carotenoids has not been selected. In organisms such as bean (*Phaseolus vulgaris*) (Ref.14) and sunflower (*Helianthus annuus*) (Ref.15) normal prothylakoids and prolamellar bodies containing protochlorophyll(ide) are formed in dark-grown plants depleted of carotenoids through germination on norfluorazon or through mutations that block carotenoid biosynthesis. Although some chloroplast development in the absence of carotenoids can occur in dim light, exposure to prolonged light or to high intensities of light rapidly inactivates such carotenoid-depleted organisms.

An unexpected effect of treatment with norfluorazon is observed in bean seedlings germinated in the presence of this inhibitor of carotenoid synthesis in darkness (Ref.14). Norfluorazon produces in darkness all of the familiar deetiolating effects of treatment with red light, such as shortening of internodes, leaf expansion, development of leaves at the second and third internodes, root development, etc. This might be due to an alteration in the biosynthesis of abscisic acid, a molecule related to the carotenoids, by norfluorazon. The effect of norfluorazon is not directly on phytochrome since treatment with far-red light does not reverse the effects of the herbicide. Confirmation of this phenomenon and some indication of its generality comes from recent work in Sweden which shows that norfluorazon acts like red light in stimulating seed germination (Ref.16).

PHOTOISOMERIZATION OF ζ-CAROTENE IN EUGLENA

Certain mutants of *Euglena* (such as W_3BUL which contain only rudimentary proplastid remnants (Ref.17)) accumulate ζ-carotene. When illuminated with blue light these mutants show peaks in the blue light minus dark difference spectrum which can be traced to a photoisomerization of *cis*-(probably 15-*cis*)-ζ-carotene to the *trans* isomer (Ref.18 & 19) (Fig. 2). The position of the absorption peaks of the *cis*-ζ-carotene and of the blue light minus dark difference spectrum in intact cells and in a cell fraction of low density floating on sucrose gradients is at longer wavelengths than observed for ζ-carotene in solvents such as acetone or ether (Fig. 2). The positions of the peaks are similar to those of ζ-carotene in solvent mixtures such as carbon disulfide/chloroform; the environment of the molecule *in vivo* may provide molecular interactions (Ref. 20) more like those in the latter solvents. The cell fractions isolated by flotation on sucrose gradients, which contain the photoisomerization activity and the *cis*-ζ-carotene, show densely-staining liposome-like bodies of various sizes on electron microscopy (Ref. 19). The relations of these bodies to other cellular structures thought to contain carotenoids will be discussed later.

The action spectrum for photoisomerization of ζ-carotene in its native cellular environment shows effectiveness in those spectral regions where ζ-carotene absorbs, but the action spectrum differs from the absorption spectrum in having a series of sharp spikes (Ref. 18) (Fig.3). Although the iodine-catalyzed isomerization of carotenoids such as ζ-carotene is well-known, (Ref. 18), ζ-carotene will undergo *cis* to *trans* photoisomerization in the absence of iodine catalysis. Acetone extracts of the floating fraction of cells of mutant W_3BUL themselves show the photoisomerization reaction in the absence of iodine (Fig. 2) as do the same extracted pigments transferred to ether (Ref. 19) or petroleum ether. *Cis*-ζ-carotene alone, purified from acetone extracts of whole cells of W_3BUL, undergoes *cis* to *trans* isomerization on illumination with blue light (Fig. 4) indicating that light absorbed by the pigment itself brings about its own isomerization. It is likely that the action spectrum already mentioned results from the kinetics governing the *cis*-*trans* photostationary state at each wavelength. This photostationary state would be expected to be governed by the extinction coefficients of the isomers at each wavelength and their concentrations. The varying kinetics of *cis* to *trans* and *trans* to *cis* photoreactions at each wavelength might result in different photostationary states leading to an action spectrum somewhat different from the absorption of either the *cis* or the *trans* form. The small peak shifts in the blue absorption peaks between *cis* and *trans* ζ-carotene might well lead to the spikes seen in the action spectrum. Other isomers of ζ-carotene are known which could be involved as well (Ref. 21).

The role of ζ-carotene photoisomerization in *Euglena* has not been determined. This reaction is not seen in dark-grown wild-type *Euglena* cells or in certain mutants, but these cells do not accumulate ζ-carotene (Ref. 18). Other mutants (such as Y_2BUL) are known which accumulate ζ-carotene but do not show the photoisomerization reaction. These mutants may contain only *trans*—ζ-carotene or may not exhibit the photoreaction for other reasons. This is not the place to enter into a discussion of the highly-branched complications of carotenoid biosynthesis (Ref.2 & 22). It remains possible, however, that the isomerization of *cis*-ζ-carotene to the *trans* form is part of the normal biosynthetic pathway of carotenoids in *Euglena* as has been suggested for *Scenedesmus* (Ref. 23). Wild-type cells may be capable of isomerizing *cis*-ζ-carotene to *trans* in darkness; mutation and loss of this enzyme activity would render the organism light-dependent for this step. If so, the pathway would have to be highly branched, the mutants leaky, or different parallel pathways present in various parts of the cells to account for the fact that mutants accumulating ζ-carotene frequently also form other carotenes and xanthophylls such as β-carotene, diatoxanthin and diadinoxanthin (Ref. 18).

CELLULAR LOCALIZATION OF CAROTENOIDS

Nonphotosynthetic cells frequently contain carotenoids. In bacteria, where the carotenoids protect the cells from deleterious photoreactions, they may be localized in the cell membrane (Ref. 2). If mitochondria arose through an endosymbiotic invasion of a primitive eucaryotic

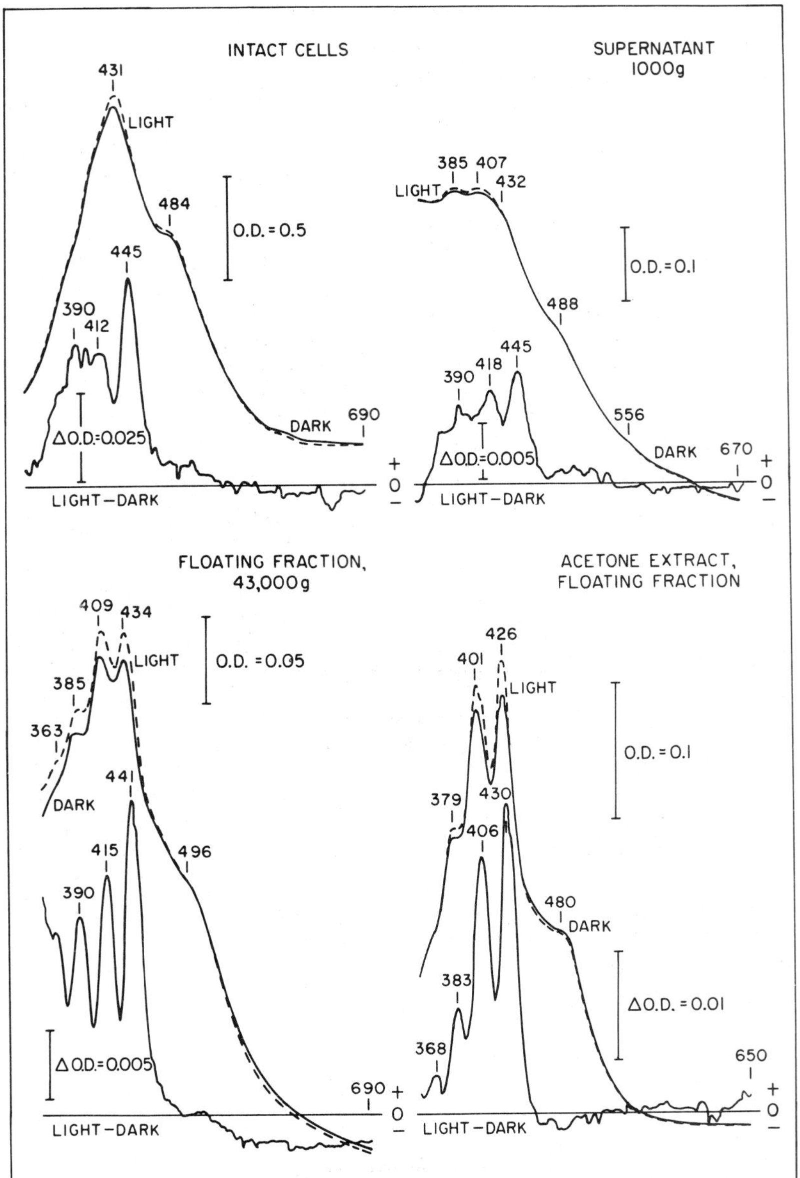

Fig. 2. Representative absorption and blue light minus dark difference spectra of various preparations from Euglena gracilis var. bacillaris W3BUL. These include whole cells, the 1000g supernatant fluid prepared from cell extracts, floating material from a 43,000g centrifugation and a 90% (v/v) acetone extract of the floating material (Ref. 19).

cell by primitive precursors of modern aerobic bacteria (Ref. 25), carotenoids might also be found in the membranes of modern eucaryotic mitochondria (Ref. 26). In the fungus Neurospora carotenoids are particularly associated with lipid globules and the endoplasmic reticulum (Ref. 27) and with the mitochondria (Ref. 28). Indeed in aerobic cells, one might expect carotenoids to be formed as a countermeasure wherever oxygen might react to form destructive radicals.

The anoxygenic photosynthetic procaryotes represented by the green and purple bacteria form carotenoids in association with the photosynthetic apparatus in the cell membranes and associated photosynthetic structures (Ref. 29). They would be used for energy transfer to bacteriochlorophyll reaction centers and as radical scavengers but probably would not be needed to deal with oxygen-generated toxic products in the light since these organisms are usually anaerobic when carrying out photosynthesis (Ref. 30). In the oxygenic/facultatively anoxygenic cyanobacteria carotenoids accompany the chlorophylls in the thylakoids and, perhaps the cell membranes of these procaryotes (Ref. 31).

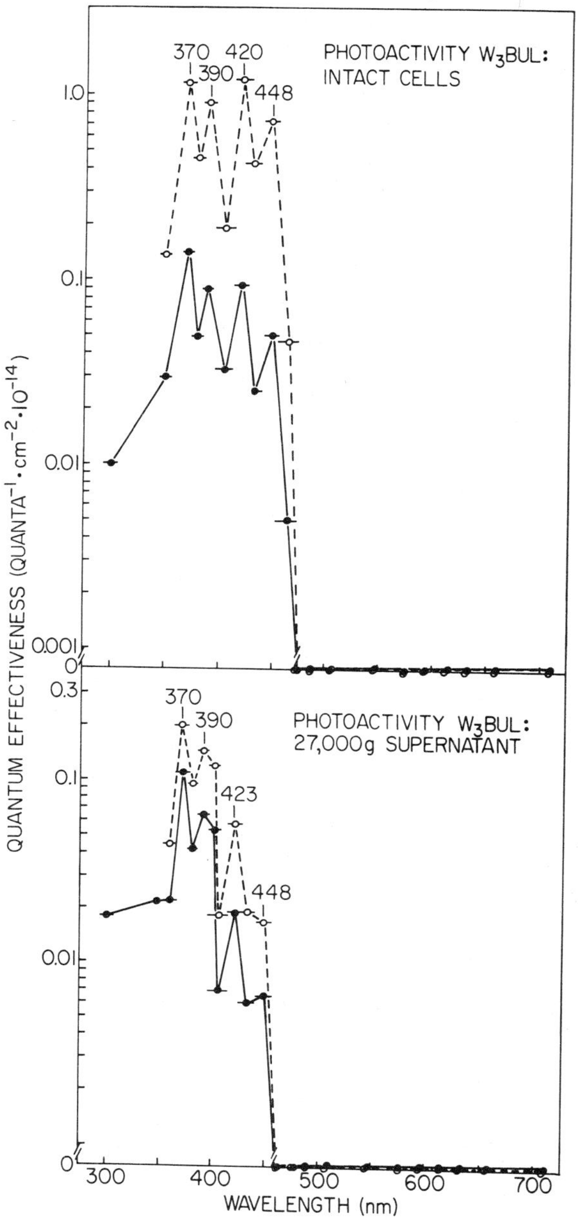

Fig. 3. Action spectra for the blue light-induced absorbance change in intact cells and in extracts of _Euglena gracilis_ W3BUL (solid lines) and with a Morowitz correction for scattering (dashed lines) (Ref. 18).

The photosynthetically oxygenic eucaryotes present more of a problem. The plastids contain high concentrations of carotenoid pigments and small amounts of carotenoids associated with other cell organelles could be ascribed to fragmentation of chloroplasts and consequent contamination of centrifugal fractions. In the eucaryotic algae, depots of carotenoids outside the chloroplast do appear to be present, for example in cell walls (Ref. 32). In the green alga _Hematococcus_ (Ref. 33) and in the red _Euglenas_ (Ref.34 & 35) the red keto-carotenoid astaxanthin occurs in cytoplasmic structures sometimes called hematochrome. In _Hematococcus_ this material appears to be associated with the endoplasmic reticulum. In the red _Euglenas_ the astaxanthin-containing structures are mobile within the cell and move in response to light and temperature. At appropriate temperatures in low light, they contract into clumps exposing the chloroplasts; in high light they expand to cover the chloroplasts and shield them from light. Pond blooms of the organism are observed to pass from a green color in low light to a red color in high light. The very crude action spectrum available indicates that this is a blue light mediated response (Ref. 35).

Less extensive red-colored flecks exist in the cytoplasm of green _Euglenas_ such as _Euglena gracilis_, but their cellular associations and composition are uncertain. No astaxanthin is

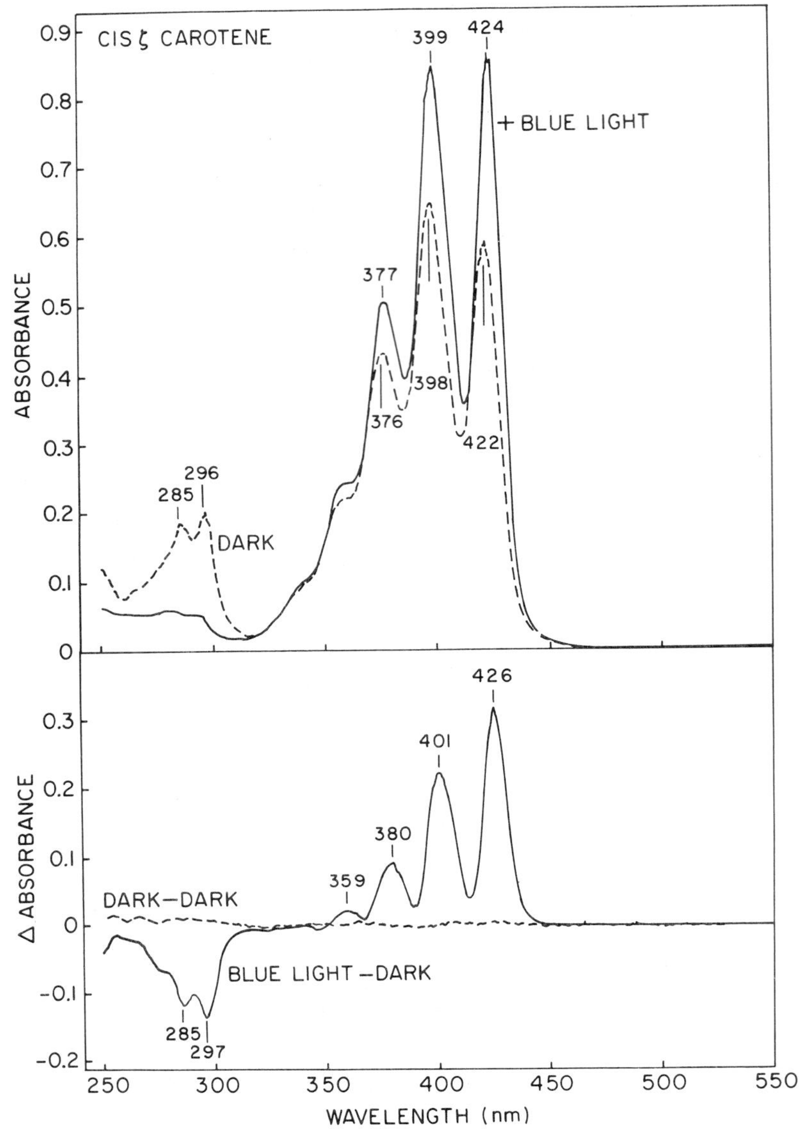

Fig. 4. Absorption spectra of purified cis-ζ-carotene from Euglena gracilis var. bacillaris W3BUL. The upper panel shows the absorption spectrum of cis-ζ-carotene in light petroleum ether before and after treatment with blue light. The lower panel shows the corresponding blue light minus dark difference spectrum. Cis-ζ-carotene was purified from dark-grown cells under green safelights on columns of activated alumina followed by thin-layer chromatography on silica gel G. The solution of cis-ζ-carotene in petroleum ether was illuminated with broad band blue light (175 w/m^2 for 5 min.) from a General Electric Quartzline Lamp DWY filtered by a Corning 5-59 filter.

detectable in Euglena gracilis (Ref. 36) suggesting that this "hematochrome" may be different in composition from that of the red Euglenas and hematochrome-containing green algae. The earlier literature suggests that the composition of the stigma and hematochrome may be related and that in some cases, hematochrome may be formed from the breaking up of the stigma (Ref.37). However, very preliminary observations using light microscopy to compare cells of wild-type Euglena gracilis containing a normal stigma and normal carotenoids with mutants that have reduced carotenoids and stigma or mutants with no stigma or carotenoids at all, indicate that the hematochrome flecks are still present when stigma and cellular carotenoids are eliminated (Ref. 38). Similar results are obtained when carotenoid levels are reduced by growing wild-type cells on norfluorazon. These results suggest that the hematochrome flecks of the green Euglenas may not be composed of carotenoids- at least not of normally extractable carotenoids. The mutants lacking carotenoids are seen by electron microscopy to contain dense bodies associated with the endoplasmic reticulum (Ref. 39) which are similar to those identified with astaxanthin-containing hematochrome in Hematococcus (Ref. 33). Taken together, the evidence suggests that "hematochrome" is a material which may or may not contain extractable carotenoids such as astaxanthin depending on the organism. A great deal more work is necessary to define this material biologically, to isolate it and determine its composition in the green Euglenas and to learn how it develops.

The stigma is the other conspicuously pigmented structure in photosynthetic cells which might contain carotenoids. In some green algae the stigma is part of the chloroplast, but in the Euglenas it is a separate organelle. The stigma in Euglena is thought to act as a shading device to cast a shadow on the paraflagellar body or swelling, the photoreceptor for phototaxis (Ref. 37). The paraflagellar body is thought to contain flavins (Ref. 40) which act as sensitizers for phototaxis. In wild-type cells and in all mutants examined, whether the cells are grown in darkness or light, the paraflagellar body is present and exhibits its normal reticulate fine structure. The form of the stigma, however, depends on whether light is available and is strongly correlated with the ability of the cells to synthesize colored carotenoids (Ref.41 & 42) (Fig. 5).

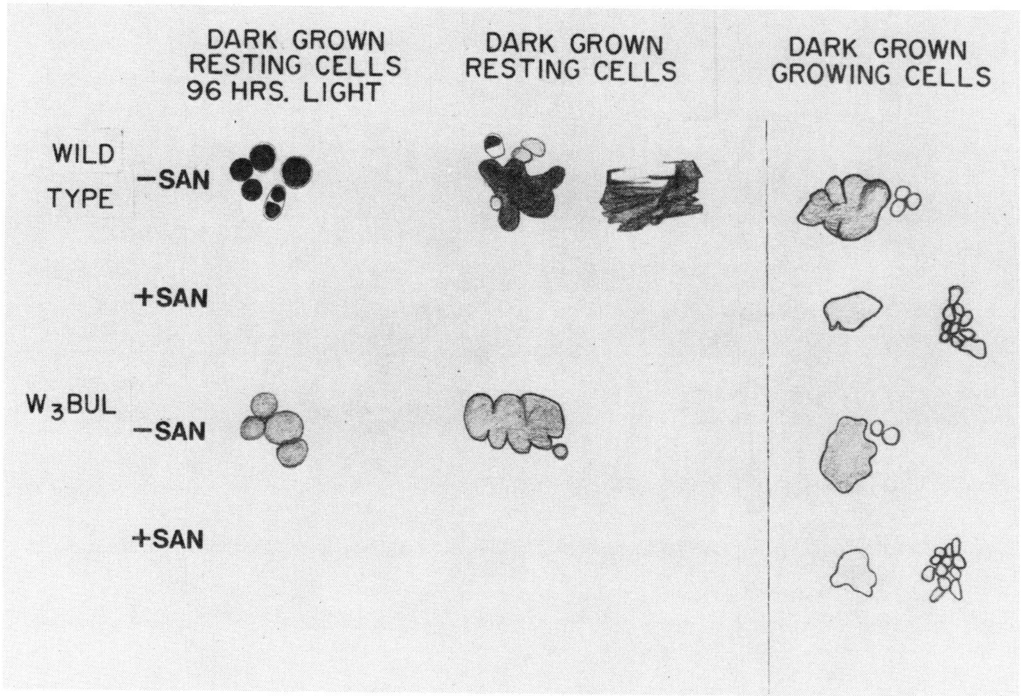

Fig. 5. Stigmas of various cells and treatments sketched to scale for comparison (Ref. 41).

Electron microscopy shows that the stigma in dark-grown wild-type cells is an amorphous densely staining structure which organizes into a group of spherical liposome-like bodies on exposure of the cells to prolonged light (Ref.41 & 43) (Fig. 6). This normal stigma of light-grown wild-type cells is brick red in color and its absorption spectrum determined in vivo by microspectrophotometry has a broad absorption in the blue and blue-green regions of the spectrum (Ref.44 & 45). The absorption in the blue region of the spectrum would be consistent with the presence of the more usual yellow-orange carotenoids, but the extended absorption in the blue-green region would have to be explained in other ways. Small amounts of unusual carotenoids might be concentrated in the stigma; astaxanthin is absent from the cells (Ref.36) but two other carotenoids, euglenone and echinenone, are present in cells lacking chloroplasts but retaining the stigma (Ref. 46). Some of the normal carotenoids might be present in an environment which shifts their absorptions to longer wavelengths. This would be similar to the shifts in ζ-carotene absorption seen in Euglena mutant W_3BUL compared with its absorption in ordinary solvents already mentioned above. Cell fractions of low density from light-grown wild-type Euglena gracilis have been isolated by flotation on sucrose density gradients (Ref.47 & 50). These pigmented fractions contain densely staining spherical particles resembling those of the stigma. However, we have found these fractions can be quite heterogeneous and similar particle fractions (although colorless) can be isolated from mutants such as $W_{10}BSmL$ that lack colored carotenoids and a stigma (Ref. 38).

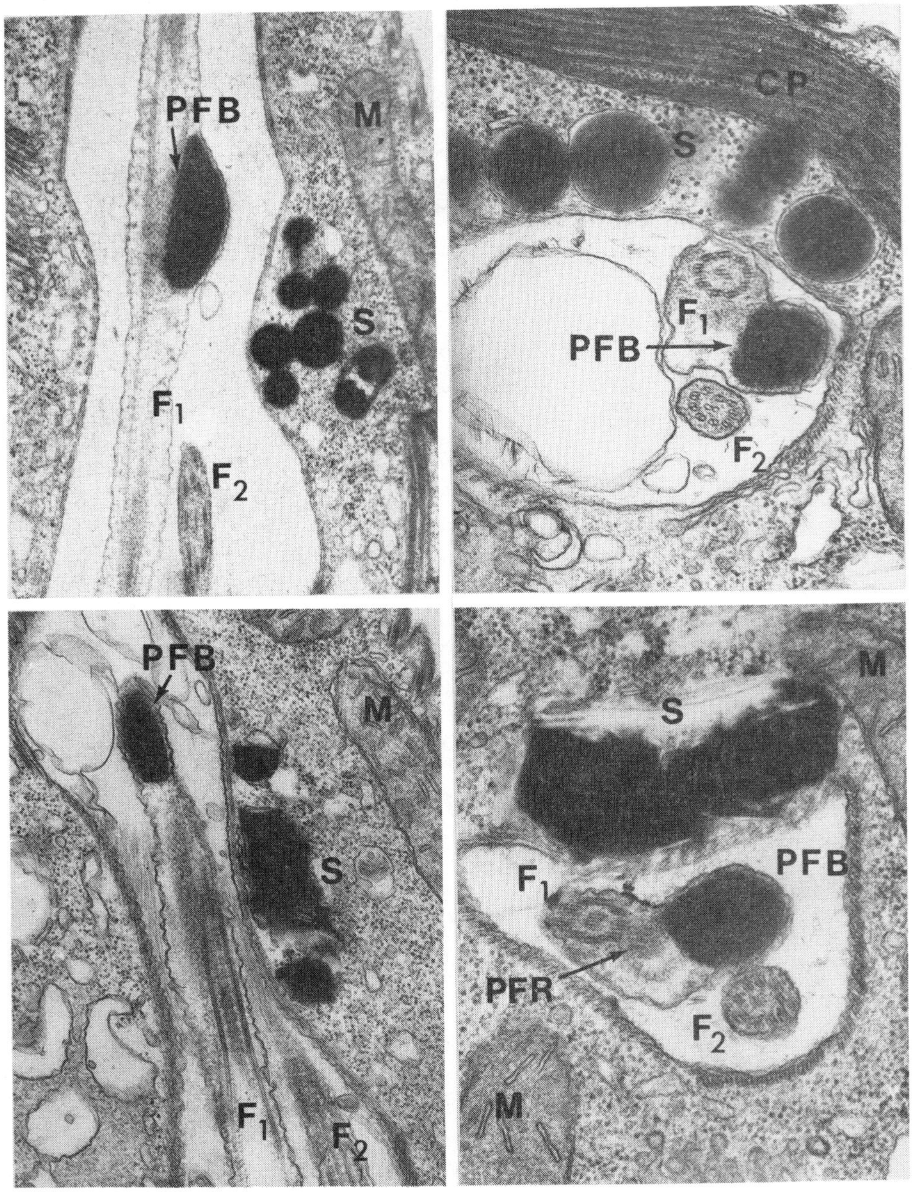

Fig. 6. Sections through the reservoir region of Euglena gracilis var. bacillaris showing: CP, chloroplast; F_1, emergent flagellum; F_2, non-emergent flagellum; M, mitochondrion; PFB, paraflagellar body (or paraflagellar swelling); PFR, paraflagellar rod; S, stigma (Ref. 41).

1) Longitudinal section through the reservoir region of a dark-grown non-dividing wild-type cell exposed to light for 96 hrs. showing stigma and paraflagellar body (37,000x).
2) Cross section through the reservoir region of a dark-grown non-dividing wild-type cell exposed to light for 96 hrs., at the level of the stigma and paraflagellar body (47,000x).
3) Longitudinal section through the reservoir region of a dark-grown non-dividing wild-type cell showing stigma and paraflagellar body (27,000x).
4) Cross section through the reservoir region of a dark-grown non-dividing wild-type cell showing stigma and paraflagellar body (47,000x).

There is no question, however, that the presence and form of the stigma correlates with the ability of the cell to make colored carotenoids (Ref.41 & 42). Cells of Euglena gracilis mutant W_3BUL, which have a lower carotenoid content than wild-type cells and a different mix of carotenoids, also (like wild-type) make an amorphous stigma in darkness which organizes into spheres on exposure to light (Ref. 41). The stigma material stains much less densely than in wild-type, however, and appears yellow in the light microscope. Mutant $W_{10}BSmL$ which cannot make colored carotenoids at all, and accumulates phytoene, does not form a stigma. Cells of wild-type or W_3BUL grown on norfluorazon to deplete carotenoids have greatly reduced stigmas (Ref. 41).

Although it is likely that the stigma of Euglena contains carotenoids, this remains to be demonstrated unequivocally along with the nature of the carotenoids present. The nature of the hematochrome flecks in the green Euglenas should also be subjected to further investigation. To our knowledge, careful carotenoid balances for various cell fractions from higher plants have not been determined, and apart from the composition of the chloroplast thylakoids and envelopes (Ref. 1) little seems to be known about other carotenoid-containing structures in these cells (Ref.2 & 26) if indeed they exist. There is much to be done if we are to understand where carotenoids are synthesized in photosynthetic eucaryotes. Is there more than one site of carotenoid synthesis? If so, are the pathways at various sites the same or different? Do intermediates in carotenoid synthesis pass from one organelle to another as other types of intermediates appear to do during chloroplast and mitochondrial development (Ref.6 & 25)?

Acknowledgement - This work was supported by a grant from the National Institutes of Health (GM 14595).

REFERENCES

1. R. Douce and J. Joyard, Adv. in Botan. Res. 7, 1-116 (1979).
2. T.W. Goodwin, The Biochemistry of the Carotenoids, 2nd ed., Chapman and Hall, London (1980).
3. A.I. Stern, J.A. Schiff and H.T. Epstein, Plant Physiol, 39, 220-226 (1964).
4. J.T.O. Kirk and R.A.E. Tilney-Bassett, The Plastids, Elsevier, Amsterdam (1978).
5. N.I. Krinsky, A. Gordon, and A.I. Stern, Plant Physiology 39, 441-445 (1964).
6. J.A. Schiff, Adv. in Morphogenesis 10, 265-312 (1973).
7. S. Klein, J.A. Schiff and A.W. Holowinsky Develop. Biol., 28, 253-273 (1972).
8. J.G. Bovarnick, Early Events in Chloroplast Development in Euglena gracilis var. bacillaris as studied with Streptomycin and Actinomycin D. PhD Dissertation, Brandeis University, (1969).
9. W.L. Butler, Biochem. Biophys. Res. Commun. 2, 419-422 (1960).
10. S. Bingham and J.A. Schiff, Biochim. Biophys. Acta 547, 512-530 (1979).
11. S. Bingham and J.A. Schiff, Biochim. Biophys. Acta 547, 531-543 (1979).
12. A.J. Vaisberg and J.A. Schiff, Plant Physiol. 57, 260-269 (1976).
13. N.I. Krinsky in Twenty-Sixth Symp. Soc. Gen. Microbiol.: The Survival of Vegetable Microbes ed. T.G.R. Gray and J.R. Postgate, pp. 209-239, Camb. Univ. Press (1976).
14. A.D. Pardo and J.A. Schiff, Can. J. Botany 58, 25-35 (1980).
15. B. Walles, Hereditas 53, 247-256 (1965).
16. C. Sundquist, K.O. Widell and H. Virgin in Abstracts, European Symposium on Light Mediated Plant Development, p. 2.4, Bishofsmais (1981).
17. T. Osafune and J.A. Schiff, J. Ultrastruct. Res. 73, 64-76 (1980).
18. F. Fong and J.A. Schiff, Planta 146, 119-127 (1979).
19. Y.L. Steinitz, J.A. Schiff, T. Osafune, and M.S. Green in The Blue Light Syndrome ed. H. Senger, pp. 269-280, Springer, Heidelberg (1980).
20. F. Feichtmayr, E. Heilbronner, A. Nurrenbach, H. Pommer and J. Schlag, Tetrahedron 25, 5383-5408 (1969).
21. G. Britton and R. Powls, Phytochemistry 16, 1253-1255 (1977).
22. R. Powls and G. Britton, Arch. Microbiol. 113, 275-280 (1977).
23. R. Powls and G. Britton, Arch. Microbiol. 115, 175-179 (1977).
24. M.M. Mathews and N.I. Krinsky, Photochem. and Photobiol. 4, 813-817 (1965).
25. J.A. Schiff in The Biochemistry of Plants ed. E.E. Conn and P.K. Stumpf, 1, 209-272 Academic Press, N.Y. (1980).
26. C. Costes, C. Burghoffer, E. Carrayol, G. Ducet and M. Diano, Plant Sci. Letts. 6, 253-259 (1976).
27. U. Mitzka-Schnabel and W. Rau, Phytochemistry 19, 1409-1413 (1980).
28. W. Neupert, G.D. Ludwig, and A. Pfaller in Biochemistry and Biophysics of Mitochondrial Membranes Ed. G.F. Azzone et al., pp. 559-568, Academic Press. N.Y. (1972).
29. S. Liaaen-Jensen in The Photosynthetic Bacteria ed. R.K. Clayton and W.R. Sistrom pp. 233-247 (1978).
30. G. Cohen-Bazire, W.R. Sistrom, and R.Y. Stanier, J. Cellular Comp. Physiol. 49, 25-68 (1957).
31. R.Y. Stanier and G. Cohen-Bazire, Ann. Rev. Microbiol. 31, 225-274 (1977).
32. J. Burczyk, H. Szkawran, I. Zontek, and F.-Ch. Czygan, Planta 151, 247-250 (1981).
33. N.J. Lang, J. Phycol. 4, 12-19 (1968).

34. J. Tischer, Z. Physiol. Chemie (Hoppe-Seyler) 267, 281-284 (1941).
35. L.P. Johnson and T.L. Jahn, Physiol. Zool. 15, 89-94 (1942).
36. N.I. Krinsky and T.H. Goldsmith, Arch. Biochem. Biophys. 91, 271-279 (1960).
37. D.E. Buetow in The Biology of Euglena ed. D.E. Buetow, I, 109, Academic Press, N.Y. (1968).
38. M. Green, The Stigma and Hematochrome of Euglena gracilis Klebs var. bacillaris Cori, Undergraduate Honors Thesis, Brandeis Univ. (1981).
39. T. Osafune and J.A. Schiff, Unpublished Results.
40. P.A. Benedetti and A. Checcucci, Plant Sci. Lett. 4, 47-51 (1975).
41. T. Osafune and J.A. Schiff, J. Ultrastruct. Res. 73, 336-349 (1980).
42. P. Kivic and M. Vesk, Cytobiology 10, 88-101 (1974).
43. P.A. Kivic and M. Vesk, Can. J. Bot. 52, 695-699 (1974).
44. P.A. Benedetti, G. Bianchini, A. Checcucci, R. Ferrara, and S. Grassi, Arch. Microbiol. 111, 73-76 (1976).
45. J.J. Wolken, J. Protozool. 24, 518-522 (1977).
46. T.W. Goodwin and J.A. Gross, J. Protozool. 5, 292-295 (1958).
47. P.P. Batra and G. Tollin, Biochim. Biophys. Acta 79, 371-378 (1964).
48. C.J. Bartlett, P.O. Walne, O.J. Schwarz, and D.H. Brown, Plant Physiol. 49, 881-885 (1972).
49. D.V. Heelis, W. Kernick, G.O. Phillips and K. Davies, Arch.Microbiol. 121, 207-211 (1979).
50. D.V. Heelis, P.F. Heelis, W.A. Kernick and G.O. Phillips, Cytobios. 29, 135-143 (1980).

THE FUNCTIONS OF CAROTENOIDS IN PHOTOSYNTHESIS

Paul MATHIS and Craig C. SCHENCK
Service de Biophysique, Département de Biologie
Centre d'Etudes Nucléaires de Saclay, 91191 GIF-SUR-YVETTE cédex, France

Carotenoids are widely present in photosynthetic structures. These hydrophobic molecules are associated with photosynthetic membranes and fulfil several functions : 1) they serve to absorb light and transmit excitation energy to a discrete site in the membrane where charge separation takes place, 2) they protect the photosynthetic organisms from photodynamic destruction mediated by singlet $(^1\Delta_g)O_2$, 3) they may be involved in electron transfer reactions in green plants. Carotenoids are evidently not essential to the function of the photosynthetic apparatus ; blue-green carotenoidless mutants of photosynthetic bacteria are vigourous phototrophs under anaerobic conditions.

CAROTENOIDS IN CHLOROPHYLL-CAROTENOID-PROTEIN COMPLEXES

Carotenoids are generally considered as lipids and older models of the photosynthetic membrane presented these pigments floating or anchored in the lipid bilayer. During the 1960s it became recognized that most of the photosynthetic pigments were inserted into the membrane as pigment-protein complexes and experimental evidence now supports the view that practically all the chlorophylls and all the carotenoids are present together in a number of well-defined integral membrane protein complexes. These complexes play the role of antenna (light-harvesting complexes) or of energy converter (reaction centers). These proteins are made of hydrophobic polypeptides and of pigments. They can be purified by detergent solubilization of photosynthetic membranes.

The antenna of purple photosynthetic bacteria contains two light-harvesting complexes LHC (1) : the B 800-850 complex whose minimum unit (MW≈20 kD) contains three bacteriochlorophylls and one carotenoid and the B 870 complex (MW≈20 kD) which contains two bacteriochlorophylls and two carotenoid. The type of carotenoid present in these two complexes varies with the strain of bacteria and also with growth conditions. In a carotenoidless mutant of Rhodopseudomonas sphaeroides a bacteriochlorophyll-protein complex named B 850, analogous to the B 870 complex, can be isolated and carotenoids (spheroidene or neurosporene) can then be incorporated in the complex. The CD spectrum of the incorporated carotenoid shows that it occupies a specific binding site. This carotenoid can sensitize bacteriochlorophyll fluorescence (2) similar to the carotenoid in light harvesting complexes of wild type bacteria.

Photoactive reaction centers were first prepared from bacterial strains devoid of carotenoids. This suggests a possible function of carotenoids in permitting a more stable structure of the photosynthetic membranes. This aspect remains rather vague in terms of quantitation and mechanism. Similar observations on a relation between the structural stability and the presence of carotenoids have also been made in higher plants (3, 4). Reaction centers from wild type purple bacteria contain about one molecule of carotenoid (spheroidene, chloroxanthin or spirilloxanthin, according to the species) (5-8). This molecule is probably bound to the small protein subunits. It can be reinserted specifically into carotenoidless reaction centers (6).

In oxygen-evolving plants and algae, all the chlorophyll is incorporated in pigment-protein complexes (9). All of them contain carotenoids. At least half of the chlorophyll is inserted in a light-harvesting complex, devoid of photochemical activity. The size, content and spectral properties of the complex depend on the method of isolation (for reviews, see refs. 10-13), but the basic pigment stoichiometry is always about 3 Chl a, 2 Chl b, 1 carotenoid. From low-temperature studies on triplet state formation, it can be inferred that each basic subunit contains one carotenoid (71). The great variety of oxygen-evolving organisms is reflected in diverse light-harvesting complexes. As an example we may mention a complex, extracted from dinoflagellates, which contains 4 peridinin and one chlorophyll a per ≈35 kD unit (14 ; see also ref. 15).

Membrane fragments enriched in Photosystem-I are enriched in β-carotene (16). Rather large fragments, with 100-150 chlorophylls per P-700, contain several xanthophylls in addition to β-carotene, probably because they include a specific part of the light-harvesting complex (13). In a more purified complex with about 40 chlorophyll a per P-700 only β-carotene is present : about 5 molecules per P-700 (15, 17), a number which is reduced to 1-2 in some preparations (11). Small particles enriched in Photosystem-II also contain β-carotene as the major carotenoid : about 4-5 molecules per reaction center (with 40 chlorophyll a) (18, 19). Two small complexes, named CP-III and CP-IV, contain 4 and 5 chlorophyll a molecules, respectively, and 1 β-carotene per protein unit (47-50 kD) (20). These complexes are probably associated with the PS-II reaction center, although they are devoid of photochemical activity.

Chloroplasts from higher plants contain, for an average photosynthetic unit of 400 chlorophylls, about 83 molecules of carotenoids (24 β-carotene, 38 lutein, 10 violaxanthin, 10 neoxanthin) (21). About half of the β-carotene molecules are rather closely associated with the reaction centers (although the specific binding that has been reported in bacterial reaction centers has not been reported in oxygen-evolving systems). All of the xanthophylls probably belong to the light-harvesting complex. If the light-harvesting system comprises 300 chlorophylls with a chlorophyll/carotenoid ratio of 5, we can thus acount for 60 carotenoids ; with 5 β-carotene associated with each reaction center, it thus appears that 84 % of the chloroplast carotenoids are found in isolated pigment-protein complexes. Some of the carotenoids may have been detached from their original structure and extracted by the detergent.

In conclusion it can be said that, in all photosynthetic organisms, practically all the carotenoids located in the photosynthetic membranes are present in the form of chlorophyll -carotenoid-protein complexes. In parallel, practically all the complexes contain at least one molecule of carotenoid. There are a few exceptions to these assertions. First, some carotenoid-protein complexes lacking chlorophyll have been extracted from photosynthetic membranes (see e.g. refs 22, 23). It is not clear whether these complexes are genuine membrane components or preparation artifacts. A second category of exception is constituted by antenna complexes which do not contain carotenoids. These complexes are often rather water-soluble and are not necessarily integral membrane constituents : phycobiliproteins, bacteriochlorophyll-protein from green sulfur bacteria, water-soluble chlorophyll protein-complexes from some higher plants.

CAROTENOIDS IN VIVO AND IN ISOLATED COMPLEXES : STRUCTURAL ASPECTS

Some structural information on carotenoids, supposedly kept in their native conformation, has been obtained in the last few years, mostly by spectroscopic methods.

- Resonance Raman spectroscopy. By this method, most of the carotenoids in light harvesting complexes of green plants and bacteria appear to be in a state similar to that attained in solution. By contrast the carotenoid of bacterial reaction centers appears to be strained in a *cis* configuration by the protein moiety. This conformation disappears upon extraction of the carotenoid, but it appears when all-*trans* spheroidene is incorporated into carotenoidless reaction centers (24, 25). A specific conformation has also been inferred from circular dichroism measurements (5).
- Measurements with polarized light. Photosynthetic sub-organelles can be oriented by various methods and pigment orientation determined by absorption or fluorescence spectroscopy. Carotenoids which belong to the light-harvesting system appear to be oriented with respect to the membrane plane (26-29) or with respect to (bacterio-) chlorophyll molecules (30-31). In general this orientation is not very strong. In reaction centers of the photosynthetic bacterium *Rhodopseudomonas sphaeroides* the carotenoid molecule is strongly oriented (5, 32). In Photosystem-I, it has also been reported that carotenoid molecules have a well-defined orientation relative to P-700 (33).
- Electrochromism. It is now well-established that photoinduced electron transfer gives rise to an electric field across the photosynthetic membrane and that the absorption spectrum of the pigments, and especially of carotenoids, is modified by electrochromism. This property has been widely used to study various aspects of electron transfer and phosphorylation (34, 35). A detailed analysis of the electrochromism gives structural information on the carotenoids (29). This problem cannot be discussed in detail here and we will focus on a few results :

1. Most of the carotenoid molecules in the photosynthetic membrane do not respond to the light-induced field. They behave like isolated molecules, the electrochromism of which varies quadratically with the field strength (36, 37).
2. A minor pool (10-30 %) of carotenoids is responsible for the light-induced electrochromism. This effect varies linearly with the field, a property which indicates that these carotenoid molecules have a component of permanent polarization perpendicular to the membrane. The permanent field (10^6 to 10^7 $V.cm^{-1}$) probably induces a red shift ($\sim$7 nm) of the absorption spectrum (29). It may have a different polarity in different bacterial species (38). It has been proposed that, in chloroplasts, the carotenoid polarization occurs through complexing with chlorophyll (39, 40).
3. In *Rhodopseudomonas* chromatophores the pigment-protein B 800-850 (or at least part of it) is responsible for the electrochromic shift (41, 42, 53). In chloroplasts, the field-sensitive carotenoids may be preferentially located close to the Photosystem-II reaction center (43).

This review is too short to discuss in detail the insertion of carotenoids in the photosynthetic membranes. The modes of approach are rather indirect and many questions are still pending. Some recent work, however, seems to indicate that there is a specific site for the binding of a carotenoid molecule in a pigment-protein complex (25, 44). This point is rather critical for future research, which should answer the questions of the structure of the binding site, the mode of binding, the structural relations between carotenoids and chlorophylls. The isolation of well-defined chlorophyll-carotenoid-protein complexes and the possibility of fixing a carotenoid on a complex from a carotenoidless mutant (2, 25, 6) will certainly be of great help for answering these questions.

LIGHT-HARVESTING FUNCTION : SINGLET-SINGLET ENERGY TRANSFER

It is well known that carotenoids function as accessory photosynthetic pigments, probably by a mechanism of singlet-singlet energy transfer :

$$\text{Car} \xrightarrow{h\nu} {}^1\text{Car}^* \qquad {}^1\text{Car}^* + (\text{B})\text{Chl} \longrightarrow \text{Car} + {}^1(\text{B})\text{Chl}^*$$

This role is manifested by a contribution of carotenoids to the action spectra of chlorophyll fluorescence (45, 46) or of photochemistry in intact organisms or in a large variety ofsub-organelles, including purified light-harvesting complexes and reaction centers. The yield of transfer varies greatly (from 0 to 100 %) from one material to another and from one carotenoid to another (see e.g. refs 2, 5, 6, 14, 45-48).

Energy transfer among photosynthetic pigments has been described in terms of physical theories, such as the dipole-dipole mechanism proposed by T. Förster. In this mechanism the yield of energy transfer from a donor D (here ^{1}Car*) to an acceptor A (chlorophyll) can be written as follows (49) :

$$\eta = \left(1 + \frac{R^6}{Bk^2\ \phi_D \Omega}\right)^{-1}$$

where R is the distance between D and A ; B is a constant ; k^2 is an orientation factor ; ϕ_D is the fluorescence yield of the donor in absence of the acceptor ; Ω is an overlap function, proportional to the spectral overlap between the emission of D and the absorption of A. In this formula, R is a key factor, but it is not well known. There is some hope to obtain a value for k^2, since there has been progress in the estimation of the relative orientations of chlorophylls and carotenoids in pigment-protein complexes (vide supra).

Most photosynthetic carotenoids are practically non-fluorescent and ϕ_D is probably smaller than 10^{-6}, based on attempts to measure fluorescence yields (50) and on picosecond resonance Raman experiments (51). The value of Ω is also not known, but it is probably not favorable. Recent work indicates that there may be a low-lying singlet state in β-carotene which may account for the low fluorescence yield and be involved in the energy transfer (52). Accepting a value $\phi_D = 10^{-6}$ and other conditions being optimum, Moore et al evaluated that $\eta = 0.5$ for $R = R_0 = 11$ Å (54). This value must be considered as an upper limit and it would be more realistic to accept a value of R_0 between 5 and 8 Å for the transfer between carotenoids and chlorophyll a. At these very short distances the dipole-dipole mechanism may be superseded by another mechanism of energy transfer, such as the electron exchange (Dexter) mechanism, as discussed by Razi Naqvi (49).

Thus, in despite of some progress, the mechanism of energy transfer from carotenoids to chlorophylls is still not well understood. A new and important tool for the research in this field is offered by the recent synthesis of covalently linked porphyrins and carotenoids, in which energy transfer takes place from the carotenoid to the porphyrin moiety (54, 55). The transfer yield varies with the geometry of the complex. It is also noteworthy that carotenoids may quench the fluorescence of chlorophyll or porphyrins in vitro (55, 56) ; thus it is necessary to understand the factors which favor the energy transfer over the wasteful quenching.The most general conclusion on this problem is that efficient energy transfer from carotenoids to chlorophylls probably requires that both molecules are kept in permanent close contact (<10 A) in a pigment-protein complex.

FUNCTION OF PROTECTION : THE TRIPLET STATE

Light is potentially harmful to all living organisms and it is a very general role of carotenoids to protect against photodamage. This function has been reviewed in detail (e.g. by Krinsky, 57) and we shall focus on recent results obtained in photosynthetic structures. The major photodamage takes place through singlet oxygen $^1O_2$; the destructive and protective processes involving chlorophyll (Chl) and carotenoids (Car) can be summarized as follows (the superscripts 1 and 3 refer to a singlet and a triplet state, respectively ; the star denotes an excited state) :

<u>Photodamage</u> :

$$^1Chl^* \xrightarrow{k_p} \text{Photochemistry}$$

$$\xrightarrow{k_F} Chl + h\nu \text{ (fluorescence)}$$

$$\xrightarrow{k_{ISC}} {}^3Chl^*$$

$$^3Chl^* + {}^3O_2 \longrightarrow Chl + {}^1O_2^*$$

$$^1O_2^* \longrightarrow \text{harmful oxidations}$$

<u>Protection</u> :

$$^3Chl^* + Car \longrightarrow Chl + {}^3Car^*$$

$$^1O_2^* + Car \longrightarrow {}^3O_2 + {}^3Car^*$$

$$^3Car^* \longrightarrow Car \text{ (radiationless conversion)}$$

The photodamage is thus supposed to be initiated by the triplet state of chlorophyll (we shall mostly consider chlorophyll <u>a</u>, but the situation is analogous with bacteriochlorophyll). In solution the rate k_{ISC} is about twice k_F. If the rates are the same <u>in vivo</u> and since the Chl fluorescence yield is 2-8 % in chloroplasts or algae, it can be assumed that the yield of ^3Chl formation is included between 4 and 16 %. Actual measurements agree with these values (58). This yield is relatively high and permits one to understand the rapid damage that occurs without carotenoids. Carotenoids exert their protection at a double level : by quenching $^3Chl^*$ and, in case of formation of $^1O_2^*$, by quenching that species. Both modes of quenching have been shown to occur with a high efficiency <u>in vitro</u> (57, see also 59).

<u>Properties of $^3Car^*$</u>

The triplet state of carotenoids remains relatively poorly known, for three main reasons ; its low energy level, its short lifetime and the fact that it cannot be populated by direct excitation. In general, direct excitation of carotenoids leads to non-radiative conversion to the ground state ; the lack of triplet state population is in agreement with the lack of fluorescence and with the very short $\leq 10^{-12}$ s) lifetime of the state $^1Car^*$. The triplet state can be populated by energy transfer from another triplet (like chlorophylls or aromatic hydrocarbons) or in the recombination of radicals produced by pulse radiolysis (60-64). A direct population of the triplet state has been reported with polyene derivatives (65). It has also been reported with carotenoids included in photosynthetic membranes or in detergent micelles (66, 67), under conditions where bimolecular processes may be favored.

The triplet state $^3Car^*$ has been mainly characterized by flash absorption spectroscopy. It possesses a strong absorption band in the visible (around 520 nm for β-carotene), the exact position of which varies greatly with the solvent and with the number of conjugated double bonds (59, 63, 68). The corresponding electronic transition is strongly allowed and is thus very probably from the lowest excited to a higher excited triplet state. The knowledge of the extinction coefficient of ^{3}Car* is of importance for quantitative studies but there is a tremendous variation among the published values. In a group of carotenoids with 9 to 11 conjugated double bonds, the values fall between 495,000 M^{-1} cm^{-1} for lycopene (69, determined by a quantitative analysis of pulse radiolysis data) and 9,500 M^{-1} cm^{-1} for spheroidene (48, in a light-harvesting complex). The pulse radiolysis experiments led to values of 420,000 and 29,000 M^{-1} cm^{-1}, respectively, for two closely related molecules : 7-7'dihydro-β-carotene and spheroidene (69). Flash photolysis measurements led to values in an average range : 62,000 or 191,000 for β-carotene in CS_2 or hexane (70). We believe that there are unrecognized systematic errors in these determinations and that these measurements should be repeated with a more critical eye.

The lifetime of ^{3}Car is in the microsecond range. It is shortened in the presence of oxygen (68). In the absence of oxygen, it is hardly affected by lowering the temperature (71). The lifetime is shorter for long chain than for short chain carotenoids (see Table and discussion in ref. 68). The short lifetime is certainly not determined by a radiative return to the ground state (phosphorescence) but rather by the rate of non-radiative intersystem crossing. A phosphorescence has not been reported for carotenoids. In the absence of this emission it is difficult to know the energy level of ^{3}Car* above the ground state, although this is a key factor in the protective mechanism which implies an energy transfer from ^{3}Chl* or from $^1O_2$* to carotenoid. The energy level of ^{3}Car* has been determined by indirect methods, based on the protective action and on the quenching of $^1O_2$* by carotenoids of different length (for a review, see ref. 57 ; more recent data, ref. 59).

TABLE

Spectroscopic and kinetic data for the lowest triplet state ^{3}Car* of β-carotene and of hydrocarbon analogs (adapted from ref. 68), in benzene at 23°C.

Number of conjugated double bonds	7	9	11	15	19
Absorption maximum (nm)	457	495	526	595	620
Lifetime (μs)	20	10	6	3.2	2.5
Rate of quenching by $^3O_2$ ($M^{-1}s^{-1}$)	$2.8x10^9$	$3.2x10^9$	$3.6x10^9$	$7.0x10^9$	$5.6x10^9$
Energy above ground state (cm^{-1})	8900	7200	6000	4700	3700

The triplet state ^{3}Car* has been studied recently by other spectroscopic methods : resonance Raman spectroscopy and electron paramagnetic resonance. Resonance Raman methods indicated that the β-carotene molecule may be twisted in the triplet state (72). The EPR spectrum of ^{3}Car* has been obtained in photosynthetic sub-organelles and *in vitro*, with β-carotene in detergent micelles or in lipid bilayers (67). Both types of study are just beginning and many developments may be expected.

In photosynthetic structures containing chlorophyll *a*, ^{3}Car* happens to be an efficient quencher of the fluorescence of chlorophyll *a* (71, 73-77). A similar phenomenon has been reported in bacterial chromatophores (78) but not in reaction centers (79).

In chromatophores the mechanism of this quenching has been shown to be singlet-triplet fusion (83, 78). A similar reaction may take place in green plant systems (71, 89). It is also possible that the quenching takes place by a rapidly reversible electron transfer reaction : $^3Car^* + {}^1Chl\ \underline{a}^* \longrightarrow Car^{+\cdot} + Chl^{\bar{\cdot}}\ \underline{a} \rightarrow Car + Chl\ \underline{a}$

Triplet-triplet energy transfer in vivo

In photosynthetic structures, the triplet state of (bacterio-) chlorophyll is populated by two mechanisms : by intersystem crossing from the excited singlet state in antenna complexes, or by the radical-pair mechanisms in reaction centers in which normal electron flow has been impeded. In both cases this is often followed by a triplet-triplet energy transfer to neighbouring carotenoids.

In bacterial reaction centers lacking a carotenoid the primary charge separation between the special pair of bacteriochlorophylls (P-870) and the initial acceptor (I) is followed, when forward electron transfer cannot operate, by several possible reverse electron transfer reactions :

$$P\text{-}870^+ \ldots I^- \longrightarrow {}^1P\text{-}870^*,\ {}^3P\text{-}870^*,\ P\text{-}870$$

These back-reactions produce both the singlet and the triplet excited states of P-870 as well as the ground state P-870. The triplet state of P-870, also named P^R, is formed with a rather high yield (≈15 %) and lasts for 6-100 μs. When carotenoids are present a rapid triplet-triplet energy transfer takes place, forming ^3Car (80, 81). The rate and the yield of formation of both ^3P-870* and ^3Car, under these conditions, are affected by temperature in a complex manner. In particular, energy transfer from ^3P-870* to Car is blocked below 20 K, maybe for energetic reasons (81). Detailed experiments by Boucher et al (6) established that the reaction center carotenoid exerts a protective role against photooxidations.

In the light-harvesting system of bacteria the triplet state $^3Car^*$ is also formed very rapidly (less than 20 ns) after a flash, probably at the expense of the triplet state of antenna bacteriochlorophylls (48, 82-84). This transfer is very probably related to the protective function (48). In higher plant chloroplasts and subchloroplast fractions, $^3Car^*$ is also formed very rapidly : the rate of transfer is about $8.10^7\ s^{-1}$ at 21°C and only slightly less at low temperature (58). There is some evidence for a transient formation of $^3Chl\ \underline{a}^*$, but it is not really compelling (58). ^3Car is formed in all types of sub-chloroplast fractions roughly in proportion to their chlorophyll fluorescence yield (71) and there is no evidence for a specific formation of $^3Car^*$ at the reaction center of Photosystem-I or II (71, 85). In greening material a long-lived chlorophyll triplet has been detected (86, 87). Under these conditions carotenoids do not sensitize the fluorescence of chlorophyll $\underline{a}$ (88) and the chlorophyll is known to be photolabile. This may indicate that carotenoids and chlorophylls are not yet incorporated together in the pigment-protein complexes. In chloroplasts and chromatophores it has been shown that, at high flash energy, only a small fraction of the carotenoids can go into the triplet state (less than 3 per reaction center) (70, 77, 78). It has been suggested that this indicates that triplet-triplet energy transfer occurs only at a limited number of sites. However a much larger fraction of carotenoid molecules can enter their triplet state in sub-organelle fractions (48, 71) and it is highly probable that the results obtained in complete organelles are due to the annihilation of excited states (singlet-singlet or singlet-triplet fusion).

DO CAROTENOIDS PLAY A ROLE IN ELECTRON TRANSFER ?

For a long time carotenoids have been implicated in photosynthetic electron transport. This view has been held predominantly by a small minority among the community of scientists devoted to the study of photosynthesis : the weakness of the experimental evidence did not permit a more general agreement. One of the reasons for the hypothesis is the possibility for conjugated polyenes to make charge-transfer complexes, for instance with iodine (90-92). Studies with oxygen-evolving systems also showed a cycle of interconversion among xanthophylls (violaxanthin, antheraxanthin and zeaxanthin) (93), which has been related to the mechanism of photosynthetic oxygen evolution. The participation of carotenoids in electron transfer was also advocated by Lundegardh who conducted parallel studies in vivo and in vitro and concluded that there was direct involvement of β-carotene in Photosystem-I (94). More recently it has been shown that removal of β-carotene from chloroplasts by extraction with organic solvents led to a loss of photochemical activity of Photosystem-II. The treatment also removes plastoquinones which are probably the key component in these experiments, although β-carotene seems to be required for the so-called C-550 shift (95 and other references therein). In relation with this possible association of carotenoids with Photosystem-II activity, it should be mentioned that an antiserum to lutein inhibits the electron transfer through that photosystem (96). A specific role of β-carotene in Photosystem-I has also been proposed recently on the basis of extraction experiments (97). It was found that complete removal of β-carotene leads to a nearly complete suppression of Photosystem-I photoactivity.

Apart from the formation of its triplet state, there has been only one well-defined photochemical reaction involving carotenoids in vitro : an electron donation from β-carotene or zeaxanthin to the flash-populated triplet state of toluidine blue (70, 98 ; see also ref. 99 for a study of the photooxidation of carotenoids). This system is rather complex since two types of reaction occur :

$$^{3}TB^{*} + Car \longrightarrow TB + {}^{3}Car^{*}$$

$$^{3}TB^{*} + Car \longrightarrow TB^{\overline{\cdot}} + Car^{\dagger}$$

In addition, toluidine blue and its photochemical products (^{3}TB, $TB^{\overline{\cdot}}$) have several protonation states and display a complex kinetic behaviour. The cation-radical $Car^{+\cdot}$ has a strong absorption band around 910 nm, with an extinction coefficient evaluated as 130,000 M^{-1} cm^{-1}. The long-wavelength absorption is approximately that predicted by comparison with other polyenic cations (98). Radical-cations and anions of β-carotene and of lycopene were also produced by pulse radiolysis (100) ; they both possess a strong absorption band in the near infra-red, at longer wavelength for the cation (∿ 1050 nm) than for the anion (820-950 nm). The species Car^{+} is able to oxidize chlorophyll a (101). This attests to the highly positive redox potential of the couple Car-Car^{+}, since the potential of the couple Chl a-Chl a$^{\pm}$ is about +0.8 V (102). Redox potential measurements have been carried out with β-carotene by polarography and the reported E_m is +0.87 V versus NHE (103).

Recently we were able to show that a carotenoid is oxidized to the radical-cation state at the reaction center of Photosystem-II. With chloroplasts the following observations were made (this work will be published elsewhere in greater detail) :

1. Excitation with short flashes induces an absorption increase in the near infra-red, with a well-defined peak around 990 nm and an absorption decrease around 500 nm.

This indicates the formation of $Car^{+\cdot}$ at the expense of the neutral species Car.

2. With untreated chloroplasts the signal size increases at low temperature. At 77 K about one $Car^{+\cdot}$ is formed in 10 % of the Photosystem-II centers by one flash and 2-3 times more by a 1 s irradiation with white light.
3. At room temperature, the $Car^{+\cdot}$ signal is dramatically increased when the chloroplasts are supplemented by chemicals such as ANT, FCCP or tetraphenylboron which are known to inhibit oxygen evolution. A single flash can then produce one $Car^{+\cdot}$ in about half of the centers. This large extent of signal is not observed in case of inhibition of oxygen evolution by Tris or by low pH.
4. The signals due to the formation of $Car^{+\cdot}$ are not formed when electron transfer through Photosystem-II is blocked by preillumination in the presence of DCMU or by addition of dithionite.
5. The formation of $Car^{+\cdot}$ is biphasic at 77 K : a small phase rises in less than 50 μs and a major phase with $t_{\frac{1}{2}}$ = 0.65 ms. This may correlate with a fraction of the decay of P-680$^+$ and indicate that Car donates an electron to P-680$^+$, but this point could not be firmly established. $Car^{+\cdot}$ is then stable over several seconds. At 21°C, with 40 μM tetraphenylboron, $Car^{+\cdot}$ is formed more rapidly ($t_{\frac{1}{2}}$≈20 μs) and decays in a few milliseconds. The re-reduction of $Car^{+\cdot}$ is accelerated by electron donors such as reduced dichlorophenolindophenol or benzidine.

Experiments with highly purified Photosystem-II particles (in collaboration with Drs B. Diner and K. Satoh) permitted a better spectroscopic and kinetic characterization of $Car^{+\cdot}$ and further established that $Car^{+\cdot}$ is formed in Photosystem-II. The species could not be detected in a light-harvesting complex or in Photosystem-I particles. In recent work (104), Velthuys also found that a carotenoid is bleached, probably by oxidation, upon excitation of chloroplasts in the presence of tetraphenylboron.

We have observed a large $Car^{+\cdot}$ signal only under conditions where the oxygen-evolving system is inhibited. A carotenoid bleaching has already been reported when chloroplasts are illuminated under oxidizing conditions, when oxygen evolution is blocked (e.g. ref. 105). $Car^{+\cdot}$ may be formed at the expense of oxidized species which would normally lead to oxygen evolution. It is also possible that $Car^{+\cdot}$ is a normal intermediate in electron transport between P-680 and the oxygen-evolving complex : its lifetime may be increased and it may become detectable after inhibitory treatments. Our experiments provide a firm basis for the association of carotenoids with primary reactions in Photosystem-II, although we still cannot decide whether they play a role under physiological conditions.

ACKNOWLEDGEMENTS

This work was supported in part by the Commission of European Communities (Solar Energy Program, Contract n° ESD-015-F).

REFERENCES

1. Cogdell, R.J. and Thornber, J.P., FEBS Lett. 122, 1-8 (1980)
2. Davidson, E. and Cogdell, R.J., Biochim. Biophys. Acta, 635, 295-303, (1981)
3. Vernon, L.P., Yamamoto, H.Y. and Ogawa, T., Proc. Nat. Acad. Sci. USA, 63, 911-917 (1969)
4. Alberte, R.S. and Thornber, J.P., FEBS Lett., 91, 126-130 (1978)
5. Cogdell, R.J., Parson, W.W. and Kerr, M.A., Biochim. Biophys. Acta, 430, 83-93 (1976)
6. Boucher, F., van der Rest, M. and Gingras, G., Biochim. Biophys. Acta, 461, 339-357 (1977)
7. Olson, J.M. and Thornber, J.P., "Photosynthetic reaction centers" in Membrane Proteins in Energy Transduction (R.A. Capaldi, ed.) pp. 279-340, Marcel Dekker, New York (1979)
8. Cogdell, R.J., Phil. Trans. Royal Soc. Lond., B 284, 569-579 (1978)
9. Markwell, J.P., Thornber, J.P. and Boggs, R.T., Proc. Nat. Acad. Sci. USA, 76, 1233-1235 (1979)
10. Thornber, J.P., Ann. Rev. Plant Physiol., 26, 127-158 (1975)
11. Thornber, J.P., Alberte, R.S., Hunter, F.A., Shiozawa, J.A. and Kan, K.S., Brookhaven Symp. Biol., 28, 132-148 (1976)
12. Boardman, N.K., Anderson, J.M. and Goodchild, D.J., Curr. Top. Bioenergetics, 8, part B, 35-109 (1978)
13. Anderson, J.M. and Goodchild, D.J., in The Biochemistry of Plants, 8 (M.D. Hatch and N.K. Boardman, eds) Academic Press (1981) (in press)
14. Song, P.S., Koka, P., Prézelin, B.B. and Haxo, F.T., Biochem., 15, 4422-4427 (1976)
15. Barrett, J. and Anderson, J.M., Biochim. Biophys. Acta, 590, 309-323 (1980)
16. Boardman, N.K. and Anderson, J.M., Biochim. Biophys. Acta, 143, 187-203 (1967)
17. Sétif, P., Acker, S. Lagoutte, B., Duranton, J., Photosynth. Res., 1, 17-27 (1980)
18. Vernon, L.P., Shaw, E.R., Ogawa, T. and Raveed, D., Photochem. Photobiol. 14, 343-357 (1971)
19. Wessels, J.S.C., van Alphen-van Waweren, O. and Voorn, G., Biochim. Biophys Acta, 292, 741-752 (1973)
20. Delepélaire, P. and Chua, N.H., Proc. Nat. Acad. Sci. USA, 76, 111-115 (1979)
21. Lichtenthaler, H.K. and Park, R.B., Nature, 198, 1070-1072 (1963)
22. Ji, T.H., Hess, J.L. and Benson, A.A., Biochim. Biophys. Acta, 150, 676-685 (1968)
23. Schwenker, U., St-Onge, M. and Gingras, G., Biochim. Biophys. Acta, 351, 246-260 (1974)
24. Lutz, M., Agalidis, I., Hervo, G., Cogdell, R. and Reiss-Husson, F., Biochim. Biophys. Acta, 503, 287-303 (1978)
25. Agalidis, I., Lutz, M. and Reiss-Husson, F., Biochim. Biophys. Acta, 589, 264-274 (1980)
26. Breton, J., Michel-Villaz, M. and Paillotin, G., Biochim. Biophys Acta, 314, 42-56 (1973)
27. Breton, J., Biochem. Biophys. Res. Comm., 59, 1011-1017 (1974)
28. Paillotin, G., Vermeglio, A. and Breton, J., Biochim. Biophys. Acta, 545, 249-264 (1979)
29. de Grooth, B.G., Thesis, University of Leiden (1980)
30. Becker, J.F., Breton, J., Geacintov, N.E. and Trentacosti, F., Biochim. Biophys. Acta, 440, 531-544 (1976)

31. Bolt, J. and Sauer, K., Biochim. Biophys. Acta, 546, 54-63 (1976)
32. Verméglio, A., Breton, J., Paillotin, G. and Cogdell, R., Biochim. Biophys. Acta, 501, 514-530 (1978)
33. Schaffernicht, H. and Junge, W., Photochem. Photobiol., (1981) (in press)
34. Junge, W., Ann. Rev. Plant Physiol., 28, 503-536 (1977)
35. Crofts, A.R., Prince, R.C., Holmes, N.G. and Crowther, D., in Proc. 3rd Intern. Congress Photosynthesis (M. Avron, ed.) pp. 1131-1146, Elsevier, Amsterdam (1974)
36. Schmidt, S. and Reich, R., Ber. Bunsengesell., 76, 1202-1208 (1972)
37. de Grooth, B.G., van Gorkom, H.J. and Meiburg, R.F., Biochim. Biophys. Acta, 589, 299-314 (1980)
38. Bowyer, J.R. and Crofts, A.R. Arch. Biochem. Biophys., 202, 582-591 (1980)
39. Sewe, K.U. and Reich, R., Z. Naturforsch., 32c, 161-171 (1977)
40. Sewe, K.U. and Reich, R., FEBS Lett., 80, 30-34 (1977)
41. Webster, G.D., Cogdell, R.J. and Gordon-Lindsay, J., Biochim. Biophys. Acta, 591, 321-330 (1980)
42. Holmes, N.G., Hunter, C.N., Niederman, R.A. and Crofts, A.R., FEBS Lett., 115, 43-48 (1980)
43. Conjeaud, H., Michel-Villaz, M., Verméglio, A. and Mathis, P., FEBS Lett., 71, 138-141 (1976)
44. Webster, G.D., Cogdell, R.J. and Lindsay, G.J., FEBS Lett., 111, 391-394 (1980)
45. Goedheer, J.C., Ann. Rev. Plant Physiol., 23, 87-112 (1972)
46. Duysens, L.N.M., Thesis, University of Utrecht (1952)
47. Goedheer, J.C., Biochim. Biophys. Acta, 172, 252-265 (1969)
48. Cogdell, R.J., Hipkins, M.F., McDonald, W. and Truscott, T.G., Biochim. Biophys. Acta, 634, 191-202 (1981)
49. Razi-Naqvi, K., Photochem. Photobiol., 31, 523-524 (1980)
50. Tric, C. and Lejeune, V., Photochem. Photobiol., 12, 339-343 (1970)
51. Dallinger, R.F., Woodruff, W.H. and Rodgers, M.A.J., Photochem. Photobiol., 33, 275-277 (1981)
52. Thrash, R.J., Fang, H.L.B, and Leroi G.E., J. Chem. Phys., 67, 5930-5933 (1978)
53. Scolnik, P.A., Zannoni, D. and Marrs, B.L., Biochim. Biophys. Acta, 593, 230-240 (1980)
54. Moore, A.L., Dirks, G., Gust, D. and Moore, T.A., Photochem. Photobiol., 32, 691-695, (1980)
55. Dirks, G., Moore, A.L., Moore, T.A. and Gust, D., Photochem. Photobiol., 32, 277-280, (1980)
56. Beddard, G.S., Davidson, R.S. and Trethewey, K.R., Nature, 267, 373-374 (1977)
57. Krinsky, N.I., Pure Appl. Chem., 51, 649-660 (1979)
58. Kramer, H. and Mathis, P., Biochim. Biophys. Acta, 593, 319-329 (1980)
59. Rodgers, M.A.J. and Bates, A.L., Photochem. Photobiol., 31, 533-537 (1980)
60. Chessin, M., Livingston, R. and Truscott, T.G., Trans. Farad. Soc., 522, 1519-1524 (1966)
61. Mathis, P., Photochem. Photobiol., 9, 55-63 (1969)
62. Land, E.J., Sykes, A. and Truscott, T.G., Photochem. Photobiol., 13, 311-320 (1971)
63. Bensasson, R., Land, E.J. and Maudinas, B., Photochem. Photobiol., 23, 189-193 (1976)

64. Jensen, N.H., Wilbrandt, R. and Pagsberg, P.B., Photochem. Photobiol., 32, 719-725 (1980)
65. Bensasson, R., Dawe, E.A., Long, D.A. and Land, E.J., J. Chem. Soc. (Faraday Trans. I) 73, 1319-1325 (1977)
66. Rademaker, H., Hoff, A.J., van Grondelle, R. and Duysens, L.N.M., Biochim. Biophys. Acta, 592, 240-257 (1980)
67. Frank, H.A., Bolt, J.D., Costa, S.M.B. and Sauer, K., J. Amer. Chem. Soc., 102, 4893-4898 (1980)
68. Mathis, P. and Kléo, J., Photochem. Photobiol., 18, 343-346 (1973)
69. Bensasson, R. and Land, E.J., Photochem. Photobiol. Rev., 3, 163-191 (1978)
70. Mathis, P., Thesis, University of Orsay (1970)
71. Mathis, P., Butler, W.L. and Satoh, K. Photochem. Photobiol., 30, 603-614 (1979)
72. Jensen, N.H., Wilbrandt, R., Pagsberg. P.B., Sillesen, A.H. and Hansen, K.B., J. Am. Chem. Soc., 102, 7441-7444 (1980)
73. Duysens, L.N.M., van der Schatte Oliver, J.E. and Den Haan, G.A., Abst. 6th Int. Congress Photobiology, (Bochum), 277 (1972)
74. Zankel, K.L., Biochim. Biophys. Acta, 325, 138-148 (1973)
75. Den Haan, G.A., Thesis, University of Leiden (1976)
76. Maroti, P. and Lavorel, J., Photochem. Photobiol., 29, 1147-1151 (1979)
77. Breton, J., Geacintov, N.E. and Swenberg, C.E., Biochim. Biophys. Acta, 548, 616-635 (1980)
78. Monger, T.G. and Parson, W.W., Biochim. Biophys. Acta, 460, 393-407 (1977)
79. Holmes, N.E., Van Grondelle, R. and Duysens, L.N.M., Biochim. Biophys. Acta, 503, 26-36 (1978)
80. Cogdell, R.J., Monger, T.G. and Parson, W.W., Biochim. Biophys. Acta, 408, 189-199 (1975)
81. Parson, W.W. and Monger, T.G., Brookhaven Symp. Biology, 28, 195-212 (1977)
82. Kung, M.C. and De Vault, D., Photochem. Photobiol., 24, 87-91 (1976)
83. Monger, T.G., Cogdell, R.J. and Parson, W.W., Biochim. Biophys. Acta, 449, 136-153 (1976)
84. Renger, G. and Wolff, C., Biochim. Biophys. Acta, 460, 47-57 (1977)
85. Satoh, K. and Mathis, P., Photochem. Photobiophys. (1981) (in press)
86. Krasnovsky, A.A., Lebedev, N.N. and Litvin, F.F., Studia Biophys., 65, 81-89 (1977)
87. Franck, F. and Mathis, P., Photochem. Photobiol. 32, 799-803 (1980)
88. Butler, W.L., Arch. Biochem. Biophys., 92, 287-295 (1961)
89. Breton, J. and Geacintov, N.E., FEBS Lett., 69, 86-89 (1976)
90. Platt, J.R., Science, 129, 372-374 (1959)
91. Lupinsky, J.H., J. Phys. Chem., 67, 2725-2728 (1963)
92. Ebrey, T.G., J. Phys. Chem., 71, 1963-1964 (1967)
93. Yamamoto, H.Y., Nakayama, T.O.M. and Chichester, C.O., Arch. Biochem. Biophys. 97, 168-173 (1962)
94. Lundegardh, H., Nature, 216, 981-985 (1967)
95. Knaff, D.B., Malkin, R., Myron, J.C. and Stoller, M., Biochim. Biophys. Acta, 459, 402-411 (1977)
96. Radunz, A. and Schmid, G.H., Z. Naturforschg., 28c, 36-44 (1973)
97. Searle, G.F. W. and Wessels, J.S.C., Biochim. Biophys. Acta, 504, 84-99 (1978)
98. Mathis, P. and Verméglio, A., Photochem. Photobiol., 15, 157-164 (1972)
99. Seely, G.R. and Meyer, T.H., Photochem. Photobiol., 13, 27-32 (1971)

100. Dawe, E.A. and Land, E.J., J.Chem. Soc. Faraday 1, 71, 2162-2169 (1975)
101. Lafferty, J., Land, E.J. and Truscott, T.G., J. Chem. Soc. Chem. Comm. 70-71 (1976)
102. Davis, M.S., Forman, A.. and Fajer, J., Proc. Nat. Acad. Sci. USA, 76, 4170-4174 (1979)
103. Mairanovsky, V.G., Engovatov, A.A., Ioffe, N.T. and Samokhavalov, G.I., J. Electro anal. Chem., 66, 123-137 (1975)
104. Velthuys, B.R., FEBS Lett., 126, 272-276 (1981)
105. Yamashita, K., Konishi, K., Itoh, M. and Shibata, K., Biochim. Biophys. Acta, 172, 511-524 (1969)

CAROTENOIDS AND HERBICIDE ACTION

Stuart M. Ridley

ICI Plant Protection Division, Jealott's Hill Research Station, Bracknell, Berkshire, England

Abstract - One of the most important functions of carotenoids in photosynthetic tissue is to protect the chloroplast against photo-oxidative damage. Interference with this function is an essential part of the mode of action of a range of herbicides, and is expressed in two principal ways : firstly, by blocking the synthesis of carotenoids in developing tissue, and secondly by inducing the destruction of pre-existing carotenoids in mature tissue. When there is an apparent direct inhibition of carotenoid synthesis, the desaturation reactions between phytoene and neurosporene are the major sites for herbicidal attack although in the absence of a direct enzyme assay the evidence for this is still essentially circumstantial. Herbicides of this type are of diverse structure but can be divided into two groups on the basis that they mainly cause a build up of either phytoene, or zeta-carotene; the activities of individual herbicides are discussed. Herbicides inducing destruction of pre-existing carotenoids act indirectly through inhibition of chloroplast electron transport and cause a breakdown of a photo-protection mechanism that is already operational. The results of a series of experiments have shown that the photodestruction of carotenoids (and subsequently, chlorophylls) is induced by the inhibition of cyclic electron flow around photosystem I and more specifically with the functioning of the reaction centre, P700. Photosystem I is a focal point for the dissipation of excess light energy and hence an essential protective mechanism (via the associated β-carotene) that herbicides destroy either directly by inhibiting carotenoid synthesis or indirectly by inhibiting electron transport.

INTRODUCTION

Carotenoids in photosynthetic tissues of plants are located in the chloroplasts, and about 50% of all herbicides interfere with the chloroplast in some way as part of their mode of action. So in reviewing carotenoids and herbicide action it will be necessary to consider not only herbicides that are believed to have a direct action on carotenoid synthesis but the discussion will also focus on the indirect effects of herbicides on carotenoids where this is thought to be an essential part of the overall mode of action. Unfortunately the distinction between what might appear to be a direct specific effect but what is in fact an indirect effect is not easily defined and this is further complicated because so many herbicides have more than one site of action. Consideration will be given initially to some general points relating to carotenoid inhibition, and then discussion will focus on experiments designed to look at the action of specific herbicides on carotenoid synthesis, and finally another important aspect of carotenoids and herbicide action will be discussed in which herbicides induce the destruction of pre-existing carotenoids.

CONSEQUENCES OF INHIBITING CAROTENOID BIOSYNTHESIS

It has been recognized for a long time from studies with various mutants (1) including those from higher plants (such as the maize mutants studied by Robertson *et al* (2)) that aberrations in carotenoid synthesis are usually lethal when the mutant is exposed to bright light. How the lethal effect is expressed in higher plants during growth depends on the particular site at which the lesion occurs, but the characteristic consequence is one of varying degrees of chlorosis. A similar situation arises when plants are treated with a variety of herbicides affecting carotenoid biosynthesis. The symptom of chlorosis is mainly brought about because the carotenoids cannot protect the chloroplast against what is known as the photodynamic effect, and this deficiency in protection is reckoned to be central to the mode of action of herbicides of this type.

Figure 1 summarizes in simple terms the way in which carotenoids protect against photo-oxidative damage in plants. When the light-harvesting chlorophylls receive more light energy than can be dissipated through the normal channels of the reaction centres and into the electron transport system, much of the excess energy is harmlessly removed by the carotenoids; β-carotene is mainly responsible for this (3). Under these saturating conditions part of the energy dissipation from excited chlorophylls is through ^{3}Chl. The chances of ^{3}Chl reacting with O_2 to produce the very reactive $^1O_2$ are limited to about 10% (4) so long as there is carotenoid in close association with the chlorophyll, because the quenching of ^{3}Chl by the carotenoid is so much faster than its reaction with O_2. During normal plant growth any $^1O_2$ produced will be quenched by the carotenoids, but following herbicide treatment, even when carotenoid synthesis is only partially inhibited, the probability of generating damaging amounts of $^1O_2$ will increase, and the extent of the damage will depend on the light intensity, or conversely, the extent of the protection will then depend not only on how much carotenoid is present but also on its specific location within the membrane with respect to the sensitized chlorophyll molecules. It will also depend, as studies with mutants have shown, on the site of the lesion in carotenoid synthesis because only carotenoids containing 9 or more conjugated double bonds can effectively quench $^1O_2$ (reviewed by Krinsky (5) & (6)).

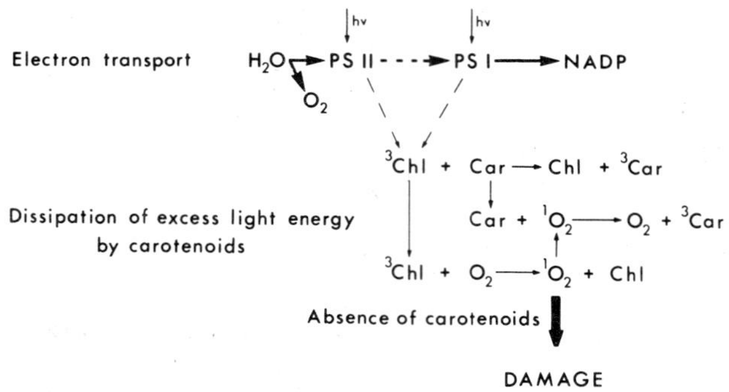

Fig. 1. A simplified scheme for the protection of photosynthesis by carotenoids against photo-oxidative damage.

So a complete inhibition of carotenoid synthesis is not necessary to produce a herbicidal state in which the $^1O_2$ generated can oxidize the membranes of chloroplasts and the components contained within them. This can be seen in the range of symptoms from yellow chlorosis through to white chlorosis that can be induced by different herbicides. The damage can be recorded by the production of malondialdehyde (7) or the generation of ethane (8) as well as by the photodestruction of chlorophyll itself. Feierabend and colleagues (9 & 10) measured destruction of ribosomal RNA and certain enzymes and it is interesting to note that catalase seems to be readily inactivated during photodestruction (9) even though the enzyme is located outside the chloroplast in the peroxisome.

As a more general observation at the whole plant level, the effectiveness of a herbicide that blocks carotenoid synthesis will also depend on the stage of growth at which it is applied. Treatment of plants which are still developing will produce chlorotic new growth but the herbicide will not affect existing green tissue where carotenoid synthesis has already taken place until the carotenoids turn over and have to be resynthesized. The effectiveness will also depend on the mobility characteristics of the compound within the plant because it must of course accumulate at the sites of carotenoid synthesis in sufficient concentration to be inhibitory. So there could be many compounds that possess an inherent ability to block carotenoid synthesis but which are not herbicidal. For the purpose of this paper only compounds that are truly herbicidal will be discussed.

HERBICIDES BELIEVED TO AFFECT CAROTENOID SYNTHESIS DIRECTLY

Of the herbicides that are believed to act by directly inhibiting carotenoid synthesis, Britton (11) has discussed three main potential processes that might by inhibited within the metabolic sequence from phytoene through to the formation of xanthophylls. These are shown in Fig. 2. Firstly, the desaturation reactions between phytoene and lycopene which are dependent on 'desaturase' enzymes. This sequence also includes an isomerization that occurs between phytoene and zeta-carotene (probably from cis- to trans-phytofluene) but there is no real evidence yet that this actually requires an isomerase which could be open to herbicide attack; secondly, the cyclization of lycopene and/or neurosporene ultimately giving α- and β-carotene; and thirdly the introduction of the oxygen function into xanthophylls.

It is perhaps not surprising that herbicides that are believed to interfere to a greater or lesser extent with carotenoid synthesis should do so at the desaturation reactions between phytoene and neurosporene because the number of conjugated double bonds in the intermediates that accumulate is below that which is needed to provide adequate protection (reviewed by Krinsky (6)).

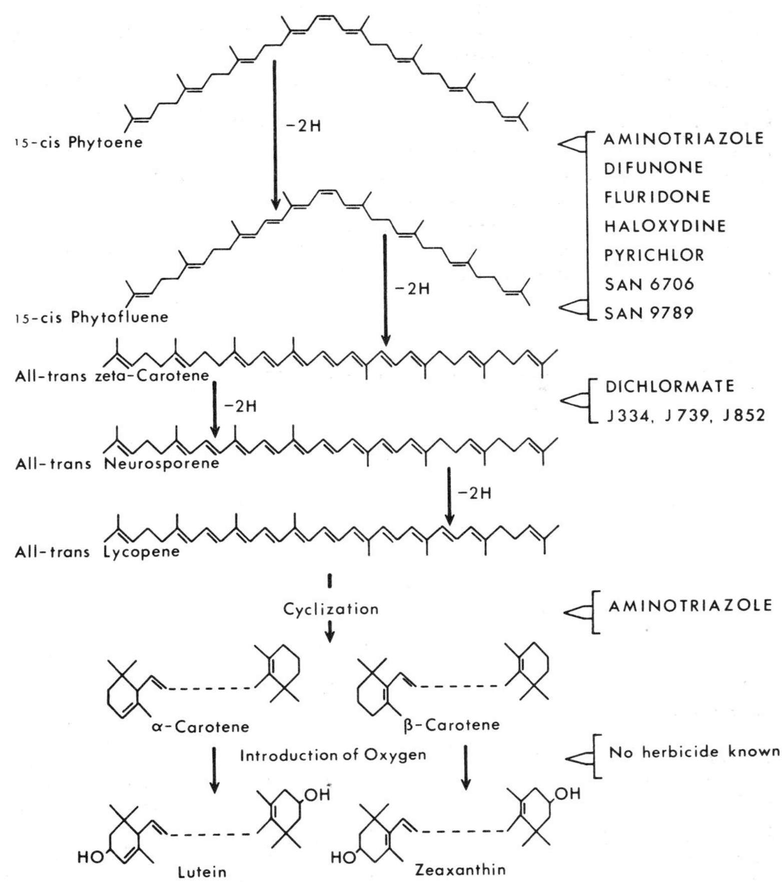

Fig. 2. An abbreviated sequence of the steps in the synthesis of carotenoids from phytoene (reviewed by Davies (12)), and the proposed sites of herbicidal attack.

In general these herbicides can be divided into two groups :

i) those that mainly cause a build up of phytoene, and
ii) those that mainly cause a build up of zeta-carotene.

However, other sites in this sequence (such as interference with cyclization) may also be affected in addition to interference with the desaturation reactions. The action of many of these herbicides will be discussed individually.

The evidence for inhibition of the desaturation reactions is circumstantial because it relies on the observed accumulation in pigment extracts of intermediates such as phytoene, phytofluene and zeta-carotene. As yet there is no specific *in vitro* assay for any of the 'desaturase' enzymes, and so long as this direct evidence is lacking the cause of the metabolite accumulation must be open to other interpretations. Doubtless this aspect will eventually be clarified to provide a more reliable basis for structure-activity studies, but now some experiments with individual chemical types that interfere with carotenoid synthesis will be discussed, starting with the substituted pyridazinone herbicides.

Substituted pyridazinones

These herbicides were introduced in the early 1960s and since then a lot of research has been done to establish the consequences of their action, much of it in fact in the last 5-6 years. They have also become widely used as research tools for studying carotenoids during chloroplast development (13, 14 & 15).

Within this series there are three principal biochemical mechanisms that are affected to different extents according to structure. Table 1 shows four of the most important structures and their relative effects on these biochemical processes.

TABLE 1. Structures and activities of some substituted pyridazinones. Carotenoids and polar lipids were extracted from wheat shoots following seed treatment and growth for 4 days under 28 klux light intensity. (Data calculated from St. John and Hilton (17) and given as percentage inhibition of the levels in untreated plants). Electron transport activity was recorded in isolated chloroplasts from barley (16) or pea (Ridley, unpublished).

			% Inhibition of synthesis in wheat by 100μM SAN 6706	
		Electron transport I_{50} (in vitro)	Linolenic acid	Carotenoid
Pyrazon	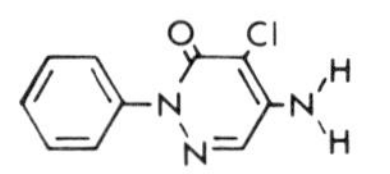	7μM	6	12
SAN 9785	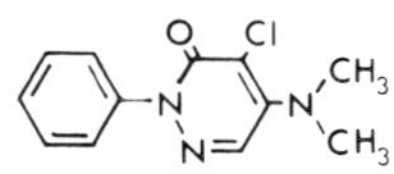	14μM	71	2
SAN 9789 (Norflurazon)	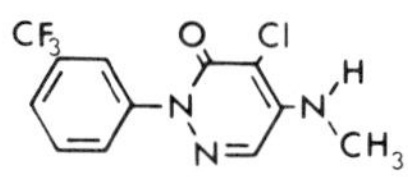	33μM	56	98
SAN 6706 (Metflurazon)	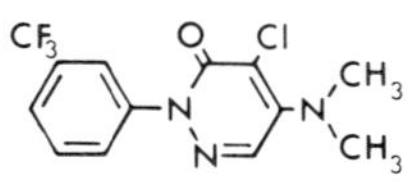	4μM	64	98

The three actions are:

Firstly, direct inhibition of electron transport in isolated chloroplasts. Pyrazon and SAN 6706 are the most effective (16) and it seems that the site of inhibition may be the same as that of DCMU (18), in other words close to the reducing side of photosystem II.

Secondly, St. John (19) has shown that the fatty acid composition in the lipids is altered which implies that there is an effect on the mechanism of fatty acid desaturation so as to produce more saturated fatty acids. Pyrazon is only very weakly active here while SAN 9785 is quite effective. St. John and Hilton (17) found that SAN 9789 did not inhibit linolenic acid formation in the dark suggesting that loss in the light is a secondary effect resulting from the lack of carotenoids since Takahama (21) has shown that carotenoids also protect lipids against photo-oxidation. However, SAN 6706 does show some direct effect on linolenic acid formation in the dark (17).

Thirdly, there is the inhibition of carotenoid synthesis which is associated mainly with an accumulation of phytoene. There is a much clearer division between structure and activity here. SAN 6706 and 9789 are potent inhibitors of carotenoid synthesis and produce a white chlorosis under glasshouse conditions while pyrazon and SAN 9785 are only weakly active (17 & 20). It seems that the trifluoromethyl substitution on the phenyl ring is a necessary requirement for carotenoid inhibition although at very high doses it is possible to induce chlorosis without the CF_3 group. In addition to this there is also a need for a methyl or dimethyl substitution on the amine because with the amine alone the compound is not active against carotenoid synthesis.

Pre-emergence treatment of plants with the electron transport inhibitor, pyrazon, or the fatty acid inhibitor, SAN 9785 does not produce the marked chlorotic action of SAN 6706 and 9789 which indicates that carotenoid synthesis inhibition is mainly responsible for the loss of chlorophyll, although the other sites of action may ultimately produce herbicidal effects. So only the action of either SAN 6706 or SAN 9789 will be considered in this paper.

The effects produced by these herbicides are dependent on the stage of growth at which they are applied. Plants grown in the dark synthesize mainly xanthophylls, so when seeds are germinated and grown in the dark in the presence of one of these inhibitors, (Table 2), it is mainly xanthophyll synthesis that is going to be inhibited (15, 22 & 23), and this is associated with a large accumulation of phytoene.

When untreated dark-grown plants are illuminated this triggers the conversion of etioplasts into active chloroplasts capable of fixing CO_2 within about 2 hr and is associated with large increases in the synthesis of carotenes and xanthophylls as well as the conversion of protochlorophyllide to chlorophyll. The effect of herbicide treatment on plants grown in the dark would appear to be specific for carotenoids because the plants in which carotenoid synthesis is impaired have normal prolamellar bodies in the etioplasts as shown by Pardo and Schiff (15) and by Walles (24) and contain the usual phototransformable chlorophyll precursors (15). When these plants are illuminated the observable effects depend on the light intensity used.

TABLE 2. Carotenoids in 6-day dark-grown wheat seed-treated with 100μM SAN 6706. (Data from Bartels and McCullough (22)).

	CONTROL	100 μM SAN 6706
	μg/g fresh wt	
CAROTENES	13·0	0·1
XANTHOPHYLLS	53·0	0·3
PHYTOENE	0	43·0
PHYTOFLUENE	0	2·4

This is shown in Table 3 in which 6-day etiolated wheat has been illuminated for 12 hours under high and low light. Under the low light of 10 lux where carotenoid synthesis is inhibited by about 95%, chlorophyll is formed to a level which is about 70% of the control, but under the high illumination of 15,000 lux, chlorophyll is less than 20% of the control. So this certainly suggests that the bulk of the chlorophyll loss is through photodestruction due to the absence of carotenoid, but there is perhaps some other factor also involved which is not entirely a consequence of photodestruction since Bartels and Hyde (25) have shown that grana stacking in the chloroplast tends to be inhibited as well even under low light.

TABLE 3. Effects on pigment formation when 6-day dark-grown wheat is illuminated for 12 hours under low or high light intensity; wheat was seed-treated with 100μM SAN 6706. (Data from Bartels and Hyde (25)).

μg/g fresh wt

	6-days dark		+ 12hr 10lux		+ 12hr 15,000 lux	
	Chl	Carot	Chl	Carot	Chl	Carot
CONTROL	0	75	55	48	62	40
SAN 6706 (100 μM)	0	3	41	2	11	1

This type of experiment with seed-treated plants can only tell us that both xanthophyll and carotene synthesis is inhibited, that phytoene accumulates, and that chlorophyll loss under high light is most probably due to photodestruction. It is possible to get further information from whole plants on how these carotenoid inhibitor herbicides act by treating the plants at a different stage of growth. As we have seen, plants grown in the dark for 6 days accumulate mainly xanthophylls, so if the treatment of dark-grown plants with SAN 6706 is delayed until the end of the period of dark growth but shortly before a period of illumination, it will be the light-dependent synthesis of β-carotene that will be mainly inhibited.

Figure 3 shows this in an experiment with etiolated barley treated before the start of illumination with 100μM SAN 6706. There is a complete inhibition of light-dependent β-carotene synthesis but the synthesis of xanthophylls does not appear to be inhibited until about 8 hours after the start of illumination. Mainly phytoene accumulates but this increases further after about 8 hours at the same time as xanthophyll synthesis is halted. So what we are seeing in this experiment is a differential effect on the synthesis of carotene and xanthophyll. One possible explanation is that there are separate groups of enzymes for the synthesis of the two carotenoid types, SAN 6706 only being accessible to one of these during the first 8 hours of illumination.

The idea can be supported through experiments that make use of the two major activities of SAN 6706, namely as an inhibitor of carotenoid synthesis and an inhibitor of electron transport, and we can do this by looking at the rates of photosynthesis in treated and untreated leaves during the period of illumination. In Fig. 4, 6-day etiolated barley seedlings have been treated before illumination with 100μM SAN 6706, and the rates of photosynthesis in whole leaves monitored at intervals. It can be seen that photosynthesis is unaffected by the treatment, except for an initial lag of 5-6 hours. (The lag is only an apparent one since it is related to a delay in the formation of Chl b and grana stacking so that the measuring light intensity became less than saturating (14)).

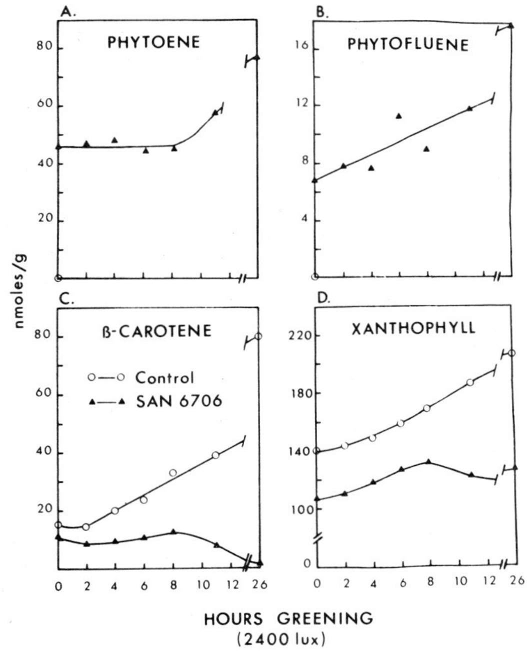

Fig. 3. Accumulation of carotenoids in barley shoots greening at 2400 lux following 6-days dark growth. Twelve hours before the start of illumination plants were treated with 100μM SAN 6706 (14).

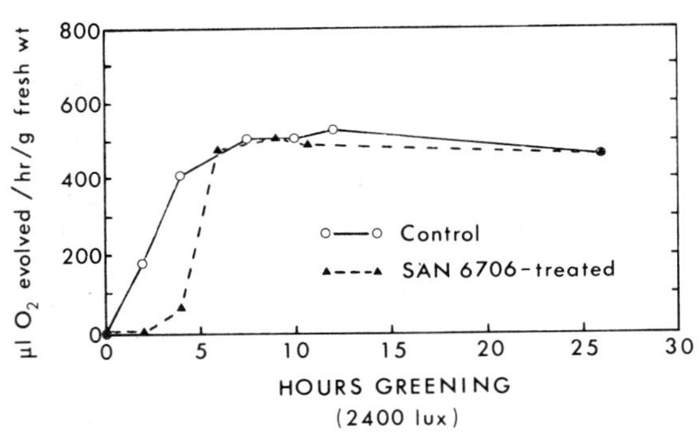

Fig. 4. Development of photosynthetic activity during greening of 6-day dark-grown barley shoots under 2400 lux illumination (14).

SAN 6706 inhibits electron transport in isolated chloroplasts with an I_{50} of 4μM, and yet treatment of leaves with 100μM SAN 6706 that causes complete inhibition of light-induced β-carotene synthesis fails to inhibit photosynthesis. This strongly suggests that SAN 6706 does not get into the chloroplast to block electron transport and so must be inhibiting carotenoid synthesis from the cytoplasm. The finding provides an explanation for the differential effects on carotenes and xanthophylls, because if the enzyme in xanthophyll synthesis which SAN 6706 inhibits is already present inside the etioplast at the time the herbicide is applied, it will not be inhibited until the enzyme turns over and has to be resynthesized in the cytoplasm. But if that enzyme for the light-dependent synthesis of the bulk of β-carotene is made de novo in the cytoplasm, it can be immediately inhibited at the start of illumination. Because these herbicides cause phytoene to accumulate it implies that the enzyme in question is phytoene 'desaturase', and its de novo synthesis is under phytochrome control, but Grumbach and Drollinger (28) and Jabben and Deitzer (29) have established that these herbicides do not interfere directly with the phytochrome system.

So there are two concepts here that arise from these studies with this pyridazinone herbicide. Firstly, that the herbicide does not get into the chloroplast but inhibits carotenoids from the cytoplasm, and secondly, that there are two separate groups of enzymes for the synthesis of carotenes and xanthophylls.

There is supportive evidence for these concepts from Dr Grumbach and colleagues (26, 27 & 28) at Karlsruhe who have shown that inhibition of cytoplasmic protein synthesis by cycloheximide completely prevents the bleaching effect of SAN 6706. The precise reason for this is not known but it does demonstrate that the bleaching effect is developed outside the chloroplast. The same group have also concluded from studies with the incorporation of radiolabelled mevalonate and acetate that β-carotene is synthesized by two independent biosynthetic pathways, one of which produces the xanthophylls. Retrospectively, this has perhaps been evident for a long time in mutants such as the yellow Helianthus annuus that lacks β-carotene and yet contains xanthophylls (30).

Other interpretations of the causes of chlorophyll loss induced by these herbicides have been put forward as alternatives to the idea of a simple block in carotenoid synthesis followed by photo-oxidation. Lichtenthaler and Kleudgen (31) have suggested that SAN 6706 blocks both chlorophyll and carotenoid formation due to interference with a basic mechanism common to both, and have speculated that the site may be the formation of chloroplast ribosomes. Kleudgen (32) later raised the possibility that the cytoplasmic ribosomes may be the common site because of the evidence that SAN 6706 does not get into the chloroplasts (14). It seems that the experimental conditions that have led to any of the alternative ideas do not completely eliminate the photo-oxidative effect and so complicate the interpretations. The maximum potential effect on carotenoid synthesis develops when plants are seed-treated, and if they are also illuminated continuously during growth then only at very low light intensity will it be possible to prevent photodestruction with a consequent chain of secondary effects. Even if these herbicides are studied using algae grown heterotrophically (33) so that chlorophyll synthesis occurs in the dark, complications arise because chlorophyll synthesis is closely regulated by carotenoid synthesis (34) which is not true of higher plants (13 & 14). So what is needed is a more direct in vitro assay to be confident about what is really the primary action. The current weight of evidence is perhaps in favour of a direct rather than an indirect action of these herbicides on the desaturation enzymes of carotenoid synthesis.

There is one further point that needs to be discussed which relates to the consequences of carotenoid inhibition. When etiolated plants are treated and then illuminated, the inhibition of light-induced carotenoid synthesis means that the bulk of β-carotene will not be formed, and yet photosynthesis appears fully operational as seen in Fig. 4. This suggests that the bulk of β-carotene is not necessary for chloroplast development, but so long as the light intensity is not too high, the small amount formed in the dark before herbicide treatment is adequate to provide protection and allow photosynthesis to develop; (the extent to which the xanthophylls are involved in protection under these conditions is not really known). β-Carotene is known to associate with photosystem I (35), but if we look at the photosystem I reaction centre complex (the P700-Chl a protein, CPI) isolated at intervals during chloroplast development from treated and control plants (Fig. 5), we can see that there is no difference in the ratio of β-carotene to P700 during that period. This means that even when β-carotene is severely limited, (but not completely absent) there is a favoured association between β-carotene and the P700 complex which is particularly essential because the long wavelength chlorophylls of photosystem I are extremely photosensitive when carotenoids are completely absent (36). This has led to the general concept that the close association of β-carotene with these reaction centre chlorophylls provides an essential mechanism for energy dissipation since the energy migration in the chlorophyll complexes is directed towards the longer wavelength forms as proposed by Seely (37). Junge and coworkers (38) have also established that the configuration of β-carotene within photosystem I is most favourable for such a protective role.

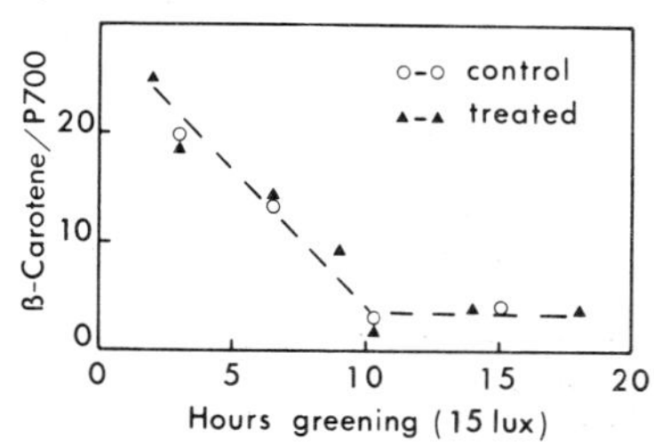

Fig. 5. The changing ratio of β-carotene to P700 in the P700-Chl a complex isolated at intervals during greening of 6-day etiolated barley under low light following treatment of shoots with 100μM SAN 6706 12 hours before the start of illumination (14).

So where there is less than total inhibition or destruction of carotenoid, as might be found with herbicides of weaker activity, or under lighting conditions that induce only moderate photodestruction, any β-carotene associated with photosystem I will provide a measure of protection which might delay the herbicidal effect or, in an extreme case, even allow the plant to recover. Therefore, an active photosystem I is likely to be an essential part of the overall protection mechanism for the plant. Another aspect of this is discussed later, but consideration will now be given to some other chemical types that are believed to inhibit carotenoid synthesis directly.

Fluridone

The structure of fluridone is shown in Table 4 and is compared with the structure and activity of one of the pyridazinone carotenoid inhibitors. Fluridone produces white chlorosis under glasshouse conditions just like the two active pyridazinones. Bartels and Watson (39) reported an accumulation of phytoene together with smaller amounts of phytofluene in pre-emergence-treated wheat, but small amounts of zeta-carotene can also be found (Table 4).

TABLE 4. A comparison between the structure and activity of fluridone and the pyridazinone herbicide SAN 6706. Barley seeds (25/sample) were treated with 20ml of 0.5μM fluridone or 0.5μM SAN 6706, and grown at 22°C for 7 days under low red light filtered through ICI Perspex No. 400 and giving 2μE/m²/sec. Shoots were harvested and extracted as in (14). (Ridley, unpublished data).

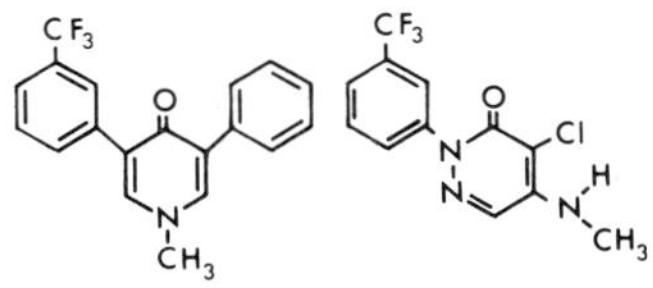

	CONTROL	FLURIDONE	SAN 6706
		nmoles/g	
PHYTOENE	0	279	286
PHYTOFLUENE	0	36	41
ZETA-CAROTENE	0	3	4
ß-CAROTENE	40	21	13
XANTHOPHYLLS	138	47	19

Also like the pyridazinones, the removal of the CF_3 group greatly diminishes its ability to inhibit carotenoid synthesis. A major difference between these two herbicides is that fluridone does not inhibit electron transport in isolated chloroplasts whereas SAN 6706 and 9789 do. Since fluridone is a relatively new herbicide there have been no reports of effects on metabolic processes other than carotenoid synthesis, but it is certainly one of the most potent carotenoid inhibitors discovered so far. Although it appears rather less active than SAN 6706 in Table 4 this is because it translocates less well by seed treatment so that the shoot tips are not affected. Figure 6 shows a Dixon plot for the inhibition of light-induced β-carotene synthesis when etiolated barley is treated and then illuminated for 10 hours. Fifty percent inhibition is given by less than 1μM and this is more potent than SAN 6706 under the same conditions.

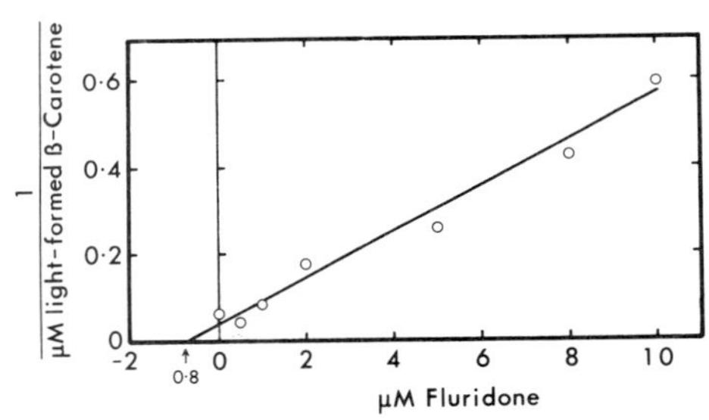

Fig. 6. A Dixon plot for the inhibition of light-induced β-carotene synthesis by fluridone. Six-day etiolated barley was sprayed with varying doses of fluridone 8 hours before illumination at 380 lux for 10 hours at 23°C. (Ridley, unpublished data).

Difunone

Difunone has a very different structure from the pyridazinone herbicides (Table 5) yet it also blocks carotenoid synthesis causing a large accumulation of phytoene with much smaller accumulations of phytofluene and zeta-carotene. Urbach and co-workers (20) initially reported the build up of intermediates in algae but Table 5 shows this also in a higher plant with the accumulation of phytoene being massive, so in spite of the apparent marked difference in structure in comparison with the pyridazinones and fluridone, difunone is probably acting at the same point. As with the other carotenoid inhibitors, chlorophyll is formed under low light (10), but Hampp and colleagues (40) have reported that difunone inhibits chlorophyll synthesis directly in a higher plant through interference with the activity of porphobilinogenase. Kunert and Boger (41) disputed this in studies with algae where they showed that chlorophyll loss is entirely due to carotenoid inhibition. Furthermore, difunone does not inhibit electron transport in isolated chloroplasts but, again, effects on other metabolic processes have not yet been reported.

TABLE 5. Structure of difunone and activity on barley seed-treated with 50μM and grown under low light (15 lux) for 6 days. (Ridley, unpublished data).

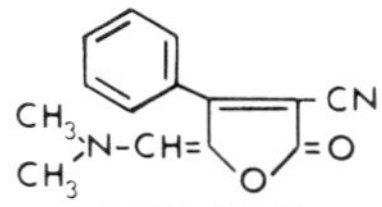

	CONTROL	DIFUNONE
	nmoles/g	
Phytoene	0	467
Phytofluene	0	26
Zeta-carotene	0	1
β-Carotene	28	3

4-Hydroxypyridines

The original herbicide of this type was pyriclor (2,3,5-trichloro-4-hydroxypyridine) which was introduced in 1965. As a chlorosis inducer, Burns et al (42) showed that it primarily blocks carotenoid synthesis causing a build up of phytoene, phytofluene and zeta-carotene and there was no direct action on chlorophyll synthesis. More recently some other 4-hydroxy pyridines have been examined and again, like the pyridazinones, these show interesting structure-activity features, but there are two main observable symptoms within the group : chlorosis, and stunting.

TABLE 6. A comparison of structures and activities of 4-hydroxy pyridines. Chlorophylls and carotenoids were extracted from oat seedlings (as in (14)) following pre-emergence treatment and growth under glasshouse conditions for 8 days (light : 100μE/m^2/sec, on an 18 hour day at 23°C). I_{50} values for inhibition of chloroplast electron transport were obtained from a ferricyanide - Hill reaction using isolated pea chloroplasts. (Ridley, unpublished data).

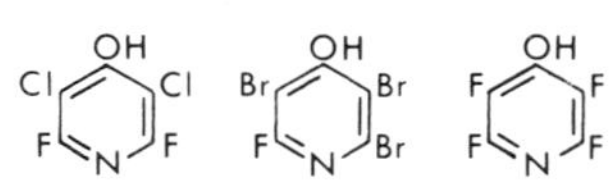

	Control	Haloxydine 0·25 Kg/ha	J 771 2·0 Kg/ha	J 481 2·0 Kg/ha
		nmoles/g		
Phytoene	0	614	99	0
Phytofluene	0	40	13	0
Zeta-Carotene	0	22	15	0
α- and β-Carotene	96	40	41	131
Xanthophylls	134	31	120	219
Chlorophylls	1068	149	701	1087
Electron transport I_{50}, μM		43	0·15	not active

Table 6 shows three closely related structures together with their effects on carotenoid synthesis during growth of oat seedlings under glasshouse conditions following pre-emergence treatment; their potency on electron transport in isolated chloroplasts is also given. The three compounds differ only in the combination of halogens around the ring. Haloxydine and J771 both inhibit carotenoid synthesis but haloxydine is more potent. There is a very large accumulation of phytoene with significant but smaller amounts of phytofluene and zeta-carotene. Although haloxydine has been applied (pre-emergence) at a low dose in this experiment, it seems to be a characteristic of the 4-hydroxy pyridines that the chlorosis tends to leave the shoots yellow, rather than white as it does with the pyridazinones. This implies that carotenoid inhibition is never complete but there is always some present that may provide a measure of protection, which could explain the reduced secondary effects on the activities of a number of enzymes that Feierabend and co-workers (9 & 10) reported, but in spite of this incomplete inhibition, Dodge and Lawes (43) showed that the general disruption of the membranes in chloroplasts from haloxydine-treated plants is still apparent in electron micrographs.

J771 is a potent inhibitor of electron transport in isolated chloroplasts but in spite of this the symptoms are more characteristic of a weak carotenoid inhibitor than of a Hill reaction inhibitor. It is quite possible that J771, like SAN 6706, fails to get into the chloroplast to exert this particular inhibition and so can be discounted as part of the overall mode of action. Substituting the two chlorines in haloxydine for two fluorines completely changes the mode of action as can be seen in plants treated with J481. There is no inhibition of carotenoid synthesis or chloroplast electron transport, but the plants are markedly stunted so the pigment levels on a fresh weight basis are raised above those in the control. The stunting is caused by action at a site that has not yet been characterized and it may be inherent in the action of the 4-hydroxypyridines generally because high doses of haloxydine and J771 also cause stunting in seedlings that are still using their seed reserves.

Aminotriazole

In the correct historical sequence, the herbicide aminotriazole (structure shown in Fig. 7) should have been considered first because reports on the compound appeared as long ago as 1953. It has been subjected to much research since that time to elucidate the primary mode of action, but it was not until 1971 that Burns *et al* (42) reported on its ability to inhibit carotenoid synthesis in dark grown plants. It is now more or less accepted that inhibition of carotenoids is the major mechanism whereby herbicidal effects are induced and accounts for most of the other inhibitions reported in aminotriazole-treated plants grown in the light (reviewed by Carter (44)) because of the consequent photo-oxidative destruction in the absence of carotenoids.

Burns *et al* (42) found that aminotriazole induced a build up only of phytoene, phytofluene and zeta-carotene in wheat while Rüdiger *et al* (46) found lycopene to be the major carotenoid intermediate to accumulate in the same species.

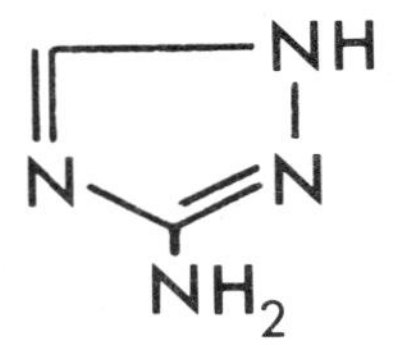

Fig. 7. Structure of aminotriazole (amitrole).

Lycopene was also noted by Guillot-Salomon *et al* (45) in aminotriazole-treated maize, and Grumbach (47) reported a specific inhibition of lycopene cyclization in radish seedlings. So here we have another structure that seems to interfere with the desaturation reactions (and lycopene cyclization as well) and yet seems to be structurally quite different from the other herbicides that are believed to act at the same point. The inhibition of carotenoids is incomplete in aminotriazole-treated plants grown under low light so that a subsequent exposure to bright light only slowly causes chlorophyll to bleach (10). Certainly if lycopene (with 11 conjugated double bonds) accumulates, this should continue to provide a significant degree of quenching of photo-oxidation and the protection may account for the weaker inhibition of some enzymes during illumination by aminotriazole found by Feierabend and Schubert (9) when compared with herbicides such as SAN 6706 and difunone.

Blockers of Zeta-Carotene Desaturation

The second general group of compounds that appear to inhibit carotenoid synthesis directly are those that mainly induce a build-up of zeta-carotene. The only herbicide about which there is published information is the N-methyl carbamate, dichlormate (42), but fairly recently another group has been discovered at Jealott's Hill which seems to act in the same way and yet appears to be structurally unrelated. These are substituted 6-methyl pyrimidines.

Figure 8 shows the structures together with some comparative histograms of total β-carotene and zeta-carotene accumulation in barley shoots after low light illumination of etiolated leaves treated with 0.1mM inhibitor. On the basis of zeta-carotene accumulation it can be seen that the two pyrimidines are more active than dichlormate, and the level of β-carotene diminishes as the zeta-carotene increases.

It is interesting to note in some of the experiments discussed in this paper that herbicides can cause a build up of an intermediate that is vastly in excess of the amount of end products (carotene and xanthophyll) in the control plants. This is seen with the build up of phytoene by fluridone and SAN 6706 (Table 4), and by difunone (Table 5) and haloxydine (Table 6), and the accumulation of zeta-carotene by J852 (Fig. 8). When β-carotene synthesis is inhibited it may at the same time remove a feed-back inhibition of one of the enzymes further back in the terpenoid pathway and so allow synthesis to proceed unchecked up to the point of the herbicide block. This by itself gives strong circumstantial evidence that the herbicides are interfering with the desaturation reactions directly, but with the build up of zeta-carotene (seen in Fig. 8) we can at least attempt to check this further by applying another herbicide assumed to block further back in the pathway, at the same time as applying one of the herbicides assumed to block zeta-carotene desaturation. The object would be to see if zeta-carotene accumulation could be diminished.

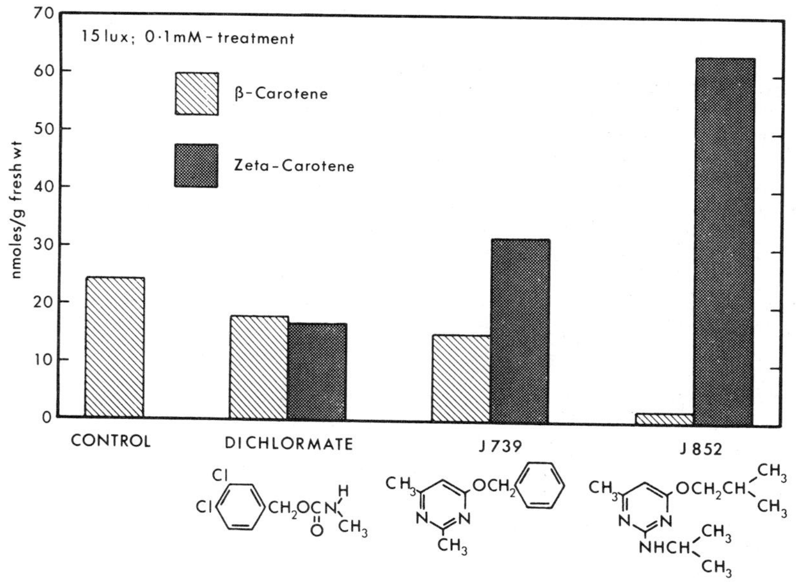

Fig. 8. Structures and activities of herbicides that induce a build up of zeta-carotene in plants. Seven-day etiolated barley was treated with 0.1mM compound 12 hours before illuminating with low light (15 lux) for 8 hours. β-Carotene is shown as the total at the end of the experiment; (7 nmoles/g were formed in the control before illumination). The very low level of β-carotene in the J852-treated shoots may have been caused by a complete inhibition of carotenoid synthesis at a time when the 'turnover' of β-carotene was quite rapid. (Ridley, unpublished data).

TABLE 7. Effects of fluridone on the accumulation of zeta-carotene in barley seedlings induced by J334. Conditions as in TABLE 4 except for the use of slightly higher light (5μE/m^2/sec). (Ridley, unpublished data).

	Control	J334 (20μM)	Fluridone (0·5μM)	J334 + Fluridone
	nmoles/g			
Phytoene	0	78	182	209
Phytofluene	0	30	25	48
Zeta-carotene	0	117	1	45
ß-Carotene	37	17	18	5
Xanthophylls	208	57	73	25

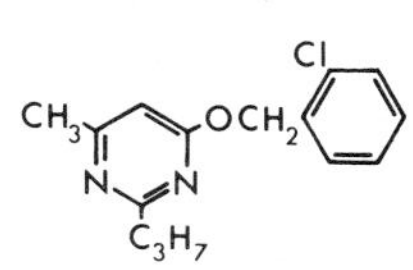

J334

In the experiment in Table 7, barley has been seed-treated and grown under low light, and we have used fluridone to try and block zeta-carotene accumulation caused by the 6-methyl pyrimidine, J334. It can be seen that the zeta-carotene level is greatly diminished and at the same time there is a large accumulation of phytoene. So this encourages the belief that these compounds are acting directly on the desaturation enzymes, but no attempt has been made in this paper to rationalize the structural diversity of herbicides that exhibit common features in their action.

HERBICIDE-INDUCED DESTRUCTION OF PRE-EXISTING CAROTENOIDS

Finally I want to turn to a rather different aspect of carotenoids and herbicide action and discuss a series of experiments relating to the herbicide-induced destruction of carotenoids which have already been synthesized in developing or developed plant shoots. In effect, this means a herbicide-induced breakdown of a photo-protection mechanism that already exists, so this must be regarded as an essential part of the mode of action of those herbicides that can do it.

The photodestruction of pre-existing chlorophyll is a characteristic symptom of herbicides such as DCMU (diuron) that block chloroplast electron transport close to photosystem II. We can do experiments to simulate this in vitro using isolated intact chloroplasts treated with herbicide (48, 49), and the sequence of events which bring about the photodestruction can then be examined in some detail.

Figure 9 shows an experiment in which DCMU is incubated with intact chloroplasts and illuminated for 24 hr during which time the pigment levels are monitored. The main feature here is the greater and more rapid loss of carotenoids over that of the chlorophylls, and the carotenoid loss actually begins about an hour before the loss of chlorophyll as previously shown by Stanger and Appleby (48) and Ridley (49). So what we are seeing are the conditions in which DCMU is inducing the photodestruction of the carotenoids and because the protective mechanism is being removed, there is a subsequent photodestruction of chlorophylls. Of course the photodestruction does not stop at the chlorophylls because lipid peroxidation occurs at the same time leading to membrane destruction as shown by Pallett and Dodge (50), and all of this ultimately produces the herbicidal state. When experiments such as that in Fig. 9 are done in vessels flushed with nitrogen, no destruction of pigments occurs.

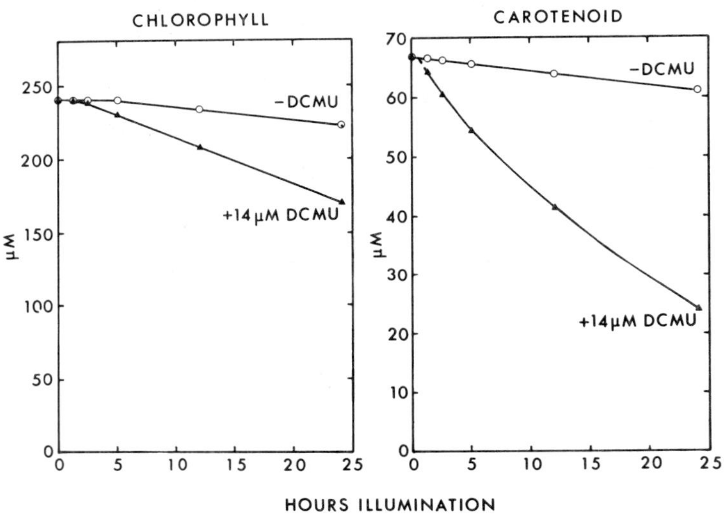

Fig. 9. Photodestruction of pigments induced by DCMU in isolated intact chloroplasts illuminated at 14,000 lux, 20°C. Conditions were the same as previously reported by Ridley (49) except that 0.1% bovine serum albumin was added to the chloroplast resuspension medium which provided a considerable degree of protection against the photo-induced destruction of pigments in the controls. The final concentration of chlorophyll in the chloroplast suspension was 240μM.

We can look at the photodestruction in more detail to see how the individual pigments are affected by the DCMU action. Table 8 shows a gross pigment analysis of chloroplasts illuminated for 20 hours in the presence and absence of DCMU. It can be seen that the greatest loss occurs with carotene, which is mainly β-carotene, but the xanthophylls are destroyed to the same extent as Chl a, and the pigment least affected is Chl b (49). So it is probably the initial loss of protection by β-carotene that is mainly responsible for the loss of the other pigments.

What is it that induces β-carotene to be destroyed? Is it simply the inhibition of electron transport with the consequent 'over-loading' of the protection mechanisms or is there some other essential process being inhibited at the same time? To try and answer this question it has been necessary to establish just what is happening with the electron transport system itself and to relate this to the pigment loss during illumination. To do this, a series of experiments has been put together in which DCMU dose-responses for the inhibition of three different processes have been recorded as far as possible under similar conditions using intact chloroplasts or freshly ruptured chloroplasts.

TABLE 8. Changing concentrations of pigments in chloroplast suspensions illuminated for 20 hours in the presence and absence of 5μM DCMU (49).

	Chl a	Chl b	Carotene	Chl a/Carotene	Xanthophylls	Chl a/Xanth
	μM		μM		μM	
− DCMU	141	68	15	9:1	31	5:1
+ DCMU	80	52	4	20:1	17	5:1

The results are shown in Fig. 10. The three processes looked at were : firstly, coupled non-cyclic electron transport measured as O_2 evolution with ferricyanide as the electron acceptor; secondly, cyclic electron transport measured indirectly by the incorporation of ^{14}C-leucine, which makes use of ATP from cyclic phosphorylation (51), and so is an indirect measure of cyclic electron flow itself (the addition of ATP can reverse this inhibition so the protein synthesis mechanism itself is not being inhibited, only the production of ATP); and thirdly, the photodestruction of pigments during 24 hours illumination. Because the DCMU inhibition varies with the chlorophyll concentration the amount of chlorophyll was kept the same (200μM) for all three processes.

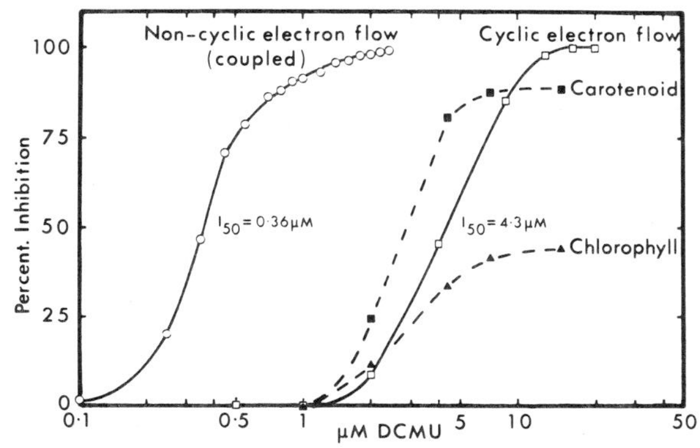

Fig. 10. Dose responses for the effects of DCMU on cyclic and non-cyclic electron transport, and on pigment photodestruction during 24 hours illumination. Coupled non-cyclic electron transport was recorded as O_2 evolution (Hansatech electrode) in a medium (1ml) containing 330mM-sorbitol, 50mM-HEPES pH 7.8, 2mM-$MgCl_2$, 2mM-EDTA, 5mM K_2HPO_4, 0.1% BSA, 450μM K ferricyanide, DCMU, and freshly ruptured chloroplasts (200μM final concn. of Chl). Cyclic electron flow was measured indirectly by ^{14}C-leucine incorporation by a suspension of intact chloroplasts (52) following 30 min incubation (20°C) and illumination (10 klux) in a medium (0.5ml) containing 0.2M KCl, 66mM-tricine-KOH, pH 8.3, 6.6mM-$MgCl_2$, 5.72μM ^{14}C-leucine (1μCi) and chloroplasts (200μM Chl). Pigment photodestruction in chloroplasts (200μM) was recorded after 24 hours illumination at 10 klux as described in (49) except with 0.1% BSA in the medium. All data as % of controls. (Ridley and Swart, unpublished data).

What is immediately apparent is that pigment photodestruction closely follows the progressive inhibition of cyclic electron transport rather than the progressive inhibition of non-cyclic electron flow. It is not until the inhibition of non-cyclic electron transport is greater than about 98% that there is any photodestruction of pigment. This corresponds to a Chl : DCMU ratio which is less than about 200:1 which agrees with what Stanger and Appleby (48) have previously reported for pigment photodestruction. The ratio is also similar to that needed to optimize fluorescence quenching by cyclic electron flow, and Mills and coworkers (53) believe that this optimization corresponds to the correct redox 'poising' of the electron carriers common to both cyclic and non-cyclic electron transport. The higher DCMU doses also progressively inhibit chlorophyll fluorescence quenching (just as they inhibit ^{14}C-leucine incorporation) presumably be causing the cyclic carriers to become overoxidized as non-cyclic flow becomes completely inhibited. So it seems that we could equate increased fluorescence in the short-term with photodestruction in the long-term, both of which are induced by the inhibition of cyclic electron flow by DCMU. In simple terms this again suggests, as it did in a rather different context with the pyridazinone studies during chloroplast development, that a functional photosystem I is an essential part of a general mechanism for protecting the plant against photo-oxidative destruction.

The extreme photosensitivity of the long wavelength forms of chlorophyll in the absence of β-carotene (36) has already been mentioned and Junge et al (38) have shown that β-carotene is closely associated with the photosystem I reaction centre complex in such a way as to be able to act in a protective capacity. So if we were able to destroy the photosystem I reaction centre selectively we should induce a similar photodestruction of pigments as found with the higher rates of DCMU needed to stop cyclic flow because this would remove more directly one of the main routes for the dissipation of excitation energy. We have managed to find conditions which achieve this in both intact chloroplasts and in the isolated photosystem I reaction centre itself using the herbicide, paraquat.

Figure 11 shows the results of an experiment in which the P700-Chl a protein (CPI), containing initially about 40 antennae chlorophylls per P700, has been isolated from the chloroplast lamellae and illuminated for 15 hours with and without a high dose of paraquat. Over this period the photodestruction of chlorophylls in the antennae occurs at the same rate in both the illuminated samples, but with paraquat present there is a much greater loss of P700 activity, although there is a lag of about 2 hours before the difference becomes noticeable. DCMU at a dose that will induce photodestruction in whole chloroplasts has no effect on the destruction of pigments in the photosystem I particles and so rules out the possibility of DCMU having a direct action on P700 to inhibit cyclic electron transport.

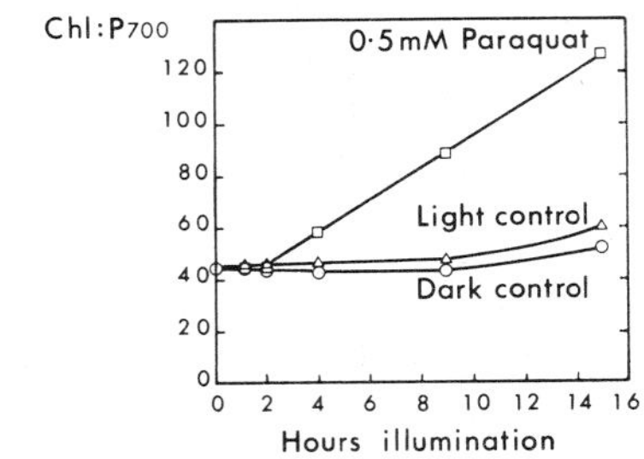

Fig. 11. The changing ratio of Chl : P700 in the isolated P700-Chl a protein complex (CPI) during 15 hours illumination at 10 klux (20°C). The P700-Chl a protein was isolated by the method of Shiozawa et al (54). Incubation as in (49). (Ridley, unpublished data).

We do not yet know to what extent the paraquat effect is relevant to its mode of action because the concentration is high, but it can provide another means of demonstrating the need to destroy a functional photosystem I in order to induce the photodestruction of pigments. Figure 12 shows an experiment in which whole chloroplasts have been illuminated in the presence of varying concentrations of paraquat. Figure 12A shows the effects on total chlorophylls and carotenoids after 24 hours during which time the capacity for O_2 evolution drops to about 10% of the rate before illumination, but this has been compared with the consequences of blocking electron transport with 5μM DCMU. Figure 12B shows the effects after 44 hours illumination during which the ability to evolve O_2 ceases altogether. It is apparent that only when electron transport from photosystem II is inhibited can paraquat induce a significant degree of pigment destruction and this is assumed to be caused by the direct action on P700. The action markedly synergizes the photodestruction of pigments caused by DCMU (Fig. 12A), and in 'aged' chloroplasts the lack of electron flow from photosystem II produces the same effect (Fig. 12B). Elstner and colleagues (55 & 56) have also reported a similar enhanced destruction of pigments by paraquat in 'aged' chloroplasts. Of course paraquat requires a functional electron transport system for its major herbicidal action which is to generate the superoxide free-radical ion, so the effect recorded in Fig. 12 is an additional mechanism that could become significant in whole plants if photosystem II activity is destroyed by the superoxide as Elstner (55) has suggested.

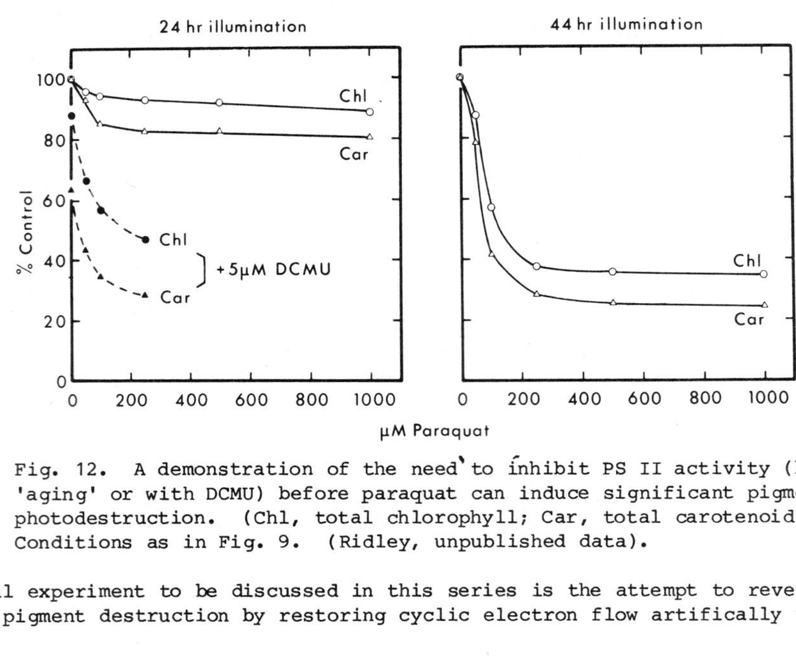

Fig. 12. A demonstration of the need to inhibit PS II activity (by 'aging' or with DCMU) before paraquat can induce significant pigment photodestruction. (Chl, total chlorophyll; Car, total carotenoid). Conditions as in Fig. 9. (Ridley, unpublished data).

The final experiment to be discussed in this series is the attempt to reverse the DCMU-induced pigment destruction by restoring cyclic electron flow artifically using suitable cofactors which short-circuit the natural cyclic flow. Phenazine methosulphate (PMS) was found to be the most effective. In Fig. 13 it can be seen that at quite low concentrations of PMS there is a remarkable degree of protection against pigment destruction in DCMU-treated chloroplasts illuminated for 22 hours. Again we see that the protection against photodestruction of carotenoids is rather less than the protection against photodestruction of chlorophyll which implies that it is the protective capacity of the carotenoids that is primarily being restored and this in turn allows chlorophyll to be protected.

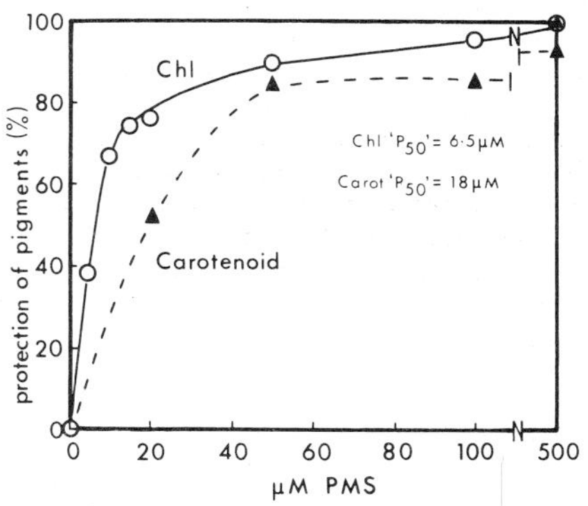

Fig. 13. Protection against pigment loss in 5μM DCMU-poisoned chloroplasts by phenazine methosulphate after 22 hours illumination. (Data from Ridley (49) but including carotenoid protection in the same experiment not given with the original data).

So what seems to be happening when herbicides block electron transport is that the means by which light energy is dissipated is altered so as to overload the protective mechanism which ultimately induces photodestruction. This can be illustrated with the aid of the diagram in Fig. 14 which is a model based on Seely's (57) concept of the photosynthetic unit but containing the tripartite pigment-protein blocks of photosystem I, photosystem II and light-harvesting Chl a/b protein established by a number of different researchers (reviewed by Thornber (35) and by Boardman et al (58)). Initially the light energy received by the light-harvesting complex is dissipated via the two photosystems through the electron transport system, but increasing doses of DCMU give a progressive inhibition so that more and more of the energy has to be dissipated by other means and much of it is channelled towards the longer wavelength forms of chlorophyll. The energy can be lost through the functioning of cyclic electron transport which will prevent the over-oxidation of P700. As cyclic flow is gradually inhibited as well, photodestruction then begins. It is likely that the destruction involves (wholly or in part) the generation of $^1O_2$ in excess of that which can be harmlessly quenched by β-carotene (see Fig. 1) so leading to its own destruction and the removal of an essential protective mechanism. The first component to suffer photodestruction is therefore the P700-Chl a complex with its attendant β-carotene molecules. We can show this by analyzing the pigment-protein complexes fractionated from chloroplasts treated with DCMU (49). For instance, when chloroplasts are treated with 5μM DCMU and illuminated in the presence of a small amount of PMS (10μM), it is possible to demonstrate as much as a 45% loss of chlorophyll from the photosystem I complex before there is any loss from the shorter-

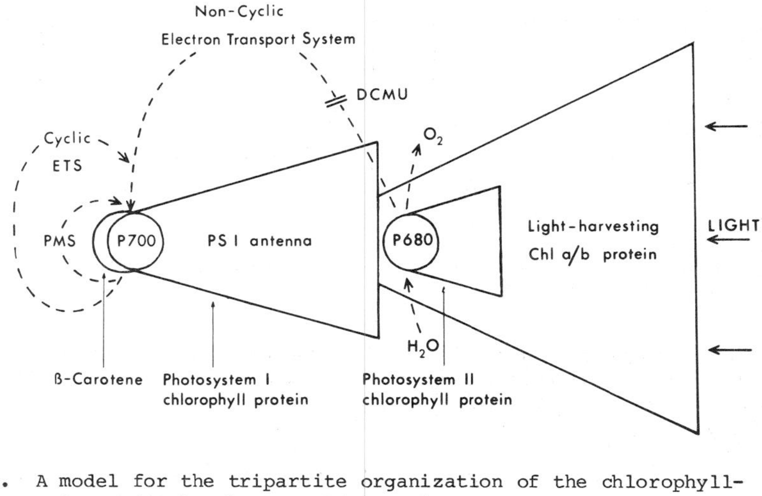

Fig. 14. A model for the tripartite organization of the chlorophyll-protein complexes in the photosynthetic unit.

wavelength chlorophylls of the light-harvesting chlorophyll protein; (analysis of the photosystem II complex has not yet been achieved). This illustrates that the light energy is being channelled towards photosystem I so that P700 becomes the focal point for energy dissipation. The mechanism has features in common with the effects of herbicides that act directly by inhibiting carotenoid synthesis because the complete inhibition of β-carotene synthesis removes the essential association of carotenoid with the photosystem I reaction centre that plays such an important role in protecting the chloroplast against photo-oxidative damage.

REFERENCES

1. W. R. Sistrom, M. Griffiths and R. Y. Stanier, J. Cell. Comp. Physiol. 48, 473-515 (1956).
2. D. S. Robertson, M. D. Bachmann and I. C. Anderson, Photochem. Photobiol. 5, 795-805 (1966).
3. H. T. Witt, Quart. Rev. Biophys. 4, 365-477 (1971).
4. C. S. Foote, Free Radicals and Biological Systems (Ed. W. A. Pryor), p85, Academic Press, New York (1976).
5. N. I. Krinsky, Pure & Appl. Chem. 51, 649-660 (1979).
6. N. I. Krinsky, Phil. Trans. R. Soc. Lond. B 284, 581-590 (1978).
7. R. L. Heath and L. Packer, Arch. Biochem. Biophys. 125, 189-198 (1968).
8. E. F. Elstner and I. Pils, Z. Naturforsch. 34c, 1040-1043 (1979).
9. J. Feierabend and B. Schubert, Plant Physiol. 61, 1017-1022 (1978).
10. J Feierabend, U. Schulz, P. Kemmerich and T. Lowitz, Z. Naturforsch. 34c, 1036-1039 (1979).
11. G. Britton, Z. Naturforsch. 34c, 979-985 (1979).
12. B. H. Davies, Lipids and Lipid Polymers in Higher Plants (Ed. M. Tevini and H. K. Lichtenthaler), p199, Springer-Verlag, Berlin (1977).
13. S. Frosch, M. Jabben, R. Bergfeld, H. Kleinig and H. Mohr, Planta 145, 497-505 (1979).
14. S. M. Ridley and J. Ridley, Plant Physiol. 63, 392-398 (1979).
15. A. D. Pardo and J. A. Schiff, Can. J. Bot. 58, 25-35 (1980).
16. J. L. Hilton, A. L. Scharen, J. B. St.John, D. E. Moreland and K. H. Norris, Weed Sci. 17, 541-547 (1969).
17. J. B. St.John and J. L. Hilton, Weed Sci. 24, 579-582 (1976).
18. W. Tischer and H. Strotmann, Biochim. Biophys. Acta 460, 113-125 (1977).
19. J. B. St.John, Plant Physiol. 57, 38-40 (1976).
20. D. Urbach, M. Suchanka and W. Urbach, Z. Naturforsch. 31c, 652-655 (1976).
21. U. Takahama, Plant & Cell Physiol. 19, 1565-1569 (1978).
22. P. G. Bartels and C. McCullough, Biochem. Biophys. Res. Comm. 48, 16-22 (1972).
23. C. Buschmann, K. H. Grumbach and T. J. Bach, Physiol. Plant. 49, 455-458 (1980).
24. B. Walles, Hereditas 53, 247-256 (1965).
25. P. G. Bartels and A. Hyde, Plant Physiol. 45, 807-810 (1970).
26. K. H. Grumbach and T. J. Bach, Z. Naturforsch. 34c, 941-943 (1979).
27. K. H. Grumbach, Z. Naturforsch. 34c, 1205-1208 (1979).
28. K. H. Grumbach and M. Drollinger, Z. Naturforsch. 35c, 445-450 (1980).
29. M. Jabben and G. F. Deitzer, Plant Physiol. 63, 481-485 (1979).
30. H. M. Habermann, Physiol. Plant. 13, 718-725 (1960).
31. H. K. Lichtenthaler and H. K. Kleudgen, Z. Naturforsch. 32c, 236-240 (1977).
32. H. K. Kleudgen, Pestic. Biochem. Physiol. 12, 231-238 (1979).
33. H. W. Kümmel and L. H. Grimme, Z. Naturforsch. 30c, 333-336 (1975).
34. A. J. Vaisberg and J. A. Schiff, Plant Physiol. 57, 260-269 (1976).
35. J. P. Thornber, Ann. Rev. Plant Physiol. 26, 127-158 (1975).
36. G. Öquist, G. Samuelsson and N. I. Bishop, Physiol. Plant. 50, 63-70 (1980).
37. G. R. Seely, J. Theor. Biol. 40, 173-187 (1973).
38. W. Junge, H. Schaffernicht and N. Nelson, Biochim. Biophys. Acta 462, 73-85 (1977).
39. P. G. Bartels and C. W. Watson, Weed Sci. 26, 198-203 (1978).
40. R. Hampp, N. Sankhla and W. Huber, Physiol. Plant. 33, 53-57 (1975).
41. K. J. Kunert and P. Böger, Weed Sci. 26, 292-296 (1978).
42. E. R. Burns, G. A. Buchanan and M. C. Carter, Plant Physiol. 47, 144-148 (1971).
43. J. D. Dodge and G. B. Lawes, Ann. Bot. 36, 315-323 (1972).
44. M. C. Carter, Herbicides. Chemistry, degradation and mode of action, Vol 1 (2nd Edition) p377, Marcel Dekker, New York (1975).
45. T. Guillot-Salomon, R. Douce and M. Signol, Bull. Soc. Franc. Physiol. Veget. 13, 63-79 (1967).
46. W. Rüdiger, J. Benz, U. Lempart, S. Schoch and D. Steffens, Z. Pflanzenphysiol. 80, 131-143 (1976).
47. K. H. Grumbach, Proc. 5th Int. Congr. Photosynth. (1981). In press.
48. C. E. Stanger and A. P. Appleby, Weed Sci. 20, 357-363 (1972).
49. S. M. Ridley, Plant Physiol. 59, 724-732 (1977).
50. K. E. Pallett and A. D. Dodge, Z. Naturforsch. 34c, 1058-1061 (1979).
51. J. M. Ramirez, F. F. del Campo and D. I. Arnon, Proc. Nat. Acad. Sci. 59, 606-612 (1968).

52. G. E. Blair and R. J. Ellis, Biochim. Biophys. Acta 319, 223-234 (1973).
53. J. D. Mills, R. F. Slovacek ane G. Hind, Biochim. Biophys. Acta 504, 298-309 (1978).
54. J. A. Shiozawa, R. S. Alberte and J. P. Thornber, Arch. Biochem. Biophys. 165, 388-397 (1974).
55. E. F. Elstner, E. Lengfelder and G. Kwiatkowski, Z. Naturforsch. 35c, 303-307 (1980).
56. E. F. Elstner, H. P. Fischer, W. Osswald and G. Kwiatkowski, Z. Naturforsch. 35c, 770-775 (1980).
57. G. R. Seely, J. Theor. Biol. 40, 189-199 (1973).
58. N. K. Boardman, J. M. Anderson and D. J. Goodchild, Current Topics in Bioenergetics, Vol 8, p35, Academic Press, New York, (1978).

CHEMICAL REGULATION OF CAROTENOID BIOSYNTHESIS

H. Yokoyama, W.J. Hsu, S.M. Poling and E. Hayman

Fruit and Vegetable Chemistry Laboratory, Agricultural Research Service, U.S. Department of Agriculture, Pasadena, California 91106

Abstract - A large number of onium compounds regulate carotenoid biosynthesis in plant tissues. Some exert their action by inhibition of biosynthetic pathways. Conversely, others stimulate the biosynthetic pathways. Research efforts involved in the development of the latter compounds have generated a substantial amount of information relative to structure-activity relationships for bioregulation of carotenoid pigments in microorganisms and higher plants. Both the trans- and cis- biosynthetic pathways can be regulated. Compounds of the general formula $(C_2H_5)_2N\ CH_2CH_2\ R$ stimulate the production of trans-carotenoids whereas compounds of the type $(C_2H_5)_2N\ R_1R_2$ regulate the biosynthesis of cis-carotenoids. The carotenoid pattern observed is determined essentially by the nature of the onium compounds employed.

INTRODUCTION

A large number of onium compounds regulate pigment biosynthesis in plant tissues. Some, such as certain pyridazinones (Ref. 1, 2, & 3), are herbicides and exert their action by inhibition of biosynthetic pathways. Conversely, others stimulate the biosynthetic pathways with no herbicidal activity.

The regulation of the biosynthesis of the carotenoids was demonstrated in the early 1950's when it was shown that β-ionone stimulated carotenogenesis in the fungus *Phycomyces blakesleeanus* (Ref. 4, 5, & 6) without itself being incorporated into the carotene molecules (7). A similar stimulatory effect of β-ionone was observed on carotene production in heterothallic cultures of *B. trispora* (Ref. 8). Effects somewhat similar to that observed with β-ionone were seen with trisporic acid (Ref. 9). The compound only stimulates carotenogenesis in the (-) strain. Both β-ionone and trisporic acid do not appear to affect carotene biosynthesis in higher plants (Ref. 11). Ninet et al. (12) investigated the biosynthesis of carotenoids by *B. trispora* in the presence of various nitrogenous compounds. Pyridine, imidazole and some of their derivatives were found to stimulate the synthesis of trans-lycopene (ψ,ψ-carotene) while isonicotinoylhydrazine, succinimide and 4-hydroxypyridine enhanced β-carotene (β,β-carotene) synthesis.

In 1969 Knypl (13) had found that an onium compound chlormequat (2-chloroethyl)-trimethylammonium chloride, causes all-trans-lycopene (ψ,ψ-carotene) accumulation in detached pumpkin cotyledons. However, no such response was observed when chlormequat was applied to other plant tissues (Ref. 14). A major step forward was observed in 1970 with the discovery that another onium compound, 2-(4-chlorphenylthio)-triethylammonium chloride (CPTA), can cause the accumulation of lycopene in a wide array of plant tissues and microorganisms. (Ref. 14)

Since the discovery of CPTA research efforts involved in the development of the onium compounds have generated a substantial amount of information relative to the structure-activity relationships for bioregulation of carotenoid pigments in higher plants and microorganisms. Both the trans- and cis-biosynthetic pathways can be regulated. The carotenoid pattern observed is determined essentially by the nature of the onium compounds employed.

BIOREGULATORS OF ALL-TRANS CAROTENES

General formula

In the regulation of the trans-carotenogenic systems the onium compounds have the general formula: $(C_2H_5)_2N\ CH_2\ R$. In general, the N,N-dimethyl analogs are less effective than the N,N-diethyl compounds. The magnitude of the stimulation, but not the general pattern of carotenoid response, depends on R (Ref. 15). The nature of R can cause modifications in the amount of the individual carotenoids. Thus when R lacks an aromatic ring, there appears to be less inhibition of the cyclase(s); consequently, more cyclic carotenoids accumulate. Examples are given in Tables 1,2 & 3. All the compounds caused lycopene accumulation in Marsh grapefruit. The untreated fruit had the normal light yellow color. After treatment the color of the flavedo ranged from light orange to an intense red. The flavedo of all treated fruit showed lycopene accumulation. Lycopene was not detected in the untreated fruits and it is not normally detected in mature grapefruit (Ref. 16). The biological activity was also correlated with the logarithm of the 1-octanol-water partition coefficient (log ρ).

Diethylalkylamines

Treatments with diethylalkylamines (Table 1) gave a fairly consistent response pattern as the length of the alkyl group was increased. The amount of any given carotene remained about the same or increased slightly with diethylpentylamine and diethylhexylamine, while diethylheptylamine caused a larger response, and diethyloctylamine and diethylnonylamine caused very large increases. Lycopene accounted for most of the increase in the total carotene content but the intermediates, ζ-carotene (7,8,7',8'-tetrahydro-ψ,ψ-carotene) and neurosporene (7,8-dihydro-ψ,ψ-carotene) also increased appreciably. Of significance are the 3.5 and 4.6-fold increases in the cyclic carotenes, γ-, α- and β-carotene (i.e., β,ψ-, β,ε- and β,β-carotene) caused by diethyloctylamine and diethylnonylamine, respectively. The increase in cyclic carotenes is much larger than that caused by compounds with aromatic rings. Butyldiethylamine has also been observed to cause the development of red color in grapefruit but only with higher concentrations and longer treatment periods. The higher members of this series, diethyldecylamine, diethylundecylamine and diethyldodecylamine, caused increasing peel injury as the length of the alkyl chain increased. The last two damaged the peel whenever they were applied. The color of the peel next to the damaged areas showed color enhancement but to a lessening degree as the alkyl chain lengthened.

Diethylaminoalkylbenzene

The responses of fruit treated with compounds in Table 2 were similar to that of fruit treated with diethylalkylamines (Table 1). There was a much larger increase in ζ-carotene and neurosporene for diethylaminobutylbenzene and diethylaminopentylbenzene while the increase in cyclic carotenes was not very great. For the diethylalkylamines lycopene increased to a very high level and then dropped for the last members of the series. The drop in lycopene accumulation was observed with diethylaminobutylamine but the amount of lycopene increased with diethylaminopentylamine although remaining less than the maximum for the series. The very large increase in phytofluene (7,8,11,12,7',8'-hexahydro-ψ,ψ-carotene), as well as ζ-carotene, caused δ-diethylaminopentylbenzene to give the greater increase in the total carotene content. Whether this was caused in part by some side effect of the extensive peel damage or entirely by the compound is not certain. A similar effect has been previously observed (Ref. 17) after treatment with [γ-(diethylamino)-propoxy]-benzene and [δ-diethylamino)-butoxy]-benzene. In these cases the increases in phytofluene and ζ-carotene were also very large but no great damage was observed. This effect may arise when the diethylamino and phenyl groups of the inducers are separated by a chain of four or five carbon atoms.

ANALOGS OF β-[(DIETHYLAMINO)-ETHOXY]-BENZENE

Substituted Diethylaminophenylethers

Treatment with analogs of β [(diethylamino)-ethoxy]-benzene (Table 3) gave a similar pattern. Neurosporene did not increase as much as previously although ζ-carotene did show a large increase. The cyclic carotenes, with the exception of γ-carotenes, did not show a significant increase. There was a general decrease, not previously observed, of all the carotenes after treatment with diethylaminoethyl-4-tert-butylphenylether as compared with diethylaminoethyl-4-iso-propylphenylether, instead of the steady increase of ζ-carotene and neurosporene observed in the other series (Tables 1 and 2). The greater biological activity of those compounds in Table 3 as compared to those in Tables 1 and 2 is probably due to a higher degree of interaction between the compound and the active site.

Generally the response increased with increasing concentration to a maximum value and further increases in the concentration of diethylaminoethylphenylether from 0.26 to 0.52M reduced the observed response (Ref. 17), while treatment with CPTA (Ref. 18) at 0.018M caused an accumulation of carotenes equal to that in Table 3. Doubling the concentration (0.2M) caused large increases for diethylaminoethylphenylether and diethylaminoethyl-4-methylphenylether while doubling of diethylaminoethyl-4-ethylphenylether had almost no effect (Ref. 15). That increasing CPTA concentrations begin to lose effectiveness in inducing greater carotene biosynthesis has also been observed in *Blakeslea trispora* (Ref. 19).

Inducers of β-Carotene (β,β-Carotene)

A series of *para*-substituted 2-diethylaminoethylbenzoates caused a much larger accumulation of β-carotene than other lycopene inducers although lycopene remained the major pigment (Table 4, Ref. 20). Table 4 gives the results of treatment with the *para*-substitued 2-diethylaminoethylbenzoates. The response is similar to that previously observed for

TABLE 1. Effect of $(C_2H_5)_2N(CH_2)_nCH_3$ on carotene content of Marsh seedless grapefruit (μg/g dry wt)[1] (Ref. 15)

	Control	Treatment[2] n=4	5	6	7	8
Phytofluene	37.3	38.6	29.0	28.3	27.8	39.5
ζ-Carotene	2.25	2.47	3.13	4.32	14.6	17.8
Neurosporene	1.72	1.28	1.37	1.38	2.94	5.16
Lycopene		1.01	6.99	59.0	143	115
γ-Carotene	0.37	0.30	0.96	1.17	2.59	3.21
α-Carotene	0.54	1.04	1.02	1.26	2.07	2.11
β-Carotene	1.72	1.41	1.20	1.35	4.73	6.75
Total	43.9	46.1	43.7	96.8	197.7	189.5
Log ρ		2.94	3.44	3.94	4.44	4.94

[1] Dried *in vacuo* at 65°

[2] Isopropanol solution at 0.2M poured over fruit, postharvest

TABLE 2. Effect of $(C_2H_5)_2N(CH_2)_nPh$ on carotene content of flavedo of Marsh seedless grapefruit (μg/g dry wt)[1] (Ref. 15)

	Control	Treatment[2] n=1	2	3	4	5
Phytofluene	23.1	25.3	29.3	37.9	38.7	86.2
ζ-Carotene	1.13	1.38	3.87	6.77	27.5	53.8
Neurosporene	0.71	0.83	1.85	1.11	7.16	12.0
Lycopene		8.62	60.5	188	104	153
γ-Carotene		0.55	0.77	1.07	0.59	1.67
α-Carotene	0.57	0.77	0.84	0.61	2.19	0.76
β-Carotene	0.95	0.56	0.46	0.95	trace	0.68
Total	26.5	37.8	97.6	235.5	180.1	308.1
Log ρ						

[1] Dried *in vacuo* at 65°

[2] Isopropanol solution at 0.2M poured over fruit, postharvest

TABLE 3. Effect of $(C_2H_5)_2NCH_2CH_2OC_6H_4R$ and CPTA at 0.1M on carotene content of flavedo of Marsh seedless grapefruit (μg/g dry wt)[1] (Ref. 15)

	Control	R=H	*p*-CH_3	*p*-C_2H_5	*p*-iso-C_3H_7	*p*-tert-C_4H_9	CPTA
Phytofluene	44.9	48.1	50.9	44.9	51.1	33.7	42.6
ζ-Carotene	2.74	5.45	19.0	13.7	20.6	4.57	10.1
Neurosporene	0.33	0.91	0.84	0.93	1.62	0.63	1.21
Lycopene		22.2	249	182	226	54.4	199
γ-Carotene	0.27	1.01	2.48	2.13	2.74	1.04	1.90
α-Carotene	0.35	0.57	0.41	0.38	0.40	0.63	0.23
β-Carotene	1.35	1.26	0.40	0.82	0.70	0.58	0.39
Total	49.9	79.5	323.0	244.9	303.2	95.6	244.4
Log ρ							

[1] Dried *in vacuo* at 65°

[2] 0.1M Isopropanol solution poured over fruit, postharvest

TABLE 4. Effect of p-R $C_6H_4COOCH_2CH_2N(C_2H_5)_2$ on the carotene content of the flavedo of Marsh seedless grapefruit (μg/g dry wt)[1] (Ref. 20)

	Treatment[2]										
	Control	R=H	NH_2	CN	NO_2	MeO	F	Me	Cl	Br	t-Bu
Phytofluene	173	191	192	229	245	199	244	234	228	233	204
ζ-Carotene	38.6	44.7	60.7	57.6	64.5	44.9	62.5	62.5	60.4	61.1	51.0
Neurosporene	1.52	0.62	0.95	1.23		1.05	1.43	2.01			1.97
Lycopene		1.14	83.6	17.5	215	170	245	285	474	507	
γ-Carotene	0.38	0.37	3.67	1.48	3.82	1.94	3.04	3.80	3.18	2.91	1.14
α-Carotene	.53	0.53	0.84	1.76	3.86	2.62	2.82	5.54	4.01	4.22	0.40
β-Carotene	1.31	1.51	27.4	12.0	25.7	6.64	13.6	25.0	17.3	32.4	2.05
Total carotenes	215	240	369	320	557	426	572	618	787	841	261
Total xanthophylls	33.7	35.9	39.8	38.7	45.0	44.6	48.5	42.8	45.3	44.6	46.5
Log ρ		1.54	2.75	3.06	3.08	3.14	3.25	3.48	3.93	4.04	4.58

[1] Dried *in vacuo* at 60°

[2] Isopropanol solution at 0.1M poured over fruit, postharvest

other triethylamines except for the much larger accumulation of the cyclic carotenes, γ, α- and particularly β-carotene.

For further examination of the β-carotene effect, the 2-diethylaminoethylesters of the shorter chain alphatic series were investigated (Ref. 21). As shown in Table 5, these esters caused significant increases in β-carotene, so that it was the major pigment, with only a small amount of lycopene. The esters were applied as free amines in isopropanol. The peel remained healthy on all the fruit except those treated with octanoate and nonanoate which damaged about 30 and 60% of the peel area respectively. The tendency to cause peel damage with increasing lipid solubility has been noted for other inducers (Ref. 22).

As shown in Table 6 ω-arylaliphatic ester, phenylacetate, more closely resembled the benzoate in its effect than the other members of the series. An increase in the chain length by one methylene group, i.e. hydrocinnamate, reversed the relation between lycopene and β-carotene and the latter became the major pigment. 4-Phenylbutyrate was the most active of the series. The most active β-carotene inducers were the hexanoate, 4-phenylbutyrate and cinnamate.

ESSENTIAL STRUCTURAL FEATURES FOR INDUCTION OF TRANS-CAROTENES

As a further elaboration on the general formula $(C_2H_5)_2NCH_2CH_2R$, given for trans-lycopene inducing bioregulators, none of the following structural alterations totally abolished the activity or changes the response pattern: (1) Replacement of O-atom of the S-atom connecting the amine portion and the benzene moiety in the CPTA moecule; (2) elimination of the substitution on the benzene ring; (3) elimination of the benzene ring itself; (4) replacement of the ethyl groups of the amine portion by other alkyl groups. However, these alterations change the effectiveness of the compound thus modified. Benzene derivatives are more effective than alkyl derivatives; and the substitutions of certain groups on the benzene ring at the para position seem to make the compounds more effective.

Table 7 shows substitution of a methyl group at the ortho position almost completely eliminates the inducing ability of the compound. Substitution at the meta position also causes a reduction in the inducing ability. With the methyl group in the para position the compound is a very powerful inducer. The same effect is observed with the strongly electron withdrawing chloro group, as compared to the electron releasing methyl groups, for p-, m- and o-chlorophenoxy triethylamine (Ref. 23). Steric hindrance may possibly play an important role in the effectiveness of the position isomers. Studies (Ref. 23) indicated that the effectiveness of the compounds does not depend solely upon the electron-withdrawing ability of the substituting groups in the benzene moiety. Also, experimental data obtained thus far do not necessarily rule out the possible induction effects of substituents on the amine portion of the molecule.

It should be emphasized that the variable effectiveness on carotenogenesis among the triethylamine derivatives suggests the possibility that certain compounds did not penetrate well into the fruit flavedo tissue. Thus, the lipophilic-hydrophilic properties of the bioregulators appear to have an influence on the effectiveness of the compounds. These characteristics are reflected in the value of log ρ , which is the logarithm of the octanol-water partition coefficient of the unionized molecule (Ref. 24, 25, 26 & 27). Log values (Tables 1-4) have proven useful, in combination with considerations of the electronic and steric states of a molecule, as a general guide in the designing of new bioregulators (Ref. 15 & 22). Thus, there is an upper limit for log ρ at which peel damage begins to occur. The compounds with log ρ greater than 4.6 probably cause peel damage by disrupting the lipid membranes of the cells. Those compounds with log ρ less than 4.6 show no damage. Certain of the compounds probably interact more strongly at the active site(s) and produce a noticeable effect on carotenogenesis at lower concentrations and for smaller values of log ρ than others. The optimum value for log ρ appears to be in the range 3.5 to 4.5.

MODE OF ACTION OF TRANS-CAROTENOID BIOREGULATORS

The fact that carotenogenic microorganisms such as Blakeslea trispora and Phycomyces blakesleeanus respond to treatment (Ref. 14) provided an opportunity to study the mechanism of action of bioregulators in carotenoid formation. Studies (Ref. 28) conducted using the mold B. trispora indicated that the bioregulators act at the enzyme level by inhibiting cyclase(s); the transformation of the acyclic lycopene to the monocyclic γ-carotene and the bicyclic β-carotene was inhibited. These studies also suggested that the bioregulators induce (derepress) a gene regulating the synthesis of a specific enzyme or enzymes in the primary biosynthetic pathway of carotenoids and thus increase net synthesis of carotenoid pigments. The nullifying action of cycloheximide on the effect of the bioregulatory agent in carotenoid synthesis indicated that the latter compounds acts as an inducer (derepressor) of enzyme synthesis rather than as activators of pre-existing enzyme(s). Once the

TABLE 5. Effect of $(C_2H_5)_2NCH_2CH_2OOC$-R on the carotene content of flavedo of Marsh seedless grapefruit (μg/g dry wt)[1] (Ref. 21)

	Treatment[2]						
	Control	R = $CH_3(CH_2)_3$-	$CH_3(CH_2)_4$-	$CH_3(CH_2)_5$-	$CH_3(CH_2)_6$-	$CH_3(CH_2)_7$-	$C_6H_5CH{=}CH$-
Phytofluene	36.6	35.9	36.6	32.4	31.2	30.7	39.2
ζ-Carotene	5.11	10.3	19.4	15.7	13.0	8.48	20.5
Neurosporene		0.55		0.61			0.62
Lycopene		9.30	11.4	21.5	8.03	2.79	9.28
γ-Carotene	0.33	1.01	5.57	3,54	2.13	2.01	3,18
α-Carotene	0.33	1.32	3.68	3.05	6.18	3.22	2.22
β-Carotene	1.61	14.2	98.3	58.3	50.5	43.0	50.4
Other carotenes	2.40	1.19	2.52	2.16	2.40	2.04	1.64
Total carotenes	46.4	73.8	177	137	113	92.2	127
Total xanthophylls	24.9	18.2	22.0	24.4	22.1	24.3	21.2

1 Dried *in vacuo* at 65°

2 Isopropanol solution at 0.2M poured over fruit, postharvest

TABLE 6. Effect of $(C_2H_5)_2NCH_2CH_2OOCR$ at 0.2M concentration on the carotene content of the flavedo of Marsh seedless grapefruit (μg/g dry wt)[1] (Ref. 21)

	Control	Treatment[2] R=-Ph	$-CH_2-Ph$	$-CH_2CH_2-Ph$	$-(CH_2)_3-Ph$
Phytofluene	47.8	43.9	47.9	35.9	34.7
ζ-Carotene	6.48	11.0	10.7	9.91	9.78
Neurosporene	0.41	1.07	0.84	1.20	1.37
Lycopene		31.6	22.9	4.72	13.1
γ-Carotene	0.34	1.10	0.86	1.04	3.90
α-Carotene	0.18	0.38	0.81	0.78	5.48
β-Carotene	0.81	1.97	3.85	23.6	93.4
Other carotenes	1.68	0.81	0.52	0.34	0.72
Total carotenes	57.7	91.9	88.4	77.5	162
Total xanthophylls	29.8	30.4	33.7	26.6	29.0

[1] Dried *in vacuo* at 65°C

[2] Isopropanol solution poured over fruit, postharvest

TABLE 7. Effect of $(C_2H_5)_2NCH_2CH_2OC_6H_4R$ at 0.1M on the carotene content of the flavedo of Marsh seedless grapefruit (μg/g dry wt)[1] (Ref. 21)

	Control	Treatment[2] R= *o*-CH_3	*m*-CH_3	*p*-CH_3
Phytofluence	40.2	39.3	36.1	52.7
ζ-Carotene	4.66	3.26	4.00	17.7
Neurosporene	0.26	0.79	1.14	1.77
Lycopene		0.43	24.4	516
γ-Carotene		0.22	0.60	0.83
α-Carotene	0.52	0.34	0.61	0.28
β-Carotene	1.25	0.86	0.59	0.48
Total carotenes	46.9	45.2	67.4	589
Total xanthophylls	21.8	21.3	24.3	25.1

[1] Dried *in vacuo* at 65°

[2] Isopropanol solution poured over fruit, postharvest

TABLE 8. Effect of dibenzylamine and substituted dibenzylamines at 0.1M on the carotene content of flavedo of Marsh seedless grapefruit (μ/g dry wt) (Ref. 31)

	Control	Dibenzylamine	Substituted dibenzylamines					
			4-F	4-Cl	4-Br	$4-CH_3$	$4-NO_2$	4-CN
Phytofluene	34.98	36.10	39.21	40.14	37.87	32.20	50.27	43.32
α-Carotene	0.14	0.11	0.10	0.16	0.12	0.11	0.14	0.09
β-Carotene	0.65	0.83	0.95	1.88	1.05	1.00	1.01	0.78
ζ-Carotene	4.37	10.12	12.64	21.16	18.64	14.03	18.71	12.45
Poly-<u>cis</u>-γ-carotene I*		0.70	1.35	3.18	3.84	2.50	1.49	0.78
Proneurosporene*	0.31	4.91	7.99	16.24	15.03	9.30	13.45	8.28
Prolycopene*	0.55	8.03	14.08	33.10	29.76	21.28	24.95	13.19
<u>cis</u>-Lycopenes*	1.21	5.12	7.58	9.69	9.31	9.45	10.10	6.00
Poly-<u>cis</u>- -carotene II*	0.87	2.35	5.48	11.94	6.81	5.55	5.91	4.50
Unknown 453	0.48	1.74	1.44	4.18	8.22	4.11	6.40	0.94
Total carotenes	43.56	70.01	90.82	41,67	130.65	99.53	132.43	90.33
Total xanthophylls	25.48	28.76	30.04	39.36	36.58	26.08	39.74	28.47

* Tentative assignment of poly-<u>cis</u> carotenes in control.

TABLE 9. Effect of substituted dibenzylamines † at 0.1M on the carotene content of flavedo of Marsh seedless grapefruit (μg/g dry wt) (Ref. 31)

	Control	1	2	3	4	5	6	7
Phytofluene	38.81	48.84	41.48	40.70	33.06	43.14	30.37	53.89
α-Carotene	0.11	0.13	0.18	0.13	0.09	0.17	0.10	0.14
β-Carotene	0.62	0.84	1.07	1.44	1.08	1.08	0.84	1.08
ζ-Carotene	5.20	11.99	10.75	18.25	10.18	11.08	8.42	15.26
Poly-cis-γ-carotene I*		0.71	1.20	3.32	1.49	1.56	2.37	1.19
Proneurosporene*	0.54	6.55	5.44	11.67	5.13	5.51	4.42	8.74
Prolycopene*	1.31	7.72	8.90	25.23	9.86	10.50	13.80	9.83
cis-Lycopenes	1.45	5.57	5.57	13.99	7.68	7.75	8.44	8.31
Poly-cis-γ carotene II*	0.80	2.45	4.12	8.37	3.67	2.42	3.71	5.05
Unknown 453		1.54	1.18	3.29	2.37	2.98	2.10	2.62
Total carotenes	43.84	86.34	79.89	126.39	74.61	86.19	74.57	106.11
Total xanthophylls	24.64	34.77	35.51	40.01	31.92	37.18	26.94	46.1±

† 1. 2- methyl 2. 3- methyl 3. 4-methyl 4. 4-chloro, 4'- methyl 5. 4-methyl, 4'-nitro 6. N-benzylphenethylamine 7. N-benzyl 1-naphthalenemethylamine

*Tentative assignment of poly-*cis* carotenes

enzymes participating in carotenoid synthesis have been formed, cycloheximide does not affect their activity. Cycloheximide is known to act at the ribosomal protein level to inhibit the formation of messenger RNA which, in turn, inhibits protein synthesis (Ref. 29). The relative effectiveness of an individual bioregulator as a cyclase inhibitor and as an enzyme inducer could lead to variations in the carotenoid pigment response patterns amongst the different bioregulators, as seen in Tables 1-6. An alternative explanation of the mode of action of CPTA, for example, in Phycomyces mutants is that of negative control by β-carotene (Ref. 30).

BIOREGULATION OF CIS-CAROTENES

All the compounds reported above cause the accumulation of the normal, all-trans carotenoids. They are of the general formula $(C_2H_5)_2NCH_2R$. The carotene content greatly increases and all-trans lycopene becomes the major pigment unless the tertiary amines are aliphatic esters of 2-diethylaminoethanol. If they are, all-trans β-carotene is the predominant carotene.

Studies of structure-activity relationships of compounds that affect carotenogenesis led to the discovery of a new class of bioregulators causing the accumulation of poly-cis-carotenoids, (Ref. 31 & 32). The natural occurrence of cis and poly-cis carotenoids has been observed, but is not very common (Ref. 32, 33, 33, 34, 35, 36 & 37).

Tables 8 and 9 show that all the substituted dibenzylamines, N-benzylphenethylamine and N-benzyl 2-naphthalenemethylamine, show that all the secondary amines stimulated the production of poly-cis-carotenes. Tables 10, 11 and 12 show the ability of substituted N-benzylfurfurylamines, N-benzyl, N-methylfurfurylamines and N-alkyl, N-methylbenzylamines to stimulate the formation of poly-cis carotenes.

The pattern of accumulation of the poly-cis carotenes is the same as that caused by the benzylamines. The N-benzylfurfurylamines are more effective than the corresponding dibenzylamines. The only anomaly is 2-(4 bromophenoxy) ethylfurfurylamines which acted as inducers of both poly-cis carotenes and lycopene. They also inhibited the cyclase(s), a characteristic of lycopene inducers, and prevented the formation of poly-cis-γ-carotenes I and II. The effectiveness of the compounds N-methyl, N-benzylfurfurylamine, N-methyl-, N-4-bromobenzyl furfurylamine and N-methyl N-benzylfurfurylamine shows that N-methylation of the corresponding secondary amines does not eliminate but tends to enhance activity. This enhancement of activity is especially evident with the N-alkyl, N-methyl, benzylamines. While N-n-hexylbenzylamine is only weakly active, N-methyl, N-n-hexylbenzylamine is a very good inducer. These compounds are not good inhibitors of the cyclase(s) as is the case with the lycopene inducers. In none of the samples was any trace of all-trans lycopene found. Prolycopene was the major pigment but there were relatively large amounts of other poly-cis carotenes. In marked contrast, the triethylamine bioregulators primarily induced the synthesis of all-trans lycopene or β-carotene. Although not experimentally determined, the increase in the total xanthophylls observed in the treated fruit could have been due to the formation of cis and poly-cis xanthophylls. cis-Xanthophylls do occur naturally in some plants (Ref. 34).

MODE OF ACTION OF CIS-CAROTENOID BIOREGULATORS

The mode of action of the poly-cis inducers is probably gene derepression, similar to that of the lycopene inducers. However, these compounds probably derepress a recessive gene controlling the biosynthesis of the poly-cis carotenoids, whereas the lycopene inducers derepress the dominant genes giving rise to the normal all-trans carotenoids. The existence of this recessive gene can only be postulated as present in grapefruit and other citrus. Important genetic studies have shown that such a gene exists in tomatoes (Ref. 33). Tangerine tomatoes, which are homozygous for the recessive allele t, accumulate the orange pigment prolycopene at the expense of lycopene. Red fruit carry the dominant allele t+. The same situation could exist in other fruit and explain the action of the poly-cis inducers. This interpretation lends support to the postulated parallel pathways for all-trans and poly-cis carotenoids (Ref. 35). If this hypothesis is true, one would also expect to find poly-cis - ζ-carotene, -phytofluene, and -phytoene present in the fruit. The poly-cis inducers appear to differ from the lycopene inducers in another respect. In addition to gene derepression, the lycopene inducers inhibit the cyclase(s), causing lycopene to accumulate at the expense of the cyclic carotenes. The accumulation of significant amounts of poly-cis-γ-carotenes I and II indicates that the cyclase(s) are not inhibited by the poly-cis inducers and whose only apparent function is to derepress the recessive gene.

TABLE 10. Effects of compounds N-R furfurylamine at 0.1M on the carotene content of the flavedo of Marsh seedless grapefruit (μg/g dry wt)[1] (Ref. 31)

	Control	R=benzyl	4-methyl-benzyl	4-chloro benzyl	4-bromo-benzyl	4-nitro-benzyl	phen-ethyl	2-phen oxyethyl	2(4-bromo)-phenoxyethyl
Phytofluene	19.78	22.03	21.17	25.03	31.03	19.44	25.63	31.70	28.32
α-Carotene	0.34	0.24	0.33	0.23	.20	0.21	0.22	0.30	0.29
β-Carotene	1.54	1.26	1.36	1.31	1.46	0.93	1.48	1.20	0.95
ζ-Carotene	2.58	11.72	6.18	18.71	27.61	2.26	22.79	12.57	14.94
Poly-*cis*-γ-carotene I		0.95	0.45	2.24	2.72		2.01	1.25	
Proneurosporene		8.41	3.42	15.17	21.42	0.44	18.30	10.56	5.07
γ-Carotene									0.36
cis-Lycopene		7.31	3.81	14.84	23.37	1.13	17.52	8.70	3,78
Neurosporene	1.17					0.72			2.64
Poly-*cis*-γ-carotene II		4.82	1.68	10.49	14.45		8.45	5.45	
Unknown 453		2.03	1.16	2.05	3.70		3.54	2.49	
Lycopene									32.39
Total carotenes	25.38	70.17	44.79	122.95	172.49	25.83	141.42	94.64	92.73
Total xanthophylls	19.13	22.18	22.40	24.78	30.85	20.62	27.09	24.73	22.14

[1] Isopropanol solution poured over fruit, postharvest.

TABLE 11. Effect of compounds N-R furfurylamine and N-methylamine and N-methyl, N-R'-furfurylamine on the carotene content of the flavedo of Marsh seedless grapefruit (μg/g dry wt)[1] (Ref. 31)

	Control	R= benzyl	R'= benzyl	R= 4-bromo-benzyl	R'= 4-bromo-benzyl	R=phenethyl	R'= phenethyl
Phytofluene	22.13	28.83	31.54	35.63	33.30	30.94	37.05
α-Carotene	0.13	0.19	0.20	0.23	0.30	0.14	0.17
β-Carotene	0.57	1.11	1.46	1.06	1.28	1.50	1.73
ζ-Carotene	2.68	20.65	29.76	21.07	21.51	36.95	35.80
Poly-cis-γ-carotene I		2.82	4.05	4.47	3.08	3.01	5.55
Proneurosporene		14.65	21.36	19.34	14.51	29.98	25.48
Prolycopene		27.59	48.15	45.04	33.30	79.52	65.32
cis-Lycopene		18.06	29.04	26.81	26.21	30.99	39.18
Poly-cis-γ-carotene II		13.56	21.03	21.74	10.08	18.09	21.38
Unknown 453		7.12	8.55	5.67	8.10	5.92	9.09
Total carotenes	25.51	134.58	195.14	179.05	151.67	231.18	240.76
Total xanthophylls	26.33	35.71	41.95	36.71	38.87	32.10	46.75

[1] Isopropanol solution at 0.1M poured over fruit, postharvest.

TABLE 12. Effect of compounds N-methyl, N-R benzylamine on the carotene content of the flavedo of March seedless grapefruit (μg/g dry wt)[1] (Ref. 31)

	Control	R=*n*-butyl	*n*-pentyl	*n*-hexyl	*n*-heptyl	*n*-octyl
Phytofluene	24.86	29.40	24.03	35.20	28.07	34.12
α-Carotene	0.54	0.36	0.23	0.23	0.21	0.31
β-Carotene	0.95	1.01	1.70	1.64	0.77	0.93
ζ-Carotene	2.73	3.85	7.26	21.24	20.86	24.99
Poly-*cis*-γ-carotene I			0.86	2.94	2.90	3.15
Proneurosporene		1.77	5.01	16.08	16.38	18.80
Prolycopene		2.66	9.45	32.57	36.06	26.44
cis Lycopenes		3.63	4.75	10.94	13.26	12.33
Poly-*cis*-γ-carotene II		0.39	3.58	11.17	8.03	9.83
Unknown 453		0.20	1.21	2.09	3.58	2.03
Total carotenes	29.04	43.27	58.08	134.10	130.12	132.93
Total xanthophylls	25.83	25.04	27.90	33.85	27.89	27.18

[1] Isopropanol solutions at 0.1M poured over fruit, postharvest

REFERENCES

1. H. W. Kummel and L. H. Grimme, Z. Naturforsch 30c, 333 (1975).
2. D. Urbach, M. Schanka and M. Urbach, Z. Naturforsch 31c, 652 (1976).
3. F. A. Eder, Z. Naturforsch 34c, 1052 (1979).
4. G. Mackinney, T. Nakayama, C.D. Buss, C. O. Chichester, J. Am. Chim. Soc. 74, 3156 (1952).
5. G. Mackinney, C. O. Chichester and P.S. Wong, J. Am. Chem. Soc. 75, 5428 (1953).
6. G. Mackinney, T. Nakayama, C. O. Chichester and C. D. Buss, J. Am. Chem. Soc. 75, 5428 (1953).
7. B. G. Engle, J. Wursch and M. Zimmerman, Helv. Chím. Acta 36, 1771 (1953).
8. C. O. Chichester, P.S. Wong and G. Mackinney, Plant Physiol. 29, 238 (1954).
9. L. Cagliotti, G. Canelli, B. Cumerino, R. Mondelli, A. Presto, A. Quilico, T. Salvatori and A. Silva, Chim. Ind. (Milan) 45, 961 (1964).
10. D. M. Thomas, and T. W. Goodwin, Phytochem. 6, 355 (1967).
11. H. Yokoyama and W. J. Hsu, Unpublished Data.
12. L. Ninet, J. Renault and R. Tissier, Biotech. Bioeng. 11, 2985 (1969).
13. J. S. Knypl, Naturwissenschafter 56, 572 (1969).
14. C. Coggins, G. L. Henning and H. Yokoyama, Science 168, 1589 (1970).
15. S. Poling, W. J. Hsu and H. Yokoyama, Phytochem 14, 1933 (1975).
16. H. Yokoyama and M. J. White, J. Agr. Food Chem. 15, 693 (1965).
17. S. Poling, W. J. Hsu, H. Yokoyama, Phytochem 2, 2665 (1973).
18. H. Yokoyama, C. W. Coggins, G. L. Henning and C. DeBenedict, Phytochem 11, 1721 (1972).
19. W. J. Hsu, H. Yokoyama and C. W. Coggins, Phytochem. 11, 298 (1972).
20. S. M. Poling, W. J. Hsu and H. Yokoyama, Phytochem. 15, 1685 (1976).
21. S. M. Poling, W. J. Hsu, F. J. Koehrm and H. Yokoyama, Phytochem. 16, 551 (1977).
22. W. J. Hsu, S. M. Poling, C. DeBenedict, C. Rudash and H. Yokoyama, J. Agric. Food Chem. 23, 831 (1975).
23. C. Hansch, R. M. Muir, T. Fujita, P. P. Maloney, F. Geiger, M. Streich, J. Am. Chem. Soc. 85, 2817 (1963).
24. C. Hansch and T. Fujita, J. Am. Chem. Soc. 86, 1616 (1964).
25. T. Fujita, J. Iwasa and C. Hansch, J. Am. Chem. Soc. 86, 5175 (1964).
26. C. Hansch, J. E. Quinlan and G. L. Lawrence, J. Org. Chem. 33, 347 (1967).
27. W. J. Hsu, S. M. Poling and H. Yokoyama, Phytochem. 11, 2985 (1972).
28. D. Boulter, Ann. Rev. Plant 21, 91 (1970).
29. S. M. Poling, W. J. Hsu and H. Yokoyama, Phytochem. 19, 1677 (1980).
30. F. S. Murillo, Plant Science Letters 17, 201 (1980).
31. S. M. Poling, W. J. Hsu and H. Yokoyama, Phytochem (In press).
32. L. Zechmeister, cis-trans Isomeric Carotenoids,Vitamins A and Arylpolyenes, Academic Press New York (1962).
33. T. W. Goodwin, in Carotenoids (Isler, O. ed.) Birkhauser-Verlag,Basel, 577 (1971).
34. B. C. L. Weedon, in Carotenoids (Isler, O. ed.) Birkhauser-Verlag, Basel, 267 (1971).
35. L. C. Raymundo and K. L. Simpson, Phytochem. 11, 397 (1972).
36. R. W. Glass and K. L. Simpson, Phytochem. 15, 1077 (1976).
37. L. Zechmeister and W. A. Schroeder, J. Am. Chem. Soc. 64, 1173 (1942).

SUBJECT INDEX

INDEX OF ORGANISMS